'This book is an authoritative resource for students and researchers
student-friendly, engaging and accessible manner, the book draws tc
academics working at the intersections of forensic psychology anc
clear and comprehensive coverage of the discipline and is a must-re

—Dr Cla

'McGuire and Duff take an original and creative approach to scaffolding the learning process for readers new to forensic psychology, which makes this book uniquely accessible. It will appeal to both students and their teachers for the way in which the authors guide us through everything we need to know to head down the road to becoming a forensic psychologist: that most exciting of future occupations.'

—Professor Devon Polaschek, The University of Waikato, New Zealand

'A well-written, engaging book which focuses on the applied nature of forensic psychology. The chapters are sensibly organised and include a comprehensive review of the key concepts. I believe researchers and students will find the content invaluable.'

—Dr Gemma Graham, University of Brighton, UK

'This is a very timely book which contains comprehensive and up-to-date information. It will be an essential text for anyone interested in current thinking and ideas in forensic psychology: students, researchers and practitioners who want an excellent overview of the state of current knowledge in the field will find it particularly helpful.'

—Associate Professor Heng Choon (Oliver) Chan, City University of Hong Kong, Hong Kong, S.A.R., China

'McGuire and Duff position forensic psychology theory and practice within a current context. They articulate not only how the discipline developed as it did, but why forensic psychology is so critical to our understanding of crime, investigation and rehabilitation within the criminal justice system.'

—Dr Emily Glorney, Royal Holloway, University of London, UK

FORENSIC PSYCHOLOGY

Routes Through the System

James McGuire & Simon Duff

macmillan education palgrave

This edition published 2018 by
PALGRAVE

Palgrave in the UK is an imprint of Macmillan Publishers Limited, registered in England, company number 785998, of 4 Crinan Street, London, N1 9XW.

ISBN 978–0–230–24909–7

This book is printed on paper suitable for recycling and made from fully managed and sustained forest sources. Logging, pulping and manufacturing processes are expected to conform to the environmental regulations of the country of origin.

A catalogue record for this book is available from the British Library.

A catalog record for this book is available from the Library of Congress.

Printed and bound in Great Britain by Bell and Bain Ltd, Glasgow.

For Emma and Jenny
J.McG.

For Mum and Dad
S.D.

Brief Contents

Long Contents

List of Figures

List of Tables

'Focus On ...' Boxes

'Where Do You Stand?' Boxes

Preface

As research and theory in psychology continue to develop at an ever-quickening pace, its applied branches benefit from this growth but sometimes lead the way themselves in opening up new areas of inquiry. Our interest in writing this book stemmed from a feeling that this has been especially characteristic of forensic psychology. Theories about human action and experience are important elements of scientific progress in themselves, but they also offer the prospect of enabling us to address the problems of living together and avoiding doing one another harm.

We have written this book in an effort to test a particular approach to thinking about what forensic psychologists need to know and understand in order to do their jobs as effectively as possible. We imagined a journey through the network of agencies that form what we loosely call the criminal justice system. That journey begins with some type of criminal offence or antisocial act, usually of a serious kind, so the book explores the best available explanations of how such events come about. From police investigation, through courts to sentences, judicial penalty or mental health treatment, the subsequent journey can be a tortuous and circuitous one, and no text can do full justice to its potential twists and turns. We have tried to focus on the decisions made at each stage, the options available, and how the information produced at a given point influences the direction taken in the next phase. As set out in the textbook, this journey is a metaphorical rather than a literal one: individual paths may each be hugely different.

In the book we also focus on the tasks forensic psychologists typically carry out. We examine their roles in carrying out these tasks, and the skills needed to perform them. We also survey possible routes into the profession. While this book is aimed primarily at those who are considering or who are already pursuing training towards a career in this field, we hope that those currently practising will also find topics in the book treated at sufficient depth to address specific problems that arise in their work.

Thus an important theme of the book is its depiction of a journey made along different possible routes. We hope that a further strength of the book lies in the links made between forensic psychology, a specific form of applied practice, and the field of psychology as a whole; and in the links made in addition with other disciplines, from law and criminology to psychiatry, which adjoin the field of forensic psychology.

James McGuire
Simon Duff
October 2017

Tour of the Book

Part 1 | Part 2 | Part 3 | Part 4

Forensic Psychology: Concepts, Methods and Theory

Forensic psychology is a broad and developing field which can have a significant impact not only on offenders but also on those who have been affected by their offences in the past or who might be at risk in the future. Part 1 introduces ideas that are central to the role of forensic psychologists when working with offenders and with colleagues in the criminal justice system.

Part introductions

Part introductions give you a flavour of the topics and the issues which will be covered in each chapter.

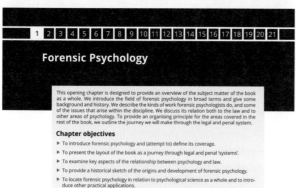

1 2 3 4 5 6 7 8 9 10 11 12 13 14 15 16 17 18 19 20 21

Forensic Psychology

This opening chapter is designed to provide an overview of the subject matter of the book as a whole. We introduce the field of forensic psychology in broad terms and give some background and history. We describe the kinds of work forensic psychologists do, and some of the issues that arise within the discipline. We discuss its relation both to the law and to other areas of psychology. To provide an organising principle for the areas covered in the rest of the book, we outline the journey we will make through the legal and penal system.

Chapter objectives

- To introduce forensic psychology and (attempt to) define its coverage.
- To present the layout of the book as a journey through legal and penal 'systems'.
- To examine key aspects of the relationship between psychology and law.
- To provide a historical sketch of the origins and development of forensic psychology.
- To locate forensic psychology in relation to psychological science as a whole and to introduce other practical applications.

Chapter objectives

Chapter objectives set out the main features of the chapter and identify the 'need to know' concepts and ideas.

Boxes to expand your knowledge:

FOCUS ON ...

Professional psychology associations relevant to forensic psychologists

Associations in the United Kingdom

British Psychological Society (BPS)
Division of Forensic Psychology (DFP)

The BPS was founded in 1901 (though the word 'British' was not added till 1906). It publishes eleven journals, and currently has ten divisions, each focused on a particular area of professional practice.

The Division of Forensic Psychology (DFP), initially established in 1977 as the Division of Criminological and Legal Psychology, changed its name in 1999. As of mid-2017 it had a membership of approximately 2,500, including 1,000 full practitioner members. the Sektion Rechtspsychologie (legal psychology section) of the Berufsverband Deutscher Psychologinnen und Psychologen (BDP, the Association of German Professional Psychologists). The Sektion publishes a house journal, *Praxis der Rechtspsychologie*, and hosts an annual conference. The BPS, the BDP and many other national associations are members of the European Federation of Psychologists' Associations (EFPA), which has a total of 36 member associations, together representing a total of 300,000 psychologists.

European Association of Psychology and Law (EAPL)

Focus on ...

Each 'Focus on ...' box looks in depth at a particular concept, topic, case study or aspect of the law.

WHERE DO YOU STAND?

Causing serious harm without committing a crime

Many kinds of avoidable harm in society are caused by actions that are not defined as crimes. Some such actions have caused more deaths and other kinds of harm than the behaviour we *call* 'crime', yet they are rarely defined as crime or included in the criminal statistics. Many do not attract the attention of law enforcement agencies. The following are examples.

Safety standards in the workplace

There are often failures to adhere to safety standards in the workplace. Few incidents of this kind result in criminal proceedings; and often, despite fatalities, no one is held respon- 2003), and there is no reason to consider that in this respect an atypical year. There is extensive evidence that tobacco companies have concealed or destroyed documents (LeGresley, Muggli and Hurt, 2005) or have sought to influence the public to disbelieve the evidence of the connection between tobacco and fatal disease (Cummings, Morley and Hyland, 2002). Those who sought redress had no recourse to the criminal law but were obliged to pursue their claims through civil litigation.

Arms sales

Arms have been sold to political regimes in circumstances where there were indications

Where do you stand?

Each 'Where do you stand?' box deals with an issue or a topic that is particularly suited to seminar debate or discussion. These boxes will encourage you to think critically.

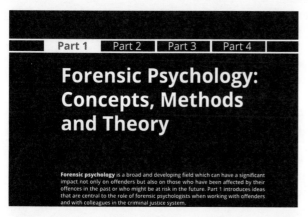

Figures and tables

Figures and tables help you to understand key points.

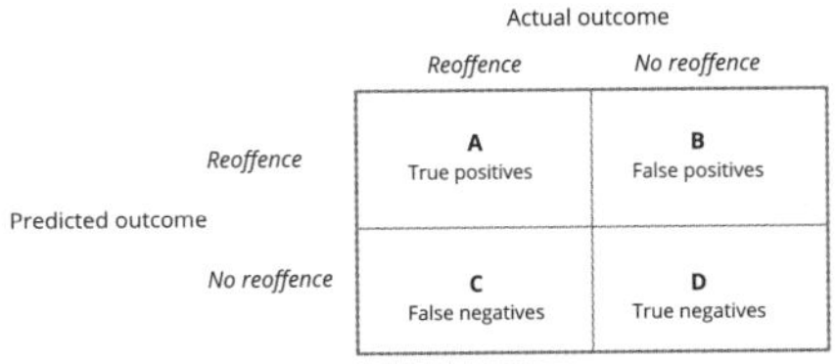

Actual outcome
Reoffence
No reoffence
Reoffence
Predicted outcome
No reoffence
A
True positives
B
False positives
C
False negatives
D
True negatives

Sensitivity = the rate of true positives (A/A+C)
Specificity = the rate of true negatives (D/B+D)

Figure 18.3
Basic terms used in studying predictive accuracy.

1 Conducting psychological applications and interventions	2 Research	3 Communicating psychological knowledge and advice to other professionals	4 Training other professionals in psychological skills and knowledge
(a) establishing requirements for, and the benefits of, applications/interventions	(a) designing psychological research activities	(a) promoting awareness of the actual and potential contribution of applied psychological services	(a) identifying and analysing needs to improve or prepare for job performance in specific areas
(b) planning applications/interventions	(b) conducting research activities	(b) providing psychological advice to assist and inform problem solving and decision-making	(b) planning and designing training and development programmes
(c) establishing, developing and maintaining working relationships	(c) analysing and evaluating psychological research data	(c) providing psychological advice to aid the formulation of policy and its implementation	(c) implementing training and development programmes
(d) implementing applications/interventions		(d) preparing and presenting evidence in formal settings	(d) planning and implementing assessment procedures for training and development programmes
(e) directing implementation of applications/interventions carried out by others		(e) responding to informal requests for psychological information	(e) evaluating training and development programmes
(f) evaluating results of applications/interventions*		(f) providing feedback to clients	

*Here 'psychological applications' refers to the 'application of psychological principles within criminal and civil legal contexts' (Division of Forensic Psychology, dfp.bps.org.uk), thus the idea is that a candidate demonstrates that they have thought through and understood the appropriateness of using psychology, and indeed specific aspects of psychology, in a particular case.

Table 21.1 Four core competences required of a forensic psychologist, and the areas they comprise.

Chapter summary

The chapter summary recaps the key issues covered in the chapter, which helps to deepen your learning.

Chapter summary

- As a unifying theme for the book, we have proposed the idea of considering the different routes an imaginary individual might make through the complex 'system' of legal, penal and mental health agencies inside which forensic psychologists work. We will follow that general direction and several others, both in the 'parent discipline' of psychology and also in other applied fields. A crucial connection, of course, is forensic psychology's relationship to law, and the chapter has mapped some of the main links that exist between the two.
- Like psychology as a whole, forensic psychology adopts a scientific

Further reading

To take your learning further, refer to these key books, online resources, journal articles or original research examples.

Further reading

- There are several major and weighty handbooks covering the connections between psychology and law, including these:
  - Irving B. Weiner and Randy K. Otto (2014), *Handbook of Forensic Psychology*, 4th edition (New York: Wiley).
  - Ray Bull and David Carson (2003), *Handbook of Psychology in Legal*
- Specifically for criminological psychology – as it pays more attention to crime and to offender rehabilitation, and less attention to forensic or psycho-legal aspects – a key source is James Bonta and Don A. Andrews (2017), *The Psychology of Criminal Conduct* (New York: Routledge).
- For a book with a more explicit in-depth legal or forensic focus, see John Monahan and Laurens Walker (2009), *Social Science*

Glossary

Key concepts and terms are printed in bold type within the chapter text. A full glossary of relevant terms can be found at the end of the book.

Glossary

Actuarial risk assessment instrument (ARAI) One of a set of methods for estimating the likelihood of future offending, in which predictions are made on the basis of a tabulation or dataset showing relationships between independent variables and outcomes on prior occasions, which when analysed yields patterns that can be used for predictive purposes. To date most ARAIs have focused on general reconviction, personal violence, partner violence or sexual reoffending.

Appeal A formal application for review of a legal decision made by a court, usually submitted to a court in a higher tier in the justice system.

Area under the curve (AUC) A statistic derived from a signal-detection model of quantifying risk which relates proportions of accurate predictions ('hits') to error rates ('false alarms'), providing a measure of the overall predictive validity of a risk assessment instrument.

Assizes These were courts held in the main county towns of England and Wales twice a

Online Resources

To access a wealth of materials to support your course and your use of the textbook, please visit: **www.macmillanihe.com/McGuire-Duff-Forensic**

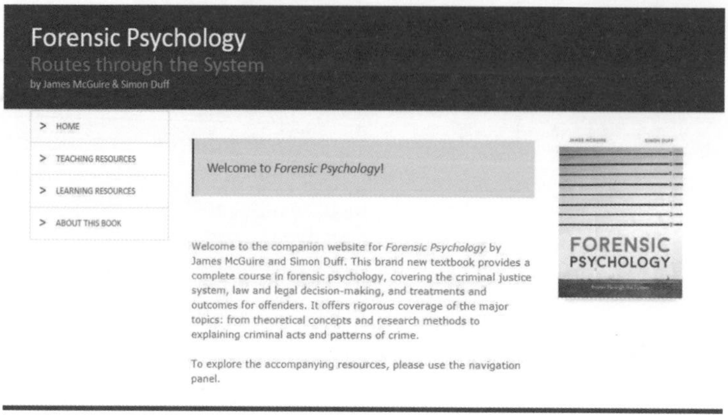
Forensic Psychology
Routes through the System
by James McGuire & Simon Duff
> HOME
> TEACHING RESOURCES
> LEARNING RESOURCES
> ABOUT THIS BOOK
Welcome to Forensic Psychology!
Welcome to the companion website for Forensic Psychology by James McGuire and Simon Duff. This brand new textbook provides a complete course in forensic psychology, covering the criminal justice system, law and legal decision-making, and treatments and outcomes for offenders. It offers rigorous coverage of the major topics: from theoretical concepts and research methods to explaining criminal acts and patterns of crime.
To explore the accompanying resources, please use the navigation panel.
FORENSIC
PSYCHOLOGY

For lecturers

» Assessment questions to accompany each chapter.

» Teaching slides which can be adapted to suit your course.

For students

» Transcripts of interviews with people involved in different 'routes through the system': a police officer; a probation officer; a clinical psychologist; and a person serving a prison sentence.

» An employability feature, which helps to map out the route to becoming a forensic psychologist.

» Online flashcards of the glossary terms in the book.

About the Authors

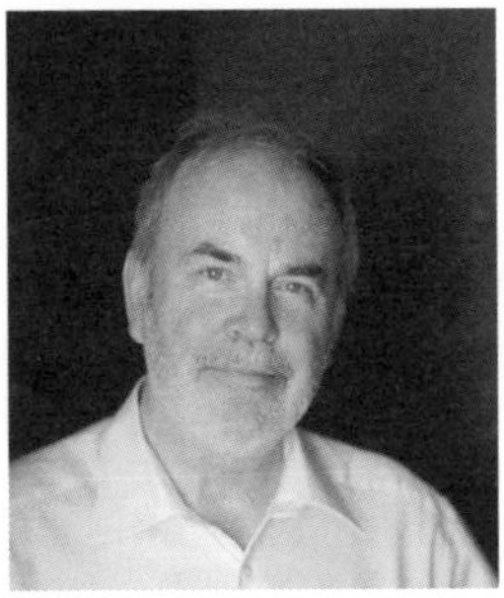

James McGuire

James McGuire, MA, MSc, PhD, is a clinical and forensic psychologist, and is Emeritus Professor of Forensic Clinical Psychology at the University of Liverpool. He obtained an MA in psychology at Glasgow University; a PhD at Leicester University, based partly on cross-cultural fieldwork carried out in Hong Kong; and an MSc in clinical psychology at the University of Leeds. He was self-employed for some time before working in intellectual disabilities services, and later worked for several years in a high security hospital. His interests include aspects of psychosocial rehabilitation with offenders, and he has carried out research in prisons, probation services, youth justice teams, addictions services, and other settings. He has conducted psycho-legal assessments for courts and for parole and review hearings; has been a member of guideline development and review groups on personality disorders for the National Institute of Health and Care Excellence (NICE); and has been a member of the Correctional Services Advisory and Accreditation Panel. He has designed and evaluated a number of intervention and staff training programmes, and has been an adviser to criminal justice agencies in the United Kingdom and several other countries.

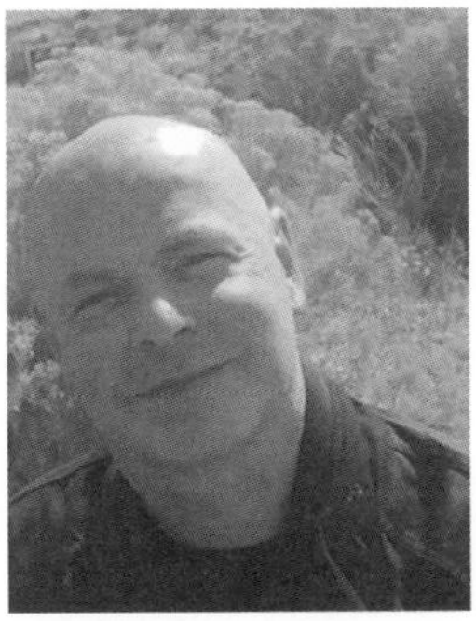

Simon Duff

Simon Duff, BSc, MSc, PhD, is a forensic psychologist. As an academic, he works at the University of Nottingham. He is currently the Director of Stage II Training in Forensic Psychology, with responsibility for the forensic doctorate programme within the Centre for Forensic and Family Psychology. He also does clinical work for Mersey Forensic Psychology Service, where he works individually and in groups with a variety of clients. His teaching covers a range of topics, including sexual offending, stalking, and working with clients with complex problems; and his research interests focus primarily on aspects of sexual offending, stalking, fetishism, and the impact of pornography. Prior to his post at the University of Nottingham, he worked at the University of Liverpool in the UK and at Bergen University in Norway; and he also undertook postdoctoral studies at UC San Diego.

Authors' Acknowledgements

James McGuire

I wish to thank Simon Duff for co-authoring this book. I also thank former and present staff of Palgrave for their patience, encouragement and support while the book was being written. Thank you to Paul Stevens, Amy Grant, Lauren Zimmerman, Tiiu Särkijärvi and Isabel Berwick. Thank you also to Andrew Nash for your meticulous work in editing the text, and greatly improving its clarity, and to Liz Holmes for overseeing text production.

Simon Duff

I wish to thank those people who have directly and indirectly, in large and small ways, been instrumental in this book existing and in teaching me so much about psychology and more. In no particular order: James McGuire; the amazing and patient Palgrave people (Paul, Amy, Lauren, Tiiu, Jamie); my family; my Mersey Forensic Psychology Service colleagues through the years; all my beautiful friends, but especially Coulson, Dorman, King, Nightingale, Scott, Tree; the bike tribe; my musician friends and tutors; SLs; forensic colleagues; Liverpool and Nottingham colleagues and associated professionals, who work so hard; all the clinical and forensic trainees with whom I have had the honour to work; and the clients who trusted enough to work with me.

Publisher's Acknowledgements

The authors and the publisher would like to thank the following people and organisations for the use of their material:

American Association for the Advancement of Science (AAAS), for the graph in the box *Evidence of a gene–environment (G×E) interaction*. From Caspi, A., McClay, J., Moffitt, T. E., Mill, J., Martin, J., Craig, I. W., Taylor, A. & Poulton, R. (2002). Role of Genotype in the Cycle of Violence in Maltreated Children. *Science*, 297 (5582), 851–854. http://science.sciencemag.org/content/297/5582/851 Readers may view, browse, and/or download material for temporary copying purposes only, provided these uses are for noncommercial personal purposes. Except as provided by law, this material may not be further reproduced, distributed, transmitted, modified, adapted, performed, displayed, published, or sold in whole or in part, without prior written permission from the publisher.

American Psychological Association, for:

» Figure 5.3. From Figure 1.3. in Sameroff, A. (2009). The Transactional Model. In A. Sameroff (ed.), *The Transactional Model of Development: How Children and Contexts Shape Each Other*. pp. 3–21. Washington, DC: American Psychological Association. Copyright © APA 2009. Reprinted with permission.

» Figure 5.4. From Figure 4 in Mischel, W. and Shoda, Y. (1995). A Cognitive-Affective System Theory of Personality: Reconceptualizing Situations, Dispositions, Dynamics and Invariance in Personality Structure. *Psychological Review*, 102 (2), 246–268, American Psychological Association. Copyright © APA 1995. Adapted with permission. DOI: http://dx.doi.org/10.1037/0033-295X.102.2.246

» Figure 11.1. From Figure 2 in Edens, J. F., Marcus, D. K., Lilienfeld, S. O. and Poythress Jr., N. G. (2006). Psychopathic, Not Psychopath: Taxometric Evidence for the Dimensional Structure of Psychopathy. *Journal of Abnormal Psychology*, 115 (1), 131–144. Copyright © APA 2006. Reprinted with permission. DOI: 10.1037/0021-843X.115.1.131

Annual Reviews, for the lower part of Figure 6.1. From Anderson, C. A. & Bushman, B. J. (2002). Human Aggression. *Annual Review of Psychology*, 53 (1), 27–51. Copyright © by Annual Reviews, http://www.annualreviews.org

Australian Bureau of Statistics, for data in Table 9.1. From Australian Bureau of Statistics, 2006, *Personal Safety Survey*, cat. no. 4906.0, viewed 07 October 2017, http://www.abs.gov.au/AUSSTATS/abs@.nsf/DetailsPage/4906.02005%20(Reissue)?OpenDocument Copyright © Commonwealth of Australia 2006, licensed under https://creativecommons.org/licenses/by/2.5/au

Birkbeck, University of London, for Figure 16.3. From World Prison Brief, Institute for Criminal Policy Research, Birkbeck, University of London.

Cambridge University Press, for Figure 18.1. From Figure 2.1 The "timelines" used in the interview. From Zamble, E. & Quinsey, V. L. (1997). *The Criminal Recidivism Process*. New York: Cambridge University Press. Copyright ©1997 Cambridge University Press.

Professor David Canter, for Figure 13.1. From Canter, D. V. (1994). *Criminal Shadows: Inside the Mind of the Serial Killer*. London: HarperCollins. Copyright © 1994 Professor David Canter.

Elsevier, for:

» Figure 9.3. Reprinted from *Aggression and Violent Behavior*, 11 (1), Ward, T. & Beech, A., An integrated theory of sexual offending, p. 51. Copyright 2006, with permission from Elsevier. DOI: https://doi.org/10.1016/j.avb.2005.05.002

» Figure 19.2. Reprinted from *Journal of Criminal Justice*, 38 (4), Lowenkamp, C. T., Flores, A. W., Holsinger, A. M., Makarios, M. D., Latessa, E. J., Intensive supervision programs: Does program philosophy and the principles of effective intervention matter?, p. 374. Copyright 2010, with permission from Elsevier. DOI: https://doi.org/10.1016/j.jcrimjus.2010.04.004

» The table in the box *Measuring the seriousness of sexual offending*. Reprinted from *International Journal of Law and Psychiatry*, 23(2), Aylwin, A. S., Clelland, S. R., Kirkby, L., Reddon, J. R., Studer, L. H. & Johnston, J., Sexual Offense Severity and Victim Gender Preference: A Comparison of Adolescent and Adult Sex Offenders, p. 117. Copyright © 2000, with permission from Elsevier. DOI: https://doi.org/10.1016/S0160-2527(99)00038-2

Guilford Publications, for Figure 6.1. From Anderson, C. A. & Carnagey, N. L. (2004). Violent Evil and the General Aggression Model. In A. G. Miller (ed.), *The Social Psychology of Good and Evil*. pp. 168–192. New York, NY: Guilford. © 2004 Guilford Publications; permission conveyed through Copyright Clearance Center, Inc.

HEUNI, for Figure 2.1. From Malby, S. (2010). Homicide. In S. Harrendorf, M. Heiskanen & S. Malby (eds.). *International Statistics on Crime and Justice*. HEUNI Publication Series No.64. pp. 7–20. Helsinki and Vienna: European Institute for Crime Prevention and Control & United Nations Office on Drugs and Crime.

John Wiley & Sons, Inc., for:

» Table 1.1. Adapted from Table 2.1: Epistemological Differences between Psychology and Law. From Hess, A. K. (2006). Defining Forensic Psychology. In I. B. Weiner & A. K. Hess (eds.). *The Handbook of Forensic Psychology*. 3rd ed. pp. 43–44. Hoboken, NJ: John Wiley & Sons, Inc. Copyright © 2006 by John Wiley & Sons, Inc. All rights reserved.

» Table 4.1. Adapted from Table 7.1 A schematic representation of levels of explanation in criminological theories. From McGuire, J. (2000). Explanations of Criminal Behaviour. In J. McGuire, T. Mason & A. O'Kane (eds.). *Behaviour, Crime and Legal Processes: A Guide for Forensic Practitioners*. pp. 135–160. Chichester: John Wiley & Sons Ltd. Copyright © 2000 by John Wiley & Sons Ltd.

» The graph in the box *Coercive family process and coercion theory*. From Figure 1 Hypothesized social interactional model of physical fighting in Patterson, G. R., Dishion, T. J. & Bank, L. (1984). Family Interaction: A Process Model of Deviancy Training. *Aggressive Behavior*, 10 (3), 253–267, Wiley-Liss, Inc. Copyright © 1984 Alan R. Liss, Inc. DOI: 10.1002/1098-2337(1984)10:3<253::AID-AB2480100309>3.0.CO;2-2

» Figure 5.2. From Figures 1 and 2 in Granic, I. & Dishion, T. J. (2003). Deviant Talk in Adolescent Friendships: A Step Toward Measuring a Pathogenic Attractor Process. *Social Development*, 12 (3), 314–334, John Wiley & Sons Ltd. Copyright © Blackwell Publishing Ltd. 2003. DOI: 10.1111/1467-9507.00236

» Figure 9.2. From Figure 14.1 The offender types in the MTC: R3 as described by Knight and Prentky (1990). From Reid, S., Wilson, N. J. & Boer, D. P. (2011). Risk, Needs, and Responsivity Principles in Action: Tailoring Rapist's Treatment to Rapist Typologies. In D. P. Boer, R. Eher, L. A. Craig, M. H. Miner & F. Pfäfflin (eds.), *International Perspectives on the Assessment and Treatment of Sexual Offenders: Theory, Practice, and Research*. pp. 287–297. Chichester: Wiley-Blackwell. Copyright © 2011 John Wiley & Sons Ltd.

» Figure 10.1. From Figure 7.4 A simplified diagram of a Choice Theory of addiction with self-control, and instrumental learning added. From West, R. & Brown, J. (2013). *Theory of Addiction*. 2nd edition. Chichester, UK: Wiley-Blackwell. This edition first published 2013, © 2013 by John Wiley & Sons, Ltd. First edition published 2009, © 2009 Robert West.

» Figure 16.6. From Figures 1, 4 & 5 in Zimring, F. E., Fagan, J. & Johnson, D. T. (2010). Executions, Deterrence, and Homicide: A Tale of Two Cities. *Journal of Empirical Legal Studies*, 7(1), 1–29, John Wiley & Sons Ltd. Copyright © 2010 by John Wiley & Sons, Inc. All rights reserved. DOI: 10.1111/j.1740-1461.2009.01168.x (The data sources are: Chan, Edna (1967–2007). *Hong Kong Police Data*. Hong Kong: Office of Commissioner of Police; Singapore Police (2005–2007). *Singapore Homicides from Police Data*. In United Nations Statistics Division, https://unstats.un.org; Statistics Singapore (1973–1982). *Homicide in Singapore*. www.singstat.gov.sg; World Development Indicators database in Nationmaster.com; World Health Organization (1984–2004). *Homicide Data from Singapore*. In Statistics Singapore, www.sing.stat.gov.sg; World Health Organization (1979–2001). *Homicide in Singapore*. www.who.int)

» Extracts in the box *Self-evaluation of reports*. Adapted from Evaluation Form for Psychological Reports in Ownby, R. L. (1997). *Psychological Reports: A Guide to Report Writing in Professional Psychology*. 3rd edition. New York, NY: John Wiley & Sons, Inc. Copyright © 1997 by John Wiley & Sons, Inc. All rights reserved.

Open International Publishing Ltd, for Figure 3.1, Table 3.1, extracts in the box *Meta-analysis and effect size*, and the graph in the box *Stability of aggressiveness*. From McGuire, J., *Understanding psychology and crime: Perspectives on theory and action*, © 2004. Reproduced and adapted with the kind permission of Open International Publishing Ltd. All rights reserved.

SAGE, for:

» Figure 9.4. Adapted from Heise, L. L. (1998). Violence Against Women: An Integrated, Ecological Framework. *Violence Against Women*, 4 (3), 262–290, SAGE. DOI: https://doi.org/10.1177/1077801298004003002

» Figure 18.2. From Figure 1 in Agnew, R. (2006). Storylines As a Neglected Cause of Crime. *Journal of Research in Crime and Delinquency*, 43 (2), 119–147. Copyright © 2006 Sage Publications. DOI:10.1177/0022427805280052

Springer, for the table in the box *Problems, risk factors, and likelihood of offending*. From Table 6 in Huizinga, D., Weiher, A. W., Espiritu, R. and Esbensen, F. (2003). Delinquency and Crime: Some Highlights from the Denver Youth Survey. In T. P. Thornberry and M. D. Krohn (eds.). *Taking Stock of Delinquency: An Overview of Findings from Contemporary Longitudinal Studies*. p. 62. New York: Kluwer Academic Publishers. © Kluwer Academic Publishers 2003.

SCSC, for the table in the box *What are the effects of psychotropic medication?* Adapted from Joanna Moncrieff, *The Myth of the Chemical Cure: A Critique of Psychiatric Drug Treatment* published 2008 by Palgrave Macmillan.

Stanford University Press, sup.org, for Figure 5.1. From *A General Theory of Crime* by Gottfredson, M. R. & Hirschi, T. Copyright © 1990 by the Board of Trustees of the Leland Stanford Jr. University. All rights reserved.

Taylor and Francis Books UK, for:

» Figure 10.2. From Figure 3.1 The etiological cycle of predatory criminality in Topalli, V. & Wright, R. (2014). Affect and the dynamic foreground of predatory street crime: Desperation, anger, and fear. In J. L. van Gelder, H. Elffers, D. Reynald & D. S. Nagin (eds.), *Affect and Cognition in Criminal Decision Making*. p. 44. Abingdon, Oxon: Routledge. Copyright © 2014 Routledge.

» Figure 14.1. From Figure 1.1 The criminal justice process and diversion mechanisms in McMurran, M., Khalifa, N., and Gibbon, S. (2009). *Forensic Mental Health*. Cullompton, Devon: Willan Pubishing. p. 3. Copyright © 2009 Willan Publishing.

Taylor and Francis Group, LLC, a division of Informa plc, for Table 3.2. Copyright © 2008. Adapted from Table 1.1 Definitions of Terms in Loeber, R., Farrington, D. P., Stouthamer-Loeber, M. and Raskin White, H. (2008). Introduction and Key Questions. In Loeber, R., Farrington, D. P., Stouthamer-Loeber, M. and Raskin White, H. (eds.), *Violence and Serious Theft: Development and Prediction from Childhood to Adulthood.* p. 9. New York, NY: Routledge.

Thomson Reuters (Professional) Australia Limited, for Table 14.2. Adapted from Freckelton, I. & Selby, H. (2002). *Expert Evidence: Law, Practice, Procedure and Advocacy.* Sydney: Lawbook Co.

University of Chicago Press, for:

» Figure 4.1. From Eisner, M. (2003). Long-Term Historical Trends in Violent Crime. *Crime and Justice*, 30, 83–142. Journal series editor: M. Tonry; Publisher: The University of Chicago Press. © 2003 by The University of Chicago. All rights reserved.

» The graph from the box *Inequality and violence.* From Fajnzylber, P., Lederman, D. & Loayza, N. (2002). Inequality and Violent Crime. *The Journal of Law & Economics*, 45(1), 1–39. Publisher: The University of Chicago Press for The Booth School of Business. Journal editors: D. W. Carlton, D. Dharmapala, J. P. Gould, R. Holden, A. Malani & S. Peltzman. © 2002 by The University of Chicago. All rights reserved.

» Table 4.2. Adapted from Pratt, T. C. & Cullen, F. T. (2005). Assessing Macro-Level Predictors and Theories of Crime: A Meta-Analysis. In M. Tonry (ed.) *Crime and Justice, Volume 32: A Review of Research.* pp. 373–450. Chicago, IL: University of Chicago Press. © 2005 by The University of Chicago. All rights reserved.

» The figure in the box *Anger dysfunctions and angry violence.* Adapted from Novaco, R. W. (1994). Anger as a risk factor for violence among the mentally disordered. In J. Monahan & H. J. Steadman (eds.) *Violence and Mental Disorder: Developments in Risk Assessment.* pp. 21–60. Chicago, IL: University of Chicago Press. Part of The John D. and Catherine T. MacArthur Foundation Series on Mental Health and Development. © 1994 by The University of Chicago. All rights reserved.

Wetenschappelijk Onderzoeken Documentatiecentrum (WODC), for Figure 2.3. From van Dijk, J., van Kesteren, J. & Smit, P. (2007). *Criminal Victimisation in International Perspective: Key Findings from the 2004–2005 ICVS and EU ICS.* Den Haag: Wetenschappelijk Onderzoeken Documentatiecentrum.

UK Parliament, for the quote on page 317 and Figure 16.4, which contain Parliamentary information licensed under the Open Parliament Licence v3.0: http://www.parliament.uk/site-information/copyright-parliament/open-parliament-licence

The UK public sector, for information licensed under the Open Government Licence v3.0: http://www.nationalarchives.gov.uk/doc/open-government-licence/version/3 Please see individual source lines for details.

Abbreviations

Note: Tests, measures, scales and interviews are marked in *italics*

AA	Alcoholics Anonymous
AASI	*Abel Assessment for Sexual Interest*
ABCs	antecedents, behaviours and consequences
ACPO	Association of Chief Police Officers of England, Wales and Northern Ireland (note: replaced from 2015 by the National Police Chiefs' Council (UK))
ADHD	attention deficit hyperactivity disorder
AERA	American Educational Research Association
AOP	Adolescent Outcomes Project (USA)
APA	American Psychological Association
APF	Arson Prevention Forum (UK)
APLS	American Psychology-Law Society
ARAI	actuarial risk assessment instrument
ASB	antisocial behaviour
ASPD	antisocial personality disorder
AUC	area under the curve
BABCP	British Association of Behavioural and Cognitive Psychotherapies
BCS	British Crime Survey
BDMA	Brain Disease Model of Addiction
BDP	Berufsverband Deutscher Psychologinnen und Psychologen (the Association of German Professional Psychologists)
BIA	Behavioural Investigative Adviser (UK)
BILD	British Institute of Learning Disabilities
BPD	borderline personality disorder
BPS	British Psychological Society
CAPS	Cognitive-Affective Processing System
CAT	cognitive analytic therapy
CBT	cognitive-behavioural therapy
CCTV	closed-circuit television
CDATE	Correctional Drug Abuse Treatment Evaluation (USA)
CEP	criminal event perspective
CICA	Criminal Injuries Compensation Authority (UK)
CIDI	*Composite International Diagnostic Interview*
CMHPs	common mental health problems
COPINE	Combating Paedophile Information Networks in Europe
CPD	continuing professional development
CPOs	child pornography offenders
CPS	Crown Prosecution Service (England and Wales)
CQT	*Comparison Question Test*
CRB	Criminal Records Bureau (England and Wales) (formerly the Criminal Records Office; subsequently incorporated as part of the Disclosure and Barring Service)

CSA	child sexual abuse
CSAAP	Correctional Services Advisory and Accreditation Panel (England and Wales)
CSEW	Crime Survey for England and Wales
CT	computerised tomography
DA	domestic abuse
DBT	dialectical behaviour therapy
DFP	Division of Forensic Psychology (of the BPS)
DNA	deoxyribonucleic acid
DOI	Digital object identifier
DPP	Director of Public Prosecutions (England and Wales)
DSM	Diagnostic and Statistical Manual of Mental and Behavioral Disorders
DT-MRI	diffusion tensor magnetic resonance imaging
DV	domestic violence
DVFRC	Domestic Violence Fatality Review Committee (USA)
DZ	dizygotic
EAPL	European Association of Psychology and Law
ECT	electroconvulsive therapy
EFPA	European Federation of Psychologists' Associations
EPM	Expository Process Model
ERG-20	*Extremism Risk Guidance* (Ministry of Justice, UK)
ES	effect size
ETS	Enhanced Thinking Skills
EU	European Union
FBI	Federal Bureau of Investigation (USA)
FIT-R	*Fitness Interview Test – Revised*
fMRI	functional magnetic resonance imaging
FRA	Agency for Fundamental Rights (EU)
FSC	Forward Specialisation Coefficient
GAD	generalised anxiety disorder
GAM	General Aggression Model
GBC	Graduate Basis for Chartered Membership (BPS)
GDP	Gross Domestic Product
GHB	gamma-hydroxybutyric acid
GKT	Guilty Knowledge Test
GLM	Good Lives Model
GNP	Gross National Product
h^2	heritability
HCPC	Health and Care Professions Council (UK)
IACFP	International Association of Correctional and Forensic Psychologists
IAPT	Improving Access to Psychological Therapies
ICC	International Criminal Court
ICD	International Classification of Diseases
ICVS	International Crime Victims Survey
IPDE	*International Personality Disorder Examination*
IPH	intimate partner homicide
IPP	Imprisonment for Public Protection (England and Wales)
IPV	intimate partner violence
ITSO	Integrated Theory of Sexual Offending

LD	learning disability
LIBOR	London Interbank Offered Rate
LSH	*Likelihood to Sexually Harass Scale*
M-TTAF	Multi-Trajectory Theory of Adult Firesetting
MAMBAC	mean above minus below a cut
MAPPA	Multi-Agency Public Protection Arrangement (England and Wales)
MBA	Master of Business Administration
MCI	*Modified Cognitive Interview*
MDS	multi-dimensional scaling
MHA	Mental Health Act
MRI	magnetic resonance imaging
MTC	Massachusetts Treatment Center
MZ	monozygotic
NCME	National Council on Measurement in Education (USA)
NCRS	National Crime Recording Standard (England and Wales)
NCS-R	National Comorbidity Survey Replication (USA)
NCVS	National Crime Victimization Survey (USA)
NDRI	National Development and Research Institutes (USA)
NEW-ADAM	New English and Welsh Arrestee Drug Abuse Monitoring study
NGRI	not guilty by reason of insanity (USA)
NHS	National Health Service
NIBRS	National Incident-Based Reporting System (USA)
NICE	National Institute of Health and Care Excellence (UK)
NIDA	National Institute on Drug Abuse (USA)
NISCALE	Netherlands Institute for the Study of Crime and Law Enforcement
NISMART	National Incidence Studies of Missing, Abducted, Runaway and Thrownaway Children (USA)
NOMS	National Offender Management Service (England and Wales)
NPS	National Probation Service (England and Wales)
NPSs	new psychoactive substances
NSCS	National Survey of Crime Severity (USA)
NSPCC	National Society for the Prevention of Cruelty to Children (UK)
NTORS	National Treatment Outcome Research Study (UK)
NVDRS	National Violent Death Reporting System (USA)
NYS	National Youth Survey (USA)
OASys	Offender Assessment System (England and Wales)
OECD	Organisation for Economic Co-operation and Development
OGRS	Offender Group Reconviction Scale (currently OGRS-3)
ONS	Office for National Statistics
ORI	obsessive relational intrusion
PACE	Police and Criminal Evidence Act 1984 (England and Wales)
PCL	*Psychopathy Checklist*
PCL:R	*Psychopathy Checklist – Revised*
PCL:SV	*Psychopathy Checklist – Screening Version*
PCL:YV	*Psychopathy Checklist – Youth Version*
PD	personality disorder
PD-TS	personality disorder – trait specified
PEACE	Planning and preparation; Engage and explain; Account, clarification, challenge; Closure; and Evaluation (interviewing model)
PIPEs	Psychologically Informed Planned Environments

PNC	Police National Computer (England and Wales)
PPG	penile plethysmography
PSI	person–situation interactions
PTSD	post-traumatic stress disorder
RCT	randomised controlled trial
RMH	response modulation hypothesis
RNR	Risk–Needs–Responsivity model
ROC	Receiver Operating Characteristics
ROIs	regions of interest
RWA	right-wing authoritarianism
SAP	Sentencing Advisory Panel (England and Wales)
SDO	social dominance orientation
SES	socioeconomic status
SHR	Supplementary Homicide Reports (FBI)
SIDS	sudden infant death syndrome
SOCs	sexual offenders against children
SOPO	Sexual Offences Prevention Order (England and Wales)
SOTP	sex-offender treatment programme (England and Wales)
SPJ	structured professional judgment
SRP	*Stalking Risk Profile*
SUDI	sudden unexplained deaths in infancy
TC	therapeutic community
TCO	threat/control override symptoms
TSI	Targeted Subject Interviewing
TUC	Trades Union Congress (UK)
UCRs	Uniform Crime Reports (US)
UN	United Nations
UN-CTS	United Nations Survey on Crime Trends and the Operations of Criminal Justice Systems
UNODC	United Nations Office on Drugs and Crime
USPO	United States Probation Service
VERA 2	*Violent Extremism Assessment protocol, Version 2*
VIM	violence inhibition mechanism
VPG	vaginal plethysmography
VPS	Victim Personal Statement (UK)
VRAG	*Violence Risk Appraisal Guide*
WAIS-IV	*Wechsler Adult Intelligence Scale*, fourth edition (psychometric test)
WAVE	Women Against Violence Europe
WHO	World Health Organization (UN)
Y-SAV	Youth Sexual Aggression and Victimization project (USA)
YOI	Young Offender Institution (England and Wales)
YOT	Youth Offending Team (England and Wales)

Forensic Psychology: Concepts, Methods and Theory

Forensic psychology is a broad and developing field which can have a significant impact not only on offenders but also on those who have been affected by their offences in the past or who might be at risk in the future. Part 1 introduces ideas that are central to the role of forensic psychologists when working with offenders and with colleagues in the criminal justice system.

1 Forensic Psychology

Chapter 1 introduces the book's main themes. As well as describing the field of forensic psychology and what forensic psychologists do, it looks at the subject's relationship with the law and with other areas of psychology.

2 Defining and Surveying Crime

Chapter 2 examines how crimes are defined, and what it means to break the criminal law. In discussing how often crimes occur and who commits them, it is important to understand and to interpret crime statistics from different sources.

3 Researching Crime: Methods and Correlates

Chapter 3 turns to ways of analysing and understanding crime, and the different research methods used in studying the subject. It also reviews some key general findings about offenders and offending behaviour, and introduces the concept of 'risk factors'.

4 Explaining Crime: Theories and Perspectives

Chapter 4 surveys the principal theories of crime and the relationship between psychology and criminology. What are the causes of crime? Criminological theory often focuses on different 'levels of explanation', from society as a whole down to the internal processes of the individual offender.

5 Understanding Criminal Acts and Actors

Chapter 5 focuses on factors that may influence the individual offender and that may potentially contribute to delinquency, antisocial or criminal behaviour, and ultimately to a criminal lifestyle. Can we learn anything about individuals' internal processes, both cognitive and emotional, as they respond to actual situations?

Forensic Psychology

This opening chapter is designed to provide an overview of the subject matter of the book as a whole. We introduce the field of forensic psychology in broad terms and give some background and history. We describe the kinds of work forensic psychologists do, and some of the issues that arise within the discipline. We discuss its relation both to the law and to other areas of psychology. To provide an organising principle for the areas covered in the rest of the book, we outline the journey we will make through the legal and penal system.

Chapter objectives

- To introduce forensic psychology and (attempt to) define its coverage.
- To present the layout of the book as a journey through legal and penal 'systems'.
- To examine key aspects of the relationship between psychology and law.
- To provide a historical sketch of the origins and development of forensic psychology.
- To locate forensic psychology in relation to psychological science as a whole and to introduce other practical applications.

Not so very long ago, few people had heard of 'forensic psychology' and it would have been difficult to find someone who described his or her job using that title. The picture of what the role entails appears to have become implanted in the popular imagination through television dramas, most notably the popular and highly acclaimed 1990s series *Cracker*, in which a somewhat eccentric (not to say maverick) psychologist enables the police to solve serious crimes, and to track down dangerous people using what at times appear to be ingenious insights. Perhaps the image has been sustained, and even amplified, by real-life media reports, which tap into the public's seemingly limitless fascination with violent and sexual crimes.

This depiction contains and perhaps also perpetuates a series of misconceptions. First, even today relatively few people who call themselves forensic psychologists work alongside the police, and those who do are unlikely to employ anything resembling the approach used by Eddie Fitzgerald, *Cracker*'s central character. The majority, in fact, work at what might be called the opposite end of the law-and-order process, in prisons and other penal agencies. Second, while bizarre crimes involving extreme violence certainly do occur, media reports are likely to leave an exaggerated impression of how often that happens, and of the psychological make-up of the majority of people who commit them. Third, the recent portrayal of forensic psychology in fictional form suggests that it is a novel invention, a recent newcomer that struggles to convey an accurate picture of what it is about. By contrast, in some respects forensic psychology is actually well over one hundred years old. It can justifiably be described as the earliest form of applied psychology to make an appearance on what we might call the 'public stage'.

This book adopts a particular approach in describing and explaining what forensic psychology comprises, what its various practitioners do, and what it can contribute to society. Given that this field is intrinsically bound up with the workings of the law, and particularly law relating to criminal behaviour and to mental health, we will follow the journey an imaginary individual might take through the intricate labyrinth of decision processes that the modern law has become. This moves in successive stages from the entry point (typically, being arrested by the police) to the exit (for example, being discharged from prison). But there are many possible entries and exits, and the transit from one to the other is by no means a uniform or linear process. The choice points and alternative pathways that might be taken along the way are numerous and multifaceted. Note that, while in the real world miscarriages of justice are known to occur, the metaphorical 'journey' examined in this book assumes that the hypothetical person we are imagining is indeed guilty of the offences that lead to her or him being prosecuted, convicted and sentenced.

The book's subtitle, *Routes Through the System*, indicates the tasks that forensic psychologists might perform in this sequence of events. Perhaps not surprisingly, the process can be confusing for everyone involved. We acknowledge from the outset that the application of psychology to law can be a subject of considerable complexity, but our prime objective is to guide those new to the area on a familiarisation trip, by the end of which, to paraphrase an old joke, you may still be confused, but at a higher level.

To get us started, this opening chapter will attempt a series of key tasks:

» The first is to consider what we mean by the term 'forensic psychology', and to examine the ways in which various competing definitions overlap or differ from one another. This will involve us in identifying some of the ways in which, despite large contrasts between the two fields, the *law* already employs numerous constructs that are essentially *psychological*. This first task will also lead us to examine the kinds of behaviour with which forensic psychologists are most frequently concerned – which are usually forms of personal violence – and how their work is informed by psychology as a whole, is connected to other forms of applied psychology, and is linked to the work of adjoining professions.

» The second task is to place these concerns in the broader context of how *psychology* itself emerged as a scientific undertaking. This entails outlining some important historical developments and landmarks; and then focusing in more detail on the background, origins and history of the field of *forensic* psychology. We will look briefly at the work of some of the discipline's earliest practitioners, which can illuminate some of its present concerns; and we will consider possible future directions in which forensic psychology may develop.

» Finally, we will look more briefly at how past trends converged into the principal ways in which most forensic psychologists work today; at how the process of 'professionalisation' within the discipline has taken shape; and at the organisational groups that have been established to support that process.

Along the way, we will also make reference to and provide a preliminary sketch of the range of work that forensic psychologists do. In the remaining chapters of the book, we will then address, expand upon and illustrate that work in the context in which it occurs.

Professional pre-qualification postgraduate training in forensic psychology has expanded enormously over the last twenty years or so, with respect not only to the numbers of people pursuing it but also to its coverage and 'knowledge base'. Such training has become established at a number of universities in the United Kingdom; in Germany, Sweden, Spain, Italy and many other parts of Europe; in the United States (where it had its origins), Canada, Australia and New Zealand; and in Japan, India and many other 'non-Western' countries. Hence it can be described as a genuinely international phenomenon, although as yet its practitioner groupings tend to be national or regional rather than worldwide in scope.

Forensic psychology: in search of a definition

Let us start from basics and consider the meanings of the constituent words. The English word 'psychology' contains two parts, both originally from the Greek language. Etymologists suggest that the word *psyche* (*ψυχή*) originally meant 'breath', but was metaphorically transmuted into the idea of 'spirit' or 'soul', and thereby 'mind'. *Logos* (*λόγος*), from the same root as the word 'lexicon', originally meant simply 'to speak', or to give an account of something. The origins of the word 'forensic', on the other hand, are Latin and have the same roots as the word *forum*, referring to a 'market': a place of talk and discussion, hence the debating chamber we call the courtroom. Does this etymology inform our concepts of what these activities consist of today? In a sense it does. Forensic psychologists collect information on individuals' behaviour and on their reported experience, and apply that information to questions that arise in the relationship between the individual and the operation of the law. What they find may then be taken into the arena of public discussion that is the courtroom. By extension, however, this could nowadays be any one of several types of legal hearing, such as a children's panel, a family court, a criminal court, an appellate court, a hearing of the Parole Board, or a Mental Health Tribunal. In Chapters 14 to 17 we will examine the specifics of what happens in several of these loci.

An indispensable and powerful element to inject into this, however, is the adoption of a scientific approach. Contemporary forensic psychology is not based on guesswork or intuition – well, not more than minimally – but on the systematic process of asking questions, gathering evidence, testing hypotheses and constructing theories that has come to be known as the *scientific method*. Hunches may at times have their place, but we should always recognise them as such and check their usefulness and value. Some people have questioned the entitlement of psychology, our 'parent discipline', to be accorded scientific status. This book is firmly grounded in the position that the questions asked by forensic psychology *can* be addressed, and most appropriately *are* addressed, through the application of scientific thinking.

What has been offered so far by way of definition? Seeking to find clarity on this issue is not aided by the fact that as yet there is no firm consensus even amongst specialists in the subject; and the available definitions, while sharing some common elements, also have important differences of emphasis.

Thus most authors writing in this area recognise the difficulty of defining forensic psychology with a precision that can demarcate it from other, related types of applied psychology. Davies (2008) used the metaphor of forensic psychology as a 'broad church' with two aisles, criminological and legal psychology. Howitt (2015) recognises a similar distinction by including both the words 'forensic' and 'criminal' in the title of his textbook. McGuire (2004a) suggested that there are three subdisciplines – legal psychology, criminological psychology, and forensic psychology – with partially distinctive but overlapping meanings, and represented this in a Venn diagram with three intersecting circles. What is now called 'forensic psychology' is fairly nuanced as there are subtle differences of focus and of emphasis between those subdisciplines, which refer to different aspects of the relationship between psychology and the legal system.

In one of the earliest British textbooks in the area explicitly using the words in its title, Haward (1981) forwarded a definition of forensic psychology as denoting:

> that branch of applied psychology which is concerned with the collection, examination and presentation of evidence for judicial purposes. (p. 1)

This conceptualisation, with its emphasis on the provision of evidence to a legal forum, was retained in subsequent proposals regarding how the field should be delineated. Writing during the period when the British Psychological Society's 'Division of Criminological and Legal Psychology' was changing its name to the 'Division of Forensic Psychology', Blackburn (1996) offered a similarly focused, some might say 'puristic' definition, oriented towards the 'front end' of the legal system. Forensic psychology was oriented towards:

> the provision of psychological information for the purpose of facilitating a legal decision. (1996, p. 7)

In the USA, Hess (2006) took a similar view. While recognising that psychologists working in almost any context can potentially come into contact with the law, and increasingly do so (to the extent that they might feel 'belegaled'), Hess described a concentration of activity in psycho-legal assessments and the provision of evidence to courts. Psychologists involved at later stages of an individual's journey through the penal system usually have other job titles, such as 'correctional psychologist'. The same distinction was later also noted by Bartol and Bartol (2014).

A quite different emphasis, which some would depict as equally narrow but for a different reason, was suggested by Huss (2009), who recognised that definitions might vary in their breadth of compass:

> Broadly speaking, forensic psychology refers to any application of psychology to the legal system. However, many refer to this broader field as *psychology and the law* or *psycholegal studies* while specifying that forensic psychology focuses on the practice of clinical psychology to the legal system. (p. 5)

Huss is primarily interested in the use of forensic psychology in the 'assessment and treatment of individuals within a legal context' (p. 6), essentially an extension of clinical psychology into the field of justice. On his own admission, such a definition thereby excludes the study of eyewitness identification, jury decision-making, evaluation of children's testimony, police and investigative psychology, and correctional and prison psychology.

Forensic psychology in practice

There seems little doubt that usage of the term 'forensic psychology' has steadily evolved and expanded to encompass a range of activity that may be some distance removed from courtrooms, and may involve little or no direct contact with legal personnel such as advocates or judges. In the UK nowadays, professionals legitimately entitled to call themselves 'forensic psychologists' pursue a wide range of activities, including assessment of individuals, preparation of reports, assisting police investigations, provision of evidence in courts and other legal hearings, treatment intervention, service evaluation, staff training, advice and consultation, and research. Taking an international perspective, the range of activities is even wider: for example, in some European countries where most forensic psychologists work in private practice (e.g. Denmark and Germany), their main focus is on child and family work. Some of these activities are outside several of the definitions itemised earlier. Nevertheless they are all interconnected with, and either lead towards or flow from, a legal process or decision. The nature and distribution of the workload differs from place to place and has gradually changed over time.

The broad spectrum of activity now indicated by the term 'forensic psychology' is reflected in other formulations. The overall picture is probably best captured in Otto and Ogloff's (2014, pp. 50–51) statement that

> there is no uniform or consensus definition of forensic psychology, and it is clear that psychologists make contributions to the legal system in a multitude of ways.

This parallels the approach taken earlier by Needs (2008), who defined forensic psychology as

> the application of methods, theories and findings from a wide range of areas within psychology to the contexts and concerns of criminal and civil justice. (p. 75)

Thus forensic psychologists practise in a wide range of settings. They work with the police; in courts, prisons, secure units, and hospitals; in probation, youth justice, and family work; and in teaching and research posts in universities. Although an exact definition remains elusive, 'forensic psychology' is perhaps more useful as a convenient umbrella term for a broad range of roles, including the use of psychological research in legal settings. This provisional, working description appears to us to be the one that best fits current practices and is the one we have drawn upon in planning the contents of this book.

Although psychologists turned their attention to legal and forensic matters over a century ago (as we will see below), for most of that period their work remained marginal to the interests of legal professionals, and was supported by very little research directly addressing the questions those professionals might want answered. Particularly during the last three decades, however, there has been vigorous and substantial growth in research. This might be illustrated with reference to the *Annual Review of Psychology* (which has the highest 'Impact Factor' of any journal in psychology, i.e. it is more frequently cited than any other source). The first overview of forensic psychology, by Tapp (1976), documented a lengthy period when psychology had played only a tangential role in the operation of law, but it discerned what appeared to be an accelerating pace of research activity and publication. Since then – and starting, admittedly, from a rather low baseline – forensic psychology has, like other fields, experienced something of a 'data explosion'. By the first decade of the 21st century, two specialised areas of research of core relevance to forensic psychology had advanced sufficiently to attract separate *Annual Review* entries. One surveyed research on eyewitness testimony (Wells and Olson, 2003); the other assessed the status of psychological evidence in (US) courts (Faigman and Monahan, 2005).

Law and psychology

Blending together the outputs from psychological science to address questions posed in law presents some potentially perplexing challenges. *Law* and *psychology* are not simply two separate disciplines, in the ordinary sense that they deal with different subject areas or lead in divergent career directions. As Brigham (1999, p. 281) has suggested, they are almost two 'different cultures'. There are some fundamental differences of perspective with respect to what each considers to be 'knowledge' and how each approaches its application. Hess (2006) identified a series of seven points of contrast between psychology and the law in philosophical and conceptual terms. They are set out in Table 1.1.

Considering the polarities shown in Table 1.1, it might be difficult to see on

Dimension	Psychology	Law
Epistemology	*Objectivity*: Focused on attaining objectivity progressively, reducing bias by methodical critique and processes of replication	*Advocacy*: Focused on promoting and testing the validity of a case in relation to the prevailing law; the strength of a case relates to its consistency with the law (higher consistency, stronger case)
Nature of law	*Descriptive*: Derives from an attempt to discover naturally occurring regularities or reliable predictions	*Prescriptive and normative*: Defines limits to behaviour, proscriptions, and the consequences of transgression
Knowledge	*Empirical*: Addressed towards collecting 'nomothetic' data, testing hypotheses in replicable ways, and developing theories	*Rational*: Based on 'idiographic' or case-generated data, making comparisons between cases, and testing against prior frameworks
Methodology	*Experimental*: Based on testing hypotheses under controlled conditions, and eliminating competing explanations	*Case methodology*: Analysis of specific instances leads to construction of a narrative with reference to a formal framework
Criterion	*Conservative*: Conclusions are dependent on comparison against a statistical standard (significance testing)	*Expedient*: Standards vary according to the context (e.g. 'balance of probabilities' versus 'beyond reasonable doubt')
Principles	*Exploratory*: Facilitates multiple theory development, each competing against an agreed standard (currently 'falsifiability')	*Conservative*: The prevailing theory in resolving cases depends on the coherence of facts in relation to legal precedents
Latitude of behaviour in legal hearings	*Limited*: Confined to observing rules of evidence and responding to judicial questioning or instruction by a lawyer	*Broad*: The capacity to operate in a flexible and creative manner, commensurate with procedural rules but allowing wide scope

Table 1.1 Differences between psychology and law – what constitutes 'knowledge', and how it may be used.

Source: adapted from Table 2.1: Epistemological Differences between Psychology and Law. From Hess, A. K. (2006). Defining Forensic Psychology. In I. B. Weiner & A. K. Hess (eds). The Handbook of Forensic Psychology. 3rd ed. pp. 43–44. Hoboken, NJ: John Wiley & Sons, Inc.

what basis psychology and law might have common ground for exchange and mutual benefit. The possibility of communicating successfully across such large conceptual chasms might seem remote. When psychologists use the term 'law' and attempt to discover patterns that fit that description, they are likely to be thinking of regularities in nature that can be discovered through experimental investigation. By contrast, criminal, civil and other types of formal law are societal constructions, arrived at through rational inquiry informed by accumulated experience from actual cases.

Notwithstanding such discrepancies, perhaps at a deeper level the two seemingly dissimilar domains of law and psychology do have some fundamental features in common. They are both concerned with human action, for example, especially as regards the impact of one person on another; and, by extension, the impact of one person on his or her community and on society as a whole. There is a sense in which the law can even be described as a form of applied psychology: it is based on the accumulation of a large number of observations of individual behaviour.

In fact, the law is replete with psychological concepts. Most fundamental of these, in criminal law, is the concept of ***mens rea***. In its most frequently used sense, this refers to the individual's state of mind at the time an offence was committed. This is usually equivalent to what is commonly called *intention*; but the term can also be used in other senses, such as recklessness, negligence and blameless inadvertence (Carson, 2000). Alongside ***actus reus*** – the crime itself – *mens rea* is a cornerstone of legal thought. For a court to convict a person of a crime, both 'blameworthy acts' and 'blameworthy mental elements' must be established (Ormerod and Laird, 2015). Whether or not a person acted with full knowledge and foresight of his or her behaviour, and was fully responsible for his or her action, are factors that lead to extensive and considered arguments in many legal proceedings. In English law, for example, *mens rea* is formalised in legal statutes such as the Homicide Act 1957, which allows for the possibility of **diminished responsibility** (the perpetrator did not knowingly plan or intend to kill, or did so as a consequence of mental disorder); and the Infanticide Act 1932, which was an acceptance into law of what is now recognised as post-natal depression. Parallel distinctions are embodied in other legal decisions, and in the penalties that accompany them. Such distinctions are made, for example, in the categories of assault defined by the Offences Against the Person Act 1861, which addresses the level of harm caused and the extent to which it was intended (Carter and Harrison, 1991).

Going still farther, law makes extensive use of what are called *legal artefacts*. These are constructions of hypothetical persons with presumed psychological capacities and culturally normative reactions. Central to them is the concept of the *reasonable person*. Eastman (2000) describes departures from this concept, which were traditionally allotted names such as: 'automatic man', 'irrational man', 'unfit man', 'mentally abnormal man', 'unbalanced woman'. We could argue, then, that the law articulated psychological constructs for some time before people calling themselves psychologists played any part in the proceedings.

At the same time, returning to Table 1.1, it could also be that Hess (2006) underestimated the importance of 'idiographic' knowledge within psychology (see below). In some respects, psychology can be described as being in a singular position as compared with the other sciences. In a sense, it is an attempt simultaneously to attain two apparently irreconcilable goals. One is to study human beings in universal terms, to discover consistent and recurrent patterns, and to arrive at meaningful generalisations about how such patterns arose and why people function as they do. Simultaneously, however, it is also applied at an individual level to produce an understanding of what makes each one of us unique.

These two approaches have attracted the widely used, but unfortunately sometimes misconstrued, terms *nomothetic* and *idiographic*. These terms come from the work of the German philosopher Wilhelm Windelband (1848–1915). Like other forms of scientific inquiry, psychology consists in part in a search for patterns that recur and of findings that can assist in the construction of theories (**nomothetic** knowledge). Complementing that, however, is a focus on the study of individuals, or of group and cultural phenomena, and on how they differ from each other, and why they are as we find them at a given moment in time (**idiographic** knowledge). Some kinds of evidence obtained from psychological research fall somewhere in the middle of this conceptual distinction: they have a restricted range of generality, applying only to certain combinations of persons and circumstances (Cronbach, 1975). In such cases, inquiry then focuses on setting the boundaries of the domain within which a particular set of findings is applicable. Working in forensic psychology, we often find ourselves involved in a process of attempting to bridge gaps of this kind.

Personal violence and harm

One concern that is undoubtedly central to forensic psychology, and that runs through almost all of its variants, is the problem of 'serious crime'. Although this might not attain the status of a defining characteristic, it is probably not unreasonable to say that the *harm* such behaviour causes, whether it can be prevented, and if so by what means, are major, perhaps universal, preoccupations of forensic psychologists. For the most part in this context, the term *serious crime*, though difficult to define formally, refers to offences of *personal and sexual violence* (homicide; serious assault; rape; abuse of children), rather than to *acquisitive or economic crimes* (theft; fraud; tax evasion; money-laundering) or other types of *organised crime* (such as drug or people trafficking, illegal arms trading, or piracy on the high seas). To date, forensic psychologists – and psychology in general – have had a fairly limited role in relation to criminal activity of the latter types. This situation may be slowly changing, however, as psychology is progressively coming to be seen as having a capacity to contribute to our understanding of many types of offence, including those acts of violence classified as *terrorism* and *genocide*. As we will see in later chapters, the rates at which violent crimes are committed vary enormously from one country to another and also over time, and the criminal justice system's response to them also differs markedly.

But the feature of paramount importance for present purposes is that it is these kinds of serious criminal acts – their causes, consequences, and how to respond to them – that constitute the primary focus of much of the activity of forensic psychologists. Whether 'helping the police with their inquiries' (e.g. assessing crime scenes, constructing psychological profiles, or offering suggestions about interview strategies), providing expert evidence in courts or tribunals, advising on the likely risk of reoffending, or making recommendations on the management of challenging behaviour, the forensic psychologist's objective is likely to be centred on the assessment or reduction of harm. Minimising harm is, understandably, a natural and recurrent preoccupation of citizens in general and of the law in particular. In the majority of cases it is the occurrence of a violent act or other type of crime that brings individuals into contact with the legal and penal system and that initiates their journey through it – a point we will expand upon in Chapter 2.

One approach to thinking about what happens from that moment onwards, one that is close to the framework adopted in this book, is to concentrate on points of discretion in the operation of the legal process (Hess, 2006). The flowchart in Figure 1.1 on the next page illustrates some of the principal pathways that might be taken and the key decision-points that occur along the way.

We freely acknowledge that this approach has some defects. It is, inevitably, a simplified version of what happens out there in that rather untidy place sometimes called 'the real world'. It refers only to adults; it maps just some of the numerous possible itineraries; it picks out only the most typical and the most busily travelled routes; and it applies in only one jurisdiction (England and Wales). Even there it does not take account of the different tiers and types of courts (Magistrates' Court, Crown Court, Appeal Court), makes no mention of plea bargaining, and does not cover many other major changes or even reversals of direction that can occur along the way (due for example to absconding or escape, to further disclosures, to appeal on various grounds, or to judicial review). As those with even the briefest experience will already know, there are individuals who spend many years going round in repeated cycles inside this 'system', like eddies at the side of a river. At almost every stage along this route there are

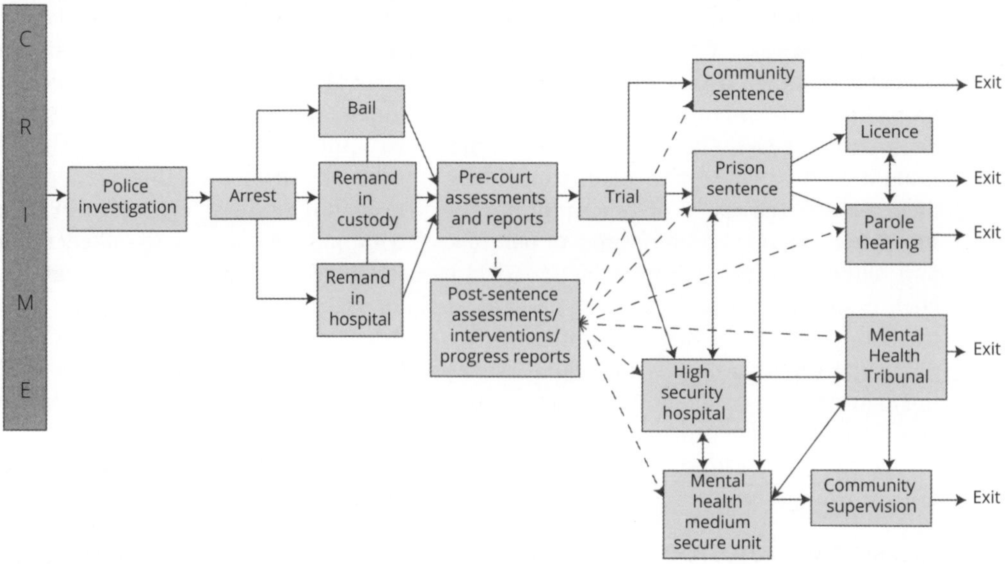
C
R
I
M
E
Police investigation
Arrest
Bail
Remand in custody
Remand in hospital
Pre-court assessments and reports
Post-sentence assessments/ interventions/ progress reports
Trial
Community sentence
Prison sentence
Licence
Parole hearing
High security hospital
Mental Health Tribunal
Mental health medium secure unit
Community supervision
Exit
Exit
Exit
Exit
Exit

Figure 1.1
Routes through the criminal justice system and decision nodes along the way. The diagram indicates possible routes for adult offenders in England and Wales. The dotted arrows identify points at which the work of forensic psychologists, through the reports they write, may have particular influence on the route someone takes.

Sources: inspired by information in National Criminal Justice Reference Service (1983). Report to the Nation on Crime and Justice. Washington, DC: US Department of Justice / National Institute of Justice, and The President's Commission on Law Enforcement and Administration of Justice (1967). The Challenge of Crime in a Free Society. Washington, DC: US Government Printing Office.

decisions to be made, and at each such decision-point there is scope for the introduction of the kinds of information that a forensic psychologist can bring to the process.

Despite the drawbacks, we believe our approach can be helpful. Just as maps are invaluable in enabling us to cross unfamiliar terrain, or a circuit diagram helps in detecting electrical faults, so an aerial view of possible pathways through the intricacies of 'the system' can assist us in understanding that system. The difference, as one eminent professor of law has remarked, is that in a sense there is no system as such at all. The network of agencies, services and decision-making procedures that now constitutes the legal framework of most countries has evolved over centuries in response to numerous demands, and in most cases with disarmingly little if any advance planning. Thus the use of the word *system* is often 'merely a convenience and an aspiration' (Ashworth, 2015, p. 75) rather than an accurate designation. In later chapters (mainly 14 and 16), we will describe some of its key features.

In successive chapters of the text, we will explore the issues that arise during various phases along the 'routes' depicted in the flowchart (and variations on them). We will discuss what factors determine the direction taken at different 'nodes', and consider the roles that forensic psychology plays during these moments. We will also suggest possible additional ways in which (from our megalomaniac perspective) forensic psychology could make further useful contributions.

Interconnectedness of forensic psychology

The evolution of forensic psychology parallels the general trajectory that psychology has travelled and the gains it has made in understanding, predicting and changing behaviour across many areas of life. That evolution reflects the extent to which findings from its research are appreciated by the legal system. In many ways the development of forensic psychology is similar to the changes that can also be found in any other area where psychology is applied, such as health, clinical, or organisational psychology.

The basic science of psychology is traditionally divided into several major branches, and its rate of growth in recent years has been such that within each of those branches even more specialised sub-branches have also emerged. If that were not already confusing enough, there are numerous cross-currents and interlinkages between many of the sub-branches. The major branches into which psychology is customarily divided include the following:

- *Biological* or *physiological psychology* focuses on the bodily processes interconnected with behaviour and experience. Psychologists study many species in addition to human beings. Specialised areas within this branch include *neuropsychology*, *comparative psychology* and *evolutionary psychology*.
- *Cognitive psychology* involves the investigation of internal ('mental') processes hypothesised to be involved in basic psychological functions and the processing of information from the external and internal environment, including perception, memory, reasoning, problem-solving, decision-making, language use and consciousness.
- *Developmental psychology* is the study of the patterns of change that occur over the human lifespan, from birth to older adulthood; and of the processes that influence continuities and discontinuities between successive phases of the life cycle.
- *Social psychology* is concerned with interaction and group processes, socialisation, interpersonal perception, interpersonal influence, attitudes, and social identity; and also with sociocultural phenomena and cross-cultural similarities and differences.
- *Differential psychology*, or the study of individual differences, is nowadays more commonly called the *psychology of personality* (what makes each one of us unique). Individual differences have also been found in a surprising variety of non-human species (Gosling, 2001) – not just dogs and horses, for example, but even fish and ants. This branch also includes *abnormal psychology*, the study of unusual experiences, and of mental and behavioural dysfunctions and disorders.

The branches distinguished above represent major sectors of activity within psychology – sectors that are identified with specialised journals and textbooks devoted to the areas named. Of course, these branches also have numerous overlaps, and trying to draw firm dividing lines around them involves a certain degree of arbitrariness. For example, many studies have investigated the relative contributions of genes and environment to different forms of behaviour. Such research inevitably crosses the boundaries between biological psychology and developmental psychology (at a minimum). Similarly, studies of the emergence of a sense of identity and selfhood are likely to combine concepts from developmental, social and differential psychology. In forensic psychology, seeking to explain a complex phenomenon such as aggression requires us to draw on studies from many areas of psychology simultaneously.

In recent years, psychology has played a major role in the emergence of *neuroscience*, an interdisciplinary inquiry also involving contributions from philosophy, physiology and computer science. Nervous systems are considered as organs that have evolved a specialised function for the processing of information about the internal and external environments that enable an organism to survive.

According to the nature of their work, forensic psychologists could view almost any part of psychology as a potential source of information and knowledge that could be applied to the questions they are trying to address. Examples of principal links between psychology and forensic psychology are given in Figure 1.2. These are only the most frequent and most likely sources that forensic psychologists use: virtually any specialised area within psychology might potentially become relevant, depending on the precise question being asked, or the individual concerning whom a report is being written or for whom services are being provided.

In addition to the subdivisions described above, which could be described as the realm of 'pure' psychology, the discipline also has a number of 'applied' fields. The most highly developed, and in terms of numbers of practitioners numerically the largest, are the following:

- *Forensic psychology* is concerned with connections between psychology and the

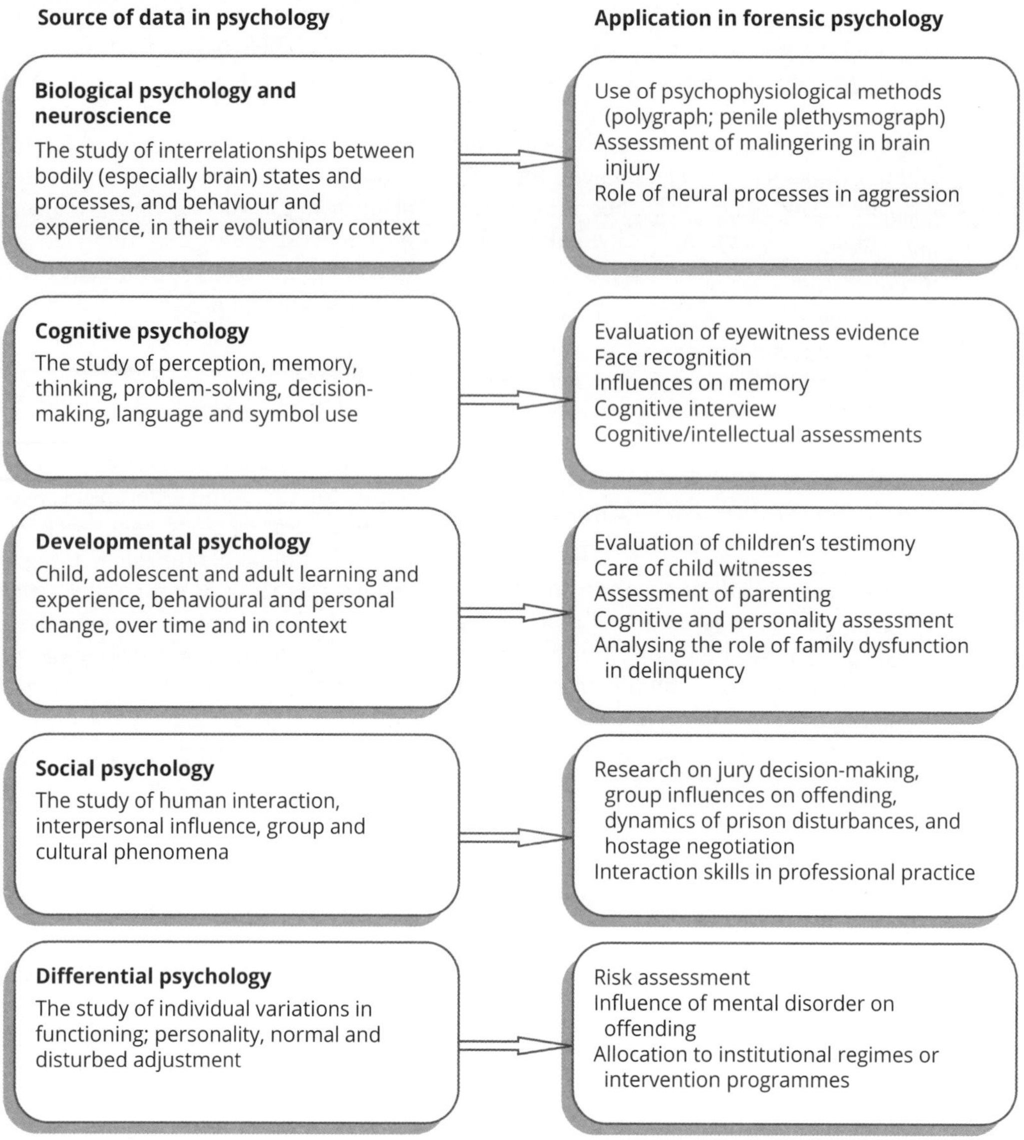
Source of data in psychology
Application in forensic psychology
Biological psychology and neuroscience
The study of interrelationships between bodily (especially brain) states and processes, and behaviour and experience, in their evolutionary context
Use of psychophysiological methods (polygraph; penile plethysmograph)
Assessment of malingering in brain injury
Role of neural processes in aggression
Cognitive psychology
The study of perception, memory, thinking, problem-solving, decision-making, language and symbol use
Evaluation of eyewitness evidence
Face recognition
Influences on memory
Cognitive interview
Cognitive/intellectual assessments
Developmental psychology
Child, adolescent and adult learning and experience, behavioural and personal change, over time and in context
Evaluation of children's testimony
Care of child witnesses
Assessment of parenting
Cognitive and personality assessment
Analysing the role of family dysfunction in delinquency
Social psychology
The study of human interaction, interpersonal influence, group and cultural phenomena
Research on jury decision-making, group influences on offending, dynamics of prison disturbances, and hostage negotiation
Interaction skills in professional practice
Differential psychology
The study of individual variations in functioning; personality, normal and disturbed adjustment
Risk assessment
Influence of mental disorder on offending
Allocation to institutional regimes or intervention programmes

Figure 1.2
Some direct connections between psychological science and its forensic applications.

law, including the provision of evidence to facilitate legal decision-making in a variety of contexts, and all aspects of the application of psychological methods, theory and research to the operation of criminal and civil justice.

» *Clinical psychology* is concerned with psychological factors that influence mental and physical health at both the individual and community levels, and with the alleviation of distress and disorder, and assessment, intervention and evaluation in healthcare settings.

» *Educational psychology* addresses issues arising in learning processes in school and allied settings, and in assessment of children and provision of support for their learning.

» *Occupational psychology* is the application of psychology to problems in the workplace, including, for example, staff selection, motivation and team working, usually in industrial or commercial settings.

Given its nature, forensic psychology also looks outward from psychology and has connections with adjoining disciplines concerned with similar problems. The very rationale for its existence depends, of course, on its relationship with *law*. This may be direct and immediate, as in the case of a psychologist who is working in a police investigation, or providing evidence to a court as an expert witness; or it may be less direct, as in the case of psychologists who work with individuals who have been subject to legal decisions such as sentences of the criminal court. Forensic psychology therefore operates constantly within a legal context, and we have seen some of the implications and ramifications of this above. Such a position obliges its practitioners to acquire some knowledge of the law, with reference both to its *statutes* (formal statements enacted by legislatures that govern particular areas of conduct) and to its *procedures* (steps involved in the practice of law, and rules and standards that regulate these).

Forensic psychology also shares common ground with the discipline of *criminology*. This is the social science most closely identified with the study of crime in all its manifestations; with analysis of official (usually governmental) statistics of crime; with the study of spatial and temporal variations in rates and types of crime; with the development of delinquency and adult criminality over the lifespan; and with the dispensation of criminal justice and the activities of police, courts and the penal system. Traditionally, given its origins and development, criminology has been dominated by *sociological* rather than *psychological* models and research (McGuire, 2004a). Thus it looks towards societal structures and environmental factors as primary influences on crime, rather than individual differences and psychological processes. Probably for this reason, the relationship between the two disciplines has not always been congenial, though this may have changed significantly in recent years (Hollin, 2012).

Forensic psychology also shares common interests with *psychiatry*, the specialised branch of medicine dedicated to the study, assessment and treatment of mental disorders. As we will see in Chapter 11, sizeable proportions of the imprisoned population in many countries are considered to suffer from one or more types of mental disorder. Furthermore, there are recurrent questions concerning the relationship between some crimes (especially personal violence) and such disorders. Given these and other findings, there are clear reasons why forensic psychologists need to be aware of basic psychiatric principles and practice and the roles of psychiatrists in the mental health and criminal justice systems. As with criminology, the relationship between psychology and psychiatry has not always been an easy one, and there are several recurrent controversies over how best to explain and respond to behaviour regarded as socially problematic (Bentall, 2009).

The foregoing comments refer principally to the network of ideas that inform the intellectual basis of forensic psychology. In everyday or routine practice, forensic psychologists will come into contact with and work alongside a wide range of other professionals. Depending on the exact worksite, these may include police officers, solicitors (or attorneys), barristers, social workers, prison officers, psychiatrists and psychiatric nurses, together with assistants and students from all of these groups. Forensic psychologists will also work alongside other applied psychologists, most frequently clinical and occasionally educational psychologists.

Overall, therefore, across the breadth of activities in which forensic psychologists are engaged, it is clear that the working context is multidisciplinary and relies upon effective collaboration with other professions. This is often missed in media portrayals, which may depict the forensic psychologist as a solitary individual operating more like a private investigator than as part of a larger unit.

Psychology as a science

How did psychology develop to a stage where a proportion of those who study it beyond secondary school then go on to become practitioners in a specialised field of application? Perhaps, to paraphrase Bartol and Bartol (2014), we need to understand where we have come from in order to assess where we are going. In any case, though, looking at our past can be illuminating in itself.

In its broadest sense, 'psychological thinking' can be said to have existed in some form or other in many cultures across many historical epochs. That description applies at least to what is commonly termed *folk psychology*, everyday human curiosity and reasoning about those around us. Folk psychology entails more or less constant discussion of our own and others' intentions (or our interpretations of them), expressed in ordinary language, and may explain the massive popularity of television 'soaps'. As a field of scientific study, however, in the form in which it is now familiar in Western societies, psychology's origins can be traced to philosophical ideas that emerged during the period beginning approximately in the late 17th century and running to the end of the 18th century, a period conventionally known as the *European Enlightenment*.

That era was characterised by a massive development of intellectual thought, and the elevation in importance of the idea of *reason*. Many thinkers sought to challenge the received, deep-rooted view of *knowledge* as deriving from the pronouncements of religious or royal authority. Such changes in thinking occurred in parallel across many fields. Progressively, the physical and biological sciences emancipated themselves from philosophy, and expended progressively more effort in empirical investigation of phenomena rather than in metaphysical speculation. In due course, although at a later stage, a similar trend took place in the social sciences, including economics, criminology, sociology and politics.

It was not until the mid-19th century that this attitude of mind had been adopted sufficiently pervasively for it to be considered possible to use the method of systematic investigation to study psychological phenomena, and then the field of *psychophysics* was established. Some physiologists considered that *conscious experience* could be studied by probing into the interrelations of *sensation* (the external, measurable stimuli impinging on the body) and *perception* (the internal experience of the subject or observer). This was seen as a purely scientific, experimentally based enterprise for which the laboratory was the obvious setting. The first laboratory explicitly designed to carry out such work was set up by Wilhelm Wundt (1832–1920), a medically trained physiologist, at the University of Leipzig, Germany, in 1879. Studies were conducted in which individuals, using a method known as 'experimental self-observation' (*selbstbeobachtung*), a controlled form of introspection, reported the contents of consciousness to the researcher under different stimulus conditions (Leahy, 2003). Other workers, such as Hermann Ebbinghaus (1850–1909), one of the first psychologists to carry out detailed study of memory and forgetting, showed how different segments of a quantity of information were retained or lost over time.

In the years following this, several psychology laboratories were established in the United States of America, at Harvard, Yale, Johns Hopkins and Clark Universities. The first doctoral research programme in psychology was launched at Harvard University in 1878, and the first independent psychology department was established at Clark University in 1887.

The late 19th century saw a period of rapid growth of interest in the still new psychological science. By the 1890s there were numerous academic psychologists, working in several countries. An association of physiological psychology was created in France in 1885, and subsequently the American Psychological Association (APA), the world's first professional grouping of its kind, was founded in 1892. Many of those who were later to become the most influential in the field obtained their PhD degrees at Leipzig. They included luminaries such as G. Stanley Hall (1844–1924), who was the first president of the APA and who in 1887 founded the *American Journal of Psychology*, the earliest scientific periodical in the field. Another was Lightner Witmer (1867–1956), the first person to practise what is now called clinical psychology.

The first psychological laboratory in the United Kingdom was set up in London in 1885 by Francis Galton (1822–1911), a cousin of Charles Darwin and an acknowledged polymath who made contributions to many fields. Although Galton did not identify himself as belonging to any single profession, psychology was one of his numerous wide-ranging interests. He undertook no work that we would now explicitly recognise as forensic psychology, but he did have a considerable impact on the science of forensics and police investigation, through pioneering methods of classifying fingerprints which advanced the acceptance of fingerprints as evidence in court. As well as publishing the world's first weather map, he developed basic concepts of *psychometrics*, including the idea of *statistical correlation*. He is also renowned for developing the study of *heredity*, including the method of comparing twins, which has had a significant influence on research in human genetics. His reputation was tarnished, however, by his promotion of the idea of *eugenics*, the view that those thought to possess superior qualities should be encouraged to have more children, and to do so earlier in life, whereas steps should be taken to discourage this amongst those of lower 'genetic worth'. Such a view, though attracting much support at the time, had far-reaching and far more sinister ramifications during the 20th century.

Psychology's first court appearance

Psychological concepts have been a component of legal deliberation for some time, and there is evidence that such ideas were introduced into consideration of cases by legal practitioners themselves. Legal psychology has had a significant history in Europe, and across a number of countries it is possible to trace the study of this area to works written in the middle of the 19th century. Traverso and Manna (1992) describe the origins of criminal psychology amongst legal academics in Italy as long ago as 1833; and Jakob (1992) outlines the development of psychological thinking amongst jurists in 19th-century Germany. Treatises on the relationship between psychology and law have also been available for many decades in other countries, including Spain and Poland. Thus psychology was being applied to law for some time before there was anything known as 'forensic psychology'.

The progressive emergence of forensic psychology as a recognisable field is usually dated to the first decade of the 20th century and to the work of a number of individuals who chose to apply psychology to the operation of law during that period. From the point at which we might identify psychology as becoming more formally involved in aspects of the legal process, it was variously labelled as *criminal anthropology*, *juridical psychology*, or *criminal psychology*, and it was not until later that the term 'forensic psychology' was coined, by Marbe (1913).

The rationale for the emergence of forensic psychology has been attributed to earlier developments, and notably to the concerns of an Austrian judge, Hans Gross (1847–1915), who criticised jurisprudence for not being based on scientific principles. Indeed he described it rather dismissively as having 'nothing scientific about it' (Gross, 1898, cited in Müllberger, 2009). The motivation for research into understanding crime and aspects of the legal process, then known as the science of *criminalistics* (of which Gross is regarded as a founder), is dated from that time, and included the development of *crime-scene photography*, which Gross considered an important innovation.

James McKeen Cattell

Perhaps the earliest significant study, now recognised as the initial seed of forensic psychology, was that of James McKeen Cattell (1860–1944) in 1895. Cattell was concerned with how well we remember information that we have observed in the normal course of our experiences, and how confident we are in our observations. He discovered that we tend not to be particularly accurate in our memories, and yet at the same time we tend to be overly confident that they are accurate. Cattell was particularly interested in the veridicality of memory with regard to courtroom testimony, and his findings shed important light on the inherent dangers of relying on witnesses' memories.

More generally, Cattell was also interested in developing psychology as a science. He wrote:

> As a last example of the usefulness of measurements of the accuracy of observation and memory I may refer to its application in courts of justice. The probable accuracy of a witness could be measured and his testimony weighted accordingly. A numerical correction could be introduced for lapse of time, average lack of truthfulness, average effect of personal interest, etc. The testimony could be collected

> independently, and given to experts who could affirm for example that the chances are 19 to 1 that the homicide was committed by the defendant, and 4 to 1 that it was premeditated. (Cattell, 1895, pp. 765–766)

Clearly, Cattell was eager to draw attention to the potential value of psychology in legal settings. This value has continued to be an area of active interest for well over a century now, from the pioneering work of Bolton (1896), through the highly influential work of Loftus (1996), and beyond to the present day.

Louis William Stern

Other researchers were similarly concerned with the role that the basic principles of psychology could play within legal settings, and with how the specifics of the legal process might impact on them. Louis William Stern (1871–1938), who studied under Ebbinghaus, is primarily noted for having devised the concept of an *intelligence quotient*. In work concerned with legal testimony (Stern, 1910, 1939) he demonstrated that as *recall* declined over time, *confidence* tends to become overinflated; and that although written reports of memory for pictures were approximately 90 per cent correct, when examined under what Stern refers to as 'cross-examination', this level of accuracy dropped to approximately 60 per cent correct.

Hugo Münsterberg

From a historical standpoint, however, the work of Hugo Münsterberg (1863–1916) is the most extensively cited as instigating a major step towards establishing the relevance of psychology to applied legal settings. After completing his PhD in Leipzig in 1885 and later spending an initial three-year period in Harvard at the invitation of William James, Münsterberg finally emigrated from Germany to the United States in 1897. He studied a number of issues in what is now the field of forensic psychology, including accuracy of memory, reliability of witnesses, false confessions, and jury decision-making.

His influential book *On the Witness Stand* was published in 1907 (Benjamin, 2007). In one chapter, 'The memory of the witness', Münsterberg provides accounts of studies which he suggests demonstrate the fallibility of memory for details that would be of use in legal settings, such as the actions of various individuals involved in a staged argument and shooting (a study attributed to Franz von Liszt and described by Müllberger, 2009). Münsterberg was a strong advocate of the usefulness of psychology to law, and fairly scathing about the lack of interest from the legal community in what he believed psychology had to offer:

> The lawyer and the judge and the juryman are sure that they do not need the experimental psychologist ... They go on thinking that their legal instinct and their common sense supplies them with all that is needed and somewhat more. (1907, pp. 10–11)

Simultaneously, he was concerned with the evidence that the courts were prepared to entertain:

> The Court would rather listen for whole days to the 'science' of the handwriting experts than allow a witness to be examined with regard to his memory and his power of perception, his attention and his associations, his volition and his suggestibility, with methods which are in accord with the exact work of experimental psychology. It is so much easier everywhere to be satisfied with sharp demarcation lines and to listen only to a yes or no; the man is sane or insane, and if he is sane, he speaks the truth or he lies. The psychologist would upset this satisfaction completely. (1907, p. 46)

Although Münsterberg has an important place in the development of forensic psychology, that position is in some ways a paradoxical one, as there are criticisms of the lack of scientific support for his conclusions, and suggestions that in fact his strident attitude was responsible, at least in part, for the legal system thereafter distancing itself from psychology. Webster, for example, contends that Münsterberg

> through his early misguided enthusiasm for applying laboratory findings and methods to court proceedings,

brought the discipline into disrepute. No doubt his near-lunatic pronouncements and utter insensitivity to colleagues learned in the law did not greatly help the cause. (Webster, 1984, p. 409)

A more sober approach to assembling psychological evidence for legal purposes was described by George Frederick Arnold, a British civil servant working in India. Arnold published *Psychology Applied to Legal Evidence and Other Constructions of Law* in 1906, before the appearance of Münsterberg's much better-known book. Bornstein and Penrod (2008) compare the two books and differences of approach, and offer reasons why Arnold's name is little known in comparison to that of Münsterberg.

William Marston and Karl Marbe

William Moulton Marston (1893–1947) was particularly interested in the possibility of discovering methods for detecting deception, or what he referred to as 'the mental attitude in deceiving' (Marston, 1917, p. 117). Like Cattell, he was convinced that for psychology to be accepted in court, the court 'must be convinced that a sufficiently sound and fundamentally scientific knowledge of all the psychological symptoms of deception is available' (Marston, 1920).

His work, which formed the basis of *polygraphy* (to be discussed in Chapter 18), led him to conclude that the effort involved in deception impacted upon systolic blood pressure and reaction time. Indeed, he suggested that the use of changes in blood pressure to detect deception in the context of probation services was 'beyond question, justified' (Marston, 1921, p. 570). As we will see in Chapter 18, the use of what became the polygraph has remained controversial since that time. Like the study of witness memory, the general theme of deception and how to detect it is another area that has continued to generate research right up to the present (Granhag, Vrij and Vershuere, 2015). Another of Marston's ventures became more successful: under the pen-name Charles Moulton, he was the originator of the cartoon and later film character *Wonder Woman*.

The above developments took place in the United States. Meanwhile, however, psychologists and the results of psychological studies were being heard in court in Europe too. In possibly the earliest work to employ such a title, Karl Marbe (1869–1953) published *Grundzuge Der Forensischen Psychologie* (*Outlines of Forensic Psychology*) in Munich in 1913. This was a collection of lectures delivered to judges in order to educate them in modern, scientific psychology, including aspects of the psychology of testimony, the frequency of criminal activity, and intelligence testing.

Webster (1984) suggests that the legal profession was for some time hesitant to embrace the research and evidence of psychologists, and he provides a number of explanations as to why this might have been the case. Notably, he suggests that by questioning the validity of witness testimony and tending to shy away from simple 'yes' or 'no' answers, psychologists put themselves in conflict with the courts. Fortunately that trend appears to have been reversed, and the provision to the courts of psychological evidence is now a well-established and steadily expanding activity (Melton *et al.*, 2018).

Criminological psychology

The main concerns of Cattell, Stern, Münsterberg, Marston and Marbe were with the evidence produced by psychological research and with its usage, implications and status in court. But there is another strand of psychology with a separate focus: the search for an explanation of the *behaviour* defined as 'crime', and for effective methods of working with those who have committed crimes. The history of psychology as an approach to studying criminal conduct, and if possible finding ways to reduce it, has separate origins from the attempts to foster psychology's role in the courtroom.

The basis of criminality

In a development that preceded some of those outlined above, during the last quarter of the 19th century Cesare Lombroso

(1835–1909) formulated his theory of 'born criminals'. Lombroso was not a psychologist but a surgeon in the Italian army who, alongside his medical work, studied the body shape, proportions and other features of over 3,000 soldiers, searching for what he thought might be an explanation of criminality in physical characteristics. He considered it important:

> to determine whether the criminal man belongs in the same category as the healthy man or the insane individual or in an entirely separate category. To do this ... we must ... proceed instead to the direct physical and psychological study of the criminal, comparing the results with information on the healthy and the sane. (Lombroso, 1876/2006, p. 43)

Few researchers would now expect to find any such clear-cut differences between the 'criminal man' (or woman) and everyone else; and whilst the precise role that heredity might play in crime remains a subject of research, most would recognise the importance of environmental factors and learning processes, not to mention social definitions, in contributing to the problem of crime. The concept of such a direct relationship between body typology or physiognomy and behaviour has since largely fallen into disrepute; indeed, the historical suggestion of a connection between them might nowadays be considered regrettable, if not downright embarrassing. Nevertheless, Lombroso can be regarded as having instigated the search for possible differences between those who repeatedly break the law and those who abide by it. As such he is a forerunner of what nowadays is called *criminological psychology*. As recently as the 1980s the view that delinquency was associated with a particular body type was still taken seriously in some quarters (Wilson and Herrnstein, 1985). Though now adopting far more sophisticated methods, contemporary studies that use computerised tomography (CT) or magnetic resonance imaging (MRI) scans and other techniques for investigating neural processes are often posing questions not dissimilar to those asked by Lombroso. Similarly, the question of what neuroscience might be able to offer the law is currently a hotly debated topic, and seems likely to remain so for some time (Pardo and Patterson, 2014).

More typically, however, forensic psychologists working within what can be called a criminological orientation have addressed issues and questions that may be less immediately applicable in the courtroom. Such work includes testing theories of offending or other antisocial behaviour; researching the development of delinquency; developing methods of assessment of individual risk and need; and exploring interventions to reduce offender recidivism (Bonta and Andrews, 2017; Craig, Dixon and Gannon, 2013). In seeking to account for the occurrence of crimes, data of these kinds are today assimilated into far more elaborate theoretical models that also include many other variables, taking account of socialisation, learning experiences, cognitive processes and situational elements. We will expand on these issues in Chapters 4 and 5.

Research and treatment

As with the use of psychology in providing evidence to courts of law, its application in the treatment of persistent offending, and in the search for means to reduce such offending, is not of recent origin.

The first usage of psychological research and principles to provide treatment to offenders is generally traced to the work of William Healy (1869–1963), a child psychiatrist who in 1909 founded the Juvenile Psychopathic Institute in Chicago. The Institute undertook medical examinations, prepared social histories, and provided treatment recommendations to the nearby court. The word 'psychopathic' did not then denote the specific combination of features that make up its definition today, a point we will discuss in more depth in Chapter 11.

Based on his work at the Institute, including assessment of over 800 young recidivist offenders, Healy went on to publish in 1915 what was received as a ground-breaking book, *The Individual Delinquent*. The findings from his assessments overturned any idea of a 'born criminal' on the lines envisaged by Lombroso. Healy later founded the USA's first child guidance clinic and is seen as an originator of the provision of those services to children and families (Levy, 1968). He is regarded as influential in criminology:

> because his theory and research helped to create a sharp and permanent break between American and European criminological thought. Until the early part of the twentieth century, American ideas on the causes of crime generally duplicated European viewpoints. The multifactor theory, and its research methodology, set American criminology on a new course, primarily by drawing attention for the first time to psychological, or emotional, etiological factors. (Snodgrass, 1984, p. 333)

Notwithstanding the wide range of factors considered, Healy's model remained fundamentally a medical one, with the role of environmental factors such as poverty remaining somewhat marginal (Snodgrass, 1984).

It is possible that Grace Fernald (1879–1950), an educational psychologist who worked for a time at the Chicago Institute, could have claimed to be the first psychologist to hold an appointment specifically attached to a court of law (Sullivan, Dorcus, Allen and Koontz, 1950). Between 1909 and 1911 she was employed in Healy's newly established Institute. The Institute operated alongside the local courts, providing diagnosis and treatment, and carrying out research with persistent young offenders. Fernald's work at the Chicago Institute was instrumental in developing a variety of methods of assessing juveniles' mental capacity. She subsequently moved to California, where she acquired a national reputation for her specialised research and practice in the field of remedial education. In 1917, dismayed by limited resources, Healy too left Chicago, but for Boston, where he helped establish a foundation for the study of 'baffling cases' involving juveniles (Snodgrass, 1984).

Notwithstanding these innovations, for a lengthy period thereafter it appears that psychologists, possibly because of their intimate and sometimes exclusive association with the development of *psychometrics* (then called 'mental testing'), were employed in the penal system mainly to diagnose 'feeblemindedness'. Over ensuing decades, some writers speculated on the potential of psychological therapies in penal institutions, and in the UK provision was made for introducing 'formal psychological treatment' in the Borstal Institution at Feltham (Field, 1932). But it was not until the late 1960s and the early 1970s that prison psychology became a distinct discipline in its own right, a change thought to have been linked to the movement in the prison system during that time towards rehabilitation (Nieberding, Frackowiak, Bobholdt and Rubel, 2000; Watkins, 1992). Psychologists in British prisons steadily began to extend their range of work – though with a ratio of psychologists to prisoners in 1970 of 1:2,569 (Donald, 1970), there were clearly formidable challenges.

Psychology as a profession

Sociologists who have studied the emergence and rise to prominence of the types of workers who together constitute what is ultimately recognised as a 'profession' suggest that such groupings have some common identifying features. Over time, whether driven by necessity or through seizing an opportunity, they form themselves into associations that represent their interests. As time proceeds, the level of formality increases: they define who they are as a group; they set standards for membership; and they regulate who can join. Equally important is the process of communicating with those *outside* the group, including of course consumers of their services, a range of other professions, the public at large and government. In principle such development should work to the advantage of everyone involved: if services are then sought from its members, the association should benefit consumers of those services by providing some guarantee of quality control and a visible entity with which they can communicate.

The development of psychology since its appearance as an independent discipline has followed just such a pattern of increasing professionalisation. Over approximately the last fifty years, the number of people studying, researching and practising some form of psychology has shown accelerating growth. Like other groups of workers, psychologists have progressively coalesced into collaborative groups, and then issued documents delineating different aspects of their work and identifying who holds the credentials to undertake it.

Over the last century or more, professional psychology associations have been established in many countries. As we saw above, the American Psychological Association (APA), founded in 1892, is the oldest and remains the largest. The British Psychological Society (BPS), founded in 1901, followed not long afterwards. A more recent development is the establishment of divisions of these national groups with a specialised interest in forensic psychology. Given that many psychological associations have a growing proportion of their membership who practise forensic psychology, there are also several supranational organisations, and some cross-disciplinary ones.

Some of the key groupings that are currently shaping the field are identified in the accompanying 'Focus on ...' box. The question of how to enter the profession of forensic psychology and some issues related to practice within the profession will be considered in Chapter 21.

FOCUS ON ...

Professional psychology associations relevant to forensic psychologists

Associations in the United Kingdom

British Psychological Society (BPS)
Division of Forensic Psychology (DFP)

The BPS was founded in 1901 (though the word 'British' was not added till 1906). It publishes eleven journals, and currently has ten divisions, each focused on a particular area of professional practice.

The Division of Forensic Psychology (DFP), initially established in 1977 as the Division of Criminological and Legal Psychology, changed its name in 1999. As of mid-2017 it had a membership of approximately 2,500, including 1,000 full practitioner members. It publishes two periodicals: *Issues in Forensic Psychology*, which is primarily research-focused, and *Forensic Update*, containing some research reports and a range of other topical material. The DFP is also linked to the BPS journal *Legal and Criminological Psychology*, published twice each year. The DFP holds an annual conference and organises a variety of training events.

Associations in Europe

Every country in Europe has a professional psychological association, and some countries have more than one. Often that is because academic and research psychologists are in one group while applied and practitioner psychologists are in another. In Germany, for example, forensic psychologists are usually members of the Sektion Rechtspsychologie (legal psychology section) of the Berufsverband Deutscher Psychologinnen und Psychologen (BDP, the Association of German Professional Psychologists). The Sektion publishes a house journal, *Praxis der Rechtspsychologie*, and hosts an annual conference. The BPS, the BDP and many other national associations are members of the European Federation of Psychologists' Associations (EFPA), which has a total of 36 member associations, together representing a total of 300,000 psychologists.

European Association of Psychology and Law (EAPL)

The EAPL is a transnational group launched at Nuremberg in 1990 and formally established at Oxford in 1992. Its objectives are stated as 'the promotion and development of research improvements in legal procedures, teaching, and practice in the field of psychology and law (e.g. legal psychology, criminological psychology, forensic psychology) within Europe; and the interchange of information throughout the world aimed toward an international cooperation'. One specific activity is an annual conference held at different venues around Europe. The majority of EAPL members are from European countries but there are also members in other continents. The EAPL's official journal is *Psychology, Crime and Law*, which is published eight times each year.

Associations in the United States of America

American Psychological Association (APA) Division 41

Having been founded in 1892, the APA is the world's oldest grouping of professional psychologists. Forensic psychologists are generally members of Division 41, also called the American Psychology-Law Society (APLS), an 'interdisciplinary organization devoted to scholarship, practice, and public service in psychology and law'. The Society's official journal, *Law and Human Behavior*, is published six times each year. The APLS also distributes a newsletter; hosts a book series published by Oxford University Press; organises an annual conference and a series of training events; and engages in consultation on a wide spectrum of issues connecting psychology and law.

American Association of Correctional Psychology

In the United States there is a separate organisation for those working in the legal and penal systems, the American Association of Correctional Psychology, which publishes the journal *Criminal Justice and Behavior*. A short history of its work has been written by Bartol and Freeman (2005).

Associations in other countries

There are professional associations of psychologists in many countries, including the Psychological Society of Ireland, the Canadian Psychological Association, the Australian Psychological Society, the New Zealand Psychological Society, the Psychological Society of South Africa, the National Association of Psychological Science of India, and the Japanese Psychological Association.

International associations

More widely still, there is an International Association of Correctional and Forensic Psychologists (IACFP), founded in 1954, which publishes a quarterly newsletter, *The Correctional Psychologist*.

There are also regional or continental groupings, such as the Federation of Iberoamerican Associations of Psychology, founded in 2002, which includes countries of Latin America, Spain and Portugal, and the Asian Psychological Association, founded in Bali, Indonesia, in 2006.

Questions

1 What in your view are the advantages of having professional associations in psychology?
2 Are there any disadvantages? If so, what are they?

Chapter summary

» As a unifying theme for the book, we have proposed the idea of considering the different routes an imaginary individual might make through the complex 'system' of legal, penal and mental health agencies inside which forensic psychologists work. We will follow that general direction and study the variations in what happens along the way.

» There is no exact definition of forensic psychology upon which everyone is agreed. Forensic psychology is an area of activity with connections to several others, both in the 'parent discipline' of psychology and also in other applied fields. A crucial connection, of course, is forensic psychology's relationship to law, and the chapter has mapped some of the main links that exist between the two.

» Like psychology as a whole, forensic psychology adopts a scientific approach to its subject matter. We have examined the nature of that approach in psychology more widely, and implications for its applied branches and fields.

» As a form of applied psychology with an identified group of practitioners, forensic psychology is often seen as a relatively young discipline, yet the application of psychology to law has in fact a quite lengthy history. We noted some key landmarks within its history that have influenced the position and status of forensic psychology in society today.

» If you work as a forensic psychologist, or wish to do so, a key message is that you are not alone. Apart from colleagues close by with similar training, there are many other professions addressing the same problems. There are also national and international associations that enable practitioners from different places to make contact with and to learn from one another. And there are many sources of information and advice to draw upon.

Further reading

» There are several major and weighty handbooks covering the connections between psychology and law, including these:

- Irving B. Weiner and Randy K. Otto (2014), *Handbook of Forensic Psychology*, 4th edition (New York: Wiley).
- Ray Bull and David Carson (2003), *Handbook of Psychology in Legal Contexts*, 2nd edition (Chichester: Wiley-Blackwell).
- Gary B. Melton, John Petrila, Norman G. Poythress, Christopher Slobogin, Randy K, Otto, Douglass Mossman and Lois O. Condie (2018), *Psychological Evaluations for the Courts: A Handbook for Mental Health Professionals and Lawyers*, 4th edition (New York: Guilford Press).
- Jennifer M. Brown and Elizabeth A. Campbell (2010), *Cambridge Handbook of Forensic Psychology* (Cambridge: Cambridge University Press).

» Specifically for criminological psychology – as it pays more attention to crime and to offender rehabilitation, and less attention to forensic or psycho-legal aspects – a key source is James Bonta and Don A. Andrews (2017), *The Psychology of Criminal Conduct* (New York: Routledge).

» For a book with a more explicit in-depth legal or forensic focus, see John Monahan and Laurens Walker (2009), *Social Science in Law: Cases and Materials* (New York: Foundation Press).

» For a quick reference guide to many topics in the field, see the approach offered by Graham J. Towl, David P. Farrington, David A. Crighton and Gareth Hughes (2008), *Dictionary of Forensic Psychology* (Cullompton: Willan).

Defining and Surveying Crime

As we noted in the opening chapter, an individual's journey into the criminal justice system usually begins with committing a crime. In this chapter we examine closely what that means. What exactly happens when someone breaks the criminal law? How do formal, legal concepts of 'breaking the law' define the behaviour that constitutes different types of criminal offence? How often do crimes occur, and who commits them? Answering these questions involves considering some key ideas in criminal law, examining surveys of crime statistics of different types, and discussing how to interpret the survey data.

Chapter objectives

- To analyse formal, legal definitions of crime.
- To compare those with broader concepts of causing harm, developed within criminology.
- To examine methods of compiling criminal statistics.

What brings a citizen to the attention of the law and sets in motion a process that at some stage involves contact with a forensic psychologist? In the vast majority of instances, it will be because the individual in question has been charged with or convicted of a criminal offence. We devote the opening chapters of this book to understanding 'crime', because it is an act considered to belong in that category that triggers someone's entry to the 'system' of legal, penal, mental health and social work services and agencies within which forensic psychologists work. Much of what happens throughout the entire process that is then set in motion will be influenced by the nature, severity and frequency of that initial offending.

Part 1 of the book (comprising Chapters 1–5) therefore gives an overview of the role that psychology plays in the study of crime and of antisocial behaviour more generally. We will draw on research, theory and practice, both in psychology itself and in the adjacent disciplines of criminology and psychiatry. We will approach our study of this in three successive stages, which we can roughly characterise as *description*, *correlation* and *explanation*.

In this chapter we will first examine some definitional issues: the 'what' and 'how' of criminal offending. While the idea of 'a crime' may initially seem simple, there are several layers of complexity it is important to appreciate in order to gain a clear understanding of crime. We then go on to describe and discuss some key aspects of the character and the numbers of different types of offences, and the factors associated with their occurrence. Those two areas are covered in some depth in the present chapter.

This will take us into a second phase, focused on correlates of crime and 'risk factors' for involvement in it. That area will be covered in Chapter 3, which also includes an account of the main methods of research used in investigating this field. Going a stage further, we then examine what factors can meaningfully be claimed to contribute to *causing* crime. That discussion takes us into a review of key theories, which are the subject matter of Chapter 4.

Defining crime: the legal approach

As an important first step in the systematic study of crime, therefore, it is necessary to address an issue that on the face of it sounds straightforward; it is not one we would expect to occupy us for very long. That is the question of what exactly we mean by 'crime'. Debates on the nature of such a definition have given rise to some basic misconceptions across the whole field of criminal justice. While the operation of the criminal law is central to any discussion of crime, to focus on the law alone, as the cornerstone of how we conceptualise crime, can result in some fairly large gaps in our understanding.

Nevertheless, it is crucial to be familiar with how crimes are defined in criminal law. The 'system' we will be discussing throughout this book revolves around that set of laws. Forensic psychology requires both a general understanding of the concepts used to define crime in legal terms, and a more detailed knowledge of how separate types of crimes are described in the legal statutes that delineate them.

The elements of a crime

While the idea of a crime as 'violation of criminal law' may seem almost facile, criminal law requires that certain features be present in order that it is perfectly clear-cut when certain actions can be considered crimes. Exactly when can something be called a crime? To pin this down, legal academics have suggested that criminal law should adhere to five principles which together define its operation (Herring, 2016).

The first is *legality*: that the law should be sufficiently well defined for citizens to know when they are abiding by it or breaking it, an idea that is embodied in the Human Rights Act 1998. A second principle, *responsibility*, requires that individuals can only be criminally culpable for actions for which they were responsible. In Chapter 16 we will consider some of the conditions under which it could be accepted that that was *not* the case. A third principle is *minimal criminalisation*: that the criminal law should prohibit an undesirable action only if there is no *other* means of stopping it from happening. There are many ways in which society controls undesirable behaviour; the criminal law should be, as it were, the last resort for that purpose. Fourth, *proportionality* demands that a sentence should correspond to the seriousness of an offence. While that may be easy to arrange in broad terms, comparing different kinds of offences in their seriousness can be an extremely challenging task, as we will see in Chapter 6. The final principle is that of *fair labelling*, which requires that the way specific acts are defined as 'crimes' should reflect the nature of the action that took place. Herring (2016) noted that in England and Wales, at the time of writing, there were 8,000 statutes defining criminal offences, and he and other experts have questioned whether the process of crime labelling has already gone too far, given that many more acts are labelled as crimes in England and Wales than in other, comparable jurisdictions.

In those legal jurisdictions that rely fully or largely on what is known as a **common law** approach (to be explained more fully in Chapter 16) – jurisdictions that include Australia, Canada, England and Wales, India, Ireland, New Zealand, Pakistan, South Africa and the United States – in order for an individual to be considered liable to condemnation for a crime, two ingredients should be present (Herring, 2016; Ormerod and Laird, 2015):

1. ***Actus reus*** The first ingredient is the *actus reus* ('guilty act'), which refers to the conduct or *external* element of a crime. This is essentially the behaviour of the individual in committing the offence: 'What the defendant must be proved to have done (or sometimes failed to do), in what circumstances, and with what consequences in order to be guilty of a crime' (Herring, 2016, p. 71). Specific statutes define precisely what the *actus reus* consists of in relation to separate categories of offence. Usually (though not always) it is necessary for there to be proof that a defendant committed a particular act, that the act had a particular result, and that the act or result occurred in certain circumstances. In most cases, for an action to constitute an *actus reus*, it must have been carried out voluntarily.

2. ***Mens rea*** The second ingredient is *mens rea* ('guilty mind'), which refers to the mental or *internal* element of a crime. This may consist of 'intention, recklessness or negligence' (Herring, 2016, p. 71).

The law recognises that individuals may sometimes commit actions without having deliberately planned or intended to do so, although *mens rea* can apply also to things they omitted to do. Whether or not individuals are shown to have acted (or failed to act) *deliberately* will have a major impact on the seriousness of any resultant conviction and the ensuing penalty.

In English and Scots law, whether or not there was conscious deliberation underlines the distinction between 'murder' and 'manslaughter', for example, or between 'assault' and 'grievous bodily harm'. In the United States, 'first degree murder' is any murder that is wilful and premeditated, whereas 'second degree murder' is not premeditated or planned in advance. There are other categories of homicide in the United States, including 'voluntary manslaughter' (sometimes called 'third degree murder'), which involves intent, but one that had not been formed previously but arose in the heat of the moment; whereas in 'involuntary manslaughter' there was no intention to cause death but there was intent to cause an act that then led to death. Thus in many jurisdictions an individual's state of mind at the time of an offence, the motive in committing it, the degree of awareness of what he or she was doing, and the level of intent in relation to the *actus reus* can all be pivotal aspects in the court's deliberations concerning the nature of the offence and the resultant penalty.

Acts of commission and acts of omission

It is worth emphasising that serious crimes, including homicide, may be the result of *acts of omission* as well as *acts of commission* – for example, they may be due to *negligence* or *recklessness*. To establish recklessness, it needs to be shown that in the situation in which an offence occurred, the accused individual was aware that there was a risk of an adverse consequence – that is, that his or her conduct could cause a particular result – and that the risk was an unreasonable one for him or her to take. Based on **case law**, this kind of recklessness is sometimes called *Cunningham recklessness* to distinguish it from a different kind of recklessness, *Caldwell recklessness*. In the latter sense, an individual was reckless *either* if he or she was aware of a risk, *or* if there was an obvious and serious risk *and* the individual failed to consider whether or not there was a risk. Caldwell recklessness was abolished by the House of Lords: it was discontinued because it covered defendants who, usually as a result of some incapacity of mind, were not aware of a risk that would have been obvious to others. Application of Caldwell recklessness had led to what were considered to be some unjust decisions, and the meaning was considered to be too wide and 'catch-all'. On the other hand, the *Cunningham* definition has been considered too narrow, and efforts have been made to find an intermediate basis for the judgment of recklessness (Herring, 2016).

There are other aspects to the idea that crime can be a result of omission as well as commission. A defendant can only be found guilty of an offence as a result of failing to act if he or she had been under a *duty* to act in those circumstances. That is, contrary to what may be general moral intuitions, under common law (see Chapter 16) there is no general legal obligation to prevent harm: if you come upon a child drowning in a pond and simply walk away, in English law there is no criminal liability. By contrast, in France, Germany and other continental European countries with civil law, there is a legal requirement to assist a person in distress (sometimes called a 'duty to rescue').

Defining offences

In addition to the general concepts of *actus reus* and *mens rea*, there are also definitions specific to each type of offence. The *actus reus* of murder is 'the unlawful killing of another person in the Queen's peace'; the *mens rea* is 'an intention to cause death or grievous bodily harm to the victim' (Herring, 2016, p. 232). The first part excludes the killing of enemy adversaries during wartime. The victim of homicide must be a person, defined with respect to the lifespan from the moment of birth to that of medically determined death; other laws protect unborn children. There are controversies over whether intent to cause grievous harm rather than to kill should be included in the *mens rea* for murder. English law also specifies a less serious form of killing known as 'manslaughter', defined in two ways. One is 'voluntary manslaughter', where both the *actus reus* and *mens rea* for murder are present but there are extenuating circumstances that lessen the defendant's culpability. The other is 'involuntary manslaughter', in which a defendant did not intend either to kill or seriously to harm the victim, but was nevertheless criminally liable for the victim's death. In 2007 a new offence of this type was defined, 'corporate manslaughter', whereby an organisation may be guilty of an offence if its activities are managed in such a way as to cause a person's death as the result of a gross breach of the organisation's duty of care to that person.

The *actus reus* of 'burglary' is to enter a building or part of a building as a trespasser, and then to steal or attempt to steal anything in, or any part of the building; to inflict grievous bodily harm or rape on anyone in the building; or to do unlawful damage to the building or any of its contents. The *mens rea* in this case comprises the intent to do any of the aforementioned things. Even if none of those things was done, a person will have committed burglary if it is shown that he or she when entering the building *intended* to commit them. In the offence of 'robbery', the elements of theft must be present, and in addition at the time of the theft the perpetrator must have used, or threatened to use, force; and the force must have been used in order to steal and not for any other purpose (e.g. to escape).

The *actus reus* of 'assault' is to cause a victim to apprehend imminent unlawful force; in other words, a person need not actually have struck someone in order to have committed assault: he or she has merely to have led that person to believe that she or he was about to be struck. This is usually called 'common assault'; and it is established in law that words, and even a silent telephone call, can amount to such an assault if it has created fear in the victim. The *mens rea* is that the defendant 'intended or was reckless that the victim would apprehend imminent unlawful force' (Herring, 2016, p. 316). Where actual physical contact is made, the offence becomes one of 'battery'. Where such battery then results in actual physical harm to the victim, different offences are defined according to the severity of the harm caused, and the level of intent involved – 'actual bodily harm', 'malicious wounding', or 'wounding with intent'.

The *actus reus* of 'rape' is that the defendant penetrated the vagina, anus or mouth of the victim with his penis, and the victim had not consented to such an act; the *mens rea* is that the defendant intended to carry out such penetration and did not reasonably believe that the victim consented. While women or men can be victims of rape, only a man can commit it – though a woman can commit other kinds of sexual assault against a man. In some other respects, however, the question of what constitutes 'rape' has been subject to considerable debate. Most people might assume that it consists of forceful penile penetration, but should the definition also extend to other objects, or should those be defined as other kinds of sexual assault? There are also numerous controversies, sometimes vociferously debated, over what constitutes consent, and the nature of deception in which defendants might engage in order to force sexual intercourse upon victims (Herring, 2016).

The detailed legal concepts associated with the above examples are contained in the Homicide Act 1957, the Corporate Manslaughter and Corporate Homicide Act 2007, the Theft Act 1968, the Offences Against the Person Act 1861 and the Sexual Offences Act 2003. While these statutes define the nature of numerous types of offence, and describe their legal elements, the implementation of the statutes in actual legal practice is highly influenced by case law, with textbooks such as that of Herring (2016) illustrating how decisions have been made in individual cases and have set precedent for subsequent cases. For some types of offence, there are also legal defences against a finding of full criminal culpability, and several aspects of this issue will be expanded on later in the chapter.

Finally, however, note that there are some offences for which it is *not* necessary to demonstrate the presence of *mens rea*. These are called offences of strict liability. They arise from situations in which an individual brings about by a voluntary act a prohibited or unlawful state of affairs. They are mainly of a less serious nature; Herring (2016) gives the example of selling a lottery ticket to a person under the age of 16. Offences of this kind are often acts against regulatory laws – laws on which society depends in order to run effectively – as contrasted with acts that are inherently likely to cause harm or that are universally regarded as morally wrong. In law this gives rise to a distinction between two kinds of illegal acts. An offence may be *malum in se* or *malum prohibitum*. The first describes a type of act that is wrong in itself, against common law, and rightfully condemned. The second describes a type of act that is wrong because it has breached regulations or has been forbidden in law through written statutes.

Measuring and recording crime

We might be convinced that the problem of defining crime is solved simply by paying attention to legal statutes and applying the definitions just outlined. However, a fundamental problem emerges from doing so, which is this: even if defined in standard and well-established ways, crime is very difficult to measure. In several important respects, the idea of 'crime' as commonly understood misrepresents the volume and patterning of behaviour that causes harm in society. The events that are recorded by the police, and which are added together in weighty tables produced by government statisticians and discussed in the media and by the public at large, are known to be only a proportion of the total volume of such events that actually occur. The resultant statistics are subject to several kinds of error. Whether or not a specific action that might constitute a crime is reported to the police can be affected by numerous factors, and precisely how the police then record that action also varies according to which laws apply and how the police interpret them. Every step of the ensuing legal process – for example, whether an individual is charged and prosecuted, and with which offence; the extent of any plea bargaining; conviction and sentencing – involves complex processes. The figure that results from this chain of decisions may bear only a loose relationship to the underlying prevalence of actions deemed illegal in society. Criminologists have expended considerable effort in trying to clarify these points, in attempting to pin down where the various kinds of error creep in, and in seeking to arrive at a consensus definition of crime.

Defining 'crime'

Equally troublesome – perhaps even more so – is the problem that there are several ways to define what we think we are measuring. Muncie (2001) counted no fewer than 11 separate definitions of crime. The most familiar and widely used one is the seemingly axiomatic idea of crime as 'the breaking of the criminal law', and probably for many people that is the beginning and the end of the story. Other definitions, however, use a wider concept of departures from moral and social codes. Such definitions could include many actions not usually reported to the police. Other commentators note that the sources of definition themselves reflect the power structures of a society. The location of power may indeed be significant, to the extent that when we study crime we need also to understand the processes whereby conventional definitions are produced. Such an approach draws on a 'social constructionist' rather than a 'realist' conception of how public knowledge is formed. Finally, the most elaborate definitions of crime focus on the concept of harm and its causation. For example, there is a wide range of circumstances in which individuals are denied rights as a result of actions or events within social systems. Definitions of this kind may encompass many types of behaviour not ordinarily recorded as crimes. Some examples are given in the 'Where do you stand?' box on the next page.

Very few of the types of acts described in the 'Where do you stand?' box have resulted in prosecution in the criminal courts. This calls into serious question the adequacy of prevailing approaches to how crime is defined. 'Legal notions of "crime" do seem to provide a peculiarly blinkered vision of the range of misfortunes, dangers, harms, risks and injuries that are a routine part of

WHERE DO YOU STAND?

Causing serious harm without committing a crime

Many kinds of avoidable harm in society are caused by actions that are not defined as crimes. Some such actions have caused more deaths and other kinds of harm than the behaviour we *call* 'crime', yet they are rarely defined as crime or included in the criminal statistics. Many do not attract the attention of law enforcement agencies. The following are examples.

Safety standards in the workplace

There are often failures to adhere to safety standards in the workplace. Few incidents of this kind result in criminal proceedings; and often, despite fatalities, no one is held responsible or brought to justice.

The worst known example of this was the chemical leak from the Union Carbide plant in Bhopal, India, in 1984, which is officially recorded as having caused 3,787 deaths, but which is unofficially estimated to have led to over 20,000 deaths, as well as hundreds of thousands of injuries.

In the UK, cases such as the Zeebrugge ferry disaster of 1987 and the Hatfield train crash of 2000 eventually led to changes in the law and the introduction of the Corporate Manslaughter and Corporate Homicide Act 2007. As of October 2016 there had been 20 successful prosecutions under that Act, with some large fines having been imposed. Most cases involved small companies, and commentators have expressed scepticism as to whether prosecutions would succeed if larger companies were involved (Rose, 2011).

Tobacco sales

Despite evidence of the harmfulness of such products, which was known to manufacturers but concealed or denied by them, tobacco products continue to be marketed.

It has been estimated that, worldwide, 4.83 million premature deaths in 2000 were attributable to smoking (Ezzati and Lopez, 2003), and there is no reason to consider that in this respect an atypical year. There is extensive evidence that tobacco companies have concealed or destroyed documents (LeGresley, Muggli and Hurt, 2005) or have sought to influence the public to disbelieve the evidence of the connection between tobacco and fatal disease (Cummings, Morley and Hyland, 2002). Those who sought redress had no recourse to the criminal law but were obliged to pursue their claims through civil litigation.

Arms sales

Arms have been sold to political regimes in circumstances where there were indications that those arms were likely to be used against civilians.

Several major arms-exporting countries have been exposed as having engaged in such sales. Examples from the recent past have included the sale by Britain to Indonesia of a wide range of military equipment, including Hawk aircraft that were then used in attacks on villages in East Timor (Curtis, 2003); and sales of arms by the United States to the government of Bahrain which were then used against civilians (*Washington Post*, 2011).

The House of Commons Committee on Arms Control Exports (2011, p. 3) has expressed concern that 'successive governments have misjudged the risk that arms approved for export to North Africa and the Middle East might be used for internal repression'. Such arms have been used by the former (Muammar Gaddafi) regime in Libya, and by the Israeli government to protect disputed settlements in the West Bank.

Where do you stand on this issue?

Should the examples above be classed as 'crime'? Or should they continue to be regarded as they are at present, classed in other ways, or best left alone?

everyday life' (Muncie 2001, p. 21). The net result of this may be that by defining crime in certain ways and directing public attention towards the acts identified by those definitions, those with the power to do so can distract attention from other acts, thereby serving the purposes and privileging the interests of some segments of society over others. Orthodox definitions of crime simply as law-breaking are therefore selective. The processes of selection and the communication of what is selected are in themselves worthy of study and analysis, and some criminologists have sought to research such questions.

As we noted earlier, the number of different types of events formally classed as crimes in England and Wales is very large. As some commentators have argued, however, most of them 'create little physical or even financial harm' (Hillyard and Tombs, 2008, p. 9). As these authors indicate, many crimes are predominantly petty events, while many other more harmful events, including corporate crime, violations of safety laws, domestic and sexual violence, and crimes committed by police are by contrast 'marginal to dominant legal, policy, enforcement, and indeed academic, agendas'. 'A focus on crime *deflects* attention from other more socially pressing harms; in many respects it positively *excludes* them' (Hillyard and Tombs, 2008, p. 10). Official or conventional definitions, it is argued, thereby reinforce and help to perpetuate long-standing power structures within society.

These considerations have an important bearing on the status of psychological research and how it is perceived, especially within criminology. As psychologists, we have to admit that in the main we have tended to accept broadly traditional and what might be called 'received' notions of what constitutes crime. By and large, therefore, we have concentrated our efforts on the study of acts customarily regarded as unlawful in Western societies, such as offences against persons, violent and sexual assaults outside the family, or the illicit use of controlled drugs. This is not to deny that these are genuine problems which do indeed cause considerable harm and distress, or that we will be doing a valuable service if we can find some means to control or reduce them. It is salutary, however, to keep our notion of 'crime' in perspective and to remain aware of the wide spectrum of harms and damage that are done to persons through other acts that are rarely prosecuted as crimes, which are often on a far greater scale, and yet which attract comparatively much less attention.

Seeking a consensus definition

At the same time, there is also research suggesting that there is fairly wide agreement on the inclusion of some kinds of acts within an agreed definition of crime, and the need to draw such acts to the attention of the police, almost regardless of the legal or cultural context. Newman (1977) reported the results of a survey conducted in five countries thought to differ markedly in culture and values: the USA, Italy, Serbia, Iran and Indonesia. Participants (n=1,844) were presented with ten brief vignettes and asked whether the acts described in them should be prohibited by law, to rate their seriousness; and to say whether they would report these acts to anyone else and, if so, to whom. The vignettes portrayed incidents in which, for example:

- One person forcefully takes money from another, who requires treatment in hospital as a result.
- A father has sexual relations with his grown-up daughter.
- A person uses heroin (or other substance prohibited in that country).
- Managers of a factory permit toxic gases to be released into the atmosphere.
- An individual appropriates government funds for his own use.

There was a generally high level of agreement that these actions were crimes, in perceptions of their relative seriousness, and that they should be reported to the police. Some other acts – which included consenting homosexual relations, abortion and protesting against the government – were regarded as crimes in some places but not others.

Is it possible, then, to arrive at a consensus definition of what constitutes a crime? In an attempt to transcend debates on how crime is conceptualised whilst also taking into account evidence that the specifics of crime vary across time and place, Ellis (1988) suggested an approach to defining crime that took account of some key features attributed to it. Ellis contended that there is a set of 'core crimes' such that they were probably condemned in human communities even before formal laws were created, and indeed that there is evidence that even non-human primates find particular behaviours repugnant. Acts in this category meet certain criteria:

- There should be an intention for the act to occur, in the sense that most people could have foreseen the consequences, and the person who carried out the act had reason to *desire* those consequences.
- There should be a specific, identifiable victim of the action.
- The victim should be of the same social group as the person judging the act.
- The act should not serve the purpose only of defence of self or of one's family or possessions.
- The crime should not threaten to overthrow an unpopular or disliked government.

Thus there is a progressive narrowing or funnelling process: from all behaviour, to intended behaviour, to actions with a victim involved, to actions in which the victim was a member of one's own social group, and where the act is not defensive of self or possessions, and is non-political. Actions meeting all of these criteria, suggested Ellis, will be universally condemned as criminal.

If an action does *not* meet all of these criteria, many people will not define it as a crime. For example, attacks on members of other groups are often not seen as crimes. Actions that are unintentional or not wholly intended, that are victimless, that are impelled by self-defence or that are politically motivated are not unanimously condemned and are not universally seen as crimes. There will be differing perspectives regarding those actions. Only where an act fulfils all of the above criteria is there likely to be consensus in calling it a *crime*.

Sources of information

Even if we confine our interests to crime defined formally as the breaking of criminal law, there are major hurdles to be overcome in trying to obtain a reasonably accurate picture of the amount and patterning of such actions within society. Crime has been recorded in some form in many societies over the course of many hundreds of years. Archaeological and historic records show that early human societies experienced what are today considered violent crimes, including homicide, sacrifice, mass killing and cannibalism (Guilaine and Zammit, 2005; McCall and Shields, 2008; Walker, 2001). Records of such acts are often taken as evidence for the role of evolution in criminal behaviour, though operating in concert with other kinds of factors.

There are three main sources of information on the amount and patterning of crime in society, each of which derives from a different approach to measuring crime: (a) official crime reports and statistics; (b) self-report surveys of offending; and (c) victim surveys. It is useful to examine in turn the advantages and disadvantages of each.

Official crime reports and statistics

As we will discover in more detail in Chapter 4, it was not until 1827 in France that the first national crime statistics were published, and the availability of such statistics gave impetus to the first modern studies of the patterning of crime. In England and Wales, statistics from police forces in different parts of the country were first collated and published centrally in 1857 (Maguire, 2012). Today, the Ministry of Justice and the Office for National Statistics together produce voluminous information in a series of quarterly and annual bulletins that cover the statistics of crime overall. Separate reports contain statistics for prisons and for probation. Data on crime in Scotland and Northern Ireland are published by the Scottish Government and the Northern Ireland Office respectively. There are many other series of publications reporting analyses of crime data, each designed to serve specific purposes. (Discussing crime statistics and legal provisions in the UK, it is important to keep in mind that there are three separate jurisdictions – England and Wales, Scotland, and Northern Ireland.)

In the USA, national crime statistics in the shape of the *Uniform Crime Reports* (UCRs) were first published by the Federal Bureau of Investigation (FBI) in 1930, to replace what prior to then had been a rather uneven picture in terms of crime recording, making comparisons between states and the detection of national trends an impossible task (Mosher, Miethe and Hart, 2009). The UCRs summarise data on two sets of crimes. Part I offences include seven major types of crime: murder and non-negligent manslaughter, forcible rape, robbery, aggravated assault, burglary, larceny, and motor vehicle theft. Part II offences include a range of less serious crimes, such as other assaults and sexual offences; forgery, fraud and embezzlement; handling stolen goods; vandalism, drug abuse violations, vagrancy, drunkenness, driving while intoxicated, and disorderly conduct. The degree of consistency of crime recording was further tightened through the advent of the National Incident-Based Reporting System (NIBRS) from 1989 onwards. The US Department of Justice also publishes detailed analyses of crime statistics and an extensive range of other reports on numerous aspects of crime. In addition, it offers an invaluable information source, the National Criminal Justice Reference Service, accessible through the internet.

Many other countries have government agencies that compile and publish national statistics, undertake statistical analyses, and produce research on numerous aspects of crime and the operation of the penal system. Such agencies include, for example, Correctional Services Canada/Service correctionnel du Canada; the Australian Institute of Criminology; the Netherlands Institute for the Study of Crime and Law Enforcement (NISCALE); and, at an international level, the United Nations Office on Drugs and Crime (UNODC), which has its headquarters in Vienna. There is no shortage of statistics in the fields of criminology and penology; it is a paradigmatic example of the modern phenomenon known as the 'data explosion'. That abundance of data notwithstanding, there are still many unanswered questions concerning how crime varies in frequency and type over time and from one location to another.

The proportions of police-recorded crimes of different types for one jurisdiction, England and Wales, for a single counting year, 2015–2016, were as shown in Table 2.1. Here we see that, in terms of sheer volume, the bulk of recorded crime,

Crime category	Number of offences	% of total
Violence with injury	431,258	10%
Violence without injury	562,615	12%
Sexual offences	106,378	2%
Robbery	50,904	1%
Burglary	400,361	9%
Vehicle offences	366,715	8%
Shoplifting	336,708	7%
Theft from person/theft of bicycle	169,931	4%
Other theft	486,590	11%
Fraud	621,017	14%
Criminal damage and arson	539,909	12%
Drug offences	147,557	3%
Public order offences	204,616	5%
Possession of weapons offences	25,502	1%
Miscellaneous crime	63,332	1%
Total	**4,513,393**	**100%**

Table 2.1 Crime categories in 4.5 million offences recorded by the police in England and Wales for the year ending 31 March 2016. Percentage figures are rounded.

Source: adapted from data from police recorded crime, Home Office. Published in Office for National Statistics (2016a), licensed under the Open Government Licence v3.0: http://www.nationalarchives.gov.uk/doc/open-government-licence/version/3

with a total of just over 4.5 million offences, consists of acquisitive offences or crimes against property, with theft, criminal damage, offences against vehicles, burglary and fraud together forming 65 per cent of the total. Violent offences constitute 22 per cent of the total; and with sexual offences and robbery added, that proportion rises to 25 per cent. The publication from which these data were drawn (Office for National Statistics, 2016a) gives a more detailed breakdown of some categories. Within violent crime, for example, there were 571 homicides. Amongst sexual offences, there were 35,798 offences of rape and 70,580 other sexual offences. Amongst drug offences, there were 122,155 offences of possession and 25,402 of drug trafficking.

Turning to international comparisons, a useful source is the United Nations Survey on Crime Trends and the Operations of Criminal Justice Systems (UN-CTS; Harrendorf, Heiskanen and Malby, 2010). Note that for statistics such as these there is often a lag before figures appear, because of the time needed to collect and analyse data from many countries. Figure 2.1 shows the rate of intentional homicide in different world regions for the most recent year for which data were available up to 2008 (Malby, 2010). This offence is sometimes taken as a useful 'proxy' indicator for crime overall, as intentional homicide is more likely to be reported and officially recorded than other types of crime. Even so, there are uncertainties: for the UN-CTS these were partly overcome by using two sources of evidence, police recorded crime and medically recorded deaths due to homicide. Furthermore, many but not all countries exclude infanticide from this figure; and whether a homicide is recorded as 'intentional' is often a matter of interpretation. Note, then, that there are larger gaps between the two information sources in some regions than in others, and we should also bear in mind

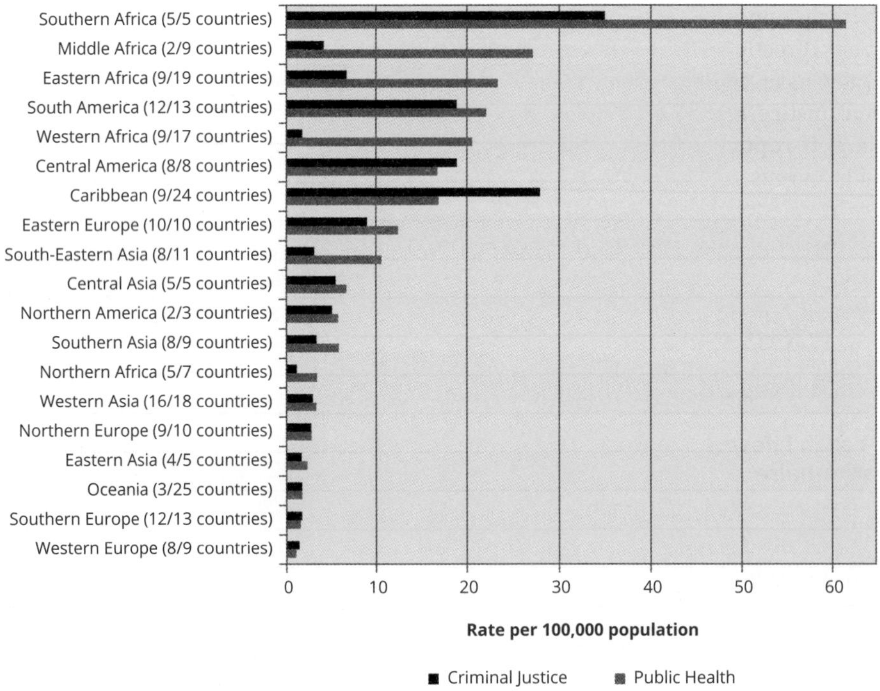

Southern Africa (5/5 countries)
Middle Africa (2/9 countries)
Eastern Africa (9/19 countries)
South America (12/13 countries)
Western Africa (9/17 countries)
Central America (8/8 countries)
Caribbean (9/24 countries)
Eastern Europe (10/10 countries)
South-Eastern Asia (8/11 countries)
Central Asia (5/5 countries)
Northern America (2/3 countries)
Southern Asia (8/9 countries)
Northern Africa (5/7 countries)
Western Asia (16/18 countries)
Northern Europe (9/10 countries)
Eastern Asia (4/5 countries)
Oceania (3/25 countries)
Southern Europe (12/13 countries)
Western Europe (8/9 countries)
0
10
20
30
40
50
60
Rate per 100,000 population
Criminal Justice
Public Health

Figure 2.1
Rates of intentional homicide per 100,000 population for different world regions. Data were extracted from two sources: police records of homicides and medical reports of deaths classed as homicides.

Source: Malby, S. (2010). Homicide. In S. Harrendorf, M. Heiskanen & S. Malby (eds.). International Statistics on Crime and Justice. HEUNI Publication Series No.64. pp.7–20. Helsinki and Vienna: European Institute for Crime Prevention and Control & United Nations Office on Drugs and Crime. Reprinted with permission.

that the proportion of countries providing data also varies by region. Clearly there are very wide variations in the figures, with the intentional homicide rate in Southern and Central Africa several times that in Europe and parts of Asia. This may be partly associated with the availability of firearms. In Central, South and North America, an average of over 60 per cent of homicides involved a gun; whereas in Western Europe and Asia the figure was approximately 15 per cent, and in Eastern and Southern Europe 10 per cent. There are also marked variations in trends over time. In some countries, for example Honduras, in the six-year period 2003–2008 the rate of intentional homicide almost doubled (a rise of 80 per cent); in others, for example Latvia, it virtually halved.

Self-report surveys

In trying to gauge the amount of crime in society, instead of starting from official figures, which inevitably can only reflect the amount of crime formally reported, a completely opposite approach is to contact citizens directly and to ask them whether or not they have committed an offence. In criminal justice research this approach is called a **self-report survey**. (Of course almost all surveys involve self-report, as they ask respondents to describe their own behaviour or attitudes.) It is on the basis of such survey work that criminologists have concluded that crime is in one sense 'normal', in that a large proportion of the population admits to having broken the law at some stage. Studies of this kind are usually done using survey methodology, mostly with quite large samples and involving interviews or questionnaires. They may be carried out face to face, by telephone, or via the internet. Respondents may be asked whether they have committed offences during a given time period, such as 'the past 12 months', or whether they have done so at any time. An example of such a questionnaire is shown in the 'Focus on ...' box below.

In trying to draw meaningful conclusions from studies of this type, one encounters the same problems as arise in almost all survey methodology. These include the difficulties of ensuring that sampling adequately reflects the configuration of the target population. In order to construct representative samples, it is important both to minimise and to be able to take account of non-responders and those who refuse to participate, as well as other methodological problems that arise from sampling error (Mosher, Miethe and Hart, 2011). Further difficulties include those resulting from measurement error; here we encounter concepts that are familiar from the field of psychometric testing (see for example Gregory, 2011): the question of whether or not responses in self-report surveys are

FOCUS ON ...

Self-reporting

The Youth Lifestyles Survey questionnaire

During the 1990s, two self-report surveys of young people investigated the possible association between offending behaviour and other aspects of 'lifestyle'. This entailed asking whether they had committed any of a list of offence types.

The following list is from Flood-Page *et al.* (2000), who expanded on the initial version by Graham and Bowling (1995). For each offence, individuals may be asked either (a) whether they have ever committed that offence at any time, or (b) whether they have done so within the last 12 months. Offences numbered 8, 9, 11, 12, 22, 23, 25, 26 and 27 are considered more serious. Participants are asked:

'Have you ...

Criminal damage

1 ... damaged or destroyed, purposely or recklessly, something belonging to someone else (e.g. a telephone box, bus shelter, car, window of a house etc.)?

2 ... set fire, purposely or recklessly, to something not belonging to you? It might be to paper or furniture, a barn, a car, a forest, basement, a building or something else.

Property offences

3 ... stolen money from a gas or electricity meter, public telephone vending machine, video game or fruit machine?

4 ... stolen anything from a shop, supermarket or department store?

5 ... stolen anything in school worth more than £5?

6 ... stolen anything from the place that you work worth more than £5?

7 ... taken away a bicycle without the owner's permission, not intending to give it back?

8 ... taken away a motorbike or moped without the owner's permission, not intending to give it back?

9 ... taken away a car without the owner's permission, not intending to give it back?

10 ... stolen anything out of or from a car?

11 ... pick-pocketed anything from anybody?

12 ... sneaked into someone's garden or house or a building intending to steal something (not meaning an abandoned or ruined building)?

13 ... stolen anything worth more than £5, not mentioned already (e.g. from a hospital, youth club, sports centre, pub, building site etc.)?

14 ... bought something that you knew, or believed at the time, was stolen?

15 ... sold something that you knew, or believed at the time, was stolen?

16 ... sold a chequebook, credit card, cash-point card (ATM card) belonging to you or someone else so that they could steal money from a bank account?

17 ... used a chequebook, credit card, cash-point card (ATM card) that you knew or believed at the time to be stolen to get money out of a bank account?

Fraud

18 ... made a false claim on an insurance policy?

19 ... claimed social security benefits to which you knew that you were not entitled?

20 ... made an incorrect tax return?

21 ... claimed more than £5 in expenses that you knew that you were not entitled to?

Violent offences

22 ... snatched from a person a purse, bag or something else?

23 ... threatened someone with a weapon or with beating them up to get money or other valuables from them?

24 ... taken part in fighting or disorder in a group in a public place (e.g. football ground, railway station, music festival, riot, demonstration or just in the street)?

25 ... beaten up someone not belonging to your immediate family to such an extent that you think or know that medical help or a doctor was needed?

26 ... beaten up someone in your immediate family to such an extent that you think or know that medical help or a doctor was needed?

27 ... hurt someone with a knife, stick or other weapon?'

Your own self-report

Take the self-report and assess your results.

1 Do you think there are any connections between offending behaviour and lifestyle?

2 What are the limitations of self-report surveys?

Reference

▸ Flood-Page *et al.* (2000). © Crown copyright 2000. Contains public sector information licensed under the Open Government Licence v3.0:http://www.nationalarchives.gov.uk/doc/open-government-licence/version/3

valid (whether they measure what they are intended to measure) and *reliable* (whether they show consistency across repeated measurement occasions) has been vigorously debated in criminology.

We may expect that people will be reluctant to confess to crimes, even petty ones, for fear of being prosecuted or because they feel ashamed, so we are unlikely to get completely honest answers in surveys of this type, even when assurances are given regarding confidentiality. The possibility of concealment can never be discounted. Nevertheless, long-term studies in which respondents have been contacted on repeated occasions suggest that what people say is often reasonably reliable as a guide to their illegal activity. However, checks against other information sources show that there are patterns of under-reporting amongst particular groups (Mosher *et al.*, 2011). Despite these obstacles, large-scale self-report studies have produced invaluable information on patterns of offending. Such studies include the US National Youth Survey Family Study (Elliott, Huizinga and Morse, 1986), a longitudinal study of 1,725 young people who have been recontacted on a series of occasions from 1976 onwards: this study has produced a plethora of research publications testing specific hypotheses. Another is the Youth Lifestyles Survey in the UK (Flood-Page, Campbell, Harrington and Miller, 2000), which examined the association between involvement in offending and other features of everyday living in a sample of 4,848 people aged between 12 and 30.

Apart from yielding information on the extent of unrecorded offending by samples of the general population, self-report surveys have also been used in research on the offence rates and patterns of *repeat offenders*, who commit the same kind of offence on successive occasions. Studies of this kind were originally carried out by the RAND Corporation in the USA in the 1970s (Visher, 1986). Prison inmates who had committed specific types of offence were asked how many similar crimes they had committed that had not been detected. This showed that the majority of offenders committed several crimes per year, but that there was a small group who committed many more such offences and who could be described as 'prolific'. For example, we can compare the median number of offences committed per annum with those for the top end of the distribution (the 'worst 10 per cent'). Here are the figures for four types of offence: for theft, median 8.59, worst 10 per cent 425; for burglary, median 5.45, worst 10 per cent 232; for robbery, median 5.00, worst 10 per cent 87; and for assault, median 2.4, worst 10 per cent 13.

Some self-report surveys have focused specifically on drug-related offending or on substance misuse more generally; we will discuss the findings of this research in Chapter 10.

Victim surveys

Victim surveys are also based on self-reporting, but in this case interviews are concerned not with involvement in offending but with whether or not the respondent has been the victim of a crime within a specified period. The first National Crime Victimization Survey (NCVS) was published in the United States in 1972, and data have been collected from a nationally representative sample twice per annum every year since then. The sample size is generally in the region of 38,000 households, with respondents aged 12 or older; this yields an annual total of approximately 136,000 interviews. Households remain in the survey for a period of three years, with new households progressively entering and later leaving the survey in an ongoing sequence (Siegel, 2012). Its counterpart in the United Kingdom, the British Crime Survey (BCS), was first produced in 1981, was then produced at irregular intervals up to 2001, and since then has been published annually, and is now known as the Crime Survey for England and Wales (CSEW) (Newburn, 2017). Sample sizes are again large, typically involving 50,000 respondents aged from 16 upwards; more recently a pilot survey was conducted with 10- to 15-year-olds. Similar surveys are conducted in a number of countries and there is also an International Crime Victims Survey (ICVS). To date there have been five 'sweeps' of the latter, in 1989, 1992, 1996, 2000 and 2005. A sixth preliminary survey was conducted for six countries in 2010 and was to be followed by more extensive data collection (ICVS, 2010), but as of 2014 there were reportedly 'no elaborate plans' to conduct further international surveys on this scale (van Kesteren, van Dijk and Mayhew, 2014, p. 66). The 2005 version covered 78 countries and involved a total of more than 320,000 respondents (van Dijk, van Kesteren and Smit, 2007).

As already noted, in many sets of crime statistics there is a gap between the official figure from police-recorded crime and the results of self-report offending surveys or victim surveys, and traditionally this has been referred to as the 'dark figure' or **hidden figure of crime** (Coleman and Moynihan, 1996). Typically, this gap represents a greater volume of crime emerging from both types of survey than is seen in the police statistics, principally of course because many offences are not reported and are therefore not recorded. The gap may be large: often more than half of assaults and thefts are not reported to the police and so do not appear in the 'official' criminal statistics. The gap is illustrated in Figure 2.2, which compares two ways of measuring crime during the period from 1981 to 2016 in England and Wales (Office for National Statistics, 2016a). The discrepancy between the two sets of statistics – police-recorded versus victim-reported crime – is sometimes even larger than that shown here.

There are several reasons for not reporting crimes. One is simply that many acts, although they are in a literal sense violations of the criminal law, are relatively trivial in their consequences, or do not involve any victimisation of others. One example would be the smoking of cannabis. Another is that the acts are so frequent as to be virtually impossible to keep track of, such as the breaking of speed limits. A third possibility is that individuals simply forget events, or misremember or misconstrue them. There are also instances where individuals do not report crimes in order to avoid drawing attention to themselves, as doing so might lead to the discovery that they had committed other crimes. Yet another reason for non-reporting is fear: particularly following violent or sexual crimes committed within households, victims may be afraid to go to the police (or indeed to tell anyone). It is often assumed that the most common type of crime is one against property, but surveys of the incidence of child abuse (e.g. Creighton, 2004) call that into question. Garside (2006, p. 23) estimates that when we extrapolate from available research on this point, 'offences such as sexual assaults and

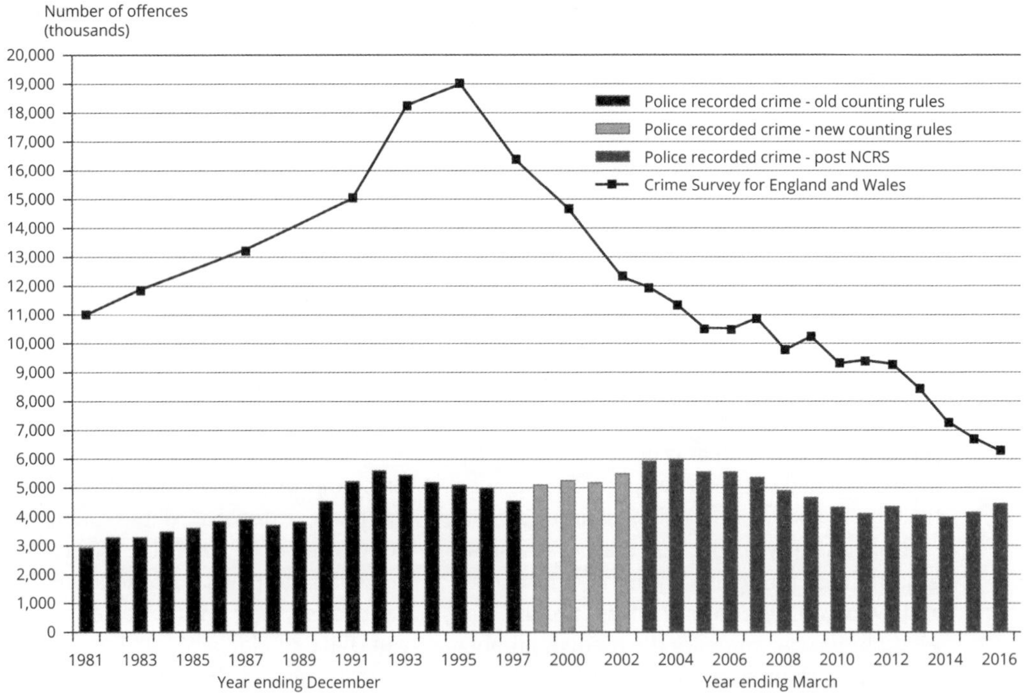
Number of offences (thousands)
20,000
19,000
18,000
17,000
16,000
15,000
14,000
13,000
12,000
11,000
10,000
9,000
8,000
7,000
6,000
5,000
4,000
3,000
2,000
1,000
0
Police recorded crime - old counting rules
Police recorded crime - new counting rules
Police recorded crime - post NCRS
Crime Survey for England and Wales
1981 1983 1985 1987 1989 1991 1993 1995 1997 2000 2002 2004 2006 2008 2010 2012 2014 2016
Year ending December
Year ending March

Figure 2.2

Crime in England and Wales, 1981–2016. The figure compares police-recorded rates with the Crime Survey for England and Wales (CSEW). During the period shown, there were two changes in methods of counting crimes, shown in the vertical bars. (The change in recording methods that occurred in 2003–2004 is also discussed in the 'Where do you stand?' box on p. 40.) Note that the vertical axis counts thousands of thousands.

Source: Crime Survey for England and Wales, Office for National Statistics / Police recorded crime, Home Office. Published in Office for National Statistics (2016a), licensed under the Open Government Licence v3.0: http://www.nationalarchives.gov.uk/doc/open-government-licence/version/3

child abuse may well be far more common than burglary or robbery'. It is quite possible that offences committed within the home are more numerous than so-called 'volume crimes' (see Chapter 6), even though the bulk of them remain invisible to outside agencies.

Like the data for officially recorded crime discussed earlier, patterns of reported victimisation also show significant international variations. As can be seen from Figure 2.3, taken from the International Crime Victims Survey, there are some quite consistent

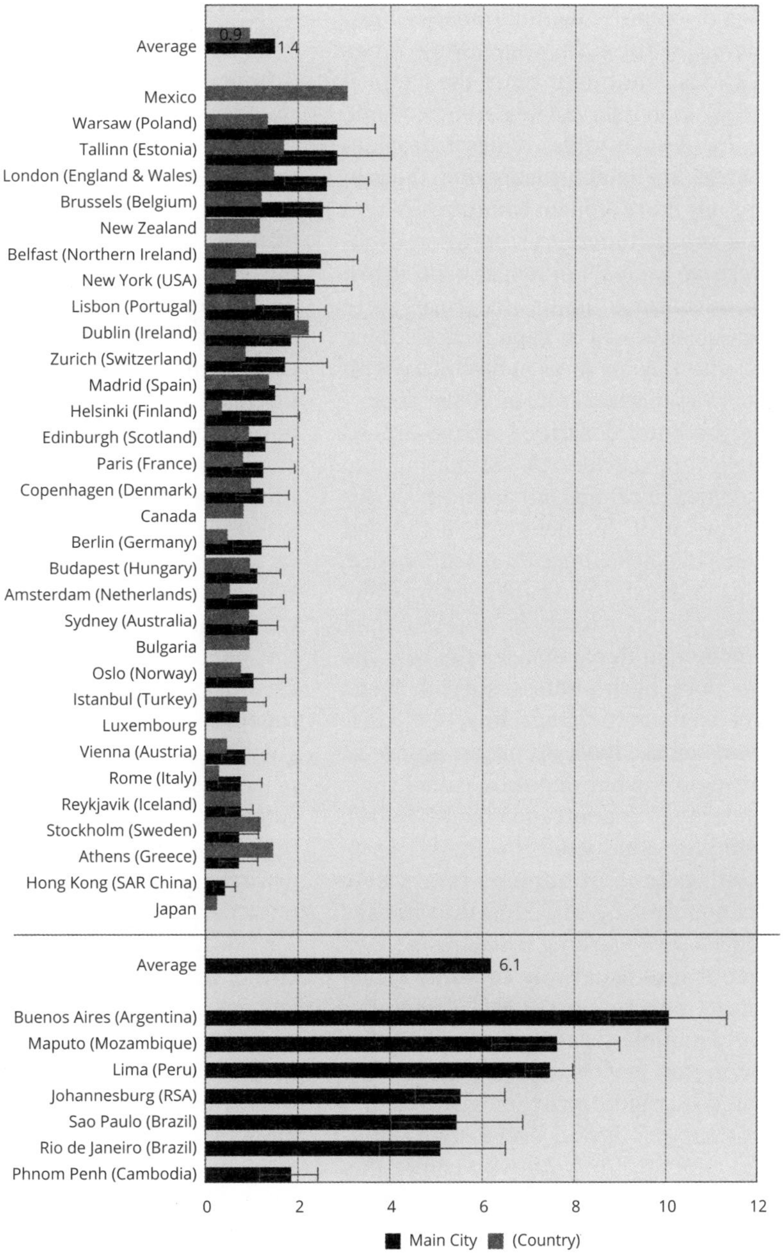

Average
0.9
1.4
Mexico
Warsaw (Poland)
Tallinn (Estonia)
London (England & Wales)
Brussels (Belgium)
New Zealand
Belfast (Northern Ireland)
New York (USA)
Lisbon (Portugal)
Dublin (Ireland)
Zurich (Switzerland)
Madrid (Spain)
Helsinki (Finland)
Edinburgh (Scotland)
Paris (France)
Copenhagen (Denmark)
Canada
Berlin (Germany)
Budapest (Hungary)
Amsterdam (Netherlands)
Sydney (Australia)
Bulgaria
Oslo (Norway)
Istanbul (Turkey)
Luxembourg
Vienna (Austria)
Rome (Italy)
Reykjavik (Iceland)
Stockholm (Sweden)
Athens (Greece)
Hong Kong (SAR China)
Japan
Average
6.1
Buenos Aires (Argentina)
Maputo (Mozambique)
Lima (Peru)
Johannesburg (RSA)
Sao Paulo (Brazil)
Rio de Janeiro (Brazil)
Phnom Penh (Cambodia)
0
2
4
6
8
10
12
Main City
(Country)

Figure 2.3

Robbery in selected countries and their main cities, 2003–2004. The figure shows one-year prevalence rates (the percentage of each sample who reported having been a victim of robbery) in the countries and cities for which these data were available.

Source: van Dijk, J., van Kesteren, J. & Smit, P. (2007). Criminal Victimisation in International Perspective: Key Findings from the 2004–2005 ICVS and EU ICS. Den Haag: Wetenschappelijk Onderzoeken Documentatiecentrum. Reprinted with permission from WODC.

trends in evidence drawn from such sources, and two in particular are worthy of comment. Findings for robbery are typical of several types of crimes. First, across almost all countries, 'robbery is one of the types of crime that is much more prevalent in larger cities than in rural areas and can therefore be characterized as a typical manifestation of urban problems of crime ... the difference is most pronounced in the USA where New York's rate (2.3%) is almost four times the national rate (0.6%)' (van Dijk, van Kesteren and Smit, 2007, p. 73). Second, rates in cities in developing countries are notably higher than those in economically more affluent countries. Within the latter group, differences between countries were fairly small. Amongst main urban centres, in contrast, the top six places were all taken up by cities in rapidly developing nations, with Buenos Aires in first place with an annual victimisation rate of 10 per cent.

The methods described above are all essentially approaches to estimating the total volumes of crime, and amounts of different types of it, in society. If in the end this seems like little more than a somewhat laborious and elaborate bookkeeping exercise, there are other methods of research in criminology that depart markedly from the need to pore over endless spreadsheets. They are used not to *count* crime, but to discover what individuals do in the course of committing it – what might be called their *modus operandi*. Bennett and Wright (1984), for example, conducted in-depth interviews with persistent burglars to ask how those contemplating breaking into houses made decisions regarding which properties to target. A less usual way to study crime is by direct observation of the crime as it happens. Examples are the work of Buckle and Farrington (1994), in which researchers waited outside department stores and surreptitiously followed every sixth shopper who entered. In two towns where this was done – Peterborough and Bedford – 1.9 per cent and 1.2 per cent respectively of those followed were observed in the act of shoplifting. Even riskier than following people is the method of *participant observation* used by Wright and Decker (1997) in their study of armed robbery in the city of St. Louis. With the permission of the city police, and the agreement of members of the criminal 'underworld', the researchers accompanied armed robbers as they went about a day's work. This yielded invaluable insights into the criminal process that could probably not have been obtained by any other means.

Methods of presenting statistics

Criminal statistics are typically reported in raw numbers on an annual (or sometimes a quarterly) basis. Typically, data will be presented in tables or graphical plots for total numbers of crimes, for different types of offence, by region, by age-group, and according to other demographics. Change over time will be reported as positive or negative percentages, with comparisons made between consecutive years or across longer periods of interest (e.g. before or after certain changes in the law or in sentencing). When comparisons are made between countries, or across time periods, or for types of offence, this is generally done by computing the respective rates per 100,000 people in the population. What are known as 'clearance' or 'clear-up' rates – the proportion of offences for which the police arrest someone and court proceedings result in a conviction (sometimes called the 'conversion rate') – are usually given as percentages. These too vary from place to place, over time, and for different categories of offence. Penal statistics such as imprisonment rates are also usually given as a proportion (the number of persons imprisoned per 100,000 population).

For the risk of becoming a victim of crime, data are usually presented as *prevalence rates*: that is, the number of people in a given population who experience a named problem (such as being a victim of robbery) within a defined time period: usually 12 months (*12-month prevalence rate*) or at some point in their lives (*lifetime prevalence rate*). These statistics can be expressed in percentage or ratio form. Prevalence statistics are also sometimes used for reporting rates of involvement in crime.

Using a combination of crime rate data and information from the penal system, it is possible to calculate the likelihood of being imprisoned for a crime. For example, the rate of incarceration for robbery in England

and Wales in 1999 was 1 in 238; whereas in the Netherlands the probability was higher, at 1 in 142, but in Switzerland very much lower, at 1 in 667 (Farrington, Langan and Tonry, 2004).

Individual criminal records

All of the statistical tables and graphs, of course, reflect the accumulated contacts of a large number of people with the criminal justice process. At the other end of the measuring rod, as it were, are individuals who have been convicted of the offences of which the output statistics are composed.

When we examine the file of an individual who has been sentenced by the court, we typically find a record of his or her previous offences and convictions alongside certain other pieces of information. In England and Wales such documents vary in format across different agencies and locations, but will almost certainly include at least the following:

» Identifying information on the individual: name; date of birth; and Criminal Records Bureau (CRB) or Police National Computer (PNC) number.

» The date of each appearance in court.

» The date of each offence.

» The name of the court.

» The type of *index offence* or *principal offence* – the most serious offence of which the individual is currently convicted – and the number of incidents of that offence.

» The sentence or penalty imposed.

In addition to the above, the typical file found in a prison or other penal setting includes numerous other documents, such as **pre-sentence reports**, prepared for the court in which the individual appeared; social work or social circumstances reports; and possibly other information on an individual's background. In secure mental health settings, there will also be psychiatric, psychology and nursing reports. Again, as with the large-scale statistics, there appears to be no scarcity of information. Often, however, a proportion of that information will be found to be repetitious; some of it may be inaccurate; and elsewhere there may be large gaps in what is available and reliably known. We will return to the issue of assessment information and discuss some of these problems in Chapters 12 and 18.

Crime, news media and public perceptions

Crime is more or less perennially in the news. As we will note at various points in this book, when discussing many questions in psychology and other social sciences, it is often difficult to keep separate the scientific knowledge available on any given issue and how that issue is understood more generally. That applies even more when the issues in question are contentious or sensitive ones on which people may hold a variety of prior beliefs. Crime is, or appears to be, an issue of prime **public interest**. Research shows that a very high proportion of printed news content – indeed, the largest single share in comparison with other topics – consists of stories about crime. Furthermore, a similar pattern can be found across all types of news media (Carrabine, Cox, Lee and South, 2002). Such stories focus disproportionately on violent and personal crimes, and on the *nature* of the incidents described rather than their possible causes (Reiner, 2007). There are discrepancies in crime literature and cinema that parallel those found in news reporting. But there is also one large difference: in fictional accounts the majority of crimes are solved.

In terms of its departures from a scientific account, discussion of crime is often highly politicised. By this we mean that – across the political spectrum – crime statistics and sometimes individual cases are used to argue for or against some pre-existing point of view, typically concerning whether or how crime is related to other social problems, what its occurrence tells us about the kind of society we live in, whose fault all of that is, and of course what needs to be done about it and by whom. How crime data are interpreted, or the perspective on them that is presented, very often feeds into an agenda promoted by one or other political party, or by the numerous 'think tanks' or pressure groups that proliferate in this field. Some instances of such crime reporting are cited in the 'Where do you stand?' box on page 40.

WHERE DO YOU STAND?

Crime: rising or falling?

Perhaps understandably, there is a widespread preoccupation amongst the news media with the overall amount of crime, and the rates of different types of crime. A core question within this discussion is whether the crime rate is stable or is rising or falling by significant amounts. The yearly publication of official crime statistics has therefore become a key fixture in the cycle of news events.

Mosher, Miethe and Hart (2011) recount several instances of quite large-scale misinterpretation or misrepresentation of crime statistics both in the United States and in the United Kingdom. In May 2001, for example, there was considerable confusion in the US media when official crime data suggested that, after a ten-year period of steady decline, the national crime rate had risen again. This was widely reported and discussed in the media, sometimes in alarmist tones. Two weeks later, however, a report of the National Crime Victimisation Survey indicated the opposite: that crime had fallen still further, and indeed that violent crime had shown its largest ever single drop, of 15 per cent. It subsequently emerged that the official report had consisted of preliminary analysis only – a point made in the report itself, but not mentioned in media coverage of it.

A similar situation arose in the UK in 2004 when, in response to the appearance of that year's crime statistics, a former Home Secretary, Michael Howard, declared that police statistics had shown that crime was rising dramatically. Again, victimisation rates, as recorded in the British Crime Survey, showed the reverse. According to a former Home Office researcher who commented on Mr Howard's claim that crime had risen:

> As a former home secretary, he must be aware that this is a gross misrepresentation of crime trends. Police statistics bear little relation to the reality. The British Crime Survey (BCS) shows unequivocally that major types of crime have fallen dramatically since 1995: vehicle crime down by half, house burglary down by 47%, assault down by 43%, wounding down by 28%, vandalism down 27%. Mugging shows a small fall that is statistically not significant.
>
> Recorded crime has gone up over the past five years because the police have changed the way that they count crime. In particular, they altered their 'counting rules' in 1998, and introduced a National Crime Recording Standard (NCRS) from 2002. They previously rejected victims' reports of crime if they doubted them; now, under the NCRS, these are taken at face value. Both sets of changes have inflated the police count of crime, and this inflation has been greatest for crimes of violence. That is the reason for the 83% rise in violence that Mr Howard cites. (Hough, 2004)

Media attention to crime figures has widespread effects. Not only does the sometimes careless or even wilful misuse of such figures provide a talking point in news programmes or political interviews; the impressions formed may also reverberate widely within society, influencing the beliefs that many citizens hold about crime, their level of concern about it, and their fear of becoming victims of it. For example, as we have just seen, all the crime statistics, regardless of method of collection, indicated that crime in England and Wales *fell* steadily from approximately 1995 onwards (the trend continued and was still doing so in 2016). Despite this, researchers at the time found that many citizens nevertheless believed the opposite: that crime had risen or was continuing to rise. Such a belief was moderated by the type of newspaper they read. Regular readers of 'tabloid' newspapers were twice as likely as those who read 'broadsheets' (43 per cent versus 21 per cent) to think the national crime rate had *increased* in the previous two years (Lovbakke, 2007).

Where do you stand on this issue?

1 Do you think that the media have a responsibility to accurately report crime figures?

2 Do you think that factors other than the media contribute to society's general impression that crime is on the increase?

The tendency of crime journalism towards selectiveness or bias in the handling of stories is illustrated in a study by Forsyth (2001) of the reporting of drug-related deaths in Scotland in the 1990s. During that decade there were 2,255 'toxicologically confirmed' drug deaths, 546 of which were reported in the four newspapers (the biggest sellers in their respective markets) that Forsyth analysed. Whereas the drug actually associated with the largest single proportion of deaths was diazepam (21.3 per cent of all deaths), the one most frequently mentioned in the newspaper reports was heroin (13.7 per cent of all stories). Of the 28 deaths associated with ecstasy, 26 were reported in the press, a ratio between forensic toxicology records and news reports of approximately 1:1. The corresponding ratio for heroin was 5:1, for diazepam 48:1, and for paracetamol 265:1. Put another way, whereas almost all of the deaths due to ecstasy received media attention, only one of the 265 deaths due to paracetamol did so. The 16 'most newsworthy' cases, as reflected in the number of column inches devoted to them, produced half as many column inches again as the remaining 530 cases; and 11 of those cases involved ecstasy (sometimes combined with other drugs). Overall, with the exception of heroin, 'the drugs which were responsible for relatively few deaths tended to receive more attention by the press than those which were responsible for the most deaths' (Forsyth, 2001, p. 447). Story content also reflected bias towards reporting deaths that involved young female recreational users. Forsyth speculated to what extent news reports may influence public opinion and thereby policy. Overall, the conclusion is inescapable that news reports, with a few exceptions, cannot be described as dependable sources of systematic information on crime and related issues.

Chapter summary

As we embarked on the journey visualised in the opening chapter, we considered the most typical way for that journey to start: when a person commits an act that is prohibited by the criminal law, an act defined as a crime.

- It is important to be aware of how specific crimes are defined in law. Legal definitions have been phrased very carefully and precisely, and we need to have a clear picture of the definition in each individual case.
- In legal terms, 'crimes' are defined as having certain elements, including those of *actus reus* and *mens rea*. The specific details of these elements are given in legal statutes for each type of act that is defined as an offence.
- There are several different ways of measuring crime and of compiling criminal statistics. These include police-recorded crime, self-report surveys and victim surveys.
- However, crime as reported in official statistics is widely viewed as representing only a part of total illegal activity and only a subset of actions that cause harm. We discussed the problems that arise when interpreting crime statistics, and considered several other perspectives on how crime can be conceptualised.

Further reading

- There are numerous, and usually compendious, textbooks on criminal law; and while they obviously cover basically the same ground, they differ in how accessible they are to a non-specialist. We have found the books by Jonathan Herring (2016) and by David Ormerod and Karl Laird (2015) particularly valuable as resources.
- The study of criminal statistics may sound rather dry! However, *The Mismeasurement of Crime* by Clayton Mosher, Terance D. Miethe and Timothy C. Hart (2011) is very clearly written and, despite its subject matter, a lively and engaging account of methods of compiling such statistics.
- There are also many excellent introductory textbooks on criminology, which discuss problems such as how to define crime.

For UK readers, Tim Newburn's (2017) *Criminology* is highly recommended, and is accompanied by a book of readings published alongside the first edition (Newburn, 2009). For readers in the USA, Larry J. Siegel's (2012) *Criminology* is hard to beat.

» For detailed analysis of a series of key issues in criminology, the *Oxford Handbook of Criminology* by Mike Maguire, Rod Morgan and Robert Reiner (2012) is an indispensable resource.

The Office for National Statistics (www.ons.gov.uk) produces a steady output of statistics covering not only criminal justice but all aspects of public life. The ONS publishes statistics related to crime and the operation of the penal system, replete with data tables, and also more focused analytic studies on specific issues. Other excellent sources include the United States Department of Justice (www.justice.gov), which produces numerous research reports; and, for international crime data, the United Nations Office on Drugs and Crime, which is based in Vienna (www.unodc.org).

Researching Crime: Methods and Correlates

The previous chapter focused on how crime is defined, contrasting formal legal concepts contained in criminal law statutes, which are the basis of 'official' crime statistics, with other ways of defining and then of measuring it. This chapter turns to other ways of analysing and understanding offending behaviour and the patterns it takes. We examine different ways of studying crime and other antisocial behaviour which open up possibilities for understanding some key factors related to crime. We review the main research methods used in that process, and identify some key findings they have produced.

Chapter objectives

- To examine methods used in the psychological study of crime.
- To become familiar with some key features of reported crime.
- To understand the concept of risk factors for involvement in crime.
- To survey key findings on the development of offending behaviour.

So far, we have discussed a general picture of crime, reviewing definitions of what crime is thought to be; and how, with reference to the most commonly used definition, it is recorded and then patterns within it are analysed. Moving on from this descriptive approach, our next step is to examine what variables are correlated with crime, an area now usually seen as the realm of **risk factors** research. This has been an area of momentous growth in psychology and criminal justice, particularly in the period since roughly 1990 onwards.

A 'risk factor' is a variable that is significantly correlated with an adverse outcome of interest – correlated to the extent that the risk factor can be used as a predictor of that outcome, though there is unlikely to be any single factor (or even a combination of factors) that can do this perfectly. The concept of risk factors and their identification through steadily mounting research has represented a major advance in forensic and other forms of applied psychology. It also underpins the process of risk assessment that we will describe more fully in Chapter 18.

However, the concept of risk factors *correlated* with outcomes does not necessarily imply any form of *causation*. Many variables that are considered to be risk factors for crime are also thought to contribute to causing it, but often evidence supporting such a causal link is lacking. For further meaningful advances to be made beyond the concept of correlates, the question of demonstrating causation – of showing *why* offences occur – needs to be addressed. This will move to centre stage later in the present chapter when we look at the findings of longitudinal and developmental research. Examining the relationships over time between risk factors and entry into offending or **desistance** from offending can also allow the testing of hypotheses about cause–effect relationships.

These concepts will then be elaborated upon in the next three chapters. Chapter 4 will survey a broad range of attempts to formulate theories of crime causation, moving through a series of levels of explanation from large-scale and societal to individual and psychological. Chapter 5 will focus more specifically on what is known about this in relation to separate types of offence, but with particular reference to offences involving aggression and violence. Chapters in Part 2 will then address the relationships between internal, mental states, both 'normal' and 'abnormal', and the committing of specific types of criminal acts. The possibility of being able to identify causes of crime or antisocial conduct opens up the prospect of being able to influence and remedy those causes, and thereby perhaps to reduce the frequency or severity of crime itself. (The latter issue is one that will be discussed in depth much later in the book, in Chapter 19.)

What place do psychologists have in how we understand crime, and what contribution can they make to the intricate systems society has set up to address it? In the first half of this chapter, we will describe the types of methods used by psychologists and other professionals in carrying out research on aspects of criminal conduct. In addition to studying or analysing data from official sources such as government statistics, or on the basis of self-report or victim surveys (of the kinds we met in Chapter 2), criminological and forensic psychologists also conduct specially designed research projects within the agencies in which they work. There are several types of research design on which psychologists and others draw in attempting to gain an understanding of the factors that influence crime. Before proceeding to discuss the findings that have been obtained, it is important to examine the different methods used in that research, as the design of studies can often have an important influence on what is found. Following this, the remainder of the chapter then summarises some of the principal findings obtained from the use of those methods, paying particular attention to the results relating to risk factors, and which of those factors may play a causal role.

Primary studies: research methods

Longitudinal research

The type of study often regarded as the most powerful and informative is one in which typically a quite large cohort of individuals is followed by researchers over an extended period of time, with data being collected at successive points on a number of aspects of those individuals' lives, including the extent of any involvement in crime. This is a type of research known as a **longitudinal study** (though sometimes called a *cohort study* or a *panel design*), and projects like this have played a major part in the formulation of theories concerning which variables can be described as risk factors for crime and which may play a part in its causation.

The advantage offered by such studies is the opportunity they afford to examine the order in which events occur, an important basis for inferring the presence of cause–effect relationships. This variety of research can be used to answer questions such as these:

» 'Is there an association between the amount or consistency of parental discipline during childhood and the likelihood of participating in delinquency?'

» 'Is there a link between not attending school and becoming involved in substance misuse?'

» 'Is cannabis use a "gateway" to the use of other drugs and to involvement in crime?'

An example of this kind of research is the Cambridge Study in Delinquent Development, a study of 411 London males begun when they were aged eight, which has now been ongoing for a period of over 40 years (Farrington *et al.*, 2006). Some longitudinal studies also incorporate an experimental element, drawing a comparison between the pathways of two cohorts known to have had different types of prior experiences, such as 'basic' versus 'enhanced' pre-school or family support (Farrington, 2006).

Experimental studies

Psychology is in large part an experimental science and *true experiments*, of the kind widely used in many of its specialist branches, must be carried out under tightly controlled conditions. In many areas of study experiments are conducted in laboratory settings. Major advances in the subdivisions of comparative, cognitive, developmental and social psychology, and in behavioural and cognitive neuroscience, have been made in this way. As we will see in later chapters, research in some areas of forensic psychology also lends itself particularly well to laboratory-based study. This includes, for example, work on face recognition, witness memory, the reliability of testimony, or the use of different types of questioning of suspects.

Unfortunately, there are limitations in the extent to which findings from highly controlled research can be extrapolated to other settings. As happens elsewhere in psychology, there is a pay-off in research designs between internal validity and external validity: achieving a high level of one often means surrendering some degree of the other. For example, the greater the similarity between the members of a study sample, the greater the extent of uniformity we will secure in features we want to control (in order to eliminate them as extraneous variables). By the same token, however, that very uniformity may make the sample less representative of the larger population from which it was initially drawn. In that case, it may not be possible to generalise the study findings to more heterogeneous samples like the ones typically seen in routine applied/service settings.

Group comparisons

Another type of research consists of cross-sectional **group comparison designs**. As used in criminological and forensic psychology, this is a type of investigation in which a sample of individuals who have a history of involvement in criminal offending is systematically compared with a sample that is equivalent in most other respects (e.g. age, gender, ethnicity and social background) but who have not been involved in offending. Designs of this kind can be used to answer questions such as: 'Do persistent offenders show different levels of impulsivity, or of moral reasoning, from a matched group of people who have not broken the law?' An example of this type of study is the work of Zamble and Quinsey (1997) on the factors that influence recidivism, or the committing of new offences by those already convicted of other crimes.

Correlational research

A fourth, related approach is the direct study of a single designated group of individuals. Psychologists are often preoccupied with the requirements of laboratory-based research methods, the use of matched comparison samples, and achieving a high level of control over extraneous variables. There are occasions, however, when that ideal is simply impracticable; and in some cases it may also be superfluous or redundant, as there are many questions that can be answered, and many hypotheses that can be tested, by studying the patterns of action, or of the relationships between variables, *within* a population.

This type of **correlational research** can answer questions such as: 'Amongst offenders who are also involved in substance misuse, are there different patterns in which this occurs, and if so what are the factors associated with them?' Examples of research adopting this format include the work of Bennett and Holloway (2007) on the relation of substance misuse to crime, to be described in Chapter 10.

Qualitative research

A fifth type of research employs *qualitative methods* rather than quantitative ones. Interviewing individuals who have broken the law, and even writing biographies of such individuals, has been a feature of criminological research for many decades (Bernard, Snipes and Gerould, 2015). In-depth interviewing can elicit information that is often far richer than that contained in any official records, and that can facilitate a fuller understanding of individuals' perceptions and their motives for action. Examples of this variety of research include the work of Willott and Griffin (1999) on reasons for continuing in offending, or of Maruna (2001) on reasons for moving away from it.

While this does not constitute formal research as such, there can also be illuminating material in a quite different source. Some individuals, who had achieved notoriety in the early phases of their lives for the crimes they committed, have later gone on to write autobiographies that may throw light on their histories and motivations in a way no researcher can (Boyle, 1977; McVicar, 2004; and see Morgan, 1999). The narrative, life-history approach to development has received increasing attention from psychologists in recent years (McAdams, 2009).

Treatment-outcome research

There is one more type of research that can be useful for testing ideas from the preceding ones. When we have identified a variable that appears to be associated with repeated involvement in offending behaviour, and if that variable is one that can be changed (such as increasing individuals' levels of self-control, or reducing their substance misuse) and we also find that altering the variable results in lowering reoffence rates, that outcome adds to our confidence that the variable concerned probably *is* a contributory factor in criminal activity. Thus, *treatment-outcome evaluations* of intervention or rehabilitation services, as well as being useful studies in themselves, also give leverage for hypothesis testing and theory construction in this area. An example of this kind of research is a review of outcome studies on the general self-control theory of crime, reported by Piquero, Jennings and Farrington (2010).

When the possibility exists of allocating participants to experimental and control samples on a random basis, a type of design known as a **randomised controlled trial** (RCT) may be carried out. RCTs are generally considered to be the most powerful designs for hypothesis-testing purposes in outcome research. Conducting such evaluations in criminal justice services, however, is not always practicable, and group membership is more often decided on some other basis; research designs are then described as **quasi-experimental designs**. (We will encounter research of both these kinds in Chapter 19.)

By combining results from these studies with other types of data described earlier, such as large-scale official crime statistics, or detailed forensic analysis of individual cases, it has proved possible to identify some of the most important variables associated with pathways into and out of crime. Doing so may focus on several key time-points. The first is the likelihood of initial involvement in offending, the *initial participatory decision*. A second, for that proportion of offenders who continue their involvement over a period of several years or in some cases longer, is the question of what accounts for its *maintenance*. A third is focused on the factors that influence *desistance* from crime, whereby individuals reduce its frequency or its dominance in their lives. This may be entirely the result of their own decisions; it may be in response to other changes in their lives or in their environments; or it may be influenced by deliberate efforts in that direction on the part of personnel within the criminal justice system.

Research synthesis: evidence review and meta-analysis

The various kinds of research just described – in which individuals are interviewed or administered questionnaires, or file data are collected concerning them, or in which they take part in laboratory experiments – are collectively known as **primary studies** or **primary research**. We can think of them as the 'basic stuff' of research investigation on which knowledge accumulation depends. As is widely known, however, the sheer volume of such research is now so great in many areas that it can be difficult to make sense of it. What we earlier called the 'data explosion' in the sciences also affects psychology and allied areas. It is vital to attempt to keep abreast of the expanding knowledge base in any field by taking stock of what has been found to date.

Hence there is another type of study, which we will encounter frequently through this book: the **systematic review**. In this kind of study, following a standard set of procedures a researcher attempts to synthesise the primary studies on a given topic, which were designed to address a selected question, in order to evaluate the *overall trends* in the results. Nowadays this task is usually undertaken using a collection of techniques communally known as **meta-analysis**. For the most part, meta-analysis is used in two main contexts. One is to integrate the findings from an assembly of cross-sectional experimental or longitudinal studies, to discover the extent to which predicted relationships between variables hold. For example, are variables such as age at first offence, consistency of parental discipline, educational level, or scores on an attitude scale or anger inventory correlated with total numbers of convictions, or with rates of disciplinary infractions while in prison? Numerous studies have been conducted to test these and other relationships, and meta-analysis can help us discern the size and consistency of any correlations that emerge, and the extent to which any correlations are influenced by other moderators. The other principal usage of meta-analysis is to collate findings from treatment-outcome evaluations, and if possible to identify which methods (and in which settings, with which groups) work best to help reduce reoffending or to engender other types of behavioural change. We will discuss the latter issues more fully in Chapter 19.

The meta-analytic approach was first used by the eminent statistician Karl Pearson, who in 1904 brought together results from several studies of the effect of inoculations on the prevalence of fevers. Discovering that the sample size in each study was too small to allow clear conclusions to be drawn, he combined data from all of the studies into a summative analysis. However, meta-analysis did not come into prominence in the social sciences until the late 1970s, when it was used to synthesise data from a large number of studies, for example on the relationship between class size and academic achievement in school (Glass, McGaw and Smith, 1981), and on the outcomes of psychological therapy for mental health problems (Smith, Glass and Miller, 1980). Since then it has been extensively used in research in many fields, including several areas of applied psychology (Lipsey and Wilson, 1993). The next 'Focus on ...' box provides information on meta-analysis and on the principal methods of reporting effect sizes.

FOCUS ON ...

Meta-analysis and effect size

Meta-analysis or *statistical review* is a form of research literature synthesis in which an attempt is made to integrate the findings of different studies numerically in order to detect trends and to examine relationships that may be difficult to discern given the complexity likely to be found in many datasets. Meta-analysis is so called to distinguish it from **primary analysis** (the original statistical treatment of results in a given primary study) and **secondary analysis** (any re-analysis of existing data carried out to check for errors or to answer questions not posed in the initial study). It has virtually replaced the traditional form of *narrative review*, although the latter is still preferable where the number of available studies is small or where studies are so diverse as to be unsuitable for statistical review.

The key output from meta-analysis of outcome literature is a statistic known as the mean **effect size** (ES), which is the mean of the individual effect sizes obtained from separate primary studies. There are reportedly more than 70 different statistics for computing effect sizes, but for simplicity they are sometimes divided into two main 'families' (Ellis, 2010). One family includes methods of comparing groups, either by examining the extent of the differences between their means, or by comparing the differences of two probabilities (e.g. success versus failure) within each group. The other family involves measuring the extent of association between an independent variable and that of a measured effect, using some form of correlation coefficient.

In reviews of research in psychology and criminal justice, generally three types of effect size statistics are employed (Lipsey and Wilson, 2001; Wilson, 2001):

- The **standardised mean difference** (known in slightly differing forms by various names, including Cohen's (*d*) and Hedges's (*g*). This difference is probably the most easily interpreted way of grasping what a meta-analysis has found. This is most often employed in treatment-outcome studies, where it compares changes in the respective means of experimental and control samples from pre-test to post-test. It allows a conclusion to be drawn such as: 'The reconviction rate of the experimental group was 15 per cent lower than that of the controls.'
- The **odds ratio** expresses the chances of one of two outcomes (such as whether or not a person has been reconvicted) for the two study groups (experimental and comparison) relative to one another. This too is intuitively appealing, as it conveys a sense of the extent to which one group outperformed the other – or not, as the case may be – and the extent to which membership of a particular group increased the chances, or odds, of a successful outcome.

- The *correlation coefficient*. There are several forms of this coefficient, the most widely used being Pearson's (r) used to compute a correlation between two continuous variables, such as scores on an attitude measure or risk assessment scale and the rate of subsequent offending (in a cross-sectional or longitudinal study), or between hours of treatment participation and subsequent rates of recidivism (in an outcome study). If the variables are *dichotomous* – assigned to two categories, such as offending versus no offending, or improvement versus no improvement – another version of this statistic, called the *phi* coefficient (Φ), is used instead. In treatment-outcome studies, correlation coefficients will be *positive* if the experimental group has done better than the controls (in other words, has lower recidivism); *negative* if the reverse is found; and *close to zero* if there is no meaningful effect ('nothing works').

When reading a meta-analysis, in addition to the mean ES it is also vital to examine the *heterogeneity* amongst the effects obtained across the individual studies reviewed. This is usually denoted by the statistics Q or I^2. If they show that heterogeneity is very large, the mean ES becomes more difficult to interpret. For example, an apparently positive overall relationship or treatment effect may be misleading if considered in isolation, just as taking the mean of any distribution but ignoring its variance could give an erroneous impression.

Questions

Apply these ideas or something similar to your research.

1. How would you decide which type of effect size statistics to apply to your research?
2. What are the limitations of each type of method?

Reference

- Partially adapted from McGuire, J., *Understanding psychology and crime: Perspectives on theory and action,* © 2004. Reproduced with the kind permission of Open International Publishing Ltd. All rights reserved.

Since in many primary studies researchers set out to test more than one hypothesis, or to report the results of several analyses (e.g. the relationships between different independent and dependent variables), meta-analysis usually generates more 'effect-size tests' than the number of original studies. It is generally accepted practice to report these under different categories of outcome, and also to attempt to take into account the impact of methodological and of moderator variables. We will refer to systematic reviews and meta-analyses at numerous points throughout this book.

Key features and correlates of crime

On the basis of all these types of research, psychologists and others have learned a considerable amount about the development of delinquency and its continuation into adult criminality; about pathways towards or away from involvement in crime; and about the factors that influence either persistence in it or desistance from it. Despite what are probably inescapable differences of detail, broadly similar results have emerged from different data sources and from different methodological approaches, though some points continue to be disputed. The following are several of the key findings that emerge with the greatest degree of consistency.

Associated factors

Gender

The majority of those who become involved in offending, those who persist in it, those who are convicted by courts, and those who are imprisoned are males. While the precise gender ratio varies across time and place, a figure in the region of 5:1 (male to female) is not unusual. There is evidence that the gender difference is less marked in self-report surveys than for recorded crimes (Mosher, Miethe and Hart, 2011). Given that the majority of those who administer the justice and penal systems are also male (from police officers and lawyers, to judges, prison wardens and law-makers), feminist criminologists see all of these features as interconnected, and as products of the system of patriarchy, a system that they therefore believe requires critical investigation as a social and psychological phenomenon (Chesney-Lind and Pasko, 2004; Daly and Chesney-Lind, 1988).

Age

In Western societies where this has been studied in some depth, the age of onset of participation in crime is on average approximately 12 years. Participation in crime peaks in the age range 15 to 19 and reduces thereafter, with desistance occurring in the majority of cases between the ages of 20 and 29. This combined set of trends is known as the **age–crime curve**, and is depicted schematically in the left-hand graph in Figure 3.1. By and large, the earlier an individual embarks on offending, the more likely it is that he or she will persist in it over a longer period. There are two points to note, however. One is that the shape of the curve may vary depending on whether police data or self-report data are used (Loeber, Farrington and Jolliffe, 2008). Another is that it is not chronological age *per se* that brings about these changes, but other factors that are correlated with it, such as biological maturity, cognitive and social development, and life events such as leaving school, associated with onset, or commencing a stable relationship, associated with desistance (Graham and Bowling, 1995).

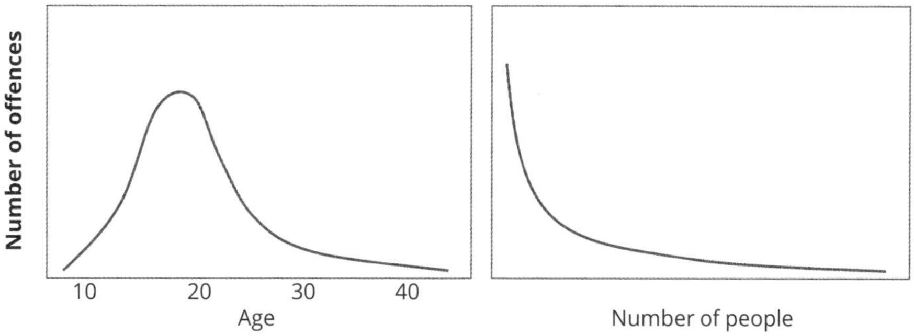
Number of offences
10
20
30
40
Age
Number of people

Figure 3.1
Some basic features of the distribution of crimes. In both cases, the vertical (*y*) axis represents numbers of offences. Left: The age–crime curve shows the likelihood of participation in crime at different ages. Right: The reverse-J curve depicts the relationship between numbers of crimes and numbers of people. Note that these are very approximate, generalised representations.

Source: adapted from McGuire, J., Understanding psychology and crime: Perspectives on theory and action, © 2004. Reproduced with the kind permission of Open International Publishing Ltd. All rights reserved.

Socioeconomic status (SES)

There has been a long-running debate over the significance and influence of social background characteristics, such as income, educational level and neighbourhood of origin, as factors contributing to risk of involvement in crime. These variables are often collectively referred to as social class, but an agreed definition of that concept has proved elusive.

Here as elsewhere it has been difficult to clarify the position because of discrepancies between police-recorded and self-reported crime rates. While the former suggests that socioeconomic status (SES) is a major determinant of criminality, the latter shows that offending occurs amongst all social groups. Dunaway, Cullen, Burton and Evans (2000) analysed the literature in this area and, noting that a majority of self-report studies are based on interviews with high-school samples, reviewed the smaller number of studies with adults. They conducted a survey of 555 adults (median age 41), who were asked to report whether or not they had committed any of a series of 50 specific offences in the past year, and since the age of 18. They found the relationship between social class (measured in a number of ways) and crime to be very insubstantial. There is, however, a recurrent finding of an association between social status and officially recorded crime (Ellis *et al.*, 2009).

Ethnicity

It has repeatedly been found that members of minority ethnic groups are over-represented amongst those who are processed by criminal justice systems (Ellis *et al.*, 2009). In the USA, for example, while African-Americans constitute only 12 per cent of the population, they are involved in 40 per cent of arrests for violent crime and 30 per cent of arrests for property crime (Siegel, 2012). In some US cities very large proportions of the African-American male population are either imprisoned or under probation supervision (Miller, 1997). Patterns not dissimilar to this can be found in many countries.

Almost certainly, several factors contribute to this. Given that self-reported rates of *offending* are similar across ethnic groups, there is some evidence of bias in the operation of the law – bias has been found both in police patrol and arrest patterns, and in the treatment of defendants in court (e.g. a lower likelihood of bail, and more severe penalties for minority group members). These factors may be superimposed on pre-existing disadvantages and hardships that result from underlying structural biases within societies (such as higher rates of unemployment, lower incomes, poorer housing, and other problems amongst minority communities), which may create conditions for crime.

Types of offending

Relatively few of those who repeatedly offend 'specialise' in a particular type of crime. Most commit several types of offence, a pattern sometimes called *generalist* or *versatile*; and the occurrence of different types of crimes tend to be correlated (Ellis *et al.*, 2009). These trends have led some theoreticians to suggest that there may be underlying psychological attributes, such as low self-control or an antisocial personality, which account for difficulties in impulse management or in rule-following across a range of situations, and which may be common to many types of crime. We will review these possibilities in Chapters 4 and 5.

Concentration

The same findings also lend support to the view that those who offend chronically (i.e. with high frequency, or with a crime career of extended duration) may be a psychologically distinct group. Numerous studies have confirmed the pattern wherein a small segment of the known offending population, which therefore comprises only a small minority of the population as a whole, is responsible for committing a disproportionately large number of crimes. This aspect of crime is depicted in the right-hand reverse-J graph in Figure 3.1. However, the membership of that group may change over time, and different factors influence the likelihood of participation in offending at different age ranges.

In large-scale **birth cohort studies**, where children born in a selected year are tracked across a sizeable segment of the lifespan, it has consistently been found that a small proportion of the cohort accounts for a large proportion of the recorded crimes. This was found, for example, in studies in Philadelphia, where 6 per cent of the sample accounted for 63 per cent of recorded crimes (Tracy, Wolfgang and Figlio, 1985); and in Copenhagen, where males with convictions for two or more violent offences formed only 0.6 per cent of the sample but accounted for 43 per cent of the violent assaults (Janson, 1983). An even more striking concentration was found in the Pittsburgh Youth Study, with a sample of 1,009 young males followed up between the ages of 7 and 25. Researchers found that just four families, with a total of 33 members, together forming 1 per cent of their research sample, accounted for 18 per cent of all convictions; while just 12 per cent of the sample contained almost half (44 per cent) of all offenders (Farrington *et al.*, 2001; Loeber, Farrington, Stouthamer-Loeber and White, 2008a). The uneven distribution of offence rates amongst repeat offenders mentioned earlier, with a small proportion offending at a far higher rate than the remainder, conforms to this broader pattern found in the community as a whole and could be considered as forming one end of the scale.

Pathways over time

In an attempt to explain some of the latter findings, Moffitt (1993, 2003) examined patterns of delinquent involvement over time, and discerned what appeared to be two main trends in, or courses of, delinquent conduct. She proposed a 'developmental taxonomy' consisting of two identifiable 'pathways':

» *Adolescence-limited* This refers to the majority of offending, for which the peak incidence occurs in the mid-to-late teenage years but which declines in frequency thereafter. During the adolescent years the rate can be so high that participation in delinquency appears almost to be a normal part of life at that stage. Most offences committed at a younger age are committed in groups, with the proportion carried out by solo individuals expanding with increasing age (Baldwin, Bottoms and Walker, 1976). The reasons for this are thought to reside partly in the conflict between members of this age-group and adults as the adolescents strive for autonomy, a struggle which progressively sharpened in the world's more affluent nations from the early part of the 20th century onwards.

» *Life-course-persistent* This refers to problem behaviour that is typically of earlier onset, is usually more serious, and persists into adulthood. Moffitt suggested that youths manifesting this pattern might sometimes serve as temporary role models for the adolescence-limited group. Moffitt and other researchers have suggested that the behaviour of this group may be indicative of psychopathology, possibly traceable to an underlying neuropsychological difference between them and the adolescence-limited majority. Indeed, some researchers have suggested that there may be neurobiological markers for this pattern, which can be detected much earlier in life in 'callous-unemotional' personality traits, and it has also been suggested that those in turn may have a partially genetic origin (Viding, Blair, Moffitt and Plomin, 2005).

Based on her analyses, Moffitt estimated that the latter group forms approximately 5 per cent of the male population, and that it is from amongst its members that a subgroup is drawn of offenders who then become long-term 'career criminals'. It is important to note, however, that not all research has confirmed this twofold taxonomy, with some studies finding three, four and even six different 'trajectories' (Lacourse, Dupéré and Loeber, 2008). Moreover, the dynamics of life events and situational influences also lead to **discontinuities** – that is, individuals do not always stay on the same pathway, or on the one we might predict on the basis of earlier indicators.

Even so, a model of this kind can help to explain the observed overall pattern whereby, as criminological surveys recurrently show, a majority of people break the law in some way at some stage of their lives, most likely in the teenage years, and then desist, whereas a smaller group of offenders commit a high proportion of the total volume of offences, and some of this group go on offending into the fourth decade of their lives. What are the features that characterise the latter group? Some of the strongest correlates of crime are to be found amongst psychological variables (Andrews and Bonta, 2010; Ellis, Beaver and Wright, 2009).

From correlation to temporal sequencing: longitudinal research

The most compelling evidence of how different factors contribute to the onset of delinquent behaviour comes from longitudinal studies of development that have addressed the problem of the emergence of crime. These have been carried out in a number of countries, including the United States (where the majority have been conducted), the United Kingdom, the Netherlands, Denmark, Sweden, Finland, Canada and New Zealand. In total, over the past half century more than 25 such studies have been reported (McGuire, 2004a; Thornberry and Krohn, 2003). Table 3.1 on the next page lists several key projects of this kind.

Some of the studies have entailed collection of data on an entire birth cohort (that is, all the children born in a selected city in a given year): for example, in Stockholm, the 15,117 new arrivals born in 1953 (Bäckman and Nilsson, 2011; Kratzer and Hodgins, 1997); or in Philadelphia, a sample of 27,160 born in 1958 (Tracy, Wolfgang and Figlio, 1985). Not surprisingly, the larger the sample, in general the less detailed will be the information obtained. Thus several of the most frequently cited birth cohort studies involving intensive data collection have sample sizes in the range 400–1,500. As we saw in the case of the Cambridge Study in Delinquent Development, some researchers have followed their target samples for periods of up to 40 years. Such projects usually have multiple objectives, incorporating

Study	Sample size(s)	Age ranges followed	Sources
Cambridge Study in Delinquent Development (UK)	411	8/9 → 40	Farrington (2006)
Stockholm Project Metropolitan (Sweden)	15,117	0 → 30	Wikström (1990)
Copenhagen Birth Cohort (Denmark)	28,879	0 → 30	Guttridge, Gabrielli, Mednick and Van Dusen (1983)
Finnish Longitudinal Study (Finland)	369	8/9 → 26	Hämäläinen and Pulkkinen (1995)
Montreal Longitudinal and Experimental Study (Canada)	1,161	6 → 22	Tremblay *et al.* (2003)
Dunedin Multidisciplinary Health and Development Study (NZ)	1,661	0 → 21	Moffitt, Caspi, Rutter and Silva (2001)
Christchurch Child Development Study (NZ)	1,265	0 → 18	Fergusson, Horwood and Nagin (2000)
Philadelphia Birth Cohorts (USA) (1945) (1958)	 9,945 27,160	 0 → 30 0 → 18	Tracy *et al.* (1985)
National Youth Survey Family Study (USA)	1,725		Elliott, Huizinga and Morse (1986)
Kauai Longitudinal Study (Hawaii, USA)	698	0 → 32	Werner (1989)
Nashville-Knoxville-Bloomington Study (USA)	585	4 → 7	Dodge, Pettit and Bates. (1994)
Denver Youth Survey (USA)	1,527	7 → 18 9 → 20 11 → 22 13 → 24 15 → 26	Huizinga, Weiher, Espiritu and Esbensen (2003)
Rochester Youth Development Study (USA)	1,000	13 → 22	Thornberry *et al.* (2003)
Seattle Social Development Survey (USA)	808	10 → 24	Hawkins *et al.* (2003)
Pittsburgh Youth Study (USA)	503 508 506	5 → 14 8 → 17 12 → 19	Loeber, Farrington, Stouthamer-Loeber and White (2008a)

Table 3.1 Key longitudinal studies on delinquent development. These studies, which are some of the most frequently cited, incorporate delinquency and crime as dependent variables.

Source: adapted from McGuire, J., Understanding psychology and crime: Perspectives on theory and action, © 2004. Reproduced with the kind permission of Open International Publishing Ltd. All rights reserved.

investigation of a wide range of areas, which might include child health, family functioning, education, employment, income, or lifestyle variables, as well as criminal history indicators such as self-reported offending, arrest, conviction, or imprisonment.

Most longitudinal studies draw on multiple sources of information. Information is likely to be obtained not only from participants themselves, but also from their parents, siblings, peers, teachers or other professionals, spouses, and, as time progresses, even their own children. In the National Youth Survey mentioned in Chapter 2, for example, interviews were also conducted with one of the young person's parents. Various methods of data collection have been used, including face-to-face or telephone interviews; access to school, health, or criminal records; psychometric assessments; and third-party observational reports. The main strength of these types of study is the possibility they open up for obtaining a picture of the *temporal sequence of cause and effect*. Thus they enable researchers to move beyond correlational analysis and to test hypotheses about possible causal relationships.

Like other kinds of research, cohort studies vary in their quality. The best are those in which data are collected *prospectively* (i.e. where a group is selected and data-gathering is planned from the outset, rather than data being collected retrospectively from files), and where the drop-out or *attrition rate* is low (as many as possible of the people who signed up at the beginning are still contactable at later stages). Perhaps their main limitation is that such studies have mostly been conducted in fairly wealthy, technologically advanced societies, although many participants come from poor neighbourhoods and from minority communities within those societies. In the longer run it will be valuable if other, similar studies can be conducted in economically more deprived, low- and middle-income nations.

Risk and protective factors

There is a consensus amongst researchers that certain variables have been fairly well established as being regularly associated with participation in offending (Bonta and Andrews, 2017; Farrington, 2007). For the most part, these factors are also correlated, though only quite weakly, with social deprivation. Such variables are called risk factors (sometimes also known as risk–need factors), and there are several that emerge with fairly high consistency from different kinds of research. They include the following:

» *Poor parental supervision* When developing children are neglected, or subject to inadequate or inconsistent parental care, this can result in low attachment to families. In part this may have the simple outcome that children are not controlled or protected and are therefore free to do as they like. But alongside this, and at a deeper level, it may also disrupt the emotional bonds that connect children to their parents, or even stop such bonds from forming.

» *Difficulties in school and employment* This might show in terms of lower levels of academic achievement, an intermittent work record, or prolonged unemployment even in economic circumstances where jobs are readily available. Success in 'meritocratic' societies is heavily dependent on satisfactory performance in these areas, and those who persistently offend are often those who do less well in this respect, and who may have a high rate of problems in basic literacy and numeracy.

» *Enmeshment in a network of 'delinquent associates'* The larger the number of peers who become involved in offending, the likelier it is that any individual will be. This is a result of what has been called *differential association*, a principle enunciated in the theorising of Sutherland (1940), whose theory we will encounter in Chapter 4, who considered this to be a key factor that led to participation in crime amongst all strata of the social 'hierarchy'.

» *Distorted or biased patterns of information-processing* Some individuals may be more likely to perceive others as having malign intent, be hypersensitive to indications of threat, focus on a narrow band of signals in an interpersonal situation, and process a limited range of options in deciding how to respond.

» *Poor personal and social interaction skills* Individuals may find it difficult to solve everyday problems, especially ones that involve relationships with others; have a limited range or level of **interpersonal skills**; have a limited ability to recognise and respond to the communications of others; have difficulties in identifying or expressing their own feelings and ideas; and have difficulties in anticipating the likely effects of their actions on themselves and others.

» *Low levels of self-control, or a tendency to act on impulses* Some individuals have difficulties in dealing with negative emotions (such as anger, anxiety, or depression), experience motor and cognitive restlessness, and have low levels of self-restraint, perhaps coupled with a sense of urgency and a felt need for action as opposed to considered reflection. Low control and impulsiveness are viewed by Gottfredson and Hirschi (1990) as the central and pivotal variable that influences involvement in crime.

» *Manifestation of antisocial attitudes or antisocial personality* Individuals may feel detached from, or hostile to, other people or systems of social rules, and be willing and ready to disregard them. They may have an unemotional or uncaring approach to personal relationships, including a preparedness to use other people for their own purposes; and in extreme cases a callous and calculating outlook, with a tendency to view people as a means to an end rather than as ends in themselves.

» *Substance misuse* This may be both a problem in itself and a factor that contributes to the added likelihood of involvement in offending. Where substance use and dependence becomes severe or chronic, it is often associated with many of the other factors above. Thus in some respects it is considered an *outcome* of many of the same risk factors as involvement in crime; while from the perspective of explaining criminality, it is itself viewed as a risk factor.

Each of the factors in the list above has both an independent and an interactive influence on the emergence of a pattern of offending. The more risk factors that are present, the higher the probability of offence participation. Some illustrations are shown in the 'Focus on ...' box below.

FOCUS ON ...

Problems, risk factors and likelihood of offending

There is an association between the number of problems that individuals experience in their lives and their likelihood of participating in illegal activity. Illustrations of this from two different studies, from separate locations and using different methodologies, are shown here. The graphs below show the relationship between the number of adverse factors or 'problems' (horizontal axis) and the rate of offending in the preceding 12 months amongst respondents in the Youth Lifestyles Survey, a self-report study, for parallel samples of boys and adult males (Flood-Page, Campbell, Harrington and Miller, 2000).

The table on the next page shows percentages from four subgroups of males identified in the Denver Youth Survey, a longitudinal study, who have different numbers

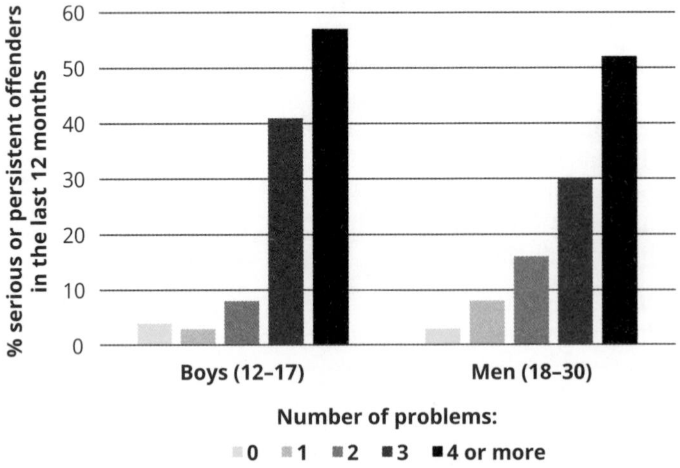
% serious or persistent offenders in the last 12 months
60
50
40
30
20
10
0
Boys (12–17)
Men (18–30)
Number of problems:
0 1 2 3 4 or more

Source: adapted from Flood-Page et al. (2000). © Crown copyright 2000. Contains public sector information licensed under the Open Government Licence v3.0: http://www.nationalarchives.gov.uk/doc/open-government-licence/version/3

3

Number of problems	Serious violent offender	Serious non-violent offender	Minor offender	Non-offender
None	2%	5%	10%	83%
One	9%	10%	24%	57%
Two	16%	19%	30%	36%
Three	32%	21%	27%	20%
Four	54%	31%	10%	5%

Source: Table 6. From Huizinga, D., Weiher, A. W., Espiritu, R. and Esbensen, F. (2003). Delinquency and Crime: Some Highlights from the Denver Youth Survey. In T. P. Thornberry and M. D. Krohn (eds) Taking Stock of Delinquency: An Overview of Findings from Contemporary Longitudinal Studies. p. 62. New York: Kluwer Academic Publishers.

of problems or risk factors (Huizinga *et al.*, 2003). The latter include difficulties in school, substance abuse, victimisation, and mental health problems. Thus amongst those facing one problem only, 19 per cent are in the two 'serious offender' subgroups (columns 2 and 3); whereas amongst those beset with four problems, 85 per cent are in these two groups. Similar patterns were reported for females, but were not presented in tabular form. (Note that percentages sum across each row in the table; except the centre row (Two problems) where there was an error in the original.)

Questions

1 Does being faced with 'adverse factors' or 'problems' in life explain someone's involvement in crime?

2 Are 'adverse factors' or 'problems' sometimes used to justify crimes?

Researchers have also discovered that the impact of some of these influences can be lessened or mitigated by the action of other variables: variables that have been called **protective factors**, sometimes resilience factors, or simply strengths. Examples might include doing well at school, or having one 'significant other' person who is a supportive attachment figure or a positive role model. Such influences can act as a buffer against the tendency of risk factors to lead into offending. Loeber, Farrington, Stouthamer-Loeber and White (2008b) have formulated more detailed definitions of the distinct categories of risk and protective factors, as shown in Table 3.2.

Type of factor	Definition	Example
Risk factor	Factor that predicts a raised likelihood of offending (in the general population or amongst offenders)	Having committed acts of violence, whether or not recorded as crimes
Aggravating risk factor	Factor that predicts a raised likelihood of later offending (in the general population)	First court appearance at an early age
Hindering risk factor	Factor that predicts a low likelihood of desistance from offending (amongst offenders)	Having no accommodation on release from custody
Protective factor	Factor that predicts a lower probability of offending (amongst youth exposed to risk factors)	Having a good relationship with a supportive adult or mentor

continued on p. 56

Type of factor	Definition	Example
Promotive factor	Factor that predicts a low probability of serious offending (in the general population or amongst offenders)	A stable intimate relationship
Preventive promotive factor	Factor that predicts a low probability of offending (in the general population)	Success in school and work
Remedial promotive factor	Factor that predicts likely cessation of offending (amongst offenders)	Participation in effective intervention programmes; investing in a close relationship

Table 3.2 Definitions of risk and protective factors.

Source: copyright © 2008. Adapted from Table 1.1 Definitions of Terms. From Loeber, R., Farrington, D. P., Stouthamer-Loeber, M. and Raskin White, H. (2008). Introduction and Key Questions. In Loeber, R., Farrington, D. P., Stouthamer-Loeber, M. and Raskin White, H. (eds), Violence and Serious Theft: Development and Prediction from Childhood to Adulthood. p. 9. New York, NY: Routledge. Reproduced by permission of Taylor & Francis Group, LLC, a division of Informa plc.

Conclusion

We suggested earlier that the advent of risk factor research and the identification of consistent correlates and predictors of offending behaviour have together represented a major advance in criminological and forensic psychology over approximately the last twenty years. However, some researchers have expressed dissatisfaction with, and criticism of, the limitations of this approach, suggesting that the study of antisocial behaviour has been 'stuck' at that stage, to the detriment of a fuller understanding of the problem (Moffitt and Caspi, 2007). In order to achieve a fuller understanding, it is argued, we need to be able to 'document causality' (p. 97).

Of course, when we come to consider causal explanations in this area, we have to bear in mind that complex behaviour such as committing a criminal offence is almost certainly **multifactorial** in origin. That is, such behaviour has numerous possible causes, and these overlap and interact with each other in various ways. Some emerge as more closely or directly associated with offending, while some act indirectly, influencing other factors rather than offending itself. Furthermore, the relationship in each case is a **probabilistic** one. That is, there are no connections between one variable and another that we can regard as being completely determined, or guaranteed to operate 100 per cent of the time. Instead, we can say that as certain factors change, the *likelihood* of involvement in offending increases (or decreases, depending on the variable selected). This creates the useful possibility of predicting its occurrence, always accepting that such predictions are unlikely to be precise, since we know that for the most part they fall some way short of this. Even so, they may be dependable enough to provide a basis for informing some kinds of legal decisions, and to supply a background for practical applications in forensic psychology.

When we have developed a proposal, or preferably a well-reasoned and soundly based account, concerning cause–effect relationships for a given phenomenon, we have what could be considered an *explanation* of that phenomenon. As explanations in science are considered to be provisional, we tend instead to call such a conceptual framework a theory. But theories are far more than abstract, academic exercises; they have inestimable value in practice as well. To quote Kurt Lewin (1951, p. 169), 'there is nothing more practical than a good theory'. It is to theoretical accounts of criminal conduct that we turn in Chapter 4.

Chapter summary

- Criminologists, psychologists and other researchers have used a wide range of methods in the study of crime. These methods include longitudinal projects, controlled experiments, quasi-experimental designs, cross-sectional group comparisons, qualitative studies, and methods of research review or synthesis.
- There are some well-established patterns within reported crime, with respect to the demographic characteristics of those involved, the *age-crime curve*, and other features. These emerge at the general level, however, and over time individuals may follow different patterns or pathways.
- By combining the findings of longitudinal research with other types of information, researchers have been able to build up a picture of the development of offending behaviour. Currently, a favoured approach to understanding this is by applying the concept of *risk factors* for involvement in crime, and that of *protective factors* which reduce the likelihood of such involvement. Drawing together findings from several sources, the chapter has reviewed evidence concerning the most prominent risk and protective factors.

3

Further reading

- Anyone seeking a book on research methods will find a wide variety available, from introductory texts to very specialised texts. To date, the most suitable one amongst them for informing forensic practice is the volume edited by Kerry Sheldon, Jason Davies and Kevin Howells (2011), *Research in Practice for Forensic Professionals* (London and New York: Routledge).
- Lee Ellis, Kevin M. Beaver and John Wright, in their *Handbook of Crime Correlates* (2009; Amsterdam: Academic Press), have assembled the results of a massive undertaking. Their book puts together a series of tables on correlates of crime, organised in sections by major category, followed by a summary of the principal findings. (This chapter has drawn extensively on their work.)
- On systematic review, see Angela Boland, Gemma Cherry and Rumona Dickson (2017), *Doing a Systematic Review: A Student's Guide* (London: Sage): particularly recommended for students undertaking reviews as part of research dissertations.
- On research review, *Introduction to Meta-analysis* by Michael Borenstein, Larry V. Hedges, Julian P. T. Higgins and Hannah R. Rothstein (2009; New York: Wiley) is a valuable 'how to' guide. For a fuller treatment of statistical issues, see Harris M. Cooper, Larry V. Hedges and Jeffrey C. Valentine (2009), *The Handbook of Research Synthesis and Meta-analysis*, 2nd edition (New York: Russell Sage Foundation).
- For more detail on longitudinal studies, the books by Terence P. Thornberry and Marvin D. Krohn (2003), *Taking Stock of Delinquency: An Overview of Findings from Contemporary Longitudinal Studies* (New York: Kluver Academic/Plenum Publishers), and by Rolf Loeber, David P. Farrington, Magda Stouthamer-Loeber and Helene R. White (2008a), *Violence and Serious Theft: Development and Prediction from Childhood to Adulthood* (New York: Routledge) are richly detailed, analytical and thorough accounts of some of the best-known studies, their findings and implications. For extensive information on the developmental approach in criminology, see Chris L. Gibson and Marvin D. Krohn (eds., 2013), *Handbook of Life-Course Criminology: Emerging Trends and Directions for Future Research*. New York: Springer

Explaining Crime: Theories and Perspectives

This chapter will introduce and survey the principal theories of crime, and discuss the interface between psychology and criminology. It will also provide an integrative overview of criminological theory, expanding upon the role that psychological factors are thought to play in the occurrence of criminal acts. We will move on, therefore, from discussing the 'what' and 'how' of crime to considering the 'why'.

Chapter objectives

- To survey theories of the causes of crime, ranging from large-scale, sociologically based explanations to individual, psychologically focused models.
- To explain historical connections between current approaches to the explanation of crime and ideas developed at earlier stages.
- To develop an integrative theory of crime, explaining the roles of psychological factors in conjunction with other types of variables.

In Chapter 2, we reviewed some of the challenges that arise in trying to define 'crime'. For practical purposes, however, we found that we needed to work within the conventional definition of criminal acts, mainly because that is the basis on which the criminal justice system operates. In Chapter 3, we reviewed evidence on the correlates of crime, and variables that can be identified as closely associated with it, some of which are regarded as 'risk factors' for criminal involvement. In this chapter, we will look more closely into debates on the 'causes of crime' and consider some important questions. Do structural factors such as unemployment, poverty or inequality play a part in criminal acts? Do rates of crime vary from one place to another, and if so what could be the reasons for that? What, if any, is the role of genetic factors in crime? Does crime run in families, and if so is that a result of inheritance or of some aspect of parenting? Are there criminal personalities? Do individuals make deliberate, calculated decisions to commit offences, or are offences the result of instant, spur-of-the-moment decisions that go badly wrong; or some mixture of the two?

The medieval era in Europe was a dangerous one in which to live. Apart from the low life expectancy, due to poor nutrition and disease, there is evidence that the level of violent crime was considerably higher than it is today. Historical research shows that in most European countries the rate of homicide has fallen steadily from the 13th century to the present. Drawing on the History of Homicide Database – a collection of 390 estimates of pre-modern homicide rates derived from court registers and other source documents – Eisner (2003) has calculated that in the 13th and 14th centuries the average annual rate of homicide was approximately 32 per 100,000. It rose to an estimated 41 per 100,000 in the 15th century, but then gradually declined to 1.4 per 100,000 in the 20th. These findings are shown in Figure 4.1. For comparative purposes, the murder rate in Dodge City, Kansas, in 1878, amidst the days of the 'Wild West', was estimated to be 160 per 100,000 (Miethe and Regoeczi, 2004).

Of course, at those points in history there were no accident and emergency facilities to which victims could be rushed for medical care that might save their lives. But this is not sufficient to explain the trend observable in these data. The high death rate following medieval assault does not seem to have been a result of citizens' inability to make 999 (or

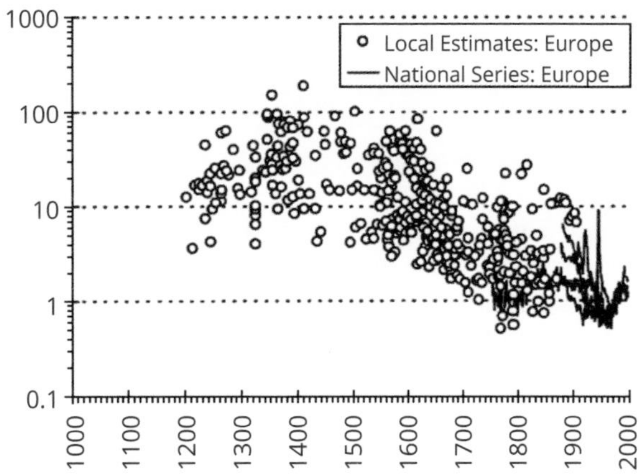

Local Estimates: Europe
National Series: Europe
1000
100
10
1
0.1
1000
1100
1200
1300
1400
1500
1600
1700
1800
1900
2000

Figure 4.1
Homicide in Europe from the medieval to the modern era. The vertical (*y*) axis denotes the rate per 100,000 population. Using a logarithmic scale, the figure plots the 390 estimates from the History of Homicide Database and four national series of statistics.

Source: Eisner, M. (2003). Long-Term Historical Trends in Violent Crime. Crime and Justice, 30, 83–142. Journal series editor: M. Tonry; Publisher: University of Chicago Press.

911) calls. A large proportion of victims died within two hours and, given the likely severity of injury, would probably not have survived even today (Eisner, 2003).

How would a citizen of that era have understood the occurrence of homicides and other violent assaults? Historians tell us that throughout the Middle Ages much human action, and certainly its moral dimension, was conceptualised in terms of supernatural forces, just as it might be in many indigenous societies today (Boyer, 2002). A Promethean struggle between good and evil was thought to pervade the universe, and when a person committed a crime, it was believed to be an effect of the Devil's power (Hanawalt and Wallace, 1998). Premeditated murders were apparently rare, the majority of homicides arising from quarrels. For example, two that occurred in London in 1276 were recorded as resulting from a dispute following a game of chess (Eisner, 2003).

It was not until the late 18th century, following the impact of the European Enlightenment and the emergence of the school of rationalist philosophy, that explanations of human misfortunes and misdeeds based on *naturalism* came to the fore. This is a way of thinking about the world around us in which attempts to explain and understand it are couched in terms of natural phenomena, rather than in terms of entities believed to exist in a different realm, such as gods, demons, or the spirits of ancestors. First the physical, then the biological, and in due course the social sciences became demarcated from philosophy and theology, and many thinkers emancipated themselves from the view that knowledge derived from the authority of monarchs, prelates, or holy books.

The growth of what we now know as the disciplines of criminology and psychology is generally traced to the period from approximately 1800 onwards. Only after then did some fundamental ideas begin to emerge that we now take for granted. They include, for example, the view that individuals can make many decisions for themselves, or that the things they do are influenced by their environments. Equally crucial was the view that these and other phenomena can be investigated empirically and systematically.

Science and values

One of the difficulties of approaching the subject matter of crime and justice scientifically, as we saw in Chapter 2 when discussing how crime is defined, is that the issues we encounter within this field are intricately entangled with many other attitudes, expectations or beliefs that people hold on the nature of society as a whole. Most of us are aware that there are highly specialised fields of study in which the methods used and the discoveries made are very difficult to understand without advanced training. Laypersons who have not studied particle physics, molecular biology or comparative linguistics accept that these are areas about which they know little. So they are unlikely to challenge, or perhaps even to question, the pronouncements of experts in these areas. That probably still applies, despite what has been described as a recent lowering of the public's confidence in science – owing, for example, to the vociferous controversies on climate change. Still, science retains a high status in society and its benefits are all around us.

When discussion turns to crime and justice, however, the parameters change markedly. Suddenly, many people have strong opinions. A few become self-appointed experts. Or perhaps they surmise that there just cannot *be* specialised knowledge on a subject as simple as crime: it seems obvious what causes it and how to deal with it. That there could be a methodical approach to the study of crime that has generated a large amount of relevant data seems an alien and highly questionable idea. If the findings of that inquiry contradict what is widely known as 'common sense', those findings can appear particularly unpalatable and might simply be rejected.

These tendencies are so powerful that it may be that the mythical war between good and evil is still alive, at least in some people's minds. When Jim Bakker, an American television evangelist, was charged with tax avoidance, his wife testified in court to say that the Devil must have got into the Revenue Department's computer (Nettler, 1984). An adviser to President Richard Nixon, Charles Colson, who was imprisoned as one of the conspirators in the 'Watergate' scandal, ascribed crime to 'sinful human nature' and believed it could only be eradicated by religious conversion (Bernard, Snipes and Gerould, 2015).

As we saw in Chapter 2, criminological research based on large-scale surveys, self-report studies and a variety of other sources shows quite convincingly that most of us commit a crime at some point in our lives. While for the majority it will be of a fairly minor type, for a by no means negligible fraction of the population it might well consist of something more serious – something that, were each of them arrested for it, could lead to a criminal charge, prosecution, a court appearance, and a penalty. In a sense, the long-standing claim made by some criminologists (e.g. Phillipson, 1971) that 'crime is normal' is supported by a great deal of evidence. It is possibly for this reason that attempts to find differences between unselected groups of 'offenders' versus 'non-offender' comparison samples have not produced especially consistent results. Any attempt to build forensic psychology on the basis that such a difference exists is unlikely to be successful.

The evidence that has accumulated, on the other hand, shows that there are more reliable and possibly more revealing differences to be discovered between those who repeatedly or persistently break the law and those who never or hardly ever do so. The material to be covered in this chapter and the next focuses our attention on that possibility, and it also provides a basis for considering how we can approach the question of whether offending behaviour can be reduced (a question to which our attention will turn in Chapter 19). Throughout the present chapter, therefore, it will be important to bear in mind that the methods described and the results reported are drawn primarily from research with those who have shown a pattern of criminal *recidivism*, or where different levels of involvement in crime have been taken into account.

The scientific study of crime

It seems very likely that human beings have been thinking about each other, pondering each other's motives, and trying to fathom the workings of each other's minds, for 50,000 years or so, and maybe even longer. Anthropologists suggest that humanity evolved into a distinct species (*Homo sapiens*) approximately 200,000 years ago, and if we look back further we seem likely to have descended from the same 'common ancestor' as some other primates over 15,000,000 years earlier.

In terms of that timescale, we have to admit, psychology was a fairly late arrival on the scene. Historians generally trace its history as a formal discipline to experimental studies that were done in the second half of the 19th century. As we saw in Chapter 1, its foundation is often dated to 1879, when Wilhelm Wundt named a room in his department at Leipzig University the 'psychological laboratory'. Applied psychology as a recognised profession, with entry qualifications, official regulations, a national governing body in each country, a code of conduct, and other accoutrements of occupational identity, is of even more recent origin than its scientific 'parent'. But as we also saw in Chapter 1, despite its somewhat eleventh-hour appearance as a recognisable independent discipline, psychology was quite rapidly pressed into practical service, and one of the earliest areas in which that happened was in presenting evidence in court.

Discussing or researching crime involves going beyond the analysis of individual cases or the study of individual differences. To engage in the enterprise sensibly requires some acquaintance with the field of criminology. As an area of formal inquiry, this is slightly older than psychology. The initial studies that today are recognised as forming part of criminology were carried out in France in 1827, after the first publication of national crime statistics. Prior to that there had been local registers, such as parish records, but this was the first time statistics were collated on a governmental scale. For most of its existence, criminology has been considerably more influenced by the neighbouring discipline of sociology than by psychology (Andrews and Bonta, 2010). Indeed, at times, as a result of very different perspectives and methods, the relationship between criminology and psychology has been tense and strained (Hollin, 2012; McGuire, 2004a).

For example, some criminologists have questioned whether psychological research and theory can play any meaningful part in helping us to understand the behaviour society defines as crime. Psychology is often viewed as 'pathologising' individuals, and as making what are actually moral rather than scientific judgments on behaviour that society has decreed to be 'deviant', often for social control rather than for any other purposes. For many criminologists, the key variables influencing what is counted as crime are societal and structural ones, such as relative poverty and wealth, social deprivation and disadvantage, and the distribution of power. Furthermore, the way laws are made and how crime is defined are **social constructs**. For the most part, the factors that drive the process of construction tend to favour some sectors of the community over others. In some countries, having much more attention paid to social security fraud than to tax evasion, for example, may be a useful distraction for those in a position to engage in the latter, despite its greater total cost to the exchequer.

Explanations of crime

In terms of understanding crime, there have unquestionably been major advances in knowledge in recent decades. That being said, many of the pivotal ideas that are familiar today in seeking to explain why crimes occur closely resemble ideas that have been in circulation since the origins of criminology itself. It is probably not inaccurate to say that over the past two hundred years attempts to explain the behaviour we call 'crime' have revolved around some fairly durable core concepts.

Essentially, there are three dominant propositions in this respect. We can set them out in the simplest terms as follows:

» *Choice* One proposition is the idea that crime is a product of individual choice. According to this view, individuals weigh up the respective costs and benefits of different courses of action, such as committing offences versus obeying the law. They calculate what will be most advantageous to them, make a decision, and act accordingly.

» *Influences* A second proposition is that crime is a function of environmental and social influences, and of each individual's position in his or her surroundings and in the social structure. This idea is related to the pressures that act on people, and also to the opportunities that are available to them. Those in turn are shaped by larger-scale societal influences outside any single individual's control.

- *Propensity* The third proposition is that crime is a result of individual differences in criminal propensity, and that this is an underlying, and relatively enduring, characteristic. Such differences may themselves derive from two kinds of sources. First, there are *biological factors* such as genes and physiological or brain processes, or some combination of those. Second, there are *psychological factors*, such as learning, personality, attitudes, patterns of thinking, or the acquisition and exercise of skills. Of course the first factor may also influence the second, and vice versa.

These perspectives can be traced back to the views of some influential 18th-century philosophers who studied human thought in general terms, and to the period in 19th-century Europe when, as noted earlier, the social sciences began to emerge as distinct fields of inquiry. The broad ideas initially formulated then later evolved into more explicit, elaborate and detailed theories (Bernard, Snipes and Gerould, 2015). The following are some key figures from that era.

Cesare Beccaria (1738–1794) was an Italian philosopher who is regarded as the founder of the school of *Classical Criminology*. According to that viewpoint, the exercise of reason is a pre-eminent force in human affairs, enabling people to calculate the outcomes of their actions by comparing likely gains with likely losses. Where someone considers that an action, even if illegal, will probably prove advantageous, and that the chance of suffering for it is low, crime is likely to result. In his landmark volume *On Crimes and Punishments* (*Dei delitti e delle pene*), published in 1764, Beccaria proposed that there should be a direct link between crime and punishment, such that the latter would deter the former by being administered promptly and in proportion to the severity of crimes. He did not, however, see the death penalty as part of this, thinking that the state should not commit a murder on the supposed grounds of preventing one. These ideas have a close affinity to those of *utilitarianism*, an approach to moral philosophy founded by the British jurist and social reformer Jeremy Bentham (1748–1832). In many respects, the modern theory of the 'reasoning criminal', more formally known as *Rational Crime*, or sometimes **Rational Choice Theory** (see below), is descended from these ideas, as is the principle of *proportionality* in sentencing.

Adolphe Quételet (1796–1874) was a Belgian mathematician and astronomer who studied the relationship between age, gender, the distribution of wealth and poverty, and the level of crime in different regions of northern France and Belgium. He also made comparisons between geographical areas, taking into account the effects of the seasons, education, and levels of alcohol consumption. He was able to do this by analysing the French national crime statistics referred to above, and in 1831 he published an influential book, *Research on the Propensity for Crime at Different Ages*. Alongside that of others, his work is sometimes grouped as part of what is called the *Cartographic School* in criminology.

Cesare Lombroso (1835–1909), whom we met briefly in Chapter 1, was a surgeon who worked for some time in the Italian army and who in the course of his duties studied the physiognomy of a large number of soldiers. On first embarking upon this work he believed that there was an important association between body typology and propensity for crime, and that the tendency to commit crime was inborn (inherited from parents). His initial thoughts were that this tendency showed itself in atavistic features: physical characteristics which suggested that some persons were at an earlier stage of evolution than others. He developed a typology of crime and criminals, and reported the findings of his research in a book *On Criminal Man* (*L'uomo delinquente*), published in 1876. These ideas were not psychological as such, but the impetus to study crime in terms of individual differences is generally traced to the impact of Lombroso's work. In his later studies, he broadened his conception of causes to include environmental and social factors.

The central concepts proposed by these key figures continue to play a major part in theory construction today, though there has of course been much refinement and recombination of ideas along the way (Siegel, 2012). What is known as Rational Choice Theory entails the view that individuals make their decisions about whether or not to commit offences based on their expectations of relative gain as compared with the relative costs likely to be incurred – perhaps most importantly, the chances of being caught. This is essentially similar to Choice Theory within economics, which sees individuals as rational consumers making decisions on the basis of their calculations, or at the very least estimates, of relative benefits and costs. Thus criminologists have studied offence decision-making and investigated, for example, how someone planning a house burglary chooses between different possible 'targets' (Bennett and Wright, 1984; Nee and Meenaghan, 2006; Wright and Decker, 1994).

Environmental and ecological theories in criminology are extensions of the fundamental notion that crime is a product of the conditions in which people live, influenced also by the resources and opportunities available to them as a function of the structure of their societies overall. Ideas similar to Quételet's were propounded and extended by members of the *Chicago School* of environmental criminology, who studied the distribution of crime within that city as crime expanded rapidly in the late 19th and early 20th centuries (Siegel, 2012). This evolved later into ideas such as **Strain Theory**, the proposal that in highly competitive societies some of those who do less well in the race for success by socially accepted means will instead resort to illegal methods.

Psychological theories take several forms, and in many respects they reflect the range of ideas we can find in other areas where psychological concepts are deployed to explain human action. Since psychology itself is a meeting point between biological and social sciences, some theories lean towards the former and see individual differences in many attributes as deriving largely from genetic influences, physiological processes, or both. These ideas are now generally stated in far less rudimentary form than the body-typology suggestions forwarded by Lombroso – though, as noted in Chapter 1, the work of Wilson and Herrnstein (1985), published not so very long ago, gave favourable coverage to the idea of a relationship between body typology and delinquency. Many contemporary research projects continue to be rooted in the notion that there are discoverable individual differences that give rise to a tendency to become involved in antisocial behaviour and later crime, and that some of those differences derive from biological, including genetic, causes. Other theories place greater emphasis on learning and on the cultural, social and family context in which crime occurs; and on how processes such as modelling, socialisation and group influence all shape the behavioural repertoires of developing individuals. Still other theories focus on the capacity of human beings to process information, and accord greater importance to cognitive events, such as how individuals appraise, construe and respond to situations (Andrews and Bonta, 2010; McGuire, 2004a).

Of course, some psychological theories are eclectic and integrative, and deploy and combine concepts from several of these directions. Today, within both psychology and criminology there are numerous specific theories that develop and extend the basic ideas outlined above, but those theories have moved forward considerably, given the now much larger volume of empirical research that has been carried out on these issues. There is also some synthesis of ideas from psychology and sociology, often focused on the observation that individuals differ in their capacity for, or exercise of, self-control. That variation may be a net result of environmental conditions, learning experiences and cognitive processes, acting in concert over an extended phase of the lifespan.

We are at a point today where a substantial amount of evidence has accumulated on the correlates of offending (Ellis, Beaver and Wright, 2009), to the extent that it is not an exaggeration to say that the phenomenon of crime, as conventionally defined, is relatively well understood. There are still numerous questions to be asked and answered, and much further progress to be made. But we have learnt enough to affirm that there is nothing supernaturally ordained, incalculably random, or in other ways impenetrably mysterious about crime.

Surveying theories of criminal behaviour

In many cases, opening a textbook of criminology can be a perplexing experience. Numerous theories have been forwarded in attempts to account for crime. The majority of them achieve at least a modicum of success in doing so; they almost all seem to have some initial plausibility. But they may also be mutually contradictory. If they all sound reasonable yet are simultaneously inconsistent with one another, how can they all be right?

There has been debate on this point within criminology for many years, with some eminent figures suggesting that theories of crime should compete with each other, and a choice made between them. This would not necessarily be done through 'critical experiments', as happens in other sciences, since this is not really feasible in criminal justice, but rather by systematic testing of which models best fit the evidence (Hirschi, 1979). Others propose that a preferable course of action, given the overlap of theories, is some form of conceptual or **theory integration**. (Bernard and Snipes, 1996).

One reason for the seeming paradox here is that separate theoretical models are often attempts to accomplish different goals: to explain different aspects of crime, or different manifestations of it. In considering the possibility of developing a comprehensive theory of crime, it can be useful to think of that process as requiring us to think on a series of different levels of explanation.

Let us look more closely at what this means. It is primarily a matter of the scope and the degree of specificity of any given explanation, and could be described as moving in stages from the 'macrocosm' to the 'microcosm'. Table 4.1 shows a series of five such stages or levels of explanation. Each level represents an attempt to account

Level	Unit of analysis	Basic question	Objective	Illustrative theories
1	Society	Why is there crime at all?	To explain why human societies experience crime, and to understand its occurrence as a large-scale social phenomenon	*Conflict theory* *Anomie/Strain theory* *Sociological control theories* *Feminist theories*
2	Localised areas, communities	Why is there more crime in some places than others?	To account for geographical variations in crime, such as urban–rural differences, or differences between districts or neighbourhoods	*Ecological/social disorganisation theories* *Differential opportunity theory*
3	Proximate social groups	Why is crime concentrated in some groups?	To understand the roles of socialisation and social influence through family, school, or peer-group	*Subcultural delinquency theory* *Differential association theory* *Social learning theory*
4	Criminal acts and events	Do criminal acts follow patterns?	To analyse and account for patterns and types of crime events, crime targets, and trends over time	*Routine activity theory* *Rational choice theory* *Situational action theory*
5	Individual offenders	What psychological factors or individual differences influence offending?	To examine patterns of individual behaviour with reference to internal, psychological factors such as thoughts, feelings and attitudes, and other recurring reaction patterns	*Neutralisation theory* *Psychological control theories* *Cognitive social learning theory* *Social information-processing theory*

Table 4.1 Major theories of crime and levels of explanation.

Source: adapted from Table 7.1 A schematic representation of levels of explanation in criminological theories. From McGuire, J. (2000). Explanations of Criminal Behaviour. In J. McGuire, T. Mason & A. O'Kane (eds.). Behaviour, Crime and Legal Processes: A Guide for Forensic Practitioners. pp. 135–160. Chichester: John Wiley & Sons Ltd. Copyright © 2000 by John Wiley & Sons Ltd.

for a different set of data concerning crime. Theories at each level have a common unit of analysis (column 2), and a shared overall objective (column 3). Some of the most widely cited models are named for illustrative purposes (column 4); we will discuss most of them in the present chapter and the remainder in the next. The 'Focus on ...' box below suggests a way of understanding this concept.

FOCUS ON ...

Levels of observation and explanation

Another way of thinking about the five levels of explanation discussed in the text is through an analogy with an optical microscope. In a *compound microscope* there are several lenses with progressively increasing powers of magnification (×100, ×300, and so on), which allow us to examine a specimen in more detail or to see smaller organisms.

To make this more concrete, here is a 'thought experiment'. Imagine you are some kind of alien looking at the Earth through a very powerful device that's a kind of combination of a telescope and microscope. You are interested in human behaviour and why members of this species seem to appropriate each other's belongings or start fights with each other. Let's assume that you have similar problems back on Planet X where you come from, and that you have been despatched on an intergalactic mission to find out how other beings deal with this behaviour.

- You look first at the patterning of crime across the Earth as a whole, and observe such behaviour happening more or less everywhere. Is it an inevitable result of human beings living together in the large conglomerations they call societies? Given that there seem to be no exceptions to the pattern – over time, as far as you can tell, having watched this planet for quite a while – it does appear to be inexorable.
- Then you switch lenses to pick up more detail, and discover that crime is unevenly distributed. There is more of it, sometimes far more of it, in some places than in others and at some times than at others. There are higher rates of crime in large cities than in smaller towns or in villages; and within cities, some urban neighbourhoods have higher rates than others – in some locations, higher rates of every type of crime; in others, higher rates of particular types of crime, for which they become 'hot spots'.
- But the problem can be even more concentrated still. With a third lens, one that lets you see right down to street level, you find certain groups – families, peer-groups, schools, or gatherings such as gangs – that are associated with particularly high rates of crime. In close groups, people who are in daily contact are likely to have a sizeable impact on each other, and some appear to influence their fellow members in a way that leads to higher rates of crime.
- Your fourth lens lets you pick out individuals. As you can track their behaviour, you see that some of them engage in a lot more of this criminal activity than others: sometimes in small groups, sometimes alone. Those patterns of persistence may account for a large proportion of the offences recorded in a given area (you can easily access their very poorly encrypted data systems) and you might search for a relationship between breaking the law and other ways in which people spend their time during an average day.
- Finally, with your most powerful and most ingenious lens (a type the humans have not yet invented, though their neuroscientists are working on it), you can look inside these beings' heads, and start to understand what is going on in there. What are the thoughts, feelings, attitudes and other internal events that may have contributed to their participation in illegal acts more often than some others?

By this stage, the urge to settle on Earth and pursue a career as a forensic psychologist has become irresistible.

Level 1: Why is there crime at all?

We can expand the content of Table 4.1 by considering in sequence the core questions that are asked, one at each of the five levels. First, why is there crime to begin with? After all, most citizens consider crime to be a major social problem, and in some countries feelings about it run so high that the issue is a standard fixture in election manifestos, with each political party saying what they will do about it.

Unlike earthquakes or volcanic eruptions, crime is not caused by something outside humanity's control but is a direct result of our own actions. Yet there is evidence from some of the earliest human remains that people met violent deaths at the hands of others. Archaeologists have found codes of criminal justice dating back to the ancient civilisations of Sumeria and Babylon, over four thousand years ago. Much more recently, the Puritan colonists, who left 17th-century Europe with the aim of setting up a better society in the New World, found that within one hundred years they were beset by a series of crime waves. This has led some sociologists to contend that crime, like other forms of behaviour that may be regarded as socially 'deviant' (the exact list varying across time and place), also serves a purpose in marking the boundaries of society, thereby supplying a target against which leaders can encourage the rest of the populace to unite (Erikson, 1966).

It might be tempting to revert to the supposed common-sense view that crime is simply caused by an ever-present minority of malevolent individuals. To some extent the language of news media perpetuates such a myth, through its references to 'mindless violence', 'evil beasts', 'feral youth', and so on. Yet when there is a breakdown in 'law and order', as occurs in conditions of political instability, sometimes quite large numbers of people break the law. Looting of stores, criminal damage and sexual assault may all proliferate. Even when governments are intact, in periods of rapid social change many more people break the law than would ordinarily do so. Such an upsurge occurred, for example, in the former Soviet Union in the early 1990s, in the years following the downfall of communism. In the social liberalisation that ensued, there was a 50 per cent rise in the crime rate in a period of just two years (Gilinskiy, 2006). Did the character of the Russian people change during that time; were there suddenly many more people with criminal personalities? That seems a fairly unlikely explanation.

We might detect in this example something that is conventionally supposed – that the front-line guardians of law and order, in the shape of the police, constantly hold back an impending deluge of crime; a proposal known as the 'thin blue line' hypothesis (McGuire, 2017a). Plausible though that can sound, it is cast into doubt by findings of several kinds. One is what happens when, as part of disputes with their employers, the police take industrial action such as 'go-slows' or strikes. Pfuhl (1983) compiled crime rate data for periods when police took such action in eleven US cities during the 1970s. The strikes that occurred ranged from 3 to 30 days in length. While there were increases in rates of some crimes in some locations, in the majority there were no changes at all. Thus, our predilections notwithstanding, there is no overall pattern supportive of police presence as a major deterrent against crime. Other researchers have explored whether variations in visible police numbers (in everyday parlance in the UK, 'bobbies on the beat') make a difference to crime rates. Using telephone survey methodology, Kleck and Barnes (2010) interviewed 1,500 people across 54 urban areas of the United States, to test whether there was a relationship between local police workforce levels and perceptions or estimates of the likelihood of arrest. They concluded that 'the evidence indicates that police manpower levels do not affect crime rates by affecting perceptions of the risk of arrest and punishment. This does not mean that prospective offenders are unaware of the risk of arrest but rather that variations in police strength do not affect perceptions of that risk' (2010, p. 20).

Findings such as these underline a fundamental point made by Tyler (2006). Much of the time, the law succeeds in its appointed purpose not because of its coercive or constraining power, but because the majority of citizens endorse its operation. Tyler adduced strong evidence to suggest that the everyday law-abiding behaviour of most people is a function of their affirmation of the law and their perception of its workings as legitimate, rather than their fear of detection and punishment if they committed crimes. In a large-scale interview study of 1,575 respondents in Chicago, Tyler discovered that the fundamental influence underpinning most individuals' adherence to lawful behaviour was their own commitment to doing so. This commitment was grounded partly in personal moral values and partly in beliefs that the laws were appropriate. Overall, where the law is perceived to have legitimacy – that is, where its rationale is considered sound and its operation is considered fair – apart from some occasional slippages, most citizens regularly and willingly act in accordance with it.

Under some other circumstances, however, this generally benign pattern can be disrupted. However unpalatable this idea may be, the capacity for committing antisocial acts appears to be present, and in certain situations can be triggered into action, amongst a very large number of people. In certain social conditions there can be outbursts of extreme and even lethal violence, as when political, religious or ethnic conflict leads to acts of genocide. On these occasions, many previously law-abiding citizens may perpetrate the most appalling crimes, even against people who have been their neighbours. Some of the horrors that occurred during the 20th century were certainly instigated or inflamed by pernicious, even megalomaniac leaders; but close analysis shows that the majority of perpetrators involved in the actual carrying out of mass murders were individuals who in other respects were what are customarily called 'ordinary people' (Staub, 1989; Waller, 2007).

Theoretical models

Several kinds of theory emerge from these observations and a number of theorists have sought to explain why crime appears to be endemic in human societies. *Conflict Theories*, which owe their origins to the philosopher Karl Marx (1818–1883) and to Marxist thought, are based on the view that economic competition determines patterns of social relations and structures of success and failure, which then become entrenched. Those at different levels of the resultant hierarchy coalesce into classes, with a more or less permanent state of friction between the classes. The dominant group institutes laws that work to its own advantage, while also serving to control the rest of the population. While Marx himself did not develop a theory of crime *per se*, several criminological theories have drawn on the idea that crime has its roots in patterns of conflict that are embedded in society.

A quite specific formulation of social conflict developed to explain crime in highly competitive, industrialised societies is *Anomie/Strain Theory*. The concept of anomie, derived from the work of the French sociologist Émile Durkheim (1858–1917), refers both to a state of *society*, in which rules and norms have broken down, and to a state of *individuals*, in which they have lost the sense of belonging to that society and allegiance to its core values. This was first proposed as a theory of crime by the sociologist Robert Merton (originator of the term 'role model'), who analysed the tension that arises between the culturally defined goals that most individuals pursue, and the socially approved, and hence legitimate, means of achieving those goals. For those who seek conventionally defined success but find that acceptable routes towards it are inaccessible to them, crime may be one result. The majority may simply conform to the expectations of society in an almost ritualistic way, accepting their limited success and abandoning the race for anything more. For others, however, crime is one type of resolution of the strain they feel when they do not succeed in achieving the most strongly favoured goals of material wealth accumulation.

Merton's ideas were later developed, with greater emphasis on their psychological aspects, by Agnew (1992, 2007; Agnew and White, 1992). Agnew's work on **Strain Theory** focused on the negative emotional states that individuals experience as a consequence of the social strain identified by Merton. With reference to crime, certain kinds of strains or stressors are more likely to lead to it than others. They are the ones that: (a) are perceived as unjust; (b) are high in magnitude; (c) are associated with low self-control; and (d) create some pressure or incentive to engage in in criminal acts, as opposed to other means of coping. Crime is particularly associated with undesirable feeling states such as anger, depression and anxiety. When asked to explain why an offence has occurred, individuals will often recount a sequence of events in a 'storyline' that begins with an adverse event and the deleterious impact it had on them (Agnew, 2006b).

Approaching the nature of conflict from a different direction, *Feminist Theory* considers that a fundamental issue that needs to be understood in criminal justice, which for a long time had been neglected, is the respective roles of women and men. Crime is profoundly 'gendered' in that not only is the bulk of it committed by males but they also dominate society in numerous other ways (Daly and Chesney-Lind, 1988). This is a function of *patriarchy*, the traditional disparity in power between males and females, which is ultimately a legacy of male ownership of property and control of inheritance, and perpetuation of a system in which women – not explicitly, but in a tacit and deep-rooted way – are viewed as a commodity (Siegel, 2012). The inequities and imbalances that derive from this, some feminist criminologists argue, may be the root causes of competitiveness, exploitation and violence. Some researchers have suggested that there is a far greater level of violence against women and children than ever becomes visible in the criminal statistics (Garside, 2006). In its most extreme form, such violence can consist of the attempted 'erasure' of unwanted women. Strong (2009) has documented a series of cases of the disappearance of women who, later research revealed, had in fact been killed by their male partners.

Yodanis (2006) compared rates of violence against women and levels of fear amongst them with their relative social status, for 27 countries. Data on crimes against women were obtained from the International Crime Victims Survey and other United Nations sources. The position of women was evaluated using the Status of Women Index, a measure of the level of advancement of women in educational, occupational and political domains. Using regression analysis, and controlling for GDP and the percentage of males aged 20–34 in the population, Yodanis found a significant association between status and the amount of sexual (but not physical) violence. Yodanis concluded that: 'The educational and occupational status of women in a country is correlated with the prevalence of sexual violence in a country, with a high status of women corresponding with lower rates of sexual violence' (2006, p. 670).

To summarise, all of the theoretical models we are considering here suggest that crime has become an integral feature of human society, which derives from its structure and the conflicts inherent within it. In one form or another, they all view crime as a product of patterns of inequality in the perennial competition for power, status and material prosperity. The next 'Where do you stand?' box provides a further example of this view in relation to income inequality.

Level 2: Why is there more crime in some places than others?

There are widely varying volumes of serious crime in different countries of the world, as shown in the statistical profiles collated by the United Nations Office on Drugs and Crime. As long ago as 1831, Quételet had confirmed that there are large regional variations in crime rates.

Systematic study of local variations in crime rates was carried out by the Chicago School of criminologists in the first half of the 20th century. As a rapidly expanding city from the 1840s onwards, Chicago had a constantly changing population. The world's first Department of Sociology was founded at the University of Chicago in 1900, and researchers there found that they had on their doorstep a natural laboratory for the study of urban change. Data collection over consecutive decades, for a period totalling 65 years, revealed how crime thrived in particular neighbourhoods; most prominently, in an area known as the *transitional zone*, which was close to the urban centre and was mostly inhabited by successive waves of migrants as they arrived from different parts of Europe (Germany, Ireland, Italy and Poland). There

WHERE DO YOU STAND?

Inequality and violence

Sociological criminologists have long contended that crime is significantly influenced by a number of structural factors in society, such as the distribution of wealth and power, patterns of social and economic inequality, and, in particular, relative deprivation (Rock, 2007).

We might expect any such relationship to show most clearly with respect to acquisitive crimes, as differences in socioeconomic status (SES) may be felt most keenly in relation to purchasing power. This would certainly be predicted by Strain Theory, and appears to hold true for the United States. However, a cross-national comparison of 62 countries by Stack (1984) found no significant association between relative income inequality and rates of property crime. Meta-analysis of risk factors for offending have generally yielded only weak associations with SES (Andrews and Bonta, 2010; Dunaway, Cullen, Burton and Evans, 2000).

More recent research has focused on offences of violence, and the question of whether a causal link to inequality can be found has become of interest within economics. In a study conducted under the auspices of the Latin American Regional Studies Program of the World Bank, one team of researchers (Fajnzylber, Lederman and Loayza, 2002) compared rates of serious violent crimes within and across societies from various regions of the world that differed in their levels of inequality of income. Elaborate analyses were undertaken to check the directionality of any causal pathway and the possible roles of other variables.

The measure of inequality employed, the *Gini Coefficient* (or *Gini Index*), is widely used in economics: it is a statistic that represents the extent of unevenness of income distribution. The coefficient is computed such that if all the income in a society were received by just one person, the coefficient's value would be 1. If, on the other hand, everyone received an exactly equal share, its value would be 0.

Using Gini coefficients, Fajnzylber *et al.* analysed rates of intentional homicide in 39 countries for the period 1965–1994, and the rates of robbery in 37 countries for the period 1970–1994. One of their findings is shown in the graph. This shows the raw results for intentional homicide, revealing a positive and statistically significant association between income inequality and violence. A similar finding, though the association was weaker, was obtained for robbery.

Fajnzylber *et al.* conducted a number of analyses of these data, controlling for level of development (measured by GNP per capita), years of education, economic growth rate, and the level of urbanisation of the countries involved. From regression and time-series analyses they concluded that there was a robust causal relationship between income inequality and the rate of violent crime; furthermore, their findings indicated that poverty reduction led to a decline in crime rates. Wilkinson (2004) reviewed other data that supported the inequality–violence link and forwarded an explanation of the trends. Wilkinson and Pickett (2009) examined correlations between inequality and a wide range of other indicators, with greater inequality being linked to a variety of outcomes including poorer physical and mental health and other social problems.

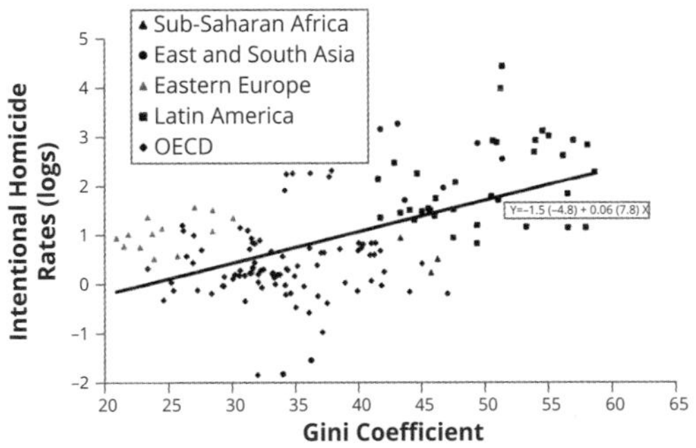
Sub-Saharan Africa
East and South Asia
Eastern Europe
Latin America
OECD
Intentional Homicide Rates (logs)
5
4
3
2
1
0
-1
-2
20
25
30
35
40
45
50
55
60
65
Gini Coefficient
Y=-1.5 (-4.8) + 0.06 (7.8) X

Source: Fajnzylber, P., Lederman, D. & Loayza, N. (2002). Inequality and Violent Crime. The Journal of Law & Economics, 45(1), 1–39. Publisher: The University of Chicago Press for The Booth School of Business. © 2002 by The University of Chicago. All rights reserved.

Where do you stand on this issue?

1 How important do you think inequality might be as a contributory factor to crime?

2 Were the 'summer riots' of 2011 in England an episode of civil unrest resulting from inequality, or did they have other explanations?

was a high level of deprivation and the population was constantly changing; the neighbourhood was felt to be perpetually on the edge of disintegration. Consistently, this area had the highest crime rate, regardless of which ethnic community lived there. Crime was generated by a social process that was independent of the characteristics of the local residents themselves: groups successively replaced each other every few years, yet the neighbourhoods into which they moved afterwards showed no increase in rates of delinquency. The Chicago researchers concluded that crime and other social ills were a function of the conditions in which communities lived, and not of the individuals who composed those communities.

Theoretical models

Ecological Theories and allied models draw on the above findings and on the concept of social organisation (or disorganisation). They have spawned a number of other theories that utilise different aspects of the urban environment as key explanatory variables. For example, *Differential Opportunity Theory* emphasises the varying positions of people in society and that they are likely to be channelled in specific directions according to what is available to them. In more deprived neighbourhoods, it is likely that gang cultures will flourish, and these provide their members both with emotional support and with the chance of recouping the self-esteem lost by lack of success in education and employment. Different types of gangs offer varied openings into illegal activity (drug dealing, property crime, or street fights). *Subcultural Delinquency Theory*, a further variant of these ideas, is the view that some types of antisocial activity represent a form of protest against mainstream values. As a result of the *status frustration* experienced by those who have little hope of success in conventional terms, delinquent groups such as gangs consciously reject the norms and expectations of law-abiding society. This may be a localised expression of the larger-scale conflicts that we saw earlier, on the first level of the conceptual scheme.

Level 3: Why is crime concentrated in some groups?

Narrowing our focus further, there is evidence that even within high crime areas there may be a concentration of delinquency in some smaller proximate groupings of people who are in regular contact – groups such as families, peer-groups, or in school classrooms or playgrounds. A striking example of this came from the Pittsburgh Youth Study, one of the longitudinal projects described in Chapter 2, in which a sample of 1,517 boys was followed up over a period of 14 years. Half of all the recorded convictions recorded for this group were accounted for by members of just 23 families, who together represented only 6 per cent of the cohort (Farrington *et al.*, 2001). We might assume that this provides evidence for criminality as a tendency that is inherited, and some researchers consider heredity to be a very important influence. A more likely explanation of these patterns, however, resides in the processes of interaction that occur inside groups. Copious amounts of research indicate that the family is the most powerful agent of socialisation in young people's lives. It is the main conduit through which society and culture are mediated to developing children, but culture is transmitted through the formative actions of parents and other family members who also bring their own personal histories and experiences to bear upon it. Thus the process of socialisation conveys general messages through which an individual is assimilated into the wider cultural group, while also inculcating habits of behaviour and of thought that bear the unique hallmarks of parents or other family members. We will discuss the role and importance of socialisation within families more fully in Chapter 5.

Theoretical models

Although dissimilar in some respects, parallel processes of mutual influence also occur within peer-groups, and these may be especially potent when those groups coalesce into the formations known as gangs. Recognition of these interactional patterns has led to the development of a number of theories. *Differential Association Theory* was formulated by Sutherland (Sutherland and Cressey, 1970) to account for the processes of mutual influence that occur inside familiar groups. In an innovative departure, however, his research suggested that this may happen not only on street corners in deprived neighbourhoods, but also in the boardrooms of large corporations and other professional settings. Sutherland (1940) coined the phrase 'white-collar crime' – referring to illegal commercial or business activities such as fraud, embezzlement, money-laundering, insider-trading and tax evasion – and conducted key research on the processes that lead to a decision to offend. According to this model, crime results from exposure to 'an excess of definitions favourable to violations of law over definitions unfavourable to it'. Putting this another way, the more people you know who say that breaking the law is a justifiable or even a desirable practice, and the fewer you know who would argue the opposite, the likelier it is that at some stage you will engage in law-breaking.

There is considerable evidence in support of the 'differential association' principle. For example, Hochstetler, Copes and DeLisi (2002) reported findings based on the US National Youth Survey, which focused on a sample of 1,492 young people followed from Wave 5 (1980) to Wave 6 (1983). (See Chapter 2 for a brief outline of the overall study.) The attitudes and behaviour of friends bore a consistently significant association with the likelihood of three different types of offence – theft, assault and vandalism – and these effects held for offences committed alone, as well as for those committed in groups. Yet the effects appeared to occur without being mediated through the individuals' own attitudes, suggesting a role for other forms of social learning than indirect attitude transmission.

Differential Association Theory can perhaps therefore be absorbed within a broader framework that in effect bridges the gap between sociologically based and psychologically based models of progressive inducement into criminal activity. **Social Learning Theory** was developed in parallel within criminology by Akers, Krohn, Lanza-Kaduce and Radosevich (1979) and within psychology by Bandura (1977). Akers and his colleagues (1979, p. 637) described their model as 'a revision of differential association theory in terms of general behavioural reinforcement theory'. Their central proposal was that crime is learned through processes of imitation and differential reinforcement by which individuals may arrive at 'evaluative definitions' (attitudes) that are supportive of antisocial action. This learning occurs in the context of social interaction, most potently within adolescent peer-groups, but it goes beyond the principle of differential association to define the processes that shape behaviour over time.

Akers and his colleagues (1979) initially tested their theory by conducting a self-report survey of involvement in substance abuse amongst a large sample of teenagers. Significant correlations were found between independent variables (measures of associative networks and opportunities for social learning) and dependent variables (levels of substance misuse). The relative balance of influences within the groups to which individuals were exposed instigated and maintained such behaviours as under-age use of alcohol and other illicit drug use. Although this study could not delineate the details of the mechanisms involved, it provided preliminary support for the importance of social learning in the onset of some kinds of proscribed behaviour.

Proponents of Social Learning Theory have surveyed relevant evidence and claim significant support for many elements of it from a wide range of research studies (Akers and Jensen, 2006; Jensen and Akers, 2003). This has reinvigorated their claim that the theory can help to explain patterns of crime 'not only at the micro-level but also at higher levels of temporal and ecological aggregation' (Akers and Jensen, 2006, p. 38). Thus in addition to the now voluminous evidence of social learning effects within the family and in peer-groups, the model might also be applied to elucidate the links between these processes and variations in social structure, again taking us back to the first level of the present schematic framework.

Pratt *et al.*, (2010) reported a meta-analysis of the status of Social Learning Theory in criminology. They reviewed 133 studies published between 1973 and 2003, which together yielded 704 effect-size tests based on a total sample of 118,403 participants. Measures of differential association, and of exposure to 'definitions' (i.e. statements made by others that were favourable to crime), showed consistently strong effects; whereas other variables in the theory, including differential reinforcement and modelling by or imitation of peers, were weaker and not entirely consistent in their effects. A possible explanation for this was thought to lie in the expanded opportunities for crime that are opened up by having delinquent associates, rather than as a consequence of their interpersonal influence *per se*. Thus support for the theory was not wholly uniform, and some key questions regarding it remain unanswered.

We will return to Social Learning Theory in Chapter 5, when we will consider it as a component of an integrative psychological theory of crime. Meanwhile, note that social learning processes have been deployed to help explain behaviour in another segment of the criminal justice system: police misconduct. In a study of 499 police officers in Philadelphia, Chappell and Piquero (2004) found a close link between patterns of peer association, shared attitudes towards certain dishonest and explicitly forbidden practices, and misconduct as measured by formal citizen complaints. It may be that this study locates an aspect of what is known colloquially (in the UK) as 'canteen culture'.

Level 4: Do criminal acts follow patterns?

As we have seen, many researchers in criminology have proposed that the specific patterning of crime in societies is influenced far more by broader social and cultural conditions than by the backgrounds or dispositions of individuals who break the law. In a variant formulation of this, some have proposed that large-scale economic and social changes also determine the range of immediate situations that individuals are likely to encounter. The same changes also influence the configuration of opportunities for offending that arise.

For example, as the availability of consumer goods has increased exponentially over recent decades, so has the rate of theft of those goods. Quite simply, there are a lot more things to steal today than there were even a generation or so ago; and while many people possess the trappings of consumer culture, many others do not. The ideal object to steal is one that is small, lightweight and portable, that can be easily concealed, and that has high resale value. Using such information sources as catalogues of department stores, Cohen and Felson (1979) analysed patterns of retail sales and unearthed relationships between the design of consumer goods and the rate at which they were stolen. For example, between 1960 and 1970 the lightest television sets fell in weight from 38 to 15 pounds (15.9 to 6.8 kilos), that is, they had been 2½ times heavier in 1960. Over successive decades, the consumer goods market has steadily produced many more items that meet the ideal conditions for theft: indeed, present-day communities are replete with such objects (wallets and purses, mobile phones, tablets, credit cards, and the like). Opportunities for theft increased. As motor vehicles multiplied and as it became increasingly possible to engage in many more attractive activities outside the home (such as visit national parks, or take holidays abroad), car theft escalated. In addition, many more households were left unoccupied and hence more vulnerable by day, thereby creating many more openings for residential burglary, which duly soared.

Further, since approximately the middle of the 20th century in Western societies, there has also been a significant change in the everyday habits and routines of large masses of people. We now spend much less time in small communal groups; we are less visible to each other; and there is less exercise of what is called 'informal social control'. (This refers to the control that is exercised through our ties to other individuals and our membership of groups, as opposed to the more formal controls that derive from the operation of law or other explicit regulatory arrangements.) Given frantic, high-density urban landscapes and widely accessible transport systems, it is possible to remain anonymous while committing an offence and then to disappear effortlessly into the crowd and make a speedy escape.

Theoretical models

The combination of these two trends – changes in the design and availability of consumer goods, and changes in the daily routines of masses of people – is held by criminologists such as Felson and Boba (2010) to explain the enormous acceleration in property crime in the modern era. Earlier, Felson and Cohen (1980) had forwarded **Routine Activity Theory**, an approach to crime analysis that relies on rigorous observation of the concurrence of different types of features in the patterning of crime. This specifies a model in which the majority of criminal offences, which take the form of what Felson and Cohen called 'direct contact predatory violations', are the outcome of the convergence in space and time of three factors: (a) a motivated offender; (b) a suitable target; and (c) the absence of capable guardians.

To some extent, this conceptualisation also converges with the ideas contained in Rational Choice Theory, which, as indicated earlier, envisages individuals as making conscious decisions as to whether or not to offend based on their assessments of the likely gains and losses on either side, and the relative risks of each course. Rational Choice Theory in turn is closely associated with concepts of deterrence, insofar as increasing the perceived likely costs of crime, or even just the effort involved in committing it, is thought to offer the most realistic prospect of influencing offence-related decisions. In conjunction, Rational Choice Theory and Routine Activity Theory have both had a significant impact on crime-prevention policies and practices in many countries – see the 'Where do you stand?' box below.

WHERE DO YOU STAND?

Situational crime prevention

The Rational Choice Theory and the Routine Activity Theory have had a notable synergy and an extensive impact on crime-prevention practices and policies throughout the world. They have led to the idea of taking steps to preclude crime from the places where it is likely to occur, a set of procedures known as **situational crime prevention**. The origins of this approach are often traced to the early 1970s and to the idea of *defensible space* forwarded by the architect and urban planner Oscar Newman (1996); as well as by the suggestion of criminologist C. Ray Jeffery that the layout of urban environments, including housing estates, can create areas that facilitate crime – and conversely, that altering the design of such areas can reduce crime opportunities. These ideas were later given impetus by some impressive outcomes that were found as the unanticipated side-effects of changes made for other reasons:

- During the 1950s, almost 50 per cent of suicides in England and Wales were committed by self-poisoning, using the domestic gas supply. From 1958 onwards, coal gas, containing highly toxic carbon monoxide, was gradually replaced first with gas manufactured from oil and then with natural gas; the latter does not contain carbon monoxide. In the period 1968–1975 during which coal gas was wholly replaced by natural gas, there was a 30 per cent drop in suicide in England and Wales, at a time when the rate continued to rise elsewhere in Europe. The proportion of suicides carried out using domestic gas fell to only 0.2 per cent. There was no reason to believe that the level of community distress had somehow fallen during that period, yet there was no evidence of individuals resorting to other means of ending their lives (a pattern sometimes called *displacement*; Clarke and Mayhew, 1988). This led to the conclusion that the change in the nature of the opportunities available, the result of removing an easily available method of carrying it out, led to more people getting through crises without resorting to suicide. A similar trend was observed in the United States between 1950 and 1960, but there (amongst males, though not females) there was displacement towards using car exhaust fumes instead (Lester, 1990).
- Another frequently cited illustration of changes in the contexts of decisions is the introduction in Germany of laws to enforce

the wearing of motorcycle helmets. This not only increased safety but also reduced the rate of motorcycle theft, from 150,000 in 1980 to 50,000 in 1986 – driving without a helmet was likely to be noticed (Mayhew, Clarke and Elliot, 1989).

These findings and others lend support to the central tenet of this combination of theories, that a large contributory cause in many social problems including criminal offences may be the availability of opportunities to act in those ways.

By analysing how offences are committed, one may identify how adjustments in the immediate environment can make the offences more difficult, or at least make it more likely that individuals committing those offences will draw attention to themselves. This kind of analysis has yielded a wide spectrum of policy directions. These have included increased security through protecting the target ('target-hardening'), but also several types of environmental redesign, for example making walkways through housing estates overlooked by others and thus events more easily seen by them.

Evaluations of situational crime-prevention initiatives have yielded many positive results. They include the following:

- *Neighbourhood Watch* Over 25 per cent of the UK and 40 per cent of the US population live in areas covered by Neighbourhood Watch schemes. Bennett, Holloway and Farrington (2008a) found that in 19 out of 25 evaluation studies there were positive outcomes. Meta-analysis of studies found reductions in crime of between 16 per cent and 26 per cent.
- *Street lighting* A review of eight US and five UK studies of improved street lighting found the American studies evenly split in their outcomes, with an average reduction in crime of only 7 per cent (statistically non-significant), whereas for the British studies the outcomes were more positive, with an average reduction in crime of 29 per cent (Welsh and Farrington, 2007). In places where this was measured, crime fell during the day as well as by night. It was suggested that this was a general effect of increased community awareness that improvements were being made, rather than a direct surveillance effect.
- *Caller ID* A study in New Jersey found that the introduction of a phone number recognition system significantly reduced hoax and obscene telephone calls (Clarke, 1997).
- *Closed-circuit television (CCTV)* A meta-analysis of 22 studies of the impact of closed-circuit television showed mixed effects. UK-based studies were all positive, whereas studies elsewhere found no benefits. Positive results applied mainly to car-related crime, and there was no impact on violent offences (Welsh and Farrington, 2003). It was estimated in 2005 that there were 4.8 million security cameras in the UK and that citizens were recorded by them on average 300 times a day. Though the number has reportedly fallen since then, the UK still has more of this kind of surveillance than any other country.

Concerns have sometimes been expressed that situational crime prevention might simply result in moving crime from one place or time to another. *Displacement* has been defined as 'the relocation of a crime from one place, time, target, offense, tactic, or offender to another as a result of some crime-prevention initiative' (Guerette and Bowers, 2009, p. 1333). However, in a review of evaluations of situational crime-prevention measures, Guerette and Bowers (2009) found that of a total of 574 observations from 102 studies, only 26 per cent showed evidence that some form of displacement had occurred. In a similar proportion (27 per cent) there was evidence that the beneficial effect had *diffused* to areas adjoining the intervention. The question then becomes one of which effect – displacement or diffusion – outweighs the other. Recent reviews have suggested that situational crime prevention results in displacement only some of the time, and that diffusion of benefits may be just as likely (Johnson, Guerette and Bowers, 2014; Telep *et al.*, 2014).

Where do you stand on this issue?

1 When crimes are prevented, which factors are most likely to have brought about the changes that occur?

2 If individuals believe they are being observed (even when they are not), what psychological process is at work that may deter them from committing crimes?

Rational Choice Theory and Routine Activity Theory are considered to have had a further resonance with each other, in that within both 'persons were treated virtually as objects and their motivations were scrupulously avoided as a topic of discussion' (Clarke and Felson, 1993, p. 2). Another approach, assembled with very little reference to the psychological dimensions of crime, is *Situational Action Theory* (Wikström, 2006; Wikström and Treiber, 2007). Wikström (2006) sets out his view of what is needed in a proper theoretical account, addressing the question of why a theory of action is important. He contends that this is so because 'it can help specify the causal mechanisms that link the individual and the environment, to action... a proper theory of action is a theory that specifies the causal processes that link the individual's characteristics and experiences (predispositions) and the features of his environment (inducements and constraints) to his acts' (p. 70). Wikström focuses on differences in morality as the core explanatory individual-level variable, and in a later study he also adds the dimension of self-control (Wikström, Ceccato, Hardie and Treiber, 2010). The latter study involves analysis of 'activity fields', the extent to which individuals move into potentially criminogenic situations during the course of an average day, by analysing 'space–time budgets' after mapping individuals' areas of movement over a four-day sampling period.

This method was applied in the Peterborough Adolescent and Young Adult Development Study, a longitudinal study of 991 young people followed from the age of 11. Offences were more likely to occur when individuals were in a situation defined as 'unsupervised with peers', and individuals with 'high criminal propensity' – a joint function of morality and the exercise of self-control – spent more time in such environments (Wikström and Treiber, 2007). This is a close parallel to the concept of 'person–situation interactions' (PSI), which we will explore more fully in Chapter 5. Strangely, however, there is no reference either to PSI or to models such as Cognitive Social Learning Theory, either of which could fill the gap in theorising that Wikström (2006) had identified.

What are we to make of the various, often perfectly credible theoretical ideas that we have considered to this point? Pratt and Cullen (2005) have reported a review of the comparative success of a series of seven 'macro-level' criminological theories, which include some of those we have scrutinised so far. Employing meta-analysis, Pratt and Cullen synthesised results from 214 studies published over a period of almost 40 years (1960–1999). Their criterion for success was the extent to which a theory accounted for a dependent variable that was a measurement of crime. Thus the effect size or measure of success of a theory was a correlation coefficient (Pearson r) between a variable used as a predictor within the theory (e.g. residential mobility in a neighbourhood, or extent of income inequality) and an outcome measure of crime or victimisation rates, both in overall terms and broken down into personal and property crimes.

This study generated a total of 1,984 effect-size estimates. Pratt and Cullen's (2005) principal conclusions, summarised in Table 4.2, were that some macro-level theories of crime were considerably better supported by evidence than others. However, some theories had been subjected to more empirical testing than others; and there were some difficulties in disentangling the effects of methodological variables in some tests, making results harder to interpret. Whereas theories concerned with Social Disorganisation or with Resource or Economic Deprivation emerged well from this exercise, Rational Choice/Deterrence and Subcultural theories did not, with other models awaiting further research or in need of clarification.

Level 5: What psychological factors or individual differences influence offending?

Some of the foregoing theories have at their centre the concept of control: the view that society is structured in such a way as to contain the urges of individuals as we pursue our own interests, regardless of whether doing so might be to the detriment of others. While this containment process succeeds with most people most of the time, there will always be a proportion of the population for whom it is ineffective. Crime is one result of this.

Theory	Adequacy of testing?	Influenced by methodology?	Level of support
Social Disorganisation	Yes	No	High
Resource/Economic Deprivation	Yes	No	High
Anomie/Strain	No	Not applicable	Moderate
Social Support/Altruism	No	No	Moderate
Routine Activity	Yes	Yes	Moderate
Rational Choice/Deterrence	Yes	Yes	Low
Subcultural	Yes	Yes	Low

Table 4.2 Results of a large-scale review of macro-level theories.

Source: adapted from Pratt, T. C. & Cullen, F. T. (2005). Assessing Macro-Level Predictors and Theories of Crime: A Meta-Analysis. In M. Tonry (ed.). Crime and Justice, Volume 32: A Review of Research. pp. 373–450. Chicago, IL: University of Chicago Press. © 2005 by The University of Chicago. All rights reserved.

Theoretical models

These *Sociological Control Theories* do not usually involve any detailed specification of psychological variables that might underlie the differences between those who conform and those who do not. *Psychological Control Theories* place more accent on the individual factors such as personality traits that may enable individuals to regulate themselves and to keep their urges, and particularly their negative emotions and reactions, in check.

What is left out of the 'routine activities' formula, for example, is the detail of what constitutes a 'motivated offender'. The psychology of criminal behaviour addresses that gap by seeking to specify the influences operating at an individual level, and this is the fifth explanatory plane in the present scheme. Several psychologically based theories have been forwarded. They have included personality theories informed by both the psychodynamic and the behavioural traditions in psychology. While the psychodynamic tradition now has little currency as an explanation of offending behaviour in general, some of its ideas have been marshalled in explaining very unusual or extremely violent types of offending (such as sexual sadism), but usually in case reports rather than more systematic research.

Other psychologically based accounts of individual differences are distant descendants of Lombroso's thought, linking aspects of bodily functioning to personality, and thereby to the potential for antisocial conduct. Even the most basic of Lombrosian ideas concerning bodily shape, personality and criminal propensity have proved remarkably durable. This is despite a large-scale research study completed in British prisons in 1913, in which Charles Goring, a medical officer, failed to find any evidence of different physical characteristics between offenders and non-offenders (Lilly, Cullen and Ball, 2014). Even so, the theory lived on, in a transformed version, in the concept of *somatotypes* proposed by psychologist William Sheldon. Sheldon developed a classification of body types (*endomorphic*, *mesomorphic* and *ectomorphic*) that depended on the overall proportions and the ratio of bone, fat and nervous tissue in the body mass. Evidence purportedly indicating an association between body build and propensity towards criminal recidivism sufficiently impressed Wilson and Herrnstein (1985) that it led to their assertion that offenders were more likely to have a mesomorphic (muscular) body type.

In an extraordinary footnote to the history of these ideas, Goode (1997) has described studies that were conducted in secret by Sheldon during the period 1940–1960. These were supposedly carried out to investigate the relationship between somatotype and intelligence. Entrants to several American 'Ivy League' universities, including Harvard and Yale, were photographed naked in order to record their body type; over a 20-year period, approximately 27,000 such images were amassed.

A number of students who later achieved considerable prominence were photographed in this way. They included future President George Bush (senior), future Secretary of State Hillary Clinton, and multiple Oscar winner Meryl Streep.

Other psychologists, however, have proposed models with somewhat greater plausibility than the notion that crime or intelligence are a consequence of body shape. Perhaps the best-known example of this genre is Eysenck's (1977) theory, in which it was proposed that individuals high on certain personality dimensions are more likely to break the law. Eysenck postulated that constitutional factors (individual differences in the functioning of the nervous system, which are presumed to be inherited) influence the effectiveness of socialisation processes. According to Eysenck, this occurs as a result of differences in the ease with which conditioned responses are established, affecting an individual's ability to learn from experience. That in turn is a result of individual variations in cortical arousal, and has implications for the learning of fear and the development of conscience. The combined effect of these factors shows through in measurable personality **traits**. Three statistically orthogonal superordinate dimensions, *extraversion*, *neuroticism* and *psychoticism*, were derived from factor analysis of psychometric test scores. Eysenck adduced some preliminary evidence that high scores on these dimensions were associated with greater likelihood of involvement in criminality. Criminological psychologists, including Hollin (2012) and Wortley (2011), have considered that the theory is coherent and has some credible evidence in support of it, but have noted that its empirical basis remains weak and inconsistent, and its explanatory power seems somewhat questionable.

There is stronger evidence of an association between some other personality dimensions and levels of persistence of criminal offending over time. One of the most widely favoured candidate variables is *low* **self-control**, pivotal to the **General Theory of Crime** (sometimes called General Control Theory) posited by Gottfredson and Hirschi (1990). Self-control is composed of six interrelated features: (a) impulsivity, an inability to delay gratification; (b) short-term horizons, and lack of diligence in pursuing tasks; (c) inclination towards risk-taking activities; (d) investing greater value in physical and less in intellectual accomplishments or ability; (e) self-centredness; and (f) poor temper control. These features were identified by Grasmick, Tittle, Bursik and Arneklev (1993), who analysed the concept and developed a scale for assessment of self-control, but found that all of the items generally measured the same underlying factor. This suggests that individuals who are involved in crime may also exercise looser control over themselves across several areas of their lives. Thus a person with generally poor self-control may also have a less reliable work record, may be more likely to misuse substances, and may more often be involved in accidents, as well as being more likely to break the law. Individual differences in self-control are held to result from patterns of early socialisation and to be relatively unchangeable beyond adolescence, though there is a gradual trend towards increasing self-control over the lifespan (Hirschi and Gottfredson, 1995).

There have been numerous attempts to evaluate the tenets of this theory. In a meta-analytic review of the evidence from 21 studies, generating 126 effect-size estimates from a cumulative sample of 49,727 individual cases, Pratt and Cullen (2000) found that poor self-control was an important predictor of crime across a broad spectrum of offence types, though it was less well supported by developmental and longitudinal research. Gottfredson (2008) summarised evidence showing the pervasiveness of the 'control variable' in studies of different age-groups, across different societies, and for different types of crimes. Noting that the majority of tests of the theory had been carried out in the United States, Rebellon, Straus and Medeiros (2008) tested the relationship between self-control and offending using data from the International Dating Violence Study (IDVS; Straus, 2008; Straus *et al.*, 2004). As part of the dating survey, respondents were asked questions that captured aspects of self-control, as well as questions that elicited information about their involvement in property and violent crime, about parental supervision and/or neglect in childhood, and about associations with criminal peers. IDVS data were collected from a total of over 22,000 participants in 32 countries located across all continents. Statistical controls were introduced for demographic factors. One difficulty is that the participants in this survey were university students, who are probably not representative of the population in general. Another is that crime self-report data were skewed, with the majority of the samples in most countries not reporting any offending history. The results were nevertheless robustly supportive of General Control Theory. Low self-control was associated with violent crime in all 32 countries and with property crime in 28. It was also significantly associated with ratings of parental neglect, although additionally (and contrary to the theory's predictions) with peer associations. The authors concluded that this provided support for the cross-cultural applicability of the self-control concept, a suggestion bolstered by a separate study conducted in Japan (Vazsonyi, Wittekind, Belliston and Van Loh, 2004). As we will see in Chapter 19, researchers have also tested whether efforts to improve self-control can be successful, and if so whether they lead to reductions in offending (Piquero, Jennings and Farrington, 2010).

General Control Theory has also been subject to some rather acerbic criticisms, however (Geis, 2000). A longitudinal study of 513 young people from the ages of 9 to 19, while showing moderate stability of self-control variables, found that their association with delinquency varied over time (Turner and Piquero, 2002). Another large-sample study of control variables alongside other factors also found them to be a relatively inconsistent predictor of criminal activity (Cretacci, 2008). The inconsistency between studies may arise from a fundamental difficulty: that any selected variable viewed in isolation is likely to explain only a proportion of the variance in offence rates and patterns. As Farrington (1996, p. 79) has noted regarding theory construction, it appears rather optimistic to expect to explain a great deal when relying on 'only one underlying construct of criminal potential'.

Perhaps, then, crime is a function of the conjoined effect of two or more personality variables. Caspi *et al.*, (1994) explored this possibility in reviewing data from two longitudinal studies, the Pittsburgh Youth Study and the Dunedin Multidisciplinary Health and Development Study. Despite differences between the samples in age, culture and social background characteristics, there were parallels in the trends observed for two personality variables. One factor to emerge was a relative absence of personal constraints, broadly commensurate with the idea of low self-control. The other was proneness to experience negative emotions, and difficulties in coping with them. The combined action of these two factors placed individuals at higher risk of involvement in delinquency.

In any study in which only a small number of variables is assessed, however, it is likely that each will explain only a proportion of the obtained variance and that probably a larger proportion will remain unexplained. This is illustrated in a large-scale transnational study carried out in the Netherlands, Switzerland, Hungary and the United States. A very large sample (7,000–8,000) of young people in the age range 15–19 took part in this research (Vazsonyi *et al.*, 2002; Vazsonyi, Pickering, Junger and Hessing, 2001). The researchers found that different portions of the variance in self-reported offending were associated with separate predictor variables. Patterns of everyday routine activities explained 16–18 per cent of the variation in offending amongst sample members. Similarly, individual differences in self-control explained 16–20 per cent of the variance. Other portions of the variance remained unaccounted for by the measures employed. Reliance on a small number of personality dimensions has largely been supplanted by more elaborate models of how individual factors relate to the risk of committing a criminal offence.

In conclusion, what we have tried to show here is that many factors contribute to crime and the patterning of crime, and that they originate from different 'levels' of causation from 'macro' to 'micro'. A full and clear picture can be obtained only by drawing on all of them in combination. It is to such an integrative approach that we turn in the next chapter.

Chapter summary

This chapter has provided a historical sketch of crime, and of some of the ideas that have been used in seeking to understand it, stretching back nearly 200 years. Many of the ideas that developed in the early phase of this attempt, albeit in modified form and using different terminology, are still applicable today.

The chapter advanced from the concepts of correlation and of risk factors, which were introduced in Chapter 3, towards the idea of causation, which is central to the task of theoretical explanation. It surveyed the principal theories that have been formulated in attempts to explain what gives rise to criminal activity.

Theories were presented in terms of a series of five 'levels of explanation':

1 Society-wide, large-scale explanation.

2 Understanding locality-based or neighbourhood-based variations.

3 Focus on proximate human groups – the influence of familiar, regular contacts.

4 Individuals seen from the 'outside' – everyday behaviour and crime opportunities.

5 Individuals as influenced by internal events and processes – the psychological level.

Further reading

» There are numerous books on criminological theories. Amongst the best for exploring the areas covered in this chapter in greater depth are those by Thomas J. Bernard, Jeffrey B. Snipes and Alexander L. Gerould (2015), *Vold's Theoretical Criminology* (New York: Oxford University Press); by J. Robert Lilly, Francis T. Cullen and Richard A. Ball (2014), *Criminological Theory: Context and Consequences* (Thousand Oaks: Sage Publications); and by Francis T. Cullen, John Paul Wright and Kristie R. Blevins (2008), *Taking Stock: The Status of Criminological Theory* (New Brunswick: Transaction Publishers).

» For a wide-ranging edited volume that includes chapters on the most prominent theories, including psychological and sociological approaches, see the book edited by Eugene McLaughlin and Tim Newburn (2010), *The Sage Handbook of Criminological Theory* (London: Sage Publications). For an extended discussion and appraisal of the General Theory of Crime, see Erich Goode (2008), *Out of Control: Assessing the General Theory of Crime.* Stanford, CA: Stanford University Press. There are also several valuable collections of readings containing key articles, such as those edited by Gregg Barak (1998), Peter Cordella and Larry Siegel (1996) and Stuart Henry and Werner Einstadter (1998).

» Unfortunately, some of these sources pay only limited attention to psychologically based theories; and even when they do, they focus on concepts that many psychologists would now consider limited or out of date. Contemporary psychological models are dealt with in greater depth by James Bonta and Don A. Andrews (2017), *The Psychology of Criminal Conduct*, 6th edition (New York: Routledge), and by Clive R. Hollin (2013) *Psychology and Crime*, 2nd edition (London: Routledge).

Understanding Criminal Acts and Actors

Following on from Chapter 4, the present chapter focuses more closely on *psychological* factors involved in the path into breaking the law. It draws on research in developmental and social psychology, as well as from criminology, to understand how variables at different levels influence the emergence of behaviour problems and later delinquency, and discusses what is known about how they interact.

Chapter objectives

- To survey research on the contribution of different sets of factors in the causation of crime.
- To focus specifically on the possible roles of several types of influences:
  - heredity or genetic endowment
  - temperament and personality
  - socialisation, via families, peers, the media and culture
  - cultural influences
  - situational influences
  - internal (cognitive-emotional) processes.
- To present an integrative model of the interaction of people and situations.

As we noted in Chapters 3 and 4, numerous influences have been associated with the occurrence of criminal acts. To put it at its simplest, there is no single variable to which we can point and say, '*That* is the cause of crime.' Like other types of behavioural and social problems, antisocial and illegal conduct is influenced by a number of variables, and is usually described as multifactorial in origin. We should also bear in mind that to qualify as a 'risk factor' (such as those we encountered in Chapter 3), a variable need only be *correlated* with offending or antisocial behaviour – that variable may or may not be causal. Moffitt and Caspi probably voiced the thoughts of many in the field when they asserted that research on antisocial behaviour is 'stuck at the "risk-factor" stage' (2007, p. 97). Nevertheless, there are highly developed theoretical accounts of the factors that influence antisocial behaviour rather than being simply correlated with it. In this chapter and in Part 2 of the book, we will take a closer look at some of them.

What should we include in such a multifactorial model? The simplest approach involves three broad categories: *biological*, *psychological* and *social*. This has led – no prizes for guessing it – to the widely referenced **biopsychosocial model**. Under each of those very capacious headings we can list subgroups of variables. For example:

» under 'biological': evolutionary, genetic, neurological, temperamental

» under 'psychological': learning, cognition, personality, attitudinal, self-regulation

» under 'social': family, neighbourhood, structural, economic, cultural.

Below each of those headings there could be a more precisely demarcated level of factors, potentially listing large numbers of more specific variables. Still further below is an extremely finely tuned level at which we can examine which variables operated for *this* person in *that* situation and led him or her to do *those* things.

While researchers have been able to distinguish some of the variables involved as triggers for illegal acts, the ways in which those variables interact are not well understood. To make matters more complicated, it is possible that the interactions themselves take several forms, suggesting that a general model of – for example – the causation of violence might remain hard to articulate and in the end prove elusive. That could require us to develop a set of interconnected models applicable to different categories of aggression or violence.

The present chapter focuses on the general types of factors that have been shown to contribute to the occurrence of crime in general, and of violent acts in particular, and to the establishment of a pattern of repeated violent conduct where that occurs. We begin with a much-debated question.

Heredity and crime

Is there a 'gene for crime' – or, more specifically, for violent crime? The court decision cited in the 'Focus on ...' item on Evidence of a gene–environment (G×E) interaction (page 85) seems to imply that potentially there might be. The question has been a controversial one for many years. Essentially, the same issue arises in many areas of psychology, in the ubiquitous 'nature–nurture' debate. Given, as we saw in Chapter 4, that there is evidence of a concentration of crime in some families, and what plausibly looks like familial transmission of crime, many people might well assume that the most likely mechanism for this is heredity. In the late 19th and early 20th century there was a widespread view that many aspects of human conduct were strongly influenced, if not wholly determined, by hereditary factors.

The most extreme manifestations of this was a eugenicist programme of enforced sterilisation of groups thought to be deficient in socially desirable properties, such as intellectual ability. This was pursued in a number of countries. The most notorious example was under the Third Reich in Germany, where it is estimated that between 1933 and 1945 as many as 400,000 persons were forcibly sterilised. Even after World War II, however, the practice continued in several countries until as recently as the 1980s. It was by no means confined to authoritarian states: those involved included some of the world's most highly esteemed open, democratic societies, such as Sweden, Switzerland, and the United States. Today, enforced sterilisation is condemned as a crime against humanity under the Rome Statute of the International Criminal Court, which became operational in 2002.

It is perhaps because of these disreputable associations that the search for the biological basis of individual differences has been seen by some as tainted, and as ideologically driven. In a survey of attitudes to this issue amongst criminologists, Ellis and Walsh (1997) found that a majority of their colleagues were avoidant of biologically based explanations of crime, and some have even been depicted as 'biosocial-phobic'. Psychologists, by contrast, more often lean towards recognising the necessity of including biological variables in our explanatory models. Part of that stance draws on research in the field of *behaviour genetics*, the study of the role of genetic factors in the formation of personality, patterns of behaviour, and other human attributes. Research in this field has generally adopted one of three principal designs:

» *Family or sibling studies* Children who vary in their degree of biological relatedness (e.g. full siblings versus half-brothers and half-sisters) are compared in their behavioural features.

» *Twin studies* Comparisons are made between the traits and behaviours of identical (monozygotic or MZ) and non-identical (dizygotic or DZ) twins.

» *Adoption studies* These take twin studies a stage further by comparing MZ and DZ twins who were brought up by their biological parents with others raised by adoptive parents.

The standard information sought from these studies is a statistic called **heritability** (h^2), which is an estimate of the amount of variation in a given attribute that is due to the action of genes. This can be expressed as a correlation coefficient or as a percentage, either of which represents a quantitative indicator across a population of the relationship between the *genotype*, which is the specific combination of *alleles* (gene variants) *carried* by each individual, and the *phenotype*, which is the resultant *expression* of an inherited trait shown in the observable characteristics of individuals (Lewis, 2011). It is important to realise that this statistic applies at the aggregate or population level, and can tell us little or nothing about the reasons why any given individual acts as he or she does. Furthermore, even when heritability has been calculated in a research study, the results 'apply only to the specific balance of genetic and environmental variation in the time and place in which its participants grew up' (Moffitt, 2005, p. 58). Carrying out a similar study in a separate population could produce a different figure for h^2.

The meaning of the heritability statistic is very often misinterpreted. The figure obtained describes the amount of variability within the selected study population that can confidently be attributed to the operation of genes. But, as Bentall (2009, p. 126) has pointed out in relation to mental health problems, 'there can be massive environmental influences lurking behind this statistic, even when it is calculated as being very high'. A heritability coefficient reflects a pattern of variation: it is not an indicator of a cause-and-effect relationship. An illustration of this can be seen in the work of Turkheimer *et al.*, (2003), who found that the extent of heritability of IQ differed as a function of socioeconomic status. Heritability was higher in families who were comfortably off, among whom there was lower environmental variation, than in families from more deprived backgrounds, whose environments were less uniform. There are also significant cross-national differences in the part played by gene–environment interactions in relation to intelligence. While such effects are positive and moderate in size in the USA, in Western Europe and Australia they are zero or reversed (Tucker-Drob and Bates, 2016). Lewontin (2006, and the accompanying commentaries) provides a more technical exposition of how to interpret the heritability statistic, and explains how even when it is high it cannot form the basis for any conclusions about cause-and-effect relationships.

The above methods have been applied in the behaviour-genetic study of crime in general, and also to specific aspects of crime such as aggressiveness. Moffitt and Caspi (2007) estimated that more than a hundred such studies had been conducted in attempts to answer this core question. Research in these areas has been reviewed in at least four meta-analyses. The first was reported by Walters (1992), who was relatively sceptical of the prospect that the gene–crime relationship might tell us anything of practical importance. What he considered to be the best heritability estimates, obtained from adoption studies, were of the order of 11–17 per cent. Reviewing twin studies with antisocial behaviour as the outcome, Mason and Frick (1994) found that the average heritability was 48 per cent. Focusing on studies of the scores of MZ and DZ twins on clinical personality inventories, Miles and Carey (1997) concluded that genetic factors accounted for as much as 50 per cent of the variance.

The most extensive meta-analysis was that of Rhee and Waldman (2002), who integrated results from 52 samples, comprising 149 groups and a total of 55,525 participant pairs. These authors reported their findings in terms of four main categories of influences on antisocial behaviour. Respective effect sizes for each of those were as follows: for additive genetic factors, 0.32; for non-additive genetic factors, 0.09; for shared environmental factors, 0.16; and for non-shared environmental influences, 0.43.

There is a wide spectrum of opinion on how to interpret the results of research in this area. According to behaviour geneticists such as Moffitt (2005), the general picture is one in which genes influence roughly 50 per cent of the variation in human antisocial behaviour; shared environmental influences within families account for a further 20 per cent or so; and unique environmental influences explain the remaining 30 per cent. Some studies have produced higher heritability estimates than this, however. One twin-based study of the genetic contribution to psychopathic traits – grandiosity, callousness, impulsiveness, irresponsibility and manipulativeness – obtained values of up to 0.56 (Larsson, Andershed and Lichtenstein, 2006). In a survey of twins by Baker *et al.*, (2007), the heritability of antisocial behaviour was estimated to be 0.96.

The opposite corner in this dispute, so to speak, has been occupied by sociological criminologists, perhaps the most prominent being Gottfredson and Hirschi (1990). These authors reviewed the evidence for the claim that genes play a significant role in the intergenerational transmission of criminal tendencies. Figure 5.1 shows their chain of reasoning. As we receive half our genes from each of our two parents, the average correlation between a father's genetic make-up and that of his son, a statistic called *relatedness* (or *coefficient of relationship*), *r*, is 0.5. If we accept median figures from behaviour genetics, the correlation between genotype and phenotype within each generation is given as 0.25. Applying these figures would result in a correlation between the father's criminality and that of his son of 0.031 ($0.5 \times 0.25 \times 0.25$). This figure would reduce rapidly in ensuing generations. Thus even with mid-range values for the elements of this equation, genetics seems unlikely to account for more than a very small proportion of the variance in the criminal behaviour of succeeding generations. On this basis Gottfredson and Hirschi, while not denying that biology may have some role to play in criminal activity, dismiss it as 'substantively trivial' (1990, p. 61).

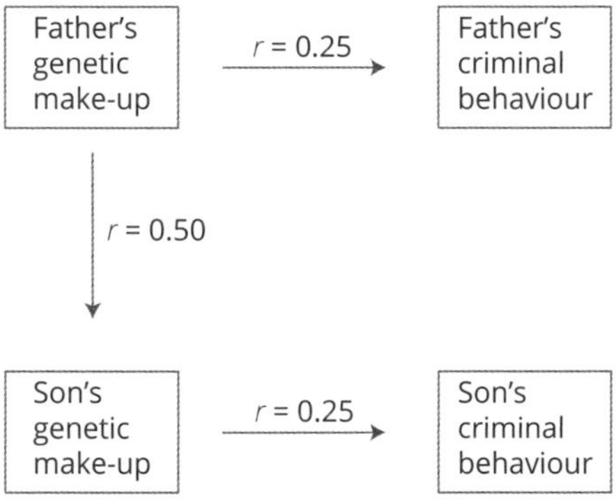
Father's genetic make-up
r = 0.25
Father's criminal behaviour
r = 0.50
Son's genetic make-up
r = 0.25
Son's criminal behaviour

Figure 5.1
Are genes involved in intergenerational transmission of criminal tendencies? Correlations necessary to produce an observed correlation of 0.031 between the criminal behaviour of fathers and sons.

Source: A General Theory of Crime by Gottfredson, M. R. & Hirschi, T. Copyright © 1990 by the Board of Trustees of the Leland Stanford Jr. University. All rights reserved. Used by permission of the publisher, Stanford University Press, sup.org

Heritability and genes

The *Human Genome Project* was a major international collaborative scientific undertaking, with the objective of mapping the sequencing of DNA of the human species – the *genome*. It involved researchers from 18 centres in 6 countries. The project was begun in 1989 and some of its work continues today. Its culminating achievement, confirmed in 2003, was the first complete mapping of the genome. It was reported that the human species possesses in the region of 23,000 genes, with a total of three billion units known as *nucleotides* which comprise the lengthy strands of the DNA molecule located within the chromosomes of each cell.

Given what is now known about the structure of the human genome, it is very unlikely that there could be any single gene that predetermined such a complex pattern of behaviour as that involved in committing a criminal offence. Most human characteristics are *polygenic* – that is, they are influenced by multiple genes whose expression and effects may vary according to the operation of other factors. As humans we have an estimated 99 per cent of our genes in common. Yet each of us is genetically unique: the small remaining fraction contributes to many of the differences between us.

A chromosome is made from a complex molecule called **DNA** *(deoxyribonucleic acid)*. A *gene* is a section of it at a fixed position on its length. Operating via intermediary molecules known as RNA (*ribonucleic acid*), each gene codes for the action of a protein or part of a protein inside the cell. This process is sometimes represented in the form: DNA → RNA → Protein, and Francis Crick, one of the scientists who discovered the structure of DNA, referred to it as the 'central dogma' of molecular biology (Baars and Gage, 2010). However, only a small proportion of our DNA consists of 'structural genes' that work in this way (Gibbs, 2003). The remainder is referred to as *noncoding* DNA (at one stage called 'junk DNA', as its function was not understood), and consists of several other types of molecules which may contribute to the functioning of *gene regulatory networks*. These operate in a number of ways to control the action of genes, and have been described as information-processing 'switches' that affect gene transcription and expression;

5

they can turn specific genes on or off according to external conditions. Thus it is possible to carry a gene that can have a specific effect, but for that not to be expressed in the phenotype. In relation to schizophrenia, for example, usually thought to be highly heritable, it is now estimated that there may be many thousands of gene variants that contribute to some genetic risk. However, there are no specific alleles that are known to present a unique risk for schizophrenia, and many of those identified to date are also part of the risk profile of several other serious mental disorders (Doherty, O'Donovan and Owen, 2011).

With respect to most complex behaviour, therefore, a direct gene influence is largely discounted. Nevertheless, there is a widespread recognition that genes play some role in complex behaviour, primarily through what are called gene–environment (G×E) interactions. An illustration of this is given in the accompanying 'Focus on ...' box. These proposals are more in accord with what we now know about the functioning of the human genome. Gottlieb (1998, 2000) reviewed evidence concerning the effects of environmental factors on gene expression in a number of different species including humans. For example, identical (MZ) twins brought up in different settings show considerable phenotypic variation. When we examine the respective roles of genes and environment in the emergence of specific problem behaviours, such as risky drinking in adolescence, research shows environmental factors are more important (Guerrini, Quadri and Thomson, 2014). Similar findings emerge across a wide range of mental disorders that are influenced by stress in the early stages of life (Cruceanu, Matosin and Binder, 2017).

While it is conceivable that G×E interactions may account for a proportion of the variance in aggression or in violent crime, even where heritability is estimated to be high, environmental and situational factors often have greater explanatory power, for two sets of reasons. First, even where behaviour is under sizeable genetic influence, this influence can fairly easily be reversed. Such an effect has been shown in research on the maze-learning abilities of rats. In what is regarded as classic work of its kind, Tryon (e.g. 1930, 1931, 1940) conducted an extended and carefully designed series of experiments over a period of 11 years. Tryon selectively bred 'maze-bright' and 'maze-dull' individuals for a series of 21 generations. After the seventh generation, there was no overlap in the error-rate of the two groups, though the gap did not continue to widen beyond that point. As the laboratory environment was kept uniform for both groups of rats, it was concluded that the difference between them was due to hereditary factors. However, in a study conducted several decades later, Cooper and Zubek (1958) found that the differences between 'bright' and 'dull' rats could become negligible within a single generation. When rats differing in selectively bred maze-running ability were placed in 'enriched' as compared to 'restricted' environments for a five-week period, their performance was altered dramatically by their learning experiences. In conditions of enriched learning opportunities, 'dull' rats equalled the performance of 'bright' rats.

Secondly, genetic factors appear unlikely to account for the large spatial and temporal variations in rates of crime. These include, for example, the international differences in rates of serious violent crimes (see Chapter 2). Genes would be fairly improbable explanations of the pattern discovered by the Chicago School, for example, in which the transitional zone showed the highest rate of all types of crime, a rate that remained higher than in other neighbourhoods regardless of the ethnic community living there, and given that the crime rate of temporary residents of the transitional zone fell after they moved elsewhere (see Chapter 4). Note, however, that at least one study has suggested that there is a relationship between the action of the MAOA gene, the level of 'youth saturation', and the amount of aggression in a neighbourhood (Hart and Marmorstein, 2009). Genes seem equally dubious as a means of explaining the decline in rates of serious crime in Europe since the 13th century (noted at the beginning of Chapter 4). And they offer very little hope of explaining cataclysmic eruptions of violence such as the genocides that took place in Cambodia (1972–1975), Rwanda (1994), or Bosnia-Herzegovina (1995).

5

FOCUS ON ...

Evidence of a gene–environment (G×E) interaction

In October 2009 it was reported in the journal *Nature* that an Italian court of law had reduced the sentence imposed on Abdelmalek Bayout, an Algerian immigrant who had been convicted of murder two years earlier (Feresin, 2009). The reason for this was that Mr Bayout had been found to have a variant gene that has been associated with a possible proclivity for aggression. This was the first occasion on which such evidence had been successfully used in a European court, though similar findings had been introduced in as many as 200 cases in the United States since the mid-1990s.

Mr Bayout was assessed as being mentally ill at the time of the offence, and so he initially received a shorter sentence than he would otherwise have done. His sentence was then commuted further following the submission of molecular biology evidence related to five different genes. The evidence that persuaded the judge to cut Mr Bayout's sentence concerned a gene known as MAOA (monoamine oxidase A).

Expression of the MAOA gene influences the level of activity of monoamine oxidase (MAO), an enzyme that in turn modulates the activity of the neurotransmitters norepinephrine, serotonin and dopamine. Low levels of MAO activity mean that these neurotransmitters are more active, a state that in turn has been associated with higher levels of aggression (Ellis, 1991).

The potential significance of this resides in findings of an association between the expression of MAOA and exposure to a specific environmental stressor: having been a victim of physical abuse in childhood. Caspi *et al*., (2002) found a striking set of results pertaining to this association.

These results emerged from the Dunedin Multidisciplinary Health and Development Study, briefly described in Chapter 3 (Table 3.1), in which individuals in a New Zealand birth cohort sample were followed up to the age of 26. From the overall pool of 1,037 participants at that stage of the study, researchers compared 163 children showing low MAOA activity with 279 children showing high MAOA activity, but also classified them into three subgroups according to suspected levels of experience of maltreatment. Of the children between the ages of 3 and 11, 8 per cent were grouped as having experienced 'Severe' maltreatment, 28 per cent as having experienced 'Probable' maltreatment, and 64 per cent as having experienced 'None'.

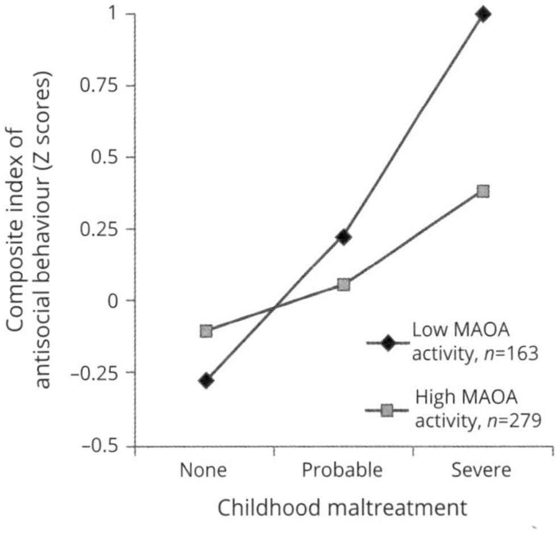
Composite index of antisocial behaviour (Z scores)
1
0.75
0.5
0.25
0
−0.25
−0.5
None
Probable
Severe
Childhood maltreatment
Low MAOA activity, n=163
High MAOA activity, n=279

Source: Caspi, A., McClay, J., Moffitt, T. E., Mill, J., Martin, J., Craig, I. W., Taylor, A. & Poulton, R. (2002). Role of Genotype in the Cycle of Violence in Maltreated Children. Science, 297 (5582), 851–854. Reprinted with permission from AAAS. http://science.sciencemag.org/content/297/5582/851

The dependent variable at age 26 was a composite index of antisocial behaviour, incorporating four measures: a record of conduct disorder in adolescence; convictions for violent crimes; symptoms of antisocial personality disorder (judged in each case by a third party who knew the sample participant well); and scores on a personality measure. What emerged was an interaction effect such that those with low MAOA activity and a history of severe ill-treatment were found to have significantly higher antisocial behaviour scores than other combinations. The levels of maltreatment varied more markedly amongst those with low MAOA activity. The results were as shown in the figure (Caspi *et al*., 2002).

Other researchers have checked whether this finding can be replicated with different samples. Some found no corresponding effect (Huizinga *et al*., 2006), but a meta-analysis supported the general trend (Kim-Cohen *et al*., 2006). Extending this across a total of eight studies, Taylor and Kim-Cohen (2007) found a significant difference between the effects of maltreatment at low and at high MAOA levels, and a later meta-analysis again confirmed the general trend (Byrd and Manuck, 2014).

For each of these patterns, a combination of social, psychological and political explanations offers a considerably more plausible account. While our cognitive and emotional processes and our social interactions are *underpinned* by biological mechanisms, they are also highly responsive to events and information in the internal and external environments. It is within those areas that we can find the 'best fit' and also the most parsimonious explanations of individual and group action.

Temperament

If inherited characteristics do play a part in the risk of someone developing a tendency to break the law later in life, it may be that this is most likely to happen distantly or indirectly through the influence of **temperament**. This term refers to biologically based individual differences in patterns of behavioural activity and emotional responding, which are evident prior to any extensive opportunity for learning and remain relatively stable, at least for the first few years of life (Kagan and Snidman, 2004; Rothbart, 2011). They may also be influenced by conditions and events *in utero* (prior to birth). The net effect is that from the moment of birth, some children appear to be more restless, fearful or anxious than others. They cope less well with short periods away from their parents (or other key caregivers). They may be more or less easy to placate when distressed; and clearly that in turn can have an impact on how caregivers respond to them. The patterning of this may change, of course, depending on the learning and socialisation experiences that ensue for any given child. The direction this development takes is largely influenced by the behaviour of caregivers, who in turn are influenced by their own circumstances, the conditions in which they themselves live, their own personalities and degree of well-being, and their own origins and developmental experiences.

The term 'temperament' is used to denote individual differences in children that are present prior to any identifiable learning experiences, and for that reason they are thought to be probably genetic in origin. Measurable variables within 'temperament' include the overall activity level, attentiveness versus distractibility, the quality and intensity of mood expression, relative proneness to distress, and adaptability to new situations (Chess and Thomas, 1990; Rothbart, Derryberry and Posner, 1994). Defined in this way, temperament has traditionally been regarded as distinct from *personality*, 'a more complex array of psychosocially shaped behavioral and cognitive preferences in adults' (Bijttebier and Roeyers, 2009, p. 306). Much research has, however, been focused on the extent of continuity between the two, and this is of particular interest in relation to the likelihood of conduct problems in childhood and of antisocial behaviour later on.

There is evidence that some early temperamental differences remain relatively stable and are maintained into the first few months and perhaps first few years of infant life, and in some cases preserved into the early adolescent years (Kagan, Snidman, Khan and Towsley, 2007). As a child grows, however, these characteristics are likely to be progressively modified or overlaid by the results of socialisation and other learning. Nevertheless, some longitudinal studies have uncovered noteworthy consistencies in temperament variables over quite lengthy periods. For example, Caspi *et al.*, (1995) compared observations of children when aged 3 with independent descriptions of them at age 15, and then with their own descriptions of themselves at age 18. Some 3-year-olds were described as 'under-controlled' and manifested irritability and impulsiveness (as rated by observers), and those were more likely to be described as having 'externalising' problems when aged 15. This term refers to aggression or other expressive or outwardly directed displays of negative feelings (colloquially, 'acting out'), as contrasted with 'internalising', which refers to changes in mood states or emotions which individuals experience within themselves, where negative reactions are inwardly focused. The pattern just described held for both girls and boys. When aged 18, children who had been described as under-controlled in infancy were more likely than others to describe themselves as reckless, careless and rebellious; and more prepared to cause discomfort or harm to others.

Lahey and Waldman (2003) proposed that there are three dimensions of temperament most relevant to the development of conduct problems: *negative emotionality*, *daring* and *prosociality*. They assembled evidence in support of these variables as fundamental factors in the emergence of persistent antisocial behaviour. Such stability as has been discovered is very likely to be a function of genotype–environmental interactions, and a **transactional model** such as that proposed by Dodge and Pettit (2003, p. 357) appears the best account of the data currently available. This incorporates the probability that certain predispositions elicit particular reactions from others. In other words, by acting in certain ways children may induce other people to respond to them in ways that are likely to reinforce how they are behaving. That may apply, for example, to a tendency towards **aggressiveness**. Where this becomes a regular or habitual feature of an individual child's interactions, it may be a function of temperamental and environmental variables acting in synergy. As illustrated in the next 'Focus on ...' box, there is evidence of some stability in the tendency towards aggressiveness over extended periods, though this declines gradually over time. There is a strong and reliable association between childhood aggression and adult criminality: the 59 studies pertaining to this that were summarised by Ellis, Beaver and Wright (2009) showed a very high degree of consistency – that is, the overwhelming majority of them showed a positive correlation between the two variables.

But we need to retain awareness of the complexity of this, and the underlying relationships are probably neither linear nor unidirectional. Researchers have concluded that it is unlikely that any single biological variable will define a temperamental bias:

> The immaturity of our current knowledge relating brain chemistry to human psychological states frustrates attempts to posit a lawful relation between a chemical profile and a particular temperament. Because genetic variation probably accounts

FOCUS ON ...

Stability of aggressiveness

Aggressiveness has been defined by Berkowitz (1993, p. 21) as 'a relatively persistent readiness to become aggressive in a variety of different situations'. Adopting a 'dispositional' perspective, we might expect such a tendency to be fairly stable over time.

This possibility has been evaluated in a number of studies. There are two reviews employing meta-analysis, the findings of which are illustrated in the graph (adapted from McGuire, 2004a). The vertical axis of the graph shows the size of correlations between measurements of aggression at two different points in time, given on the horizontal axis and varying from one to 21 years apart.

Olweus (1979, 1988) reported a review of 16 longitudinal studies that examined levels of consistency in aggressive behaviour over those time periods. The average size of samples in the studies he reviewed was 111.

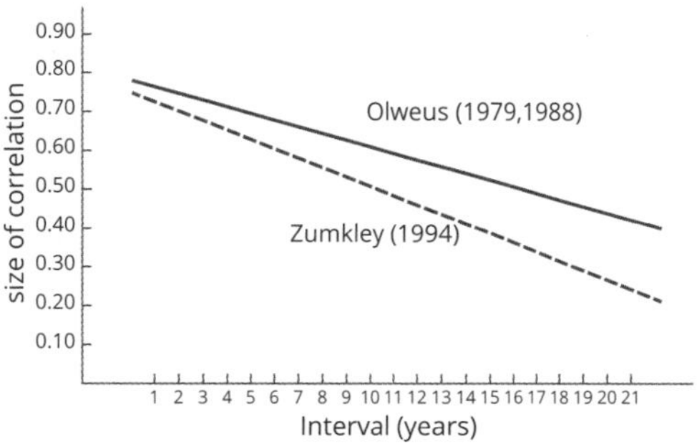
size of correlation
0.90
0.80
0.70
0.60
0.50
0.40
0.30
0.20
0.10
Olweus (1979,1988)
Zumkley (1994)
1 2 3 4 5 6 7 8 9 10 11 12 13 14 15 16 17 18 19 20 21
Interval (years)

Source: McGuire, J., Understanding psychology and crime: Perspectives on theory and action, © 2004. Reproduced with the kind permission of Open International Publishing Ltd. All rights reserved.

The dependent variables in the studies were not self-reports but nominations or ratings of aggressiveness by peers, teachers or other observers. From this dataset Olweus extracted a total of 24 correlation coefficients and plotted their interrelationships on a regression line. The results showed a striking degree of consistency over time, though, as we might expect, the correlations decreased with increasing intervals (e.g. reducing from 0.76 across one year to 0.36 across 21 years). In a later review, Zumkley (1994) analysed a further 10 studies, with an average sample size of 159, generating a further 34 correlation coefficients. As shown in the graph, this broadly confirmed the pattern found by Olweus.

In a study not included in these meta-analyses, Eron and Huesmann (1983; Huesmann, Eron and Dubow, 2002) reported a 22-year follow-up of a group of 409 individuals, and found 'moderately good predictability', though more so for men than for women. Peer-rated aggressiveness at age 8 was significantly correlated with measures of aggression at age 30 – including both self- and other ratings of aggression, numbers of convictions, seriousness of convictions, and driving while intoxicated – though the highest correlation obtained was 0.30, similar to the pattern in the graph.

In a study in Finland with 145 women and 154 men, Kokko and Pulkkinen (2005) found similar levels of stability for both groups, though slightly higher for males. Participants were assessed at ages 8, 14, 36 and 42. Ratings at earlier ages were by peers, and at later ages by self-report; 120 women and 122 men took part at age 42. There was higher stability within the two younger (8–14) and the two older (36–42) age ranges than between childhood and adulthood. Nevertheless, a latent variable measure of childhood aggression 'explained 18% of the variance of adult aggression and the stability estimate was 0.42 in both genders' (p. 494).

These findings are reinforced by others which show that bullying others in school is predictive of later antisocial outcomes, including adult criminality. This has been found over 8–10-year follow-up intervals in Germany and Sweden (Bender and Lösel, 2011; Olweus, 2011); and over a longer period in the UK, where bullying at age 14 predicted a variety of adverse outcomes up to 34 years later (Farrington and Ttofi, 2011) in the Cambridge Study in Delinquent Development. In a meta-analysis of 15 longitudinal studies, Ttofi, Farrington, Lösel and Loeber (2011) found that bullying was a significant risk factor for later offending, independently of other factors.

In the Concordia Longitudinal Risk Project, Temcheff *et al.*, (2008) reported a 30-year follow-up of 1,770 children from French-speaking, lower socioeconomic districts of Montreal. This study found a significant association between childhood aggression and self-reported violence towards a spouse amongst both males and females during adulthood.

The variations in these findings, with evidence of stability but some findings that run counter to that picture, might be best explained by the suggestion that there are subgroups within the study populations. Many individuals rarely if ever display marked aggression; a proportion are aggressive in childhood or adolescence but then desist; for others it emerges only in adulthood, while there is also a group that remain prone to aggression across all stages (Piquero *et al.*, 2012).

> for less than 10 per cent of the variation in most human behaviours, it is unlikely that any single allele for a neurotransmitter or receptor distribution will be the basis for a temperamental type. (Kagan and Snidman, 2004, pp. 69–70)

The self-regulatory aspect of temperament, as defined by Rothbart (2011), is likely to be closely linked to a personality variable that has been almost invariably associated with later offending: **impulsiveness** (sometimes called **impulsivity**). This has been described by Farrington (2007, p. 611) as 'the most crucial personality dimension that predicts offending'. It is not very well defined, however, and has been linked to a cluster of tendencies, listed by Farrington as including 'hyperactivity, restlessness, clumsiness, not considering consequences before acting, a poor ability to plan ahead, short time horizons, low self-control, sensation-seeking, risk-taking, and a poor ability to delay gratification' (2007,

p. 611). Numerous studies have found significant correlations between aspects of these variables, measured in childhood or adolescence, and criminality at various stages of adulthood. For example, longitudinal research in Sweden found close associations between *hyperactivity* (attention difficulties and motor restlessness) in the early teenage years (ages 13–15) and alcohol problems and violent offending up to the age of 35 (Eklund and Klinteberg, 2003; Klinteberg, Andersson, Magnusson and Stattin, 1993). In their overview of the correlates of crime, Ellis *et al.*, (2009) found 86 studies on the relationship between impulsivity and criminality, with a very high level of concordance amongst them. Note that impulsiveness also bears some strong resemblances to the self-control variable as conceptualised in the General Theory of Crime (which we encountered in Chapter 4), though Gottfredson and Hirschi (1990), the originators of that theory, traced individual differences in self-control almost exclusively to the effects of parenting. This has been challenged, however: although likelihood of involvement in crime may not be subject to direct genetic influence, a temperament variable such as self-control may well be. In a twin-based study, Beaver, Wright, DeLisi and Vaughn (2008) found evidence of a large genetic role in the variance of self-control and in its stability over time.

Other studies, however, have shown that impulsiveness is likely to have a mixture of determinants. Another candidate is the possibility that low self-control is at least in part a function of neuropsychological deficits. Ratchford and Beaver (2009) reported findings from the National Survey of Children, a large-scale follow-up study in the United States (with a sample size of 1,423). In relation to a picture vocabulary test regarded as a measure of neuropsychological functioning, children's performance in the age range 6–12 was found to be the strongest predictor of low self-control ten years later. Despite this, and despite a significant association between low self-control and involvement in delinquency, the strongest predictor of the latter was an index of parental punishment in childhood, with neuropsychological deficits proving non-significant.

Socialisation

The next major category of variables that influences the developing human organism derives from the actions of other people in the infant's immediate surroundings, through the process known as **socialisation**. This occurs both within individuals' families-of-origin, and also in many other contexts through all phases of the lifespan. Defined most broadly, it refers 'to the way in which individuals are assisted in becoming members of one or more social groups' (Grusec and Hastings, 2015, p. 1). The word 'assisted' is important here, because it suggests that those to whom this process is happening are not merely passive recipients but also play an active part in it themselves. In its more commonly used, narrower sense, however, 'socialisation' usually refers to 'processes whereby naïve individuals are taught the skills, behaviour patterns, values and motivations needed for competent functioning in the culture in which the child is growing up' (Maccoby, 2015, p. 3).

Family and upbringing

In most people's lives, the family is by far the most common context in which the processes of socialisation occur, and it is widely considered to be the most powerful influence on the course of socialisation, with a foundational, pervasive and even lifelong effect. The family in turn is subject to local neighbourhood conditions; and it is also the conduit of culture, through which the general expectations of a society are mediated to the developing individual. Families also have unique features derived from the histories of the parents and other members, and of the interactions between them. As Tolstoy observed in the celebrated opening lines of *Anna Karenina*, while 'all happy families resemble one another, each unhappy family is unhappy in its own way'. This was not intended to mean that all happy families are the same: just that they have some basic features in common.

Socialisation processes

Research findings suggest that socialisation processes within families are possibly the largest single source of variation with respect to a child's future risk of involvement in criminal conduct. Drawing on several types of research, including the longitudinal studies surveyed in Chapter 3, it has been possible to identify some of the main aspects of socialisation that are risk factors for such involvement. You may recall from Chapter 3 the recurrent finding that a comparatively small proportion of those individuals who break the law are responsible for a far larger proportion of recorded crimes (represented in simplified graphical form in Figure 3.1). That pattern applies also to families, and it is useful to understand what features of families may be most closely associated with an increased risk for delinquent conduct.

First, some broad structural features of families are correlates of participation in offending. They include parental criminality: having a father or mother with a history of offending predicts a heightened risk of arrest for young people. So too does having other close relatives - siblings, uncles and aunts, or grandparents - who have had offending careers. Ellis and his colleagues (2009) found 69 studies of this association, with a high level of consistency emerging. However, the most important individual relative in this respect appears to be the father (Farrington, 2007). A second correlate is larger family size: in the Cambridge Study in Delinquent Development, having four or more siblings was associated with a doubling of the risk of being convicted in the teenage years, and similar findings have been obtained in several other longitudinal studies (Farrington, 2007). Here too Ellis *et al.*, (2009) found a large amount of agreement among the 64 studies they surveyed. This trend is generally thought to be an effect of the lesser amount of attention that parents can give to each child as the number of children increases, though it could also be a result of overcrowding and stress, or other resource limitations. Stress may give rise to internal family conflict, or may be an indirect index of broader socioeconomic disadvantage, or both. Family dysfunction and conflict are very significantly associated with children's later involvement in delinquency, producing one of the highest consistency scores in the review by Ellis *et al.*, (2009) for the 55 studies they list that addressed this question.

Aspects of parenting

Several specific aspects of parenting or child-rearing have been found to be associated with an elevated risk of later criminal involvement. Consider the period from the moment of birth until the day, typically approaching 20 years later, when the individual, having reached early adulthood, leaves the family home. During those years he or she will probably have spent more time being influenced by and interacting with his or her parents (or their equivalent) than anyone else. Those exchanges will have had a profound formative impact on how the developing child perceived and learned to respond to the surrounding world. The influence of parents will have extended to periods when they were not physically present, because of their role as the main decision-makers concerning the type of home the family inhabits, the neighbourhood where they reside, the school the child attended, and the range of opportunities to gain independence that have been allowed and encouraged - or, alternatively, frowned upon or forbidden. Parents, and the home environment they create, are thus of paramount importance in shaping how an individual develops.

The Millennium Cohort Study (Sabates and Dex, 2012) followed up a sample of 18,818 children born in the United Kingdom in 2000–2001. Developmental disadvantages faced by these children were quantified in terms of ten risk indicators, according to whether one or both of the parents manifested or was experiencing: (a) depression; (b) disability or long-term illness; (c) substance abuse; (d) alcohol dependence problems; (e) domestic violence; (f) financial stress; (g) worklessness; (h) teenage parenthood; (i) lack of basic skills; and (j) overcrowding. There was clear evidence that the larger the number of risk factors to which a growing child was exposed, the greater the likelihood of adverse consequences in the child's life. Of greatest relevance here was the finding that children subject to more risks were significantly likelier to have conduct problems and hyperactivity, two characteristics that are generally amongst the firmest predictors of later delinquency. Those in the lowest of six income bands also showed significantly higher levels of these problems than those in the other five bands. There were also sizeable differences in risk exposure between ethnic groups. Within the study sample, 27–28 per cent of families faced two or more risks; extrapolating from this, the authors estimated that these conditions applied to approximately 192,000 children across the UK.

In general terms, studies confirm that the larger the number of factors such as these that are present in adverse form earlier in life, the greater the likelihood that a young person will later be convicted of a criminal offence (Snyder, Reid and Patterson, 2003). One particularly striking result from the Pittsburgh Youth Study was that young males with four or more risk factors were 14 times more likely that those with fewer than four to go on to commit homicide (Loeber *et al.*, 2005). These results notwithstanding, we should keep in mind that there are still many sources of uncertainty when attempting to use data of this kind for predictive purposes, for example in risk assessment.

The actions and attitudes of parents, and the prevailing pattern of care or supervision they provide, are major determinants of the growing person's experiences. This has been analysed into a number of separate factors or dimensions. They include, in early childhood, the consistency of parental supervision; the quality of the parent–child relationship; and the development of attachments or bonds, influenced by the level of warmth (versus coldness or aloofness) in the relationship. Later, the methods used to control or discipline the child, and the frequency of punishment, are important factors. Later still, as the child spends periods at school or with friends, the extent of the parents' monitoring of what he or she is doing becomes progressively more important. If children are left to their own devices and if parents do not know where they are, whom they are with or what they may be getting up to, there is an increased risk of possible involvement in mischief and later in delinquency. This is not merely a hand-wringing mantra of worried social commentators but has some empirical support. In a survey of 1,170 middle school pupils (mean age 12.7 years), Flannery, Williams and Vazsonyi (1999) found that low levels of parental monitoring were strongly associated with higher levels of aggressive and delinquent behaviour and substance misuse. This applied to both males and females.

Throughout development, the amount of time parents spend with a child, and the clarity or consistency of the messages they give about the world the child is growing into, will affect what he or she comes to expect, to believe or to value. Each of these has been associated with later participation in juvenile offending, both separately and in combination. This has emerged from several of the classic longitudinal studies, such as the Cambridge-Somerville Youth Study (McCord, 1979, 1992), the Pittsburgh Youth Study (Loeber *et al.*, 2005), and the Cambridge Study in Delinquent Development (Farrington, 2007), amongst others.

Two meta-analyses have examined the strength of associations between aspects of parenting and later delinquent involvement. Leschied, Chiodo, Nowicki and Rodger (2008) integrated data from 38 prospective longitudinal studies incorporating a total sample of 66,647 participants. Hoeve *et al.*, (2009) synthesised results from 119 independent studies, some employing longitudinal designs, but also including a larger batch of 88 cross-sectional studies. Given the different methodologies used, it is reassuring that the findings from these two reviews show a high level of agreement.

Leschied *et al.*, (2008) found that the influence of family processes increased according to the age of the child (i.e. those operating in adolescence had larger effects than those for early and middle childhood). 'Dynamic' family factors that were identified as significant included coercive, inconsistent parenting; structural variables, such as the marital status of the parents and involvement of the child in the welfare system; and family violence (the last irrespective of the age of the child). Hoeve *et al.*, (2009) studied parental support for and control of children and analysed these into several dimensions.

5

They found that parental affection and positive support were associated with lower rates of delinquency, while neglect, rejection and hostility were associated with higher rates. On control, they found that while this was generally linked to lower likelihood of delinquency, some dimensions of it were associated with the reverse. Notably, higher delinquency rates were linked to inconsistent discipline and use of psychological methods of control. Such methods referred to 'parents who keep their child dependent, try to change the feelings of their child, use guilt to control the child or ignore the child as a form of punishment' (2009, p. 757). One particular aspect that emerged from early research in this area, and one that has been studied fairly intensively, is a pattern of coercive interaction that occurs within some families and is particularly associated with the development of aggressiveness in children. This is described more fully in the 'Focus on ...' box below.

Family disruption

Where there is disruption in families, there are heightened risks of adjustment problems and of delinquency amongst children. Thornberry *et al.*, (1999) analysed the

FOCUS ON ...

Coercive family process and coercion theory

One of the most thorough, intensive and fruitful programmes of research on patterns of interactions in families, and of their effects on child behaviour, has been conducted at the Oregon Social Learning Centre (OSLC) over a more than 30-year period. This has made key contributions to knowledge and understanding in this field, and was one of the origins of the idea of parent training as a means of improving the behaviour and well-being of troubled children.

In the course of many separate studies, researchers at the OSLC were able to carry out direct observations of family interactions in the natural setting of the home, working with 200 families of children who had been identified as aggressive, and a comparison sample of 60 families. These observations led to the formulation of a model of **coercive family process** (Patterson, 1982; Patterson, Dishion and Bank, 1984). This describes a cyclical process of 'negative microsocial exchange', whereby a parent and child reciprocally influence each other's behaviour. Their responses are mutually interdependent and result in 'mixed schedules of *positive* and *negative* reinforcement plus frequent punishment' (Patterson *et al.*, 1984, p. 256).

Initially, in such a sequence, the child might engage in minor aversive behaviours such as belligerence towards a sibling. This elicits attention from an irritated parent, followed by a reprimand, but the parent's attention soon turns elsewhere again. To regain attention, the child then escalates the behaviour (or another more problematic action), even where this might provoke a sharper reaction from the parent. The response and feedback loop continues in an ascending spiral, until eventually the parent focuses more attention on the child. Alternatively, a parallel cycle may enable children to terminate unwanted intrusions by parents, for example when they ask a child to carry out a household chore (Reid, Patterson and Snyder, 2002). Even where these actions involve some punishment along the way, ultimately the achievement of a desired outcome reinforces the aggressive behaviour. The net effect is that parental reactions intended to reduce the likelihood of a behaviour they find aversive (such as child aggression) may work in the short term but may inadvertently serve to increase its likelihood in the long term.

Patterns like this that are learned within a family can carry into situations outside it (Dishion, Patterson and Kavanagh, 1992). Essentially, through this process parents are unwittingly training their children to fight, and this training is transferred to the children's interactions with others outside the home, as illustrated in the figure (Patterson, Dishion and Bank, 1984).

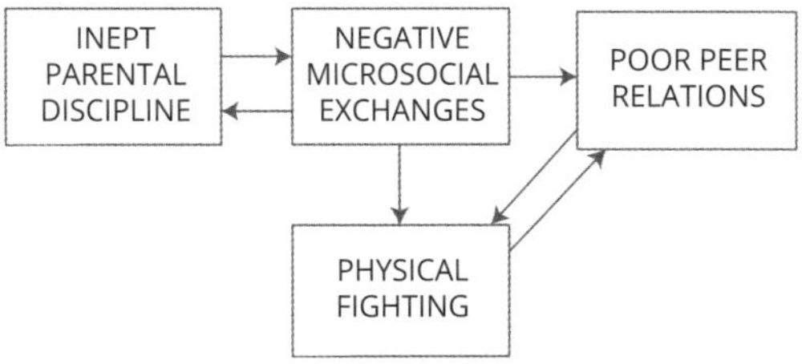
INEPT PARENTAL DISCIPLINE
NEGATIVE MICROSOCIAL EXCHANGES
POOR PEER RELATIONS
PHYSICAL FIGHTING

Source: Figure 1 Hypothesized social interactional model of physical fighting. From Patterson, G. R., Dishion, T. J. & Bank, L. (1984). Family Interaction: A Process Model of Deviancy Training. Aggressive Behavior, 10 (3), 253–267, Wiley-Liss, Inc. Copyright © 1984 Alan R. Liss, Inc. DOI: 10.1002/1098-2337(1984)10:3<253::AID-AB2480100309>3.0.CO;2-2

There is evidence that these patterns are worsened by economic hardship within families, which causes additional stress (Conger *et al.*, 1994). This is thought to operate through a series of causal connections between financial pressure, parents' low mood and marital conflict. Parents and children may argue over money issues, with growing antagonism between them. Later, during adolescence and adulthood, what might be described as the individual's 'traits' are in part the outcome of a lengthy series of numerous parent–child micro-exchanges within a process of accumulated social learning.

The coercive family process model has been extensively tested and numerous confirmatory findings have been obtained (see, for example, Eddy, Leve and Fagot, 2001). The model was also extended and formally restated as *Coercion Theory* (Reid, Patterson and Snyder, 2002).

possible impact of *transitions* on young people's behaviour, by combining data from three longitudinal studies with an aggregate sample of over 4,000 young people. 'Transition' refers here to a change in the family composition within the four-year period studied, due, for example, to the breakdown of the parental/caregiver relationship, the separation of parents, or the arrival of step-parents. At two of the sites (Rochester (NY) and Denver), there was a clear and statistically significant association between the number of transitions and levels of self-reported delinquency and substance use; and there was a similar but non-significant trend in the third (Pittsburgh), where the level of family disruption was considerably lower than in the other two. This relationship held when other factors (e.g. family poverty or initial family structure) were controlled and tests were run to ensure the temporal ordering of events (i.e. that transitions preceded delinquency involvement).

These findings are echoed by others related to the much-debated question of whether growing up in a single-parent family places a youth at higher risk of becoming involved in delinquency. Demuth and Brown (2004) studied a sample of 16,304 participants from the US National Longitudinal Survey of Adolescent Health (*Add Health*), begun in 1994–1995. They compared rates of delinquency amongst adolescents from four configurations: with two biological parents, with a single mother, with a single father, and with a step-family. Dual-parent families had significantly lower rates of delinquency than the other three clusters. However, when family-process variables (parental involvement, supervision, and monitoring of the child) were added to the statistical model, the family structural variables were reduced to non-significance.

Maltreatment and neglect

Parental conflict and poor or inconsistent supervision are associated in overall terms with higher risks for later delinquency. If difficulties of these kinds are overlaid with neglect, or with emotional, physical or sexual abuse, the risk that a child will later develop problems of various kinds is increased substantially. These links have been extensively studied, and a strong pattern emerges from the review of crime correlates by Ellis *et al.*, (2009). Of the 54 studies they found where this association was examined, 52 showed that maltreated children were more likely to be involved in crime. Childhood victimisation and neglect are associated not only with elevated risks of antisocial behaviour, but also with later involvement in substance abuse, experience of psychological distress, and development of serious mental health problems such as schizophrenia (Min, Farkas, Minnes and Singer, 2007; Read, van Os, Morrison and Ross, 2005). Maltreatment of children is usually divided into four broad categories; the following draws on the definitions used by the World Health Organization (Butchart, Harvey, Mian and Fürniss, 2006, p. 10):

» *Physical abuse* The intentional use of physical force against a child that results in, or has a high likelihood of resulting in, harm to the child's health, survival, development or dignity. This includes hitting, beating, shaking, and the many other forms of assault.

» *Sexual abuse* The involvement of a child in sexual activity that he or she does not fully comprehend, to which he or she is unable to give informed consent, or for which the child is not developmentally prepared; or that violates the laws or social taboos of society.

» *Emotional and psychological abuse* This involves 'both isolated incidents as well as a pattern of failure over time on the part of a parent or caregiver to provide a developmentally appropriate and supportive environment' (Butchart et al., 2006, p.10). Abuse may include restriction of movement, belittling, blaming, threatening, frightening, ridiculing, or other forms of rejection or hostile treatment.

» *Neglect* This involves 'both isolated incidents, as well as a pattern of failure over time on the part of a parent or other family member to provide for the development and well-being of the child' (Butchart et al., 2006, p.10) in relation to health, education, emotional development, nutrition, or shelter and safe living conditions.

Survey data reviewed by the WHO (Butchart *et al.*, 2006) and by the International Society for the Prevention of Child Abuse and Neglect suggest that between 25–50 per cent of all children report severe and frequent physical abuse, and 20 per cent of women and 5–10 per cent of men report having been sexually abused as a child. Gilbert *et al.*, (2008) reported a review of the data on prevalence of different forms of child maltreatment in high-income countries. They discovered large differences between the officially recorded rates of maltreatment and those obtained from self-report studies. It seems almost certain that the former significantly underestimate the extent of the problem. Collating the evidence, Gilbert and her colleagues (2008) concluded that there are strong indications of a long-term harmful effect of childhood victimisation, increasing the likelihood of involvement in delinquency and violence in later years. Evidence concerning the prevalence and the impact of childhood maltreatment has led governments of many countries to implement special policies to tackle the problem. It appears difficult, however, to detect clear-cut effects of such policy initiatives. A study of this in six of the world's most affluent nations found 'no clear evidence for an overall decrease in child maltreatment despite decades of policies designed to achieve such reductions' (Gilbert *et al.*, 2012, p. 770). Large differences that exist between countries – such as child poverty and child mortality being three times higher in the USA than in Sweden, and rates of violent deaths also being very much higher – remain stubbornly impervious to child protection measures.

This is not an encouraging outlook. Apart from its numerous other sequelae, there is consistent evidence that childhood maltreatment is a precursor of later aggression and of involvement in violent crime. To understand the connections, it may be important first to examine the factors thought to be associated with child maltreatment itself. In an effort to accomplish this, Stith and her colleagues (2009) integrated findings from 155 studies of the association between 39 risk factors for child maltreatment and its actual occurrence. The review and its results were conceptualised within a *microsystem* comprising the interplay of four main categories of variables: characteristics of parents, of children, and of families; and features of parent–child interactions. Their study generated a total of 656 effect sizes. The largest to be found for physical abuse were parental anger and hyperactivity, and also two family-process features – high levels of conflict, and low levels of cohesion. For neglect, parent–child interactions and the parent's perception of the child as a problem showed the largest effect sizes. There were moderate effect sizes for several other factors. Some caution should, however, be exercised in interpreting these results. As the authors indicate, the necessity of confining their literature search to a single database (PsycINFO), even if this is the one most likely to access the key research in this area, together with other exclusion criteria they employed, may mean that their final set of studies is unrepresentative of the field as a whole.

Moving to the further link between exposure to abuse or neglect and later involvement in criminal offences, including violence, several studies have obtained very similar findings. One of the earliest and still one of the best known is that of Widom (1989), who compared official arrest records of a sample of 908 abused and neglected children with those of 667 matched controls. Followed up over a 20-year period, the former were 55 per cent more likely to have had a record of juvenile delinquency, 35 per cent more likely to have an adult criminal record, and 42 per cent more likely to have been arrested for a violent crime. Later violence was associated with physical but not sexual abuse during childhood. Concerning what was then known as the 'cycle of violence' hypothesis, however, Widom (1989) was careful to point out that these were *risk factors* for later violence (i.e. the associations were probabilistic), and while 11 per cent of the abused and neglected individuals were later arrested for violence, eight times as many – 89 per cent – were not.

Lansford *et al.*, (2007) reported results of the Knoxville-Nashville-Bloomington Child Development Project, a longitudinal study of 574 children followed between the ages of 5 and 21. Those who had been physically abused during the first five years of life were significantly more likely to be convicted of an offence over the ensuing 17 years, and while this was far more likely to be a non-violent than a violent offence, the latter difference was also significant. Those who had suffered abuse also reported other difficulties more often, such as having been dismissed from a job. Maas, Herrenkohl and Sousa (2008) reviewed findings from eight longitudinal studies (including the work of Widom, but not that of Lansford *et al.*) with a cumulative sample of 8,659. They reported 'compelling evidence of a link between child maltreatment and later violence in youth' (p. 62), though this was often moderated by other factors and, as in other studies, the strongest effects were for physical abuse. The authors considered that physical abuse may be the most consistent predictor of youth violence.

Maltreatment may also have a particular association with the likelihood of carrying a weapon. Self-protection theory is a model designed to explain the links between previous experiences of threat, perceived vulnerability, having witnessed violence, and the felt need to have a means of protection available. As part of a longitudinal study (the LONGSCAN project; Runyan *et al.*, 1998), T. Lewis and her colleagues (2007) investigated this in a large sample (n=797) of 12-year-olds. The strongest effect was for gender, with boys being eight times more likely than girls to carry a weapon. Regardless of gender, however, those who had been physically or sexually abused were respectively 2.7 and 4.2 times more likely to perceive the need to carry a weapon, and 2.8 and 4.4 times more likely to actually carry one, than those with no abuse history. Similar findings have been obtained in other studies on this issue. Note, however, that of those who had experienced abuse, the majority did *not* carry a weapon, so other factors must be involved in mediating that outcome.

There are multiple causal interconnections between the variables we have reviewed so far. An accumulation of risk factors linked to low socioeconomic status (social deprivation, low income level and poor housing) places families and parents under significant strain. This is thought likely to affect the emotional states and everyday behaviour of parents or other caregivers, and the manner in which they respond to children. Some studies have illuminated the intermediate links in a chain of processes through which economic hardship may be associated with problem behaviour and in due course involvement in delinquency.

To illustrate this, consider some other findings from the Knoxville-Nashville-Bloomington Project (mentioned above). Dodge, Pettit and Bates (1994) tracked the progress of 585 children involved in the study over a four-year period from age 4 to age 7. Information was collected from their parents concerning the family's economic circumstances, typical socialisation practices, and other conditions in the home; and from teachers and classmates concerning the children's behaviour in school. The latter was described mainly in terms of the presence or absence of 'externalising' problems, one aspect of which was the extent to which a child was involved in fighting, or in threatening, others. The best prediction of the level of a child's externalising or aggressive problems came not from direct socioeconomic indicators, but from a set of pathways involving intermediate events, including patterns of interaction within the family. The latter included harsh disciplinary methods, exposure to violence, low maternal support or warmth, maternal endorsement of aggressive values, transient contacts with people outside the family, and low levels of cognitive stimulation. Thus the association between family hardship and the child's behaviour was mediated through aspects of interactional processes inside the family.

Peer influence

The process of socialisation is essentially one of learning: basic mechanisms such as **modelling** and observational learning play a direct part in the shaping of it. As suggested earlier, that process is not confined to families but occurs in many other contexts as well. As development proceeds, individuals have increasing amounts of contact with people outside the family home, including neighbours, teachers, friends and, in due course, partners. All these interactions have an influence. Also influential are the formations known as peer-groups; and where their members experiment with delinquency and gradually become entrenched on the wrong side of the law, peer-groups may evolve into gangs.

The role of peer influence raises important questions, because there is considerable – some might say voluminous – evidence that the preponderance of offending by young people is committed in groups, and such involvement typically represents the major arterial route into crime. There are variations in pathways within this; and also after the age of (approximately) 20, when differences between 'adolescence-limited' and 'life-course-persistent' offenders (see Chapter 3) emerge more clearly (Piquero and Moffitt, 2005). But numerous studies, whether in-depth and cross-sectional (Baldwin, Bottoms and Walker, 1976) or longitudinal (Reiss and Farrington, 1991), attest that co-offending is the modal pattern amongst young people who break the law. Some individuals may of course falsely claim in mitigation that they 'fell in with a bad crowd', but there is evidence that this kind of transmission genuinely does occur. For example, exposure to the acts of a violent accomplice during a first joint offence increases an initially non-violent individual's likelihood of offending violently later (Conway and McCord, 2002).

Findings from the National Youth Survey (NYS), a longitudinal study in the USA following a large sample of young people between the ages of 11 and 17, have thrown light on several aspects of this. Studies suggest that social reinforcement, whether vicarious or direct, is a crucial influence on the establishment of patterns of antisocial behaviour. Warr and Stafford (1991) analysed data from 1,726 respondents to the NYS, concerning participation in three types of illicit behaviour: cheating in exams; using marijuana; and theft. The behaviour of friends proved to be a stronger predictor of individuals' own actions than either their friends' or even their own expressed attitudes.

These social influences are not, of course, the sole determinants of delinquent involvement, but interact with pre-existing tendencies that are manifested at the individual level. In another study based on NYS data, Matsueda and Anderson (1998) followed a sample of 1,494 youths over a two-year period, examining levels of property offences (minor and serious theft, and burglary from a building or a vehicle). This study was designed to set two competing hypotheses against each other and to test their relative strengths. One is the view that individuals who are prone to offend will selectively associate with each other (the 'birds of a feather' hypothesis). An alternative view is that offending is largely a product of social influence in small groups (the 'bad company' hypothesis). In a careful analysis designed to eliminate methodological artefacts and other sources of error, these authors found that *both* numbers of delinquent peers *and* individual predispositions were associated with observed rates of offending. While results suggested that the latter had the more significant effect, 'delinquent peers and delinquency are reciprocally related in a dynamic process' (Matsueda and Anderson, 1998, p. 301).

These observations link to other findings concerning the role of peer influence, interpersonal reward and perceived status in groups where high appreciation is given for breaking rules or for appearing to act recklessly. Also using data from the NYS, Rebellon (2006) found close associations between the extent of an individual's socialising amongst groups of young people who approved of petty theft, school vandalism, truancy, drunkenness, and hitting others, and the likelihood that he or she would engage in comparable behaviour. The findings emerged similarly for both males and females, and suggested that delinquent acts make an individual socially attractive to others, rather than there being a straightforward effect of social reinforcement on delinquency. The effect of reinforcement was thus vicarious rather than direct. In a large-scale review of 273 studies relating to status and its potential role in the genesis of youthful offending, Ellis and McDonald (2001) obtained extensive confirmation of the hypothesis that individual status has an important role in maintaining involvement in delinquency. Furthermore, even romantic partners may contribute to these processes, as reported by Haynie, Giordano, Manning and Longmore (2005), who found such an effect operating when peer influence and other factors were taken into account. While these studies do not directly address the motivations that might induce people to offend in the beginning, they demonstrate that social and peer reinforcement may be powerful factors in continuing to do so.

The communication sequences through which processes of interpersonal influence take place have been investigated in studies such as one by Granic and Dishion (2003), who studied social interactions in a sample of 102 early adolescents (average age: 12.4 years). Participants were classified as 'high risk' for future involvement in delinquency on the basis of a series of relevant indicators. As part of the study, individuals nominated the person with whom they spent most time, and the resultant pairs were videotaped having conversations. The tapes were coded for episodes of 'deviant talk', defined as the proportion of time their discussion focused on 'rule-break' (RB). This consisted of 'utterances that had antisocial or norm-breaking elements' (2003, p. 315). It was hypothesised that this type of exchange was attractive and congenial for some dyads, to an extent that they became absorbed in it and the amount magnified over time. The most striking finding was that scores derived from the trend of RB talk (measured by the slope of the line averaging its change over time) significantly predicted antisocial and conflict behaviour – arrest records, exclusion from school and drug use – three years later (average age: 15.2 years). When evidence of family coercion, prior antisocial behaviour, and number of deviant affiliations were controlled, the effect held. Figure 5.2 on the next page illustrates the very different conversational patterns of interaction sequences for antisocial and 'normal' youth respectively.

On the basis of this and related research, Granic and Patterson (2006) elaborated a *dynamic systems model* in which successions of interaction episodes, beginning within the family but continuing into exchanges with peers, are viewed as the principal factor driving the establishment of aggressiveness. This appears as though it were a trait as conceived in traditional personality psychology, but it is better understood as a product of an extended series of learning experiences.

Correlates of crime

To recapitulate the findings reviewed in this section and the preceding one, Table 5.1 displays a summary of some of the outcomes of the very wide-ranging, almost panoramic literature review by Ellis, Beaver and Wright (2009) of correlates of crime. Table 5.1 focuses specifically on the areas of temperament and socialisation with the highest consistency scores – that is, where

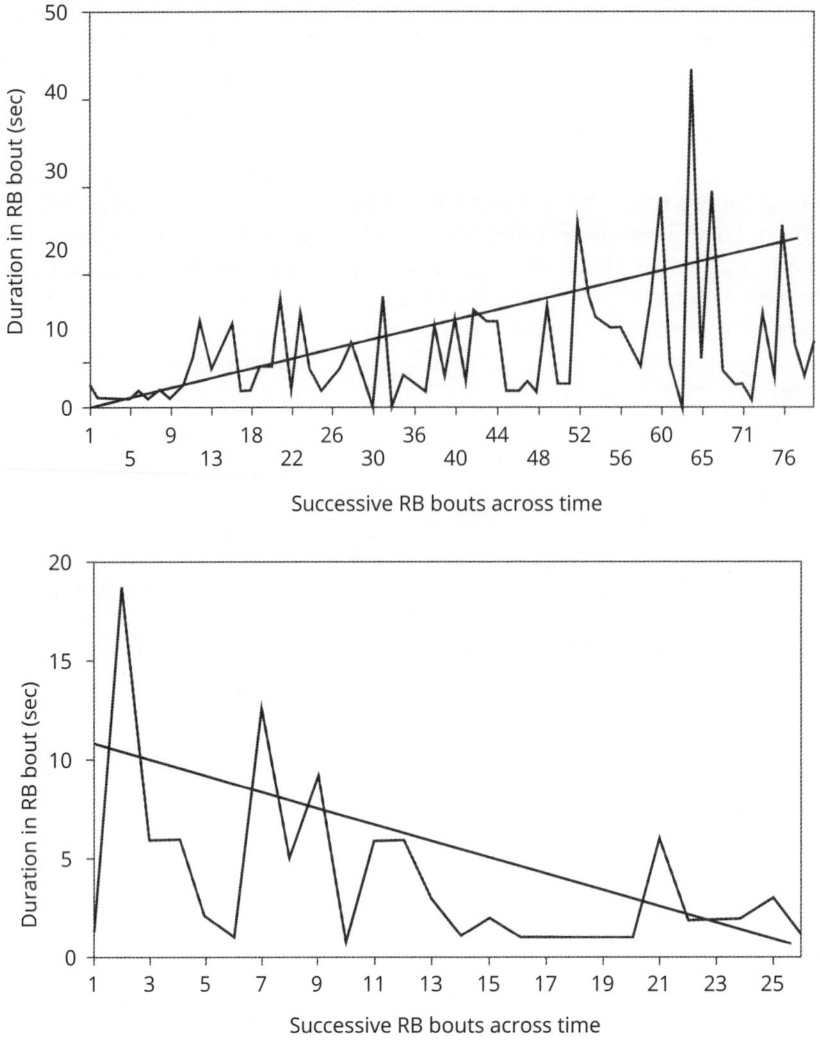

50
40
30
20
10
0
Duration in RB bout (sec)
1 5 9 13 18 22 26 30 36 40 44 48 52 56 60 65 71 76
Successive RB bouts across time
20
15
10
5
0
Duration in RB bout (sec)
1 3 5 7 9 11 13 15 17 19 21 23 25
Successive RB bouts across time

Figure 5.2
Conversational patterns among antisocial and among 'normal' youth. Speech sequences with 'rule break' (RB) conversational episodes. *Upper figure*: Time series for antisocial youth. *Lower figure*: Time series for non-delinquent youth.

Source: Figures 1 and 2. From Granic, I. & Dishion, T. J. (2003). Deviant Talk in Adolescent Friendships: A Step Toward Measuring a Pathogenic Attractor Process. Social Development, 12 (3), 314–334, John Wiley & Sons Ltd. Copyright © Blackwell Publishing Ltd. 2003. DOI: 10.1111/1467-9507.00236

the largest proportion of the available studies showed support for an association between the highlighted variables and later criminal conduct.

Culture

The behaviour of parents, teachers, peer-groups and other socialising agents takes place within the larger context of society and culture. Within this, too, there may be influences which, contrary to the formal pronouncements of society's spokespersons, may well subvert this and be indirectly supportive of crime. We are accustomed, for example, to hearing the idea that violence is not a type of behaviour of which society approves. There is no public support for violence; it is perennially described as abhorrent; and its use is denounced (other than in certain specified circumstances such as self-defence or sanctioned military operations). To advocate it in other circumstances would be seen as antisocial. In

Variable	Number of studies	Consistency score
Temperament		
Impulsivity	86	0.981
Sensation-seeking	60	0.905
Childhood aggression	59	0.950
Family socialisation		
Parent–child attachment	72	0.950
Parental supervision/monitoring	70	0.833
Larger family size	64	0.904
Marital/family discord or dysfunction	55	1.000
Childhood maltreatment by parents	54	0.978

Table 5.1 The association of temperament and socialisation with later criminal conduct. The table shows childhood variables that are positively associated with criminal convictions in adulthood. The 'consistency score' relates to official records of criminal offending; where possible, a separate score was also reported in relation to self-reported offending (not shown here). The score was calculated by first obtaining the total number of findings available (shown in the central column); then the number of findings in the majority direction (in all cases here, showing a positive association) was divided by the total number available, with the number of any findings in the opposite direction being doubled. The score has a maximum value of 1, which signifies complete consistency. Note that these data do not show actual effect sizes, nor the relative strengths of the associations found.

Source: data compiled from Ellis, Beaver & Wright (2009)

parallel, however, but on a more tacit level, there is subtle support for the expression of masculinity, and for values associated with some versions of it in which the boundary between them and the display of its more repugnant side is not always carefully drawn. Portrayals of cool-talking, no-nonsense toughness abound in the shared Euro-American cultural ethos and probably elsewhere. In another sense, then, society is replete with violent imagery (for example, in films and computer games) and with implicit endorsement of attributes linked to aggressiveness. Some possible consequences are suggested by the research findings described in the 'Focus on ...' box below.

As can be seen from those studies, there is evidence that culture may have an indirect

FOCUS ON ...

Culture and violence

We have encountered (in Chapter 2) some of the difficulties of defining the word 'crime'. A satisfactory definition of the concept of 'culture' is even harder to obtain. Nevertheless, some studies have succeeded in tracing a connection between these two extremely complex clusters of variables, with particular reference to rates of sexual and violent crimes.

Baron, Straus and Jaffee (1988) tested a *Cultural Spillover Theory* of the relationship between society-wide attitudes concerning sexual aggression and the rates of serious sexual assaults. They collected data from each of the 50 states of the USA and developed a composite measure, the Legitimate Violence Index. This combined various indirect indicators of the extent of apparent social approval of violence. The Index included measures of: (a) the proportion of violent content on television programmes; (b) rates of readership of magazines with a high violence content; (c) the existence of laws permitting corporal punishment in schools; (d) numbers of hunting licences issued; (e) levels of National Guard enrolment; and (f) the numbers of incidents of lynching per million population, in the period 1882–1927.

Scores on the Index were then compared with recorded rates of rape in each state. There was sizeable variability within this: the lowest and highest varied by a factor of eight. Broadly speaking, central and mountain states such as Wyoming, Montana, Mississippi, Utah and Idaho had high scores on the Legitimate Violence Index. Eastern and north-eastern states such as Rhode Island, Massachusetts, New Jersey, Maryland and New York came at the bottom of the scale. Several types of demographic information were also entered into the analysis; for example, information concerning each state's level of urbanisation; the degree of income inequality; the age distribution; and numbers of single and divorced males in the population.

A parallel analysis was conducted using another measure, the Violence Approval Index. Data for this were generated through an attitude survey in which citizens were asked their views regarding the use of violence in certain situations. For example, would it be permissible to punch a stranger under certain circumstances, such as an adult male who was drunk and bumped into you in the street?

Demographic variables, including the level of urbanisation and the percentage of divorced males in a state, were the strongest predictors of the rate of rape. But there was also a highly significant correlation between that rate and the Legitimate Violence Index, and a lower but still significant correlation with the Violence Approval Index.

Nisbett and Cohen (1996) focused on rates of violent crimes, including homicide. Their starting point was the finding that, excluding the largest urban areas, cities of comparable sizes in different parts of the USA have markedly different murder rates. The highest rates are in the states of the south and south-west; the lowest in the New England and Mid-Atlantic regions. Their research discovered that in the south and south-west homicides were more likely to result from arguments than to be committed in the course of other crimes (such as robbery). In surveys of social attitudes, there was: (a) greater endorsement in those regions of a shoot-to-kill policy in law enforcement; (b) stronger backing for the exercise of violence in the defence of a man's reputation; (c) a greater tendency to ruminate over personal insults; and (d) more support for physical discipline of children.

In a series of specially designed experiments, Nisbett and Cohen (1996) set up a situation in which participants were subjected to a contrived insult. They then provided blood samples for testing. The researchers found significantly higher increases in the levels of some hormones (cortisol and testosterone) amongst residents of high-homicide regions than was the case for citizens from other parts of the USA. Nisbett and Cohen forwarded the view that these differences are a function of a historical attachment to values that flow from a culture traditionally centred on the herding of animals, traceable to the high proportion of the population in some states of Scottish and Irish lineage. In such economies, a community's livelihood is dependent on the rearing and control of their herds. This, it was argued, engendered a need for individuals to present themselves as intimidating, signalling a readiness to use violence for the protection of property and of personal honour.

What has been called the 'culture of honour' thesis has been subjected to some tests. Baller, Zevenbergen and Messner (2009) analysed historical and crime data from 479 counties in the 13 states of the US 'old South' and found firm support for the thesis. In an analysis of international homicide data for 51 nations, Altheimer (2013a) also found support. However, when this dataset was extended to include 186 nations, no relationship emerged, though the latter analysis used data on modern nation-states rather than cultural sub-groups within them (Altheimer, 2013b).

but nevertheless critical influence on some types of serious violent crime. This most likely occurs via messages that are communicated through socialisation and the media, and the kinds of attitudes and expectations that are inculcated in individuals. On the basis of their findings, Baron *et al.*, concluded that 'the social approval of nonsexual and noncriminal violence has a significant relationship to rape' (1988, p. 95), and this emerged independently of other effects that were controlled for.

Such findings are convergent with others from a very different field, that of social anthropology. Although rape occurs in all societies, there are places where its rate of occurrence is reportedly very low. Sanday (2004) has described its almost complete absence amongst the Minangkabau people of Western Sumatra, which she ascribes to the structure of male–female relations within that group. Minangkabau culture has been described as the most matrilineal form of society on earth. That is, in contrast to the conventions of many other societies, land and property are passed on through female lineage, and there is a pattern of near-symmetrical male–female status and relationships, which differs considerably from that found elsewhere. Sanday (2004) ascribes the lower rate of male-to-female violence to this fundamental difference in power relations and the greater respect in which women are held.

Situational and contextual influences

The research findings discussed up to this point demonstrate the existence of some kinds of **continuity** in temperament, socialisation, or a combination of the two that are linked to the occurrence of offending, including aggression and violence. To obtain a fuller understanding of the patterning of this, we have to supplement the picture we have obtained with information on the immediate precursors of offending. Considering crime in general, criminologists have focused attention on the availability of *opportunities to offend*, and on 'opportunity structures' within society. This aspect of crime is little discussed within psychology. Changes in those structures are thought to play a focal part in the evolving contours of crime over time, viewed at least from the perspective of Routine Activity Theory (Felson and Boba, 2010), which we discussed in Chapter 4. Focusing more specifically on the events likely to *precede* aggression, extensive findings have come from laboratory and field research in social psychology (Berkowitz, 1993). This shows that there is a considerable range of situational factors that can influence aggression. They include almost any physical stimulus conditions that induce stress and increase arousal, as well as critical interpersonal 'trigger' events such as provocations or threats, and the presence of an observer 'audience'.

5

According to the social learning model (Bandura, 1977, 2001), much aggression is accounted for by determinants that arise in specific times or locations: 'what appears to be trait-like may in fact be situational, relationship-specific, and "functional"' (Snyder *et al.*, 2003, p. 30). Furthermore, 'social contingencies and experiences that foster antisocial behaviour often simultaneously mitigate the acquisition of capacities to self-regulate emotions, deploy attention, problem solve, engage in autonomous rule following, and relate effectively to others. Antisocial and skilled behaviours are "opposite sides of the same coin"' (Snyder *et al.*, 2003, p. 31).

Certain categories of events are fairly well established as likely precursors of aggression. They could be subtle non-verbal exchanges, such as fleeting eye contact, glances, facial expressions ('dirty looks'), offensive gestures, or whole bodily movements that convey hostility or contempt. While some fights are the result of an upward spiral of verbal exchanges, others may be precipitated by what appear to be the flimsiest of pretexts. The appraisal or interpretative process may be vital, but there are some signals that, for evolutionary or cultural reasons, fairly reliably instil fear and escape reactions, or elicit placatory responses to avoid adverse consequences. In a study by Ellsworth, Carlsmith and Henson (1972), researchers waited by traffic signals at road junctions, either sitting on a motorcycle or standing on the street corner. When motorists or pedestrians stopped at red lights, the experimenters either stared straight at them or looked at them but without staring. When they measured the time taken to cross the intersection after the lights had changed to green, those who had been stared at sped off significantly faster than those who had not. Rapid escape would be the normative reaction here, suggesting that the stare is a 'stimulus to flight'; but in a fraction of people such a stimulus would elicit anger and aggression, or perhaps be perceived as a challenge.

Several of the most renowned research studies in the history of psychology are illustrations of the power of situational determinants of human behaviour. They include the conformity studies of Asch (1956), the obedience experiments of Milgram (1963), the classic work on the tenuousness of psychiatric diagnosis by Rosenhan (1973), and the Stanford prison experiment by Haney, Banks and Zimbardo (1973). Some social psychologists have suggested that factors within situations have a more influential impact on behaviour than is generally realised (Ross and Nisbett, 1991/2011), and may be more potent than the personal variables involved – this is a stance known as *situationism*. Social psychologists Ten Berge and De Radd (1999) developed a taxonomic system for classifying social encounters with respect to the different rules and conventions at work within them. According to this viewpoint, behaviour changes in predictable ways that can be described in terms of ten types of situation: interpersonal conflict; joint working and exchanges of ideas; intimacy and personal relationships; recreation; travelling; rituals; sport; excesses (a term not explained by the authors); serving; and trading. Each of these carries fixed expectations regarding how we will act when we are in them, and these are forceful enough to ensure our compliance for a large proportion of the time.

Internal (cognitive-emotional) processes

The combined effects of biological endowment (expressed in temperament), of socialisation (shaped by its cultural context), and of the immediate situation are of course mediated through the internal processes of cognition, emotion, attitudes and beliefs operating within each individual. If temperament, socialisation and environmental factors separately have adverse impacts, in combination they may mean that a child's prospects for future life stability become progressively less favourable.

In relation to aggressiveness, for example, through the constantly repeated interplay of adverse factors over time, 'Eventually, the child acquires knowledge structures that include relational schemas of hostility, aggressive scripts, working models of hostile interpersonal relationships, heuristics involving rapid defensive responding rather than slower reflection, and self-defensive goals' (Dodge and Pettit, 2003, p. 363). The individual's internal processes may predispose him or her more readily than others towards antisocial behaviour. That process can occur on one or more of several levels.

Hostile beliefs

As a result of experiences while growing up, some young people may see the world as a threatening place or one where people cannot be trusted. They may develop a tendency to infer that others have an antagonistic attitude, or are about to act in a malign way towards them. De Castro *et al.*, (2002) reviewed 41 studies of the relationship between aggression and the attribution of hostile intent in children aged between 6 and 12. Effect sizes for this relationship were significantly associated with severity of behaviour problems. In a subsequent eye-tracking study, Horsley, de Castro and Van der Schoot (2010) found that even though they looked at non-hostile cues for longer than non-aggressive peers, aggressive children nonetheless ascribed hostile intent to them. A tendency towards hostile attributions may later be reinforced by repeated exposure to violent media, as Bushman (2016) found in a meta-analysis of 37 studies.

Moral reasoning and disengagement

Developing individuals acquire a set of beliefs about the rightness and wrongness of actions (moral development). Several measures have been devised for assessing levels of this development at different ages. A meta-analysis of 50 studies by Stams *et al.* (2006) found a large effect-size difference between children involved in delinquency and non-delinquent peers in their levels of moral development, with other factors including intelligence and socioeconomic status controlled. In a meta-analysis of 19 studies, extent of moral development has also been found to be significantly associated with rates of recidivism (Van Vugt *et al.*, 2011). In a separate strand of research, Bandura (1990) introduced the concept of *moral disengagement*, suggesting that individuals' levels of moral conduct are not invariant across situations, but that they self-regulate degrees of activation or withdrawal from moral standards. A review of 27 studies (cumulative sample size 17,776; age range 8–18) found significant associations between moral disengagement and a number of types of aggressive behaviour (Gini, Pozzoli and Hymel, 2014).

Automatic and controlled thoughts

Statements that individuals make to themselves in the moments leading towards a crime opportunity, or in the course of committing an offence, may reinforce the commencement and continuation of the behaviour. For example, in a seminal study in Chicago, Carroll and Weaver (1986) used a newspaper advertisement to recruit a sample of acknowledged regular shoplifters. Their participants admitted to having committed thefts on an average of 100 previous occasions. Whilst walking through department stores for a period of one hour, accompanied by a researcher, these volunteers were asked to speak their thoughts aloud, these being recorded via a lapel microphone. When compared with a group of 'novice' shoplifters, the self-confessed 'expert' group had a very different pattern of self-talk. While the minds of the novices were dominated by images of being arrested and prosecuted, members of the experienced group were analysing the store environment for opportunities to steal and to escape undetected.

Similar findings have been obtained in studies of other types of offence. Corbett and Simon (1992) investigated attitudes towards a variety of road traffic offences (speeding, going through red lights and drink-driving). High-frequency offenders focused their minds on their beliefs about the relatively low risk of being arrested, which enabled them to carry through their decisions to break the law. Wright and Decker (1994) interviewed active, high-rate house burglars in St. Louis. Most of their interviewees described themselves as deliberately focusing their minds on how they would carry out an offence, and consciously excluded other thoughts that might lead them to think about the possibility of arrest. They realised that anxiety over this could prevent them from committing the offence. In an interview-based study with 50 offenders in Britain, Nee and Meenaghan (2006) found that in the course of carrying out their offences 'expert' burglars adopted an automatic search strategy and a sequence of decision-making procedures. Parallel results have been obtained in interviews with offenders who have committed armed robbery, by Wright and Decker (1997) in St. Louis and by Morrison and O'Donnell (1994) in London.

Neutralisations

Having already committed offences, if asked why they did so, there is evidence that some frequent offenders respond in ways that enable them to endorse an accepted code of conduct while also explaining their own departures from it. In criminology, **Neutralisation Theory** was developed in an attempt to understand this. Sykes and Matza (1957) proposed that in order that individuals can tolerate incongruity or dissonance in their feelings and their attitudes related to offending, they resort to a set of internal mechanisms that reduce the emotional conflict between deviant and conformist standpoints. The resultant *techniques of neutralisation* are self-statements that permit or justify behaviour that they themselves would otherwise consider objectionable. There are several processes of this kind, which Maruna and Copes (2005) called the 'famous five', corresponding to types of statements these individuals might make to themselves:

- *Denial of responsibility* 'It wasn't my fault.' 'Someone else planned it – I just followed along.'
- *Denial of injury* 'They can afford it, they're well off. Besides, they'll claim it on insurance.'
- *Denial of victim* 'He or she ... deserved it'; '... was from a rival gang'; '... was from another ethnic group' (named abusively); '... supported the other team'; '... was gay'; '... was scantily dressed'.

» *Condemning the condemners* 'The police are corrupt.' 'The system's rotten.' 'I'm no worse than them.'

» *Appeal to higher loyalties* 'You should stand by your friends and be ready to lie [*or* say nothing, *or* fight] if you have to.'

As Maruna and Copes (2005) noted, though, this theory is unlikely to be able to explain the onset of crime, so it is of limited value *aetiologically*. However, it might help to clarify the continuation and maintenance of a pattern of offending.

The above are several examples of cognitive-emotional processing, occurring at different levels of awareness, that have been found to be associated with a likelihood of involvement in crime or antisocial behaviour. In later chapters, as we discuss different types of offence, we will consider available evidence of any links with specific patterns of cognition.

Integrative models: transactions and interactions

To comprehend the various kinds of evidence reviewed in this chapter, broad-ranging integrative models are invaluable. In addition to incorporating the major sets of factors just outlined, they also take account of the potency of *situations* in shaping specific events (such as involvement in a fight), and more importantly show how a *succession* of such occasions during her or his development channels an individual towards one pathway rather than another.

Transactional model of development

Variables associated with the developing child, his or her parents or caregivers, and the interactions between them are all engaged in a process of dynamic interaction over time. Each affects the other in a multiplicity of ways. It is very difficult to capture this in a model that specifies precise connections, because their specific patterning is likely to differ in every case.

The most simplified version of this, from the work of Sameroff (2009; Sameroff and Chandler, 1975) is shown in Figure 5.3. This tracks three principal sets of interdependent variables. Temperamental or constitutional variables are influenced by the genotype; environmental and situational variables (to which Sameroff gives the label 'environtype') are influenced by family, peers and culture; and all have an impact on the behaviour of the person himself or herself (the phenotype) – while he or she also concurrently shapes some aspects of them. This was exemplified earlier, with reference to the work of Turkheimer *et al.* (2003) on social class influences on the heritability of IQ. These processes are not simply an additive or multiplicative function of different 'inputs'. On the contrary, the variables respond to each other and are themselves altered over time. For example, children affect their parents or caregivers and to some extent mould *their* behaviour, as well as the other way round. The growing child is not merely a passive recipient of parental actions; rather, his or her temperament and reactions to caregivers may elicit certain responses from them, and there is a progression in how they respond to one another that is negotiated over consecutive encounters. In most cases a balance is achieved, but in some there is an ongoing struggle and the result may be dysfunctional over a protracted period. Overall this process is best conceptualised using a transactional model of development.

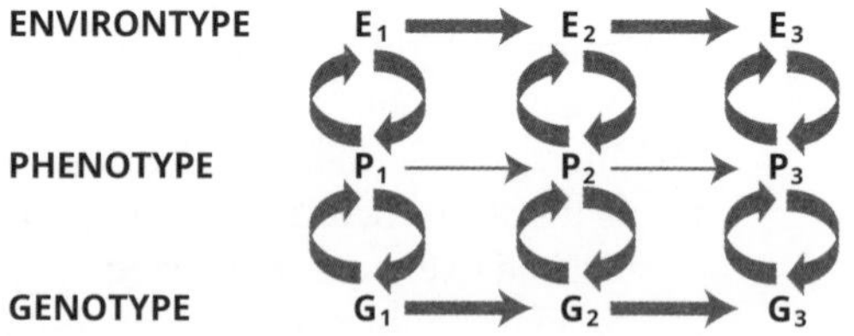
ENVIRONTYPE
E1
E2
E3
PHENOTYPE
P1
P2
P3
GENOTYPE
G1
G2
G3

Figure 5.3
The transactional model of development. This representation shows continuing dynamic interplay of genotype, phenotype and 'environtype'.

Source: Figure 1.3. From Sameroff, A. (2009). The Transactional Model. In A. Sameroff (ed.), The Transactional Model of Development: How Children and Contexts Shape Each Other. pp. 3–21. Washington, DC: American Psychological Association. Copyright © APA 2009. Reprinted with permission.

From birth to the onset of adulthood, such transactions are repeated, in a progressively evolving way, probably many thousands of times. Frequently reiterated interactional cycles reinforce learning in neural networks, connections strengthened through repeated use; the more often this happens, the more firmly established they become. Highly practised and rehearsed sequences come to dominate an individual's reactions in selected situations. 'Consistency in individual behaviours is not necessarily evidence for personal traits but rather consistency in the processes by which these traits are maintained in the interactions between child and environment' (Sameroff, 2009, p. 10).

One of the challenges in the field of developmental psychopathology is the sheer complexity of the routes through these processes. This presents some apparently intractable problems, such as those identified by Dodge and Pettit (2003). One is that of **equifinality**, whereby 'the same antisocial outcome can accrue from disparate sources' (p. 354). Another is that of **multifinality**, whereby 'specific risk factors can be associated with a variety of outcomes' (p. 354). This may make development sound almost chaotic; but there are trends within the very high level of informational 'noise', some of which we have examined in this chapter.

Person–situation interactionism

The interactional approach posits that the most soundly evidence-based account of action emerges from examining how persons and situations interact with each other, and that what occurs at any point is a product of that conjoint process.

A central concept within a model of **interactionism** is that of **reciprocal determinism**. This captures the bidirectional flow of causes and effects, in this case between personal variables and the features of immediate situations. Individuals synchronously show some patterns that are more stable, but also variability in their behaviour across situations, in a way that has been described as displaying an interactional 'signature' or profile.

Cognitive-Affective Personality System

To put all these kinds of evidence together, possibly the best candidate as an integrative model is the **Cognitive-Affective Personality System (CAPS)**, developed over a number of years by Walter Mischel and his colleagues (Kross, Mischel and Shoda, 2010; Mischel, 2004; Mischel and Shoda, 1995). While CAPS has not been explicitly applied to the problem of crime, an important advantage and strength of this approach is that its analysis of problem behaviour employs the same explanatory constructs that are used to understand other modes of action generally considered non-deviant – that is, modes that are conventional, conforming, healthy and functional. There is no fixed demarcation line between the two categories 'normal' and 'abnormal': these are **social constructions** that do not exist independently or objectively. The capacity to render offending and other forms of 'deviance' comprehensible within a model that bridges that divide is a major conceptual asset.

The core of the CAPS model is illustrated in Figure 5.4. The model encompasses biological, sociocultural, personal and situational variables. Figure 5.4 is a notional magnification of the central psychological feature, the internal information-processing or cognitive-affective component, conceptualised as being accomplished in a series of interconnected structures known as neural networks.

This chapter has reviewed evidence for the impact of different factors on the development of the tendency to act in antisocial ways, and we have discussed genes, temperament, socialisation, culture and situational variables. When we add to this list the range of information-processing capacities and other cognitive attributes through which human beings engage with their surroundings, the role of psychological factors becomes even more obvious. In Chapters 6–10, we look more closely at how they influence specific types of criminal offences.

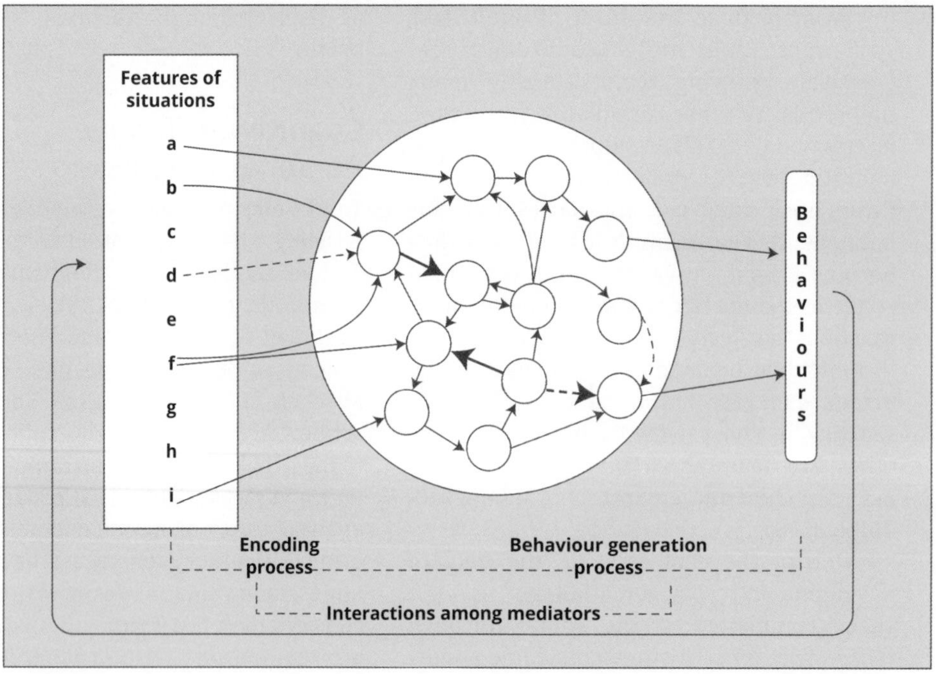
Features of situations
a
b
c
d
e
f
g
h
i
Behaviours
Encoding process
Behaviour generation process
Interactions among mediators

Figure 5.4

The Cognitive-Affective Processing System (CAPS). The figure shows a schematic representation of the operation of neural networks in CAPS.

Source: Figure 4. From Mischel, W. and Shoda, Y. (1995). A Cognitive-Affective System Theory of Personality: Reconceptualizing Situations, Dispositions, Dynamics and Invariance in Personality Structure. Psychological Review, 102 (2), 246–268, American Psychological Association. Copyright © APA 1995. Adapted with permission. DOI: http://dx.doi.org/10.1037/0033-295X.102.2.246

Chapter summary

This chapter reviewed the major variables that are believed, on the basis of extensive evidence, to be those that have the closest association with the emergence of antisocial or criminal behaviour, and with its maintenance over time in a criminal lifestyle. The variables fall under several headings:

» *Genetic* Individual inheritance plays a prominent part not only in our physical attributes, but also in our psychological make-up. Rather than having a direct impact, however, genes operate in complex pathways, such as through gene–environment (G×E) interactions.

» *Temperament* Some patterns of reaction, strongly influenced by genes, are present in newborn children, and the interaction between those patterns and the early environment influences habitual tendencies collectively called 'temperament'.

» *Socialisation* This is a broad category of influences from parents (or other direct caregivers), family, peers, teachers and other figures who have an important impact in shaping a child's learning and change.

» *Culture* Although it is difficult to define and to detect, the impact of culture is pervasive. A small amount of research has demonstrated its potential influence on patterns of some serious types of crime.

» *Situations* Individuals adapt to situations and their behaviour varies in some recognisable patterns between them. An interactional model that combines this kind of variation with personality variables provides a significant advance in seeking to explain patterns of individual behaviour.

- *Internal (cognitive-emotional) processes* All of the variables subsumed under the above headings come together at the level of each individual in the thoughts and feelings that he or she experiences, and responds to or acts upon. Actions are a product of long-term developmental factors that have shaped the person, of immediate or situational factors operating in the moment, and of the individual's acquired pattern of appraisals.

Although the ideas and findings described in this chapter are drawn from other areas of psychology, they can be used to explain criminal behaviour as one pattern that can emerge as a result of events and experiences in the lives of developing individuals.

Further reading

The following books are particularly recommended as fuller sources on the areas covered in this chapter.

- For an overview of behaviour genetics, see Terence J. Bazzett (2008), *An Introduction to Behavior Genetics* (Sunderland, MA: Sinauer Associates); and for detailed coverage of temperament, see the books by Mary K. Rothbart (2011), *Becoming Who We Are: Temperament and Personality in Development* (New York: Guilford Press) or Patricia K. Kerig, Amanda Ludlow and Charles Wenar (2012), *Developmental Psychopathology*, 6th edition (New York: McGraw-Hill).
- On socialisation, see the *Handbook of Socialization: Theory and Research*, 2nd edition, edited by Joan E. Grusec and Paul D. Hastings (2015; New York: Guilford Press); and on the transactional model, Arnold Sameroff (2009), *The Transactional Model of Development: How Children and Contexts Shape Each Other* (American Psychological Association).
- Some general texts on personality address many of the areas discussed here, but do not focus much attention on delinquency or crime; a particularly good one nevertheless is Daniel Cervone and Lawrence A. Pervin (2013), *Personality Psychology* (New York: Wiley).
- The 'classic' and frequently cited work on the psychology of situations is Lee Ross and Richard Nisbett's *The Person and the Situation*, first published in 1991 but updated in 2011 (London: Pinter & Martin).
- The review of research presented in the *Handbook of Crime Correlates* by Lee Ellis, Kevin M. Beaver and John Wright (2009; Amsterdam: Academic Press) contains useful summary tables on many of the variables discussed in this chapter.

Offences: Types of Crime and Influencing Factors

Offenders are drawn into the criminal justice system by carrying out what society has deemed to be criminal offences. Part 2 explores different kinds of crime, and considers what research has revealed about those who commit crimes and the factors that may lead to crimes and influence their nature.

6 Assault and Hate Crimes

Chapter 6 looks in detail at the factors involved in personal but non-lethal violence, including grievous assault and wounding, and hate crimes. It distinguishes between different kinds of aggression, and considers the interaction between personal characteristics and aspects of the situation.

7 Single-Victim Homicide

Chapter 7 focuses on the most serious form of personal violence at an individual level – that in which one person deliberately kills another. It examines the factors believed to precede and to influence such offences, and considers whether those who have committed this offence are likely to do so again.

8 Multiple Homicide

Chapter 8 discusses crimes in which more than one person is killed, including serial killings by one or more perpetrators, and mass killings such as familicides, massacres, terrorism and genocide. Such crimes may seem incomprehensible, but research has thrown some light on personal, political, racial and religious motivations for such acts.

9 Sexual Offences and Partner Assault

Chapter 9 discusses sexually motivated aggression and violence, and offences within close personal relationships (including harassment and stalking). It considers psychological and other factors in these offences; risk factors for further offending; and potential escalation to new kinds of offending or different victims.

10 Other Serious Crimes

Chapter 10 surveys other crimes, including robbery, arson, kidnapping and serious economic crimes. It begins by looking at the misuse of alcohol or other substances, which is widely implicated in offending behaviour. Throughout, the chapter focuses on what is known about psychological factors.

11 Mental Disorder and Crime

Chapter 11 is concerned with the impact of mental health problems on criminal or antisocial behaviour, especially offences involving violence. Many offenders have major problems of this kind, sometimes compounded by substance abuse, and may be particularly vulnerable, but many also respond to psychological therapies.

Assault and Hate Crimes

This chapter provides a more in-depth analysis of the factors involved in some of the more serious kinds of personal but non-lethal violence, including grievous assault and wounding, and hate crimes.

Chapter objectives

- To describe a range of methods that have been proposed for comparing the seriousness of crimes.
- To survey what is known about psychological factors and processes in the causation of crimes of violence against the person.
- To examine variables associated with several types of serious crimes against the person, including violent assault, wounding, and offences motivated partially or wholly by hatred of a particular group.

There are large numbers of 'ordinary' crimes – crimes that the majority of citizens say are of the most frequent concern to them, and that take up the biggest single share of most police officers' time. On account of their sheer number they are broadly termed *volume crime* by the police, who have defined the category as including offences of street robbery, burglary (dwelling and non-dwelling), theft (including shoplifting), theft of and from vehicles, criminal damage, and drug offences linked with acquisitive crime (Association of Chief Police Officers of England, Wales and Northern Ireland, 2001, p. 9). Those who have committed only these kinds of offences – which survey evidence suggests at one time or another includes a large segment of the population – are very unlikely ever to encounter a forensic psychologist. The group of people with whom our profession works may well have committed these offences at some stage, but by and large they will also have committed others of a graver nature, usually involving personal or sexual violence, or some other type of significant harm.

In this chapter and the three to follow, therefore, we begin to look more closely at the different varieties of offence in this more serious category. However, we will first consider a number of methods that have been devised in trying to measure the *seriousness* of crimes. We then turn to consider the factors that influence crimes of violence as currently defined. While some of the underlying causal processes are similar to those found in volume crimes, we will focus on the other features that differentiate them, for a number of major types of offence. There is no completely satisfactory way of dividing these, but this chapter will focus on direct personal violence, examining non-fatal assault and the factors associated with it, then turning attention to hate crimes. In Chapters 7 and 8 we will turn to crimes of violence that result in death, considering homicides with single victims and with multiple victims respectively. In Chapter 9 we will turn our attention to crimes of sexual and partner violence.

Crime seriousness

Despite several approaches from different directions, 'level of harm' remains difficult to define. Clearly, in some cases there is no doubt that major harm has been done: for example, where a crime results in death, life-threatening injury, or severe disability. But there are also many cases where the amount of harm can be hard to quantify even with medical expertise, and others where it is a matter of subjective experience. Thus while people might agree in broad terms that, for example, assault is more harmful than theft, depending on the type of injury or the value of goods stolen that might not always be true.

In some respects, legal statutes themselves classify certain crimes according to the amounts of harm caused and also take into account the extent to which that effect was intended (*mens rea*). This is codified, for example, in the Offences Against the Person Act 1861 in English law. This classifies *assault occasioning actual bodily harm* (Section 47); *malicious wounding*, also called *grievous bodily harm* (Section 20); and *malicious wounding with intent* (Section 18) (Herring, 2016). These three offences vary significantly in seriousness and lead to different penalties. When sentencing individuals to life imprisonment, judges specify the minimum term (years) to be served – the 'tariff' – which is usually intended to reflect crime seriousness and the extent of society's revulsion at the acts committed. Something similar can be seen in the distinction between *first-*, *second-* and *third-degree murder* in the United States.

In many respects, however, both seriousness and harm involve complex judgments. The role of the latter has been given considerable sway through the introduction in various jurisdictions of Victim Impact Statements, or **Victim Personal Statements**, in which individuals explain to the court the effects that a crime has had on their lives. Individuals' *reactions* to being a victim will be influenced by their prior experiences and expectations, the ramifications of the crime in their lives, the attributions they make regarding the offender's motivation, their personal fragility or resilience, and many other factors.

In Chapter 2 we saw that Newman (1976) found a fairly high level of agreement on the seriousness of crimes across five nations. Yet the offence descriptions used in that study were quite different from one another. When we try to fine-tune such judgments, the findings are less clear-cut. Criminologists, psychologists and others have attempted to develop more refined scales for measuring seriousness – for examples, see the 'Focus on ...' box below.

FOCUS ON ...

Is it possible to measure the seriousness of crimes?

Many proposals have been made for systems of grading the seriousness of crimes or the level of harm they cause. The following are examples of the methods that have been devised.

Judgments of seriousness

One plausible approach is to ask members of the public to rate the seriousness of crimes. Although this works at a general level, it is not as simple as it sounds. Crimes might be judged in terms either of their *properties* (the nature of the act) or their *effects on victims*.

In a large-scale study, the *National Survey of Crime Severity* (NSCS), Wolfgang, Figlio, Tracy and Singer (1985) asked a sample of 50,000 respondents to rate the severity of 204 crimes. However, Parton, Hansel and Stratton (1991) questioned the validity of this method, noting that judgments are readily influenced by different details given in offence vignettes.

Monetary values

Cohen (1988) attempted to assign monetary values to crimes. Some costs are, of course, difficult if not impossible to quantify. Nevertheless, Cohen considered that, using different sources, it was possible to calculate the costs of crimes to victims. Three types of costs were taken into account: (a) sums directly caused by loss of property or wages, or medical costs for treatment of injury; (b) amounts of compensation awarded for pain and suffering, obtained from study of cases of accidental personal injury; (c) an additional amount for the perceived risk of death, where the value of a life was set at US $2 million (at 1988 prices).

The resultant rankings were compared with seriousness ratings from the NSCS: they were similar for the ordering of violent offences, but differed for non-violent ones.

Living standard

Von Hirsch and Jareborg (1991) proposed a method of evaluating the seriousness of crimes by setting them against a common yardstick of 'living standard'. This refers to more than just someone's level of income. The authors identified four 'dimensions of interest' within it: (a) physical integrity (health, safety, avoidance of pain); (b) material support and amenity; (c) freedom from humiliation; and (d) privacy/autonomy. They used this conceptual framework to examine a series of nine offences and graded their seriousness on one of five levels. The question to be asked is then: 'How much does being a victim of crime detract from an individual's living standard, as defined in these ways?'

Court decisions

Francis, Soothill and Dittrich (2001) employed an approach based on analysis of courtroom decisions in which the same offender had been convicted of two different kinds of offences on the same occasion. Using data from the Home Office Offenders' Index, they tracked the criminal careers of a cohort of 7,442 offenders who had been convicted of sexual offences, and who in 1973 were serving sentences that began or ended within the 32-year period from 1963 to 1994 (inclusive). During that time, of 31,135 further court appearances, there were 8,209 such dual sentencing occasions. The authors then used paired-comparisons methodology to examine the sentences imposed for each of the two offences. The results showed a delineation of what was regarded as the 'principal' offence in each pair. This enabled compilation of a list of the 20 most serious offences as regarded by sentencers (judges and magistrates).

Increasing seriousness

Ramchand, MacDonald, Haviland and Morral (2009) proposed a developmental approach, based on the general finding that amongst those who pursue a 'criminal career' there is generally a progression from less serious to more serious crimes. These authors interviewed 1,725 young offenders from the *National Youth Survey* (NYS), and 574 under supervision in an *Adolescent Outcomes Project* (AOP) in Los Angeles. They then undertook an elaborate statistical analysis in which, for any specific type of offence, a score was derived based on the number of times it occurred for the first time *before* and *after* the first occurrence of each of the other types of offence recorded. This produced a graph of relative severity for 21 offences for the NYS group and 14 offences for the AOP group.

Harm matrix

Other proposals have emerged from a more broadly 'harm-based' approach to the field of criminal justice. Greenfield and Paoli (2013) outlined a procedure for the assessment of harm involving a number of stages. This first involves developing a taxonomy of harm, together with methods of estimating the extent of four kinds of damage (the ones specified by von Hirsch and Jareborg, noted above). Amounts of harm are estimated using severity benchmarks in five categories ('marginal' to 'catastrophic'). These were then combined with frequency to form a matrix which Greenfield and Paoli applied to analysis of cocaine trafficking in Belgium. This enabled them to formulate recommendations for law-enforcement agencies towards policies most likely to succeed in harm reduction.

6

Another possibility for gauging seriousness of assaults may be to base it on the amount of compensation offered to victims following a detailed assessment of the impact of a crime. Many legal systems make provision for this. In England and Wales, the process is managed by the Criminal Injuries Compensation Authority (CICA). Its objective is to compensate blameless victims of violent crime by making a payment in 'recognition of public sympathy' with the victim (CICA, 2012, p. 1). Payments can be made for physical or mental injury, either to the direct victim of an assault or abuse, or to a close relative if the victim was murdered. The CICA publishes a guide document which lists the types of payments that can be claimed for, and lists fixed sums for different types of injury to different body parts. In principle it would be possible to convert this 'tariff of injuries' into a method of grading crimes according to their seriousness.

Crime seriousness is a major issue that is taken into account in sentencing, but decisions regarding amounts of compensation are made some time after the court hearing, and by a separate agency. Thus the two sets of decisions are not linked.

Crimes of personal violence

As we saw in Chapter 2, official criminal statistics and self-report surveys both show that violent crimes generally form between one-fifth and one-quarter of crimes overall (e.g. Office for National Statistics, 2016a). Those proportions apply in England and Wales (as we found in the statistics for 2015–2016), but a similar pattern can be found in most economically comparable countries. By their nature, however, when violent offences occur, they understandably draw media attention and can induce a great deal of public anxiety. Offences in this category include *homicide*, *assault*, *robbery*, *family violence* and *sexual violence*. These types of offences are the most extensively researched from a psychological standpoint. They are also the types of offence in which investigation, assessment or subsequent treatment are most likely to involve a forensic psychologist.

As discussed in earlier chapters, there are large variations between countries in total amounts of serious violence. Aspects of this violence were described in a major report produced by the United Nations World Health Organization (WHO; Krug *et al.*, 2002). This suggested that during the year 2000 there were 1.66 million violent deaths worldwide. The total included 815,000 suicides; 310,000 deaths due to war; and 510,000 homicides, which corresponds to roughly one every minute. The numbers of war deaths have fluctuated markedly over time; but the other statistics have remained comparatively stable – in 2011 the figures for suicide and homicide were 798,000 and 486,000 respectively (WHO, 2013).

The 2002 WHO report also includes data on different types of violence, including some, such as domestic violence, that are notoriously difficult to measure accurately because of factors that often lead to their remaining concealed or unrecorded, such as fear on the part of victims or police reluctance to be involved (an issue discussed in Chapter 9). Problems such as these may partly explain the large between-country differences that are found in the rate of reported intimate partner violence, ranging for instance from 10 per cent in Paraguay and the Philippines, through 22 per cent in the United States, to 34 per cent in Egypt. There were even larger variations for rates of fighting in school, ranging from 22 per cent in Sweden, to 44 per cent in the United States and 76 per cent in Israel. It is very likely that some part of these variations will be due to methodological factors influencing data collection.

Specially focused *Statistics Bulletins* are published annually by the Office of National Statistics based on the Crime Survey for England and Wales (CSEW). In 2014–2015, an estimated 1.3 million violent incidents in England and Wales were reported, with 1.8 per cent of the adult population (defined as those aged 16 or over) becoming a victim (Office for National Statistics, 2016b). This is less than a third of the number (4.2 million) found in 1995, which was the point at which, after having risen steadily for many years, numbers of most types of crimes began to fall. The largest proportion of the 2014–2015 incidents (48 per cent) resulted in no physical injury, with another 27 per cent causing only minor injury; but a further 24 per cent were more serious offences of wounding. No weapon was used in most incidents (78 per cent), even in cases of robbery (72 per cent). Just under a quarter (24 per cent) of reported violent incidents were repeat victimisations.

The CSEW reports also show that, in addition to physical injuries sustained, most respondents (81 per cent in 2014–2015) were emotionally affected by violent incidents. The CSEW for 2011–2012 gave some details on the nature of those effects. In descending order of frequency, they included: anger, annoyance, shock, fear, a loss of confidence, crying, difficulty sleeping, depression, and anxiety or panic attacks.

Aggression and criminal violence

There are complex multi-layered patterns of cause and effect in most violent crimes, and while many individual factors associated with violence have been identified, the specific ways in which they interact are so far only poorly understood. It is likely that such interactions take multiple forms, suggesting that an all-purpose model of violence causation could remain hard to articulate other than in very loose terms. Such an attempt has nevertheless been made, taking a form known as the *General Aggression Model* (GAM), shown in diagram form in Figure 6.1.

The GAM represents the major sets of distal, or background, factors that influence individual development (Anderson and Bushman, 2002). In combination, following patterns such as those outlined in Chapter 5, the GAM then considers the factors that affect the developing individual in situations where his or her internal processes respond to adverse events and circumstances. The learned mode of interplay between thoughts, feelings and behaviour influences the likely pattern of responses, which – acting on the environment, and particularly on the other person or persons in it – then bring about consequences that in turn present a new situation, with that cycle being repeated as an encounter proceeds.

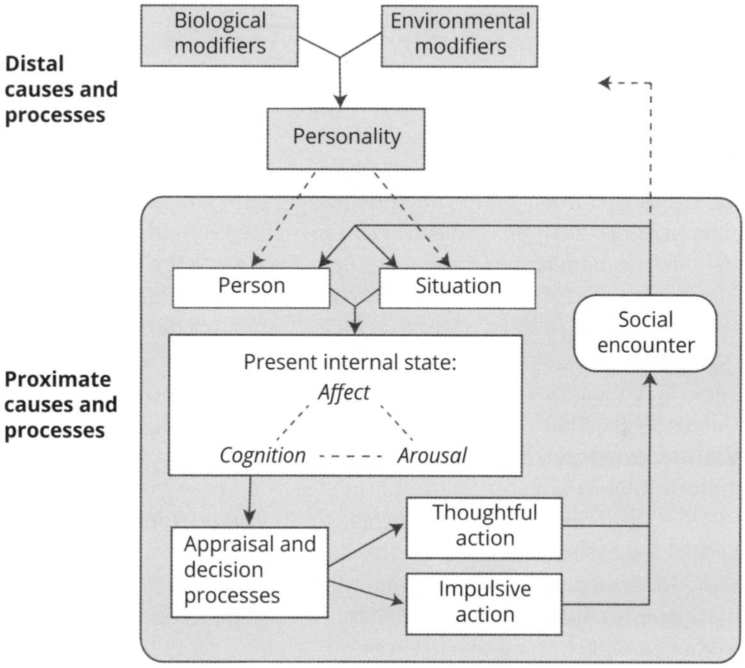
Distal causes and processes
Biological modifiers
Environmental modifiers
Personality
Proximate causes and processes
Person
Situation
Present internal state:
Affect
Cognition
Arousal
Social encounter
Appraisal and decision processes
Thoughtful action
Impulsive action

Figure 6.1
The General Aggression Model.

Source: republished with permission of Guilford Publications, from Anderson, C. A. & Carnagey, N. L. (2004). Violent Evil and the General Aggression Model. In A. G. Miller (ed.), The Social Psychology of Good and Evil. pp. 168–192. New York, NY: Guilford. © 2004 Guilford Publications; permission conveyed through Copyright Clearance Center, Inc. The lower part of the figure is reproduced with permission of Annual Review of Psychology, Volume 53 © by Annual Reviews, http://www.annualreviews.org, and is taken from Anderson, C. A. & Bushman, B. J. (2002). Human Aggression. Annual Review of Psychology, 53 (1), 27–51.

The GAM can be a useful framework for thinking of the range of factors that influence **aggression** at a very broad level. It has mainly been used, however, in accounting for a range of findings from laboratory experiments in social psychology, and has played a major part in debates concerning the role of media in the causation of aggressive moods and reactions. DeWall, Anderson and Bushman (2011) discuss how it can be made applicable to understanding offences of violence, including partner assaults and intergroup conflict, and also how it might alert us to the likelihood of increased violence as a result of global climate change.

However, the GAM's breadth and scope can also be seen as a weakness. At this level of conceptualisation, it can lack the specificity needed to explain dissimilar patterns of aggression and violent behaviour. Given the ways in which offences differ, using the GAM to understand violent crime might require researchers to develop a portfolio of interconnected models applicable to different categories of violent offence.

Differing patterns of aggressiveness

Aggressive behaviour not only varies in its seriousness but also takes numerous forms, and various distinctions have been offered in efforts to classify it – direct versus indirect, physical versus relational, active versus passive, and so on (see Parrott and Giancola, 2007). Violent offences are just one manifestation of the phenomenon of aggression. Most forms of aggression that constitute criminal offences are of the *direct* type, though they can be *physical* (assault) or *verbal* (threats). Violence can also be *passive* (e.g. negligence or recklessness as to likely harm); and it can be *indirect* (e.g. paying a third party to attack or kill someone). Social and relational forms of aggression, which may also cause considerable distress to victims, are identified in legal statutes as crimes of *harassment* (discussed more fully in Chapter 9). In its most frequent form in criminal offences, aggression is expressed when one person directly attacks an adversary, most often by making immediate bodily contact, or from a distance by throwing an object or using a firearm.

One of the most durable distinctions, and one that is incorporated in the GAM, is between *reactive* and *instrumental* aggression, which focuses on its motivational aspects. The former refers to aggression that is part of an emotional reaction, and so it is variously called 'reactive', 'expressive', 'impulsive', 'hostile', 'angry', 'retaliatory', or sometimes 'hot' aggression. The protagonist is in a state of high physiological arousal, senses mounting physical tension, and experiences a discharge of energy when the violent act is committed. The descriptive language is replete with vivid metaphors – 'heated exchange', 'flaring up', 'seeing red', 'lost my cool', 'explosive outburst'. In this form of aggression, 'harm or injury to the victim reduces an aversive emotional state' within the aggressor (Blackburn, 1993, p. 211). While at present there are no data that can completely confirm this, what is available suggests that most assaults, fights and other violent offences – including the majority of homicides, as we will see later – fit this pattern. The second, 'proactive' or 'instrumental' type of aggression refers to actions where aggressive behaviour serves some purpose other than expression of negative affect and has often been referred to as 'cold'. This usually forms part of a premeditated series of actions. That is, the objective is not to discharge pent-up feelings but to achieve a goal for the purpose of which there is a preparedness to use force. The foremost example is the offence of *robbery*.

Within psychology, considerably more attention has been paid to the first of these types of aggression than to the second. The view that emotional aggression results from a loss of ability to contain strong feelings corresponds to some major theories in both psychology and criminology (control theories). A large proportion of violent crime is a product of conflicts in which the outcome was unplanned and unforeseen. One factor contributing to this is *anger*. Novaco (1975, 2007) developed a model of anger that incorporates cognitive, emotional and behavioural elements. This has been widely applied for the purpose of devising treatment interventions that can help individuals reduce the frequency and intensity of their anger, as described in the 'Focus on ...' box on page 117. The model has stimulated the development of structured programmes that have been widely used in prison, probation, youth justice and secure mental health settings to help individuals increase their capacity for self-control. (The effects of interventions based on this model will be discussed in Chapter 19.)

Nevertheless, some researchers, including the authors of the General Aggression Model (Bushman and Anderson, 2001), have questioned the value of the hostile/instrumental distinction, mainly because many aggressive acts contain elements of both types. For example, Barratt and Slaughter (1998) devised a short self-report screening survey (the *Aggressive Acts Questionnaire*)

FOCUS ON …

Anger dysfunctions and angry violence

As noted in the text, aggression is often divided into two types, *reactive* and *instrumental*. The former has been the focus of much more research than the latter, and much of that research has been concerned with the emotion of anger.

While anger has many negative connotations, it is now widely accepted that anger is a normal adaptive response to certain events, a response that motivates or energises an individual's coping strategies (Novaco, 1975). In certain circumstances, therefore, anger can be *functional*. Under certain circumstances, feeling angry and displaying signs of anger can indicate sound psychological health. There is even evidence that in some cases angry exchanges can actually *strengthen* close relationships (Averill, 1983).

Research by Kassinove and Tafrate (2002) suggests that only 10 per cent of angry incidents are followed by actual aggression. For some people, however, anger can be dysfunctional and can become a serious problem. Such people might be angered by events that others regard as trivial, or find themselves feeling angry many times a day. They might experience their anger very sharply, and find it difficult to control. The result can include destructive or abusive behaviour, and in some cases acts of violence. In severe cases, an individual might meet the criteria for a diagnosis of Intermittent Explosive Disorder, classified in psychiatric terms as a mental illness.

Novaco (1975) worked with individuals who were experiencing repeated problems with anger, and developed a model of anger that includes cognitive, physiological, behavioural (motor) and environmental components, as shown in the diagram. The cognitive appraisal process is of crucial importance in the model. External events are not inherently provocative; they become so only when filtered through the cognitive apparatus of a perceiver. Thereafter, cognitive, emotional and behavioural events are set in motion in interconnected ways. Far from being adaptive, anger can become *dysfunctional* when it is inappropriate in terms of the interpersonal context or the prevailing value system – or when it is out of control. Thus an individual's response may be quite disproportionate relative to the provoking agent. Anger may then give rise to other problems, including violent assaults or homicides.

As an extension of his initial model, Novaco (1975, 1997, 2007) developed an intervention known as **anger control training**. This can enable individuals first to understand, and then to learn to regulate,

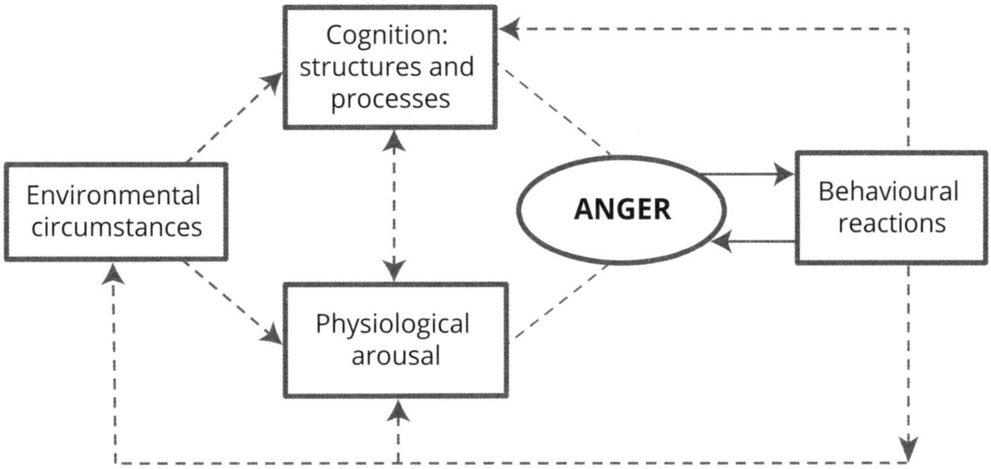
Cognition: structures and processes
Environmental circumstances
ANGER
Behavioural reactions
Physiological arousal

Source: Novaco, R. W. (1994). Anger as a risk factor for violence among the mentally disordered. In J. Monahan & H. J. Steadman (eds.). Violence and Mental Disorder: Developments in Risk Assessment. pp. 21–60. Chicago, IL: University of Chicago Press.
Part of The John D. and Catherine T. MacArthur Foundation Series on Mental Health and Development.

their degree of physical arousal and related anger behaviour. A first step in this training is to explain the model to the person concerned: to provide an *understanding* of anger and of how the above components interact. The intervention then combines *relaxation training* (which helps to reduce bodily tension) and *cognitive self-instructions* (to counteract ruminative thoughts that activate or escalate states of anger). In an experimental trial with four conditions, these two methods were compared separately and in combination with a no-treatment control group. The separate components each enabled individuals with chronic anger problems to gain some control over their anger, as compared with no treatment. Importantly, the combination of *both* relaxation training *and* cognitive self-instructions resulted in more improvement than that obtained from either method alone.

The resultant model is shown in the figure from Novaco (1994) on the previous page. There are now several large-scale reviews that show positive benefits from anger control training for a wide range of groups. As we will see in Chapter 19, however, results with people convicted of violent offences, while promising, are more mixed, and a number of questions remain to be answered.

for use with prisoners, on the basis of which they suggested that while 25 per cent of a sample of aggressive acts can be classed as impulsive and another 25 per cent as premeditated, the remaining 50 per cent were a mixture of the two, were 'medically related', or were indeterminate in nature.

The bulk of evidence, however, suggests that the distinction remains a meaningful one. Several studies using factor and cluster analyses have found clear differentiation between impulsive and premeditated aggression (Barratt *et al.*, 1999; Tharp *et al.*, 2011). Baker, Raine, Liu and Jacobson (2008; Tuvblad, Raine, Zheng and Baker, 2009) reported evidence of the validity of the distinction, making the additional suggestion that the difference can be traced to genetic components. Bobadilla, Wampler and Taylor (2012) used both psychometric and psychophysiological data, and concluded that the reactive/proactive distinction is valid. Cornell *et al.* (1996) found that while there was a high degree of overlap between instrumental and reactive violence, it was nevertheless possible to distinguish characteristics of individuals with histories of either pattern of offending. Those with a history of instrumental violence showed higher levels of psychopathy. Polman *et al.* (2007) reported a meta-analysis of 51 studies of reactive and proactive aggression in children and adolescents (aggregating data from 17,965 participants), and concluded that they 'are clearly distinct phenomena' (p. 530). However, it should be kept in mind that participants in these studies were not convicted offenders, and 80–85 per cent of the adult samples were female, meaning that extrapolation to the most frequent types of violent offending should remain provisional.

It is possible to acknowledge this and still to find the terms useful in making distinctions regarding how an act of violence was committed. This could have implications in forensic assessment and in recommendations regarding treatment. At the same time, it should also be recognised that the reactive/instrumental distinction does not directly correspond to the distinctions made in law between impulsive and premeditated homicides or other serious violent offences (Fontaine, 2007). The latter distinction is crucial in other contexts, especially in relation to the question of whether or not a defendant was provoked, and to the distinction between murder and manslaughter (an issue to which we will return in Chapters 11 and 16).

Personal variables

To what extent do individual variables such as personality contribute to explaining violent offences? If there are *specific* factors that predict involvement in assaults and other violent crimes, they have proved difficult to differentiate from the risk factors associated with crime in general. Yet as we have seen elsewhere, there is some evidence of stability and continuity in aggressiveness across sizeable segments of the lifespan – although over time, the level of aggression shown by the same individuals and the proportion of those who remain likely to be aggressive both gradually reduce. Piquero *et al.* (2012) reviewed a collection of studies that showed different types of pathways in aggressiveness over time, and found evidence of both stability and change across the successive stages of development (childhood, adolescence, adulthood). These authors also found that, on average, aggression decreases over the lifecourse, and more markedly amongst females. Nevertheless, there are a number who repeatedly engage in aggressive conduct. It seems not unreasonable to expect that there might be some features of personality that are consistently associated with this.

Jones, Miller and Lynam (2011) have reported a meta-analysis of 53 studies examining aspects of relationships between the Five-Factor Model of personality – the factors being *Neuroticism*, *Extraversion*, *Openness*, *Conscientiousness* and *Agreeableness* – and antisocial behaviour and aggression. The cumulative sample size ranged between 8,837 and 10,311 participants. Effect sizes were calculated as Pearson (*r*) correlations. For antisocial behaviour (ASB), there were low but statistically significant negative correlations with *Agreeableness* (−0.308) and *Conscientiousness* (−0.234), and a significant positive correlation with *Neuroticism* (0.092). For aggression, all five factors were significant, though the highest correlations were still rather low: *Agreeableness*, −0.327; *Conscientiousness*, −0.176; and *Neuroticism*, 0.169.

Jones *et al.* (2011) combined their results with those of DeCuyper *et al.* (2009), who had conducted a meta-analysis of studies on the relationship between the Five-Factor Model, antisocial personality disorder, and psychopathy. The resultant comparison showed a close correspondence between the 'effect-size profiles' found in the two sets of studies. This strengthens the view that the features identified here do have important predictive power in relation to continuities in aggressive and antisocial behaviour. However, the amount of variance that is explained remains fairly modest.

The psychological variable that has emerged with perhaps the firmest links to criminal violence is that of impulsiveness. Jolliffe and Farrington (2009) reported a meta-analysis of data from six longitudinal studies, focusing attention on the links between impulsiveness in childhood and later violence in adolescence and adulthood. The timescales and average follow-up periods covered by these studies varied widely. Impulsiveness was measured along two principal lines. Some assessments used *cognitive* measures, such as distractibility or difficulty in concentrating on tasks. Others used *behavioural* indicators, such as motor restlessness and levels of daring or risk-taking. Violent offending was measured both from officially recorded convictions and from self-reports. For official convictions, the results for the association over the longest time-gap were highly significant and suggested that 'between 73–76% of violent offenders would be considered impulsive as compared to 50% of those without violent offences' (Jolliffe and Farrington, 2009, p. 54). But there was sizeable heterogeneity in the results, suggesting that other, unmeasured factors were also affecting the outcome. The effect sizes for self-report were on average lower, though they were still statistically significant, and showed more homogeneity. Overall, therefore, the largest effect sizes were found for measures of *behavioural* impulsiveness, which predicted recorded convictions over shorter periods; in contrast, *cognitive* impulsiveness predicted self-reported violence over longer periods.

As a supplement to these findings, it is worth noting that in the meta-analysis by DeCuyper *et al.* (2009) just discussed, impulsiveness – which in the Five-Factor Model is one of the facets of *Neuroticism* – showed one of the highest correlations to emerge both with antisocial personality disorder and with psychopathy. At the same time, and contrary to expectations, evidence of an association between impulsiveness and violence in people suffering from psychosis has proved much more elusive (Bjørkly, 2013).

Violence and cognition

There is tentative evidence that the likelihood of involvement in violent offending is associated with some aspects of the content of thoughts and with patterns of cognitive processing. The role of hostile attributions in influencing aggression amongst children and adolescents has been illustrated in reviews such as that of de Castro *et al.* (2002), discussed in Chapter 5. It has also emerged in studies such as those of Barriga, Hawkins and Camelia (2008) with adolescents, where 'self-serving' cognitive distortions were more closely associated with externalising behaviour such as aggression, whereas 'self-debasing' distortions were more closely associated with internalising problems such as social withdrawal, anxiety and depression. It is less clear, however, whether similar processes occur amongst convicted adult offenders, as research on this has relied on some fairly transparent self-report questionnaires, which are of questionable usefulness when trying to detect attitudes that may be subject to social desirability effects (Collie, Vess and Murdoch, 2007).

Lopez and Emmer (2000, 2002) used qualitative methods in two studies with high-risk adolescent offenders (ages 14–20) in the United States. Analysing interviews through use of a grounded-theory approach, they found a distinction between attitudes to violence that mirrored the reactive/instrumental division. Young offenders believed that violence was of two main kinds: belief-driven and emotion-driven. The former was wholly condoned for some purposes: for example, when used to protect peers (a 'vigilante' function), when used to maintain a peer-group's honour, or when justified as revenge. Those who committed acts on that basis felt satisfaction, had no regrets, and gained enhanced status afterwards. In contrast, emotion-driven violence was seen as undesirable, and reactions to using it were negative, including regret, distress and denial. This value system was linked to a concept of 'hypermasculine' identity. In a similar study, based on narrative interviews with 125 active violent offenders aged 16–24 in New York City, Wilkinson (2001) obtained analogous findings. A great deal of violence served the purpose of preserving or enhancing social identity. Use of violence was 'the single most critical resource for gaining status' and was a core aspect of a culture of 'compulsive masculinity' (p. 264).

Beesley and McGuire (2009) tested the possible role of masculine identity in a cross-sectional comparison study with two groups of UK prisoners, one with and one without previous histories of violence, and a non-offending group matched in socioeconomic background variables. Participants completed assessments of gender-role identity and an attitude scale focused on hypermasculinity (Zaitchik and Mosher, 1993). Of the three groups, violent offenders showed the highest endorsement of attitudes indicative of masculine identity. On a subscale designed to measure the belief that this included use of violence, their scores were significantly higher than those of the other two groups.

Other findings suggestive of an important role for cognition have come from laboratory-based experimental research. In two studies with Canadian prisoners, Seager (2005) used a binocular rivalry task (see below), and James and Seager (2006) a dichotic listening task. Both studies used vignettes of social encounters, followed by questions designed to elicit any hostile attributions. The binocular rivalry paradigm involves simultaneous presentation of two distinct images, one to each eye. Rather than blending the two images or focusing alternately on each, most individuals perceive one as predominant. In Seager's (2005) study, violent images (involving a weapon being used in a crime) were compared with non-violent ones. If the participant reported that the former predominated over the latter, this was taken as an indicator of hypervigilance to threat cues. A history of violent offending, having convictions for assault, and reported participation in fights were all significantly correlated with hostile attributions, hypervigilance to threats and impulsivity. Gray *et al.* (2003) used the Implicit Association Test, a measure drawn from psychological research on prejudice, which is designed to access processing that occurs at an automatic level (i.e. outside conscious awareness). They found that some homicide offenders had 'diminished negative reactions to violence' (p. 497), which would probably not have been detectable using self-report measures.

Overall, the best interpretation of the available evidence appears to be that, in general terms, personality correlates of violent offending are difficult to isolate when we examine a mixed group of offenders with varying levels of violent history. Focusing on a smaller group that commits violence more frequently, and who persist in that tendency over a lengthy period, we are more likely to find personality features that include high impulsiveness, low *Agreeableness*, and low *Conscientiousness*. Within that group, some will meet criteria for diagnosis with a personality disorder. Where individuals have histories of involvement in violent crime, that may also be influenced by patterns of hostile attribution, expectation of threat, and support for, or even an openly expressed belief in, the value of violence. While at the moment these conclusions remain to some extent speculative, such cognitive patterns could be crucial in predisposing individuals towards acting violently in encounters they perceive as hostile.

Regarding other personal variables associated with violence, all the factors we reviewed in Chapter 5 may contribute in varying amounts to the occurrence of an assault. There may be genetic factors expressed through temperament that result in higher levels of impulsiveness. Socialisation processes may have excluded opportunities to acquire skills for **self-management**. Individuals may have developed belligerent or antisocial attitudes and beliefs as a function of the family environments to which they were exposed. Their self-image may be fragile and susceptible to insult; or may be inflated and linked to a sense of entitlement (Bushman *et al.*, 2009). Individuals may have absorbed 'scripts' telling them that it is vital not to back down. Finally, they may have experienced emotional degradation, or suffered physical or sexual victimisation.

The risks of acting aggressively will be elevated if an individual has consumed alcohol or drugs, and elevated further if he or she has become a regular user of them. They may also be elevated if he or she has recently been deprived of sleep, possibly through the impact of sleep deprivation on the functioning of the pre-frontal cortex (Kamphuis, Meerlo, Koolhaas and Lancel, 2012). All of these factors, in various potential combinations, could incline an individual towards resorting to violence in a stressful situation. Previous use of violence could have been reinforced in a way that makes it likelier on subsequent occasions. A reputation arising from this could be difficult to escape from or to put into reverse. Overall, the larger the number of risk factors present, the higher the probability that an individual will embark on and then remain entrenched in a crime career that includes violent offending.

Situational factors in confrontations and assaults

To obtain a fuller picture of why violent assaults happen as and when they do, however, it is also important to examine the role of *situational* variables. Given that violence represents a small proportion of all the social exchanges in which people engage, it may be that there are only certain circumstances in which it is likely to occur. Those situations may even follow standard sequences and predictable rules. This view is compatible with the general framework of person–situation interactions that we highlighted in Chapter 5 as an approach to understanding personal violence.

The neglect of situational factors has also been recognised within criminology. LaFree and Birkbeck (1991) compared patterns of violent offences (assaults, robberies and pickpocketing or 'snatch') in the USA and Venezuela. They found that, despite cultural differences, there were structural similarities between the patterning of some features of offences across the two countries. Horney, Osgood and Marshall (1995; Horney, 2001) studied the relationship between violent offences and events and circumstances in offenders' lives. Using statistical modelling, they found that the crime events were systematically preceded by changes in the offenders' lives; some events doubled the chances of offending, while others halved it. This appeared to hold irrespective of each individual's overall level of offending. On the basis of these and other studies, some criminologists have forwarded a 'criminal event perspective' (CEP) to correct the overemphasis on individual variables that dominates both criminological and psychological theorising (Meier, Kennedy and Sacco, 2001).

Can features of situations that are regularly associated with some forms of crime be identified on a smaller scale, a more 'molecular' level? Collins (2008, 2009, 2013) has collated an extensive range of observational data relating to the situational factors that are associated with many types of violence. Collins (2008) accessed film and video footage, police recordings, CCTV surveillance, forensic reconstructions, news photographs and mobile phone images of a wide range of violent episodes, including military combat, political demonstrations and riots, fights at sports matches, robbery and assault. He subjected this to 'micro-sociological' analysis, using close-ups of individual faces and bodily movements.

On the basis of this research, and the work of Ekman (2003) and others on the expression of emotions, Collins (2008) concluded that most people in potentially violent confrontations are in states of *fear* rather than *anger*. These two emotions can be clearly differentiated in human facial expressions, voice and body movements; and in most of the recorded material Collins examined, indicators of fear predominate. He suggested that this is so because the majority of people have no wish to initiate violence or to inflict harm on others, even in these extreme circumstances. Furthermore, he argues, most of us are poorly coordinated and incompetent when very highly aroused. Even when trained soldiers or police fire their weapons at close range, they miss their targets a large proportion of the time.

This research suggests that there are specific pathways along which violence becomes more likely to erupt. Collins developed a model for such situations which he calls *interaction ritual chains*. These are identifiable sequences through which the confrontational tension and fear that most parties experience in a conflict may be circumvented, enabling conflicts to intensify into physical attack. There are several ways in which this can happen, but the crucial issue in whether or not disputes spiral into violence is a function of the ongoing exchanges between the antagonists, and their perceptions of each other's emotional states. This applies in many assaults and affrays, in robbery and **aggravated** burglary, and may also underpin many instances of intimate partner violence. Even the most habitually aggression-prone individual is not violent at every opportunity. Indeed, from Collins's standpoint, it is a 'false lead' to look for types of violent individuals, as features of situations have a more potent effect on whether or not acts of violence occur.

On this basis, Collins offers an additional level to the risk factors approach. Thus as he puts it, 'crime is not easily predictable from background variables such as poverty, race, or family background. There are far more persons who fit the crime-prone pattern than those who actually commit such crimes, because initial motivations or opportunities for crime and violence are still a long way from the interactional competence to carry them out' (Collins, 2009, p. 575). Some psychological variables are probably pivotal here in enabling us to move from demographic features to risk factors for aggressiveness. As we saw earlier, they include impulsiveness (low self-control) and attitudes supportive of violence, amongst others.

The approach developed by Collins has been criticised as too anecdotal, and as not sufficiently differentiating between types of violence (Cooney, 2009). Mazur (2009) adds a biological perspective to the interactional sequences outlined by Collins, by emphasising the role of hormonal changes, especially in cortisol and testosterone, as levels of fear and aggression fluctuate in rapidly changing conflictual encounters. Levels of cortisol increase in response to stress, and there is evidence that 'heightened testosterone can promote dominant and assertive behavior' (Mazur, 2009, p. 442); but these changes are not thought to contribute directly to male violence, so the part played by hormonal changes remains poorly understood. Klusemann (2010, 2012) has applied Collins's model to an analysis of the emotional dynamics of the period immediately preceding atrocities such as the Rwandan genocide of 1994 and the Srebrenica massacre of 1995. Examples such as these illustrate how, in the midst of conflict, fear and anger can further escalate in a community as a result of broadcast messages affecting how an entire group of people is perceived, and can lead to drastic and lethal action. However, the precise roles of the different factors operating in such situations can be difficult if not impossible to disentangle.

Criminologists such as Bernard (1990) have argued that there are 'rules of anger' that define both the social circumstances in which anger is deemed appropriate and also how to respond to anger. Where individuals are in a disadvantaged social position, experiencing discrimination and other life stresses that exacerbate interpersonal tensions, such rules may help to create particularly aggressive environments. The possibility of violence is greater amongst those living certain lifestyles, and living a large portion of life 'on the street' increases the risks of becoming either a victim or a perpetrator of violence (and sometimes both). In a series of studies conducted in the 1990s, Kennedy and Baron (1993; Kennedy and Forde, 1996) analysed violent incidents involving homeless youths who were part of a 'punk rocker' culture. These individuals claimed not to be violence-prone but to have been drawn into violence by situations that arose in that environment.

In a later study, Forde and Kennedy (1997) conducted a large-scale telephone interview survey. This led to the development of a model in which individuals' involvement in crime was not a direct result of a psychological variable (low self-control), but this did influence their likelihood of engaging in 'imprudent' (i.e. risk-taking) behaviour. Actual crimes were a function of these factors in combination with proximate causes (situational factors). The resulting theory involved 'the integration of offenders' characteristics with aspects of situations to place the criminal event in the context of a situated transaction' (p. 285).

The proximate causes (or situational factors) that typically lead to violence have been studied by Felson and Steadman (1983), who analysed homicides and serious assaults, focusing on detailed descriptions of what had happened when these crimes were committed. They suggested that 'the successive behaviors of a participant are more a function of the antagonist's behaviors than they are of his or her own earlier actions' (1983, p. 69). This demonstrates the importance of the interaction sequence. Using a similar approach, Luckenbill and Doyle (1989) suggested that physical fights followed from a similar series of stages. The escalation of ill-feeling that results from such a sequence sets the scene for a violent encounter.

Other broader proximal factors have been found to influence the likelihood that people will feel and act in an aggressive manner. It is not suggested that these are direct *causes* of violence. One such factor is general conditions of physical discomfort, which have been associated with heightened levels of aggression. For example, Anderson (1989, 2001) reviewed evidence for the *heat hypothesis*, the proposal that 'hot temperatures increase aggressive motivation and (under some conditions) aggressive behavior' (2001, p. 33). This is well supported by field studies; but less well by laboratory studies, where findings are more mixed.

Drinking environments

How does this translate to everyday settings where violence is known to occur? One recurrent pattern in many assaults is an association with the consumption of alcohol. Apart from the possible role of alcohol itself in this (which we will discuss in Chapter 10), the places where drinking is done may also have a contributory role. Some features of the environment in drinking establishments have been found to be associated with increased risks of aggression and violence. Graham, Bernards, Osgood and Wells (2006) undertook a series of 1,334 observational assessments in 118 bars in Toronto, measuring aspects of the surroundings and management of each venue, and analysing their relationships with levels of recorded aggression. The frequency and severity of aggression was associated with the rowdiness of bars and with the extent of their sexual permissiveness. When people still had several drinks left as closing time approached, or when they stayed afterwards, aggression was more likely. A lower number of staff was linked to more severe aggression by *customers*, whereas a higher number was associated with more aggression by *staff*. Homel *et al.* (2004) conducted a similar study in Queensland, Australia, and examined changes over time as bars attempted to reduce the level of violence. Reductions were associated with the overall level of comfort in a bar, the availability of public transport, the frequency of 'flagrant fondling' by female customers, and the level of male drunkenness.

A study by Quigley, Leonard and Collins (2003) gives a practical illustration of the interaction between personal and situational variables in producing violence in drinking contexts. As part of their study these authors administered the *Five-Factor Personality Inventory*, the *State-Trait Anger Expression Inventory* and other measures to a community sample (n=327, 56 per cent males). Participants were also interviewed about their patterns of alcohol use, and physical aspects of the venues in which they regularly drank. Results supported the authors' hypothesis that 'violent and heavy-drinking people are attracted to bars with physical and social conditions that promote aggressive behaviour' (2003, p. 770). Based on descriptions of bars that participants provided, the bars were classified into violent or non-violent environments. The former had poorer ventilation, more noise, higher temperatures, more male employees, and more other forms of illegal activity than the latter. Individuals who frequented these bars were younger, had higher alcohol dependence scores, and higher levels of trait anger than those who frequented the non-violent bars. Thus there was an interaction between the characteristics of the individuals and the characteristics of the drinking places, though the analysis suggested that the latter were the stronger predictors of bar violence.

To summarise, then, the fullest understanding we can obtain of how and why a violent assault has occurred will be one in which we combine information about the offender with information about how the event itself unfolded and the context in which it occurred. In Chapter 18 we will discuss methods that can be used for assessment and offence analysis in efforts to obtain the clearest picture possible of why an individual acted as he or she did at the time when a violent assault took place.

Hate crime

In recent years there has been growing recognition that some violent offences, and also other crimes, are directed towards members of particular groups in society. Tensions and antipathies between different communities are of course nothing new. Almost any difference that appears to exist between people has the potential to create social distance, and therefore can be a source of suspicion and anxiety. When magnified for any reason, such a predisposition can lead to strong feelings of animosity, with results that range from individual 'hate crimes' to riots or other forms of large-scale public unrest.

As with many other terms in this area, while it might sound straightforward, **hate crime** is not easy to define. Hatred is a raw human emotion, but its expression in the form thought to constitute a type of crime is a social construction. As Gerstenfeld (2013) points out, a 'hate crime' is not simply a crime in which one person hates another: that probably applies to many kinds of offence. The phrase is reserved for a criminal act that is 'motivated, at least in part, by the group affiliation of the victim' (p. 11). The term 'hate crime' was first introduced into law in the United States in 1990 (the federal Hate Crimes Statistics Act; though some individual states had introduced similar laws before then) in order to set up a system whereby crimes against minorities could be recorded. In the official statistics for England and Wales, a 'hate crime' is considered to be 'any criminal offence committed against a person or property that is motivated by hostility towards someone based on their disability, race, religion, gender-identity or sexual orientation, whether perceived to be so by the victim or any other person' (Office for National Statistics, 2013, p. 7).

The Association of Chief Police Officers (ACPO) in England and Wales began monitoring the frequency of racially motivated murders in the period 1986–1999 (Hall, 2013). None of the legal systems in the UK employs the phrase 'hate crime'; this is colloquial rather than legal language. In England and Wales, the legislation that governs these offences is contained in three different statutes: the Crime and Disorder Act 1998; the Anti-Terrorism, Crime and Security Act

2001; and the Criminal Justice Act 2003 (Hall, 2013). They do not define hate crime as such, but specify where an offence may be considered to be 'motivated and aggravated by racial and religious prejudice' (Hall, 2013, p. 8). The offences covered by these Acts, including property damage, harassment and violence, are also defined in other Acts, but with the added provision that if a motive of hatred is established, a more severe penalty can be imposed.

Some criminologists make the definition of 'hate crime' more specific by adding that many of those likely to be victims of it are affiliated to groups that are in other ways already discriminated against or marginalised in society (Hall, 2013). Such groups include, amongst others, racial, ethnic or religious minorities; people who are gay, lesbian, bisexual, or transgender; people with disabilities; and members of travelling communities. While there have been racial tensions in many parts of Britain for some time, consciousness of them was heightened particularly in 1993 by the murder in south London of a young black man, Stephen Lawrence, by a group of white youths; and subsequently by the revelation of profound flaws in the police investigation of his death, and the conclusion of a Judicial Inquiry that the Metropolitan Police was affected by 'institutional racism' (Home Office, 1999; the Macpherson Report).

The numbers of crimes classified as having a racist element rose dramatically in the period following the publication of the Macpherson Report, which drew attention to the issues highlighted by the Lawrence case. Collating the figures, Ray (2013) found a sharp rise in the numbers of racist incidents reported in England and Wales, from 25,000 in 1999 to 57,902 in 2001. In 2011–2012, the police recorded 43,748 hate crimes, which were classified as motivated thus: related to race, 82 per cent; related to sexual orientation, 10 per cent; related to religion, 4 per cent; related to disability, 4 per cent; and related to transgender people, 1 per cent (Home Office, 2012). The European Union (EU) Agency for Fundamental Rights (FRA, 2014a) has documented the reported rates of victimisation of different ethnic minority and immigrant groups across 27 EU countries. The average rates were: Roma, 18 per cent; Sub-Saharan African, 18 per cent; North African, 9 per cent; Turkish, 8 per cent; Central and East European, 7 per cent; Russian, 5 per cent; and former Yugoslav, 3 per cent. In the United States, national data on hate or 'bias crimes' have been assembled by the Federal Bureau of Investigation (FBI), but they are thought to be a considerable underestimate of the 'true' volume as many cities do not participate in the required survey. However, in the data successfully collected for 2011, the proportions of crimes attributable to different forms of bias were: racial, 46.9 per cent; sexual orientation, 20.9 per cent; religious, 19.8 per cent; ethnicity/nationality, 11.6 per cent; and disability, 0.9 per cent (Hall, 2013).

Factors linked to hate crimes

Numerous factors contribute to offences that fit the description of hate crimes, yet – and perhaps more so than any other offences – these contributory factors are almost impossible to extract from their social context. That context may consist of beliefs that are consciously articulated by political factions or in extremist ideologies (such as Holocaust denial, or insistence that immigrants 'go home'). More often, though, it reflects constellations of attitudes that are held to varying degrees by many members of a society, as is demonstrated by the need to introduce legislation against those attitudes (as in the Equality Act 2010). Biased belief systems in turn are often influenced by the almost ubiquitous stereotyping of some communities in media portrayals or reporting of them. Content analysis of UK newspaper reports shows predominantly negative representation of a range of social groups, for example Muslims (Moore, Mason and Lewis, 2008) and disabled people (Briant, Watson and Philo, 2013), to cite just two illustrations.

It is widely supposed that resentment of some minority groups intensifies during periods of economic downturn. Research on economically deprived youths from the majority community has sometimes shown that they feel threatened when they perceive minority communities as being afforded special advantages (for example, through 'reverse discrimination' policies). Pinderhughes (1993) found this in a study of race-related violent crimes (including some notorious murders) in predominantly white neighbourhoods of Brooklyn, New York. He suggested that while other factors also operated, 'bleak structural economic conditions have laid the foundation for racial conflict by leaving some young people with extremely uncertain futures' (1993, p. 479). More recently Falk, Kuhn and Zweimüller (2011) analysed the relationship between numbers of right-wing extremist crimes and levels of unemployment in different regions of Germany. They found that a relationship emerged strongly from both time-series and cross-sectional data. Other research has not confirmed this relationship consistently (Gerstenfeld, 2013), but the evidence that fits less well concerns homophobia rather than ethnic tensions. It may be that economic factors influence the latter more than the former, as immigrants or ethnic minorities are perceived as undermining the employment prospects of citizens of the host country or ethnic majority. Even when these impressions are shown to be inaccurate (Devlin *et al.*, 2014), perceptions of outgroups as a serious threat still persist.

Ezekiel (2002) gives an account of interviews with members of white supremacist groups (Ku Klux Klan and neo-Nazi) in the United States and develops a model of the factors at work when individuals join in such alliances. However, of the crimes committed against ethnic minorities or marginalised groups, only a small proportion are committed by members of extremist political parties who have formulated an ideology or launched a campaign to further their views. More often, individuals who commit hate crimes may never have fully endorsed such an agenda. McDevitt, Levin and Bennett (2002) developed a typology of hate crimes on the basis of their analysis of police case files in Boston. They classed hate crimes into four groups. Their smallest category, 'mission' hate crimes, committed by those who had a major preoccupation with a detested group, account for less than 1 per cent of the total. Craig (2002) also found that few perpetrators were members of 'hate groups' as such.

The influence of social and cultural factors on these offences is evidently strong. But it is puzzling to suggest, as Iganski does (2010, p. 354) that hate crime can only be understood 'once free of the confinement of offender psychology'. In addition to social processes, this type of offence also contains an individual component, given that part of its motivation resides in feelings of bitterness towards members of a specific outgroup. On a psychological level, hate crime is thought to have its origins, at least in part, in *prejudice*. There has been extensive social psychological research carried out in efforts to understand sets of beliefs that lead someone, solely on the basis of another person's membership of a given group (often judged by a single attribute, such as skin colour or accent), to ascribe numerous other characteristics to that person. Gerstenfeld (2013) reviews research on the factors contributing to such prejudice. They include the transmission (explicit or tacit) of parental attitudes and beliefs. Later, the influence of peer-group membership may be crucial in a context in which a superficially different group is defined as alien and threatening.

There is evidence that some attitudinal biases hold together as clusters, and Sibley and Duckitt (2008) have identified two that are closely connected to prejudice. They are respectively called *Right-Wing Authoritarianism* (RWA) and *Social Dominance Orientation* (SDO). RWA is associated with social conformity, adherence to conventions, submission to authority, and aggression towards outsiders. Meta-analysis showed a strong negative correlation with *Openness to experience* and a positive association with *Conscientiousness* (from the Five-Factor Model). SDO is associated with a drive for one's ingroup to dominate other groups; it was negatively correlated with *Agreeableness* and less so with *Openness*. Sadly, while programmes for reducing prejudice through initiatives such as diversity training are widely disseminated, a review of the literature in this area concluded that as yet we cannot say with any certainty which interventions are most likely to work (Paluck and Green, 2009).

In addition to the aforementioned factors, there are probably ingroup dynamics at work whereby individuals with nascent views of these kinds coalesce as a result of shared attitudes. Craig (2002) reviewed research on hate crimes and found that in two-thirds of assaults there were two or more attackers involved. In addition, a larger proportion of assailants were unknown to their victims than in equivalent offences without the bias element (90 per cent as opposed to 65 per cent). Many offences served a 'symbolic' function. Those found guilty of hate crimes are often found to have consumed high levels of alcohol beforehand (Parrott, Gallagher, Vincent and Bakeman, 2010).

There is evidence that victims of hate crime experience more severe emotional reactions than those who are victimised in similar ways without the element of bias against their group. The sense that they have been targeted *because* of that membership – that they could be picked on at random, that they are in a sense interchangeable with other group members, and thus that it is an attack on their very identity – leads to a heightened sense of vulnerability, in addition to the trauma resulting from the crime itself (Herek, Gillis, Cogan and Glunt, 1997; Iganski, 2001). It is partly for this reason that legislators have introduced new laws or increased penalties for crimes driven by group hate. However, steps in that direction have been controversial, for reasons that range from the assertion that such measures infringe rights of self-expression to the suggestion that they are counterproductive and can lead to further blaming of the community they are intended to protect (Ezekiel, 2002; Hall, 2013; Iganski, 2001; Gerstenfeld, 2013).

In sum, while a proportion of those convicted of violent hate crimes might be members of extreme groups, a far larger proportion will probably not. The offence may have resulted from prejudicial beliefs, but factors not dissimilar to those associated with other types of offence will probably also have played a part. Examination of the circumstances and the context will potentially be even more important here than with other types of violent offence.

Conclusion

The simple conclusion of this chapter, if this does not sound too much of a contradiction, is that violent crime is complex. While many offences are brief in duration – as perpetrators may be keen to escape once they have carried out the offence – the sequence of events that *precede* them may present a convergence of several different kinds of influence. A possible predisposition to resort to violence may have developed as a product of the kinds of factors we examined in Chapters 4 and 5. Internal factors, such as uncontrolled emotional states, hostile attitudes and cognitive rehearsal, and situational factors may then combine to increase the risk of aggression being acted out, in the form of a physically violent assault.

Some assaults may be sustained or repeated, and a proportion have fatal results, an outcome to which we will turn next: Chapters 7 and 8 focus on homicide involving single and multiple victims respectively. Then in Chapter 9 we will turn our attention to sexual crimes and intimate partner violence; and in Chapter 10 we will examine the relationship between violence and the abuse of alcohol and other substances.

Chapter summary

The core focus of this chapter has been on serious assault and hate crimes.

» We began by considering whether or how it is possible to measure the seriousness of crimes, and described a number of proposals for carrying this out.

» We then turned attention to violent crime as defined in law, and reviewed a range of variables thought to be associated with its occurrence. This led to discussion of the distinction between instrumental and reactive aggression, and related research. We considered personal variables, cognitive processes, situational factors, and the role of alcohol in the occurrence of violent assaults, paying particular attention to some antisocial attitudes that are manifested in hate crimes.

» The occurrence of a violent offence is usually a function of several factors operating in concert. At the broadest level, these can be described as consisting of *personal* and *situational* variables, with *the interaction between them* often being the most prominent component.

Further reading

A number of excellent books have been drawn upon in preparing this chapter. They are invaluable sources of further information on specific topics covered within the chapter, although the subject is so large that no single book can cover all aspects of it.

- On aggression and violence in general, the books by Margaret A. Zahn, H.H. Brownstein and S.L. Jackson (2004), *Violence: From Theory to Research* (London: Matthew Bender); Phillip R. Shaver and Mario Mikulincer (2011), *Human Aggression and Violence: Causes, Manifestations, and Consequences* (American Psychological Association), and Barbara Krahé (2013), *The Social Psychology of Aggression*, 2nd edition (Hove: Psychology Press) provide well-researched and clearly explained accounts of both psychological research and other kinds of theory and evidence.
- For a useful and broad-ranging source on several types of serious crime, including those covered in this chapter, the edited volume *Handbook on Crime* by Fiona Brookman *et al.* (2010; Cullompton: Willan) is a valuable place to start. The compilation *Aggressive Offenders' Cognition* by Theresa Gannon, Tony Ward, Anthony R. Beech and Dawn Fisher (2007; Chichester: Wiley) contains more detail on cognitive processes associated with aggression and violence.
- Two different approaches to the study of hate crime are presented in the books by Phyllis B. Gerstenfeld (2013), *Hate Crime: Causes, Controls, and Controversies* (Thousand Oaks: Sage) and by Nathan Hall (2013), *Hate Crime* (London: Routledge).
- The Ministry of Justice (London) has been in the process of developing a *Crime Severity Tool* (Office for National Statistics, 2016e). Weights are attaching to offence types according to the resource demands they make on the police, and the level of penalty imposed (prison or community sentence, or fine). This involves comparing different categories of crimes rather than the details of individual offences within a category hence it is designed for a different purpose from the measures described here.

Single-Victim Homicide

The most serious form of personal violence at an individual level is where a single person intentionally kills one or more other people. This chapter looks closely at what is known about how and why such severe acts of violence take place, in relation to offences in which there is one victim and (for the most part) one perpetrator. We examine the factors believed to influence such offences and the different patterns they take; whether there are separate influences operating in each; and whether those who have committed such offences are likely to do so again. Chapter 8 considers homicides with two or more victims, which often have different motives.

Chapter objectives

- To consider the nature of homicide and the different patterns it takes.
- To examine factors involved in the occurrence of homicides of different types, with a particular focus on motives.
- To review evidence on rates of homicide recidivism.

In everyday language, people who have killed someone may be described as being 'killers' or 'murderers'. In legal terms and in psychological and criminological research, the terms used are more precise. The suffix-*cide* denotes the killing of the named category of people to which it is attached. *Homicide* is the general term for killing a person; *femicide* refers to the killing of women; and *eldercide* to the killing of an older adult. On a different scale entirely, there is also *genocide*, though defining what that is raises complexities we will consider in the next chapter.

Killing another person can sometimes be lawful, as, for example, in the slaying of an enemy combatant in battle, in justifiable self-defence, or in an accidental death that an inquest accepts could not have been foreseen. The *actus reus* of homicide is the unlawful killing of another person, and the law in England and Wales defines three principal categories: murder, manslaughter and infanticide. The current statutory framework governing homicide is provided by the Homicide Act 1957, the Coroners and Justice Act 2009, and the Infanticide Act 1938.

The *mens rea* of each category of homicide is different, and is dependent on a legal determination. Where a court finds that there was an intention to kill or to cause grievous bodily harm, the offence is one of *murder*, and the mandatory penalty is life imprisonment. Where a court accepts that killing was *not* intentional – which it may do on the grounds of diminished responsibility, loss of control, or (in rare cases) a suicide pact in which one of the parties survived – the finding will be one of *voluntary manslaughter*. A third category, *involuntary manslaughter*, arises when it is shown that there was no intention to kill but that death was a result of negligence or recklessness of action. In England and Wales *infanticide* is the killing by a mother of her child less than one year old, as a result of an imbalance of the mother's mind arising from the childbirth. For all of the offences that are less than murder, a life sentence can be imposed, but the penalty is often lower than this.

There are many complexities within the above definitions, which are beyond the scope of this book to cover and beyond the competence of its authors to address. On average in the years from 1998 to 2008, 35–40 per cent of those charged with homicide were convicted of murder, roughly one-third of manslaughter, approximately 20 per cent were acquitted, and the remainder were made subject to lesser charges (Brookman, 2010). There were very few cases of infanticide.

As already illustrated in Chapter 2, rates of intentional homicide vary considerably worldwide (Malby, 2010). In England and Wales, after rising steadily from 1961 to 2002–2003 (when there was an unusually high figure resulting from the inclusion of 172 murders attributed to Harold Shipman), the number of homicides has fallen. The figure for the year ending June 2016 was 681 (ONS, 2016c), though as a result of inquests completed that year this included the 96 victims of the events at Hillsborough football stadium in 1989. Excluding those victims, the then prevailing rate of 10 homicides per million people for England and Wales was lower than the rates for both 5 and 10 years earlier. Putting this in a wider context, in European Union countries the average homicide rates per million vary considerably. Pooling data across the years 2008–2010 shows a range from 3.1 (Iceland) to 77 (Lithuania). During the same period, the rates for France, Germany, Italy, Netherlands, Norway, Spain, Sweden and some other countries were all lower than that for the United Kingdom.

The majority of homicides involve a single victim. Most (80 per cent) are committed by males, and most victims (69 per cent in 2012–2013) are *also* male. Statistics show that 75 per cent of female victims are acquainted with the perpetrator, who in nearly half of cases (45 per cent) is a partner or ex-partner; the corresponding figures for male victims are 49 per cent and 4 per cent. Because the detection and clear-up rate for this type of crime is very high, and because most perpetrators are given lengthy prison sentences (or in some jurisdictions, are executed), it is likely to be the only crime of its kind that the perpetrator will ever commit.

The most common method of killing someone in England and Wales remained consistent in the period 2005 to 2015 (ONS, 2016b), and involved the use of a knife, a broken bottle or some other sharp instrument. In the year ending March 2015, for male and female victims, the proportions were 35 per cent and 38 per cent respectively. In the same year this was followed by kicking or by hitting without a weapon (25 per cent of male victims), and by strangulation or asphyxiation (18 per cent of female victims). In a smaller proportion of cases (8 per cent) a blunt instrument was used; and the numbers killed by shooting were lower still, at 21 (4 per cent). Quite small fractions involved burning, poisoning, drowning, or administration of drugs. There was also a small 'Other' category. These figures fluctuate somewhat, but this overall pattern holds for different parts of the UK and for several other countries. However, there are some countries where a far larger proportion of homicides involve firearms.

Homicide motives and dynamics

Why do people kill? Criminal justice statistics for Scotland (Scottish Government, 2003) reported some analysis of the motives for homicide, which showed some similar patterns over time. Taking 2002 as an example, there were 127 homicides recorded. The largest proportions committed by men resulted from a quarrel (35 per cent) or were attributed to rage or fury (21 per cent). Gradually decreasing percentages were attributed to feuds or factional rivalries (7.2 per cent), financial gain (7.2 per cent), jealousy (4 per cent), and insanity/mental disorder (3.2 per cent). There was one sexual murder, and there was one contract killing. A further nine homicides were unclassified and for fourteen there was no known explanation. For *female* perpetrators, five of the thirteen homicides were classified as resulting from a fight or quarrel, two as a result of rage or fury, two financial, one due to insanity, and three unknown. Two crimes remained unsolved. A similar distribution of motives could be seen ten years later, in the statistics for 2012–2013, when the number of homicides (62) was less than half that recorded in 2002 (Scottish Government, 2013). As the overall amount of homicide in Scotland is comparatively low, however, it may not produce a picture that can be generalised to other places.

Studies of the dynamics of homicidal events suggest that some of the disputes that end in a fatal assault may have a number of features in common. Luckenbill (1977) reported a study of homicides selected from those committed during a ten-year period in one county of California. He identified a six-stage dialogue between the parties who would eventually become perpetrator and victim:

1. The victim insults or disparages the offender, or refuses to comply with a request.
2. The offender interprets this as personally offensive.
3. Instead of excusing it or leaving the scene, the offender retaliates with a challenge, or an attempt to restore face; in 14 per cent of cases the victim was killed at this point.
4. In most cases the victim rebuts the offender's challenge and may add a further insult; both parties acknowledge that violence might be needed to resolve their differences.
5. There is a 'commitment to battle', and a physical attack ensues, with lethal results.
6. The perpetrator either flees (58 per cent), remains voluntarily while police are called (32 per cent), or is forcibly restrained by third parties (10 per cent).

In a study discussed briefly in Chapter 6, Felson and Steadman (1983) analysed a series of homicides and assaults not committed in conjunction with other offences (e.g. burglary or robbery). In several respects, there were similarities between homicides and assaults and the offenders in the two groups were close in age, background and prior criminal histories. However, victims of homicide were more likely to engage in 'identity attacks', physical attacks and threats than were victims of assault; they were more likely to have brandished a weapon; and they were more likely to have been intoxicated. Offenders in homicides were less likely to have threatened victims.

The largest proportion of homicides between acquaintances began as 'identity attacks' or 'character contests'. In contrast to Luckenbill, Felson and Steadman suggest three stages to homicides and assaults:

1. There is verbal conflict and a personal attack, with one person trying and failing to dissuade the other from this.
2. Threats follow, and evasive action; and sometimes efforts are made to mediate.
3. A physical attack ensues, with lethal results.

The presence of attempts at mediation led Felson and Steadman to doubt Luckenbill's suggestion that the antagonists reached a 'working agreement' that violence between them was inevitable. It is important to emphasise that while some of this may appear as if it is 'blaming the victim', it is not our intention here to assign moral or legal responsibility for a killing to anyone other than the perpetrator: our aim is simply to understand how the event occurred. Savitz, Kumar and Zahn (1991) compared the Luckenbill and Felson-Steadman models using homicides committed in Philadelphia in 1978. Of the 197 murders about which there was thought to be enough information available, just under 61 per cent fitted the transactional pattern found by Luckenbill (1977).

Athens (1997) interviewed individuals who had committed violent offences, focusing on the details of the criminal act and exploring how the perpetrator (offender) had construed the situation as it developed. Athens divided offenders' interpretations into four groups:

1. *'Defensive' interpretation* The offender assumed that the victim was planning to attack.
2. *'Frustrative' interpretation* The offender believed that the victim was purposefully resisting an action that the offender wanted to take, in a way that the offender believed could only be dealt with by violence.
3. *'Malefic' interpretation* The offender believed that the victim was deriding him or her, and in a way that suggested malicious intent.
4. *'Frustrative-malefic' interpretation* A hybrid category combining elements of the previous two.

During the encounter, the interpretation may change, leading to self-restraint – and indeed this was the commonest outcome.

Many interviewees saw themselves as having a violent disposition, and gave accounts of violent periods in their lives. This perception had a pivotal influence on their manner of interpreting the intentions of others, and on the likelihood of their acting violently in a conflict.

In the largest study of its kind, Miethe and Regoeczi (2004) analysed a voluminous database of homicide information, the FBI's *Supplementary Homicide Reports* (SHR) from 1976 to 1998. This contained details of a total of 439,954 homicides committed during that period. Miethe and Regoeczi extracted 'structural elements' of each offence, such as the number, age, gender and ethnic group of offenders and victims; the offender–victim relationship (family, acquaintance, stranger), the weapon used, the primary motive, whether an urban or a rural location, and the region of the USA. While some features changed over time, most patterns remained broadly similar. For 1990–1998, 50.8 per cent of the victims were acquaintances of the offender – 24.9 per cent were family members, and 18.2 per cent strangers. The majority of victims (70.4 per cent) were killed with a firearm. Most motives were classed as *expressive* (53.4 per cent), and others as *instrumental* (28.3 per cent), while 18.2 per cent were grouped as having other motives. The expressive group included personal confrontations and character contests, and 'defence of significant others'. Amongst the instrumental offences, the commonest motives were robbery or drug-related, with smaller proportions committed in the course of burglary, arson, or rape. Miethe and Regoeczi suggested that the expressive/instrumental dichotomy did not properly work for these offences; even so, their data collection suggested regularities in the ways in which the events that result in a homicide unfold, adding further weight to the findings of Luckenbill and others. A separate study of the FBI *Supplementary Homicide Reports*, by Fox and Allen (2014), supported the value of the instrumental-expressive distinction. They examined relationships between the gender of the victim and that of the offender, their relationship (family, acquaintance, stranger), and the type of weapon used; and their results suggested a further useful distinction, between *expressive-offensive* and *expressive-defensive* homicides.

Structural factors and homicide

Variations in homicide and other crime rates, both between places and over time, provide an opportunity to study what other factors might be associated with them. Some demographic and structural factors have been found to be closely associated with these variations. These have been studied most extensively in the USA, and there are analyses of homicide in various American cities going as far back as the 1920s (Smith and Zahn, 1999). Possibly the most frequently cited research is that of Wolfgang (1958), who analysed homicides committed in Philadelphia from 1948 to 1952. The majority of victims (73 per cent) and of perpetrators (75 per cent) were African-American, even though this group formed only 18 per cent of the population. The peak age bands for committing homicide were 20–24 and 25–29, whereas victims were more numerous in the 25–29 and 30–34 bands. The commonest methods of killing were stabbing (38.8 per cent) and shooting (33 per cent). More recently in the USA, the latter has considerably overtaken the former. Half of the homicides studied took place between 8.00 p.m. and 2.00 a.m. In 63.6 per cent of cases, either the victim or the offender had been drinking; and in 43.5 per cent, *both* had been. Although most perpetrators had criminal records (66 per cent involving assault), almost half (48.3 per cent) had only one or two prior convictions.

Land, McCall and Cohen (1990) analysed US homicide rates for the years 1960, 1970 and 1980. Larger urban populations and higher densities, greater resource deprivation, and a larger proportion of divorced males were all associated with higher rates of homicide. Unemployment and the percentage of the population aged 15–29 were also significant, but not at all levels of analysis. There were also regional variations, with the south-western states having the highest levels of homicide (see 'Focus on ... Culture and violence' in Chapter 5 for possible reasons for this).

In a later study, McCall, Parker and McDonald (2008) undertook a similar exercise. Here the factors found to be significantly associated with the variations included the rate of overall population change, the relative size of the cohort aged 15–29, and the arrest rate for sales of illicit drugs. Resource deprivation and other indicators of income inequality – including the percentage of families living in poverty, the numbers of children not living with both parents, and the proportion of African-Americans in the population – also emerged as significant. But some other factors that had been expected to emerge, such as the rate of unemployment and the proportion of divorced males in the population, proved not to be significant. Also surprisingly, changes in the numbers of police per capita had no effect on the homicide rate; and the incarceration rate, despite rising very steeply from 1980, had only a marginal effect.

Other researchers have reported international comparisons. Cutright and Briggs (1995) investigated a number of candidate predictor variables in 21 economically advanced countries over five-year periods (1955–1989). Multivariate analysis found similar strongest predictors for both males and females, with the largest coefficients being those for the gender ratio of enrolment in education (as the proportion of women rose, there were more female homicide victims); the relative sizes of age cohorts of males (34 years or younger versus 35 years or older); the rate of rape; numbers of battle deaths (reflecting a country's involvement in wars in the years 1900–1980); economic inequality; the number of divorced males aged 15–64; and cultural heterogeneity.

Given the sheer amounts of data aggregated in these studies, and the complex relationships between predictor variables, it is unlikely that any single model will emerge with very high explanatory power. Several research studies have identified different subgroups within the datasets, following separate pathways over time, and these can provide a clearer picture once disaggregated. Fox and Piquero (2003) pursued the idea that fluctuations in the American homicide rate over time were partly a function of changing proportions of different demographic groups within the population. They considered that this contributed to the drop in homicide in the 1990s, and suggested that a model could be developed to forecast homicide rates up to 20 years in advance. McCall, Land and Parker (2011) suggested that there was 'hidden heterogeneity' in the homicide-rate data they analysed (1976–2005), and that the cities studied could be divided into four subgroups, each with its own trajectory. The cities with the highest homicide rates were on average larger and more likely to be in the southern states. They had higher levels of unemployment, economic deprivation and inequality; a higher proportion of divorced males, of black citizens, and of children not with both parents; more police per capita; and a higher incarceration rate.

7

We have seen that the twenties is the peak age for committing homicide, but there is also some evidence that this differs by ethnic group. Feldmeyer and Steffensmeier (2012) disaggregated age and ethnicity data for California. Whereas for white and Native Americans, 60–70 per cent of homicides were committed by those aged 15–34, for black and Hispanic Americans the figure was 80 per cent. Correspondingly, the fraction of homicides committed by those aged 55–74 was nearly 10 per cent for whites but below 4 per cent for blacks. Amongst whites, those aged 35–54 committed a larger proportion of the homicides than the same age band in other ethnic groups. These differences remained fairly stable over the period 1985–2009.

Beeghley (2003) summarised social and structural factors associated with homicide, with particular reference to the USA. The USA's rate has been a focus of extra attention because it is considerably above that for other countries at comparable levels of economic prosperity. Key variables affecting the difference include the ready availability of firearms; the growth of illegal drug markets; racial and ethnic discrimination; exposure to violence through media and cultural influences; and substantial inequality of wealth. Each is thought to contribute separately to the scale of US homicide, but in combination they also produce very high figures in particular neighbourhoods.

Developmental patterns and crime careers

Can the likelihood of committing homicide be predicted from the pattern of other offences in an individual's 'criminal career'? There have been several attempts to answer this question. Soothill, Francis and Liu (2008; Soothill, Francis, Ackerley and Fligelstone, 2002) analysed the criminal histories of those convicted of four serious 'focus offences' in England and Wales – arson, blackmail, kidnapping, and threats to kill – between 1979 and 2001. The overall rate of reconviction for any of the four offences was relatively low (5–10 per cent), and that for committing a homicide was very low (less than 1 per cent). There was evidence that committing multiple offences of arson doubled the risk of later committing homicide. The biggest increases in risk were for those whose first serious offence was either kidnapping or threats to kill, followed by a later offence of arson. For those combinations, the risk of a subsequent homicide far exceeded that in the general population.

Most of us probably cannot imagine killing another person, so the question naturally arises, even if situational factors play a part, does it also take a particular kind of person to do it? Can the potential for an individual to commit a homicide be predicted from other factors at any prior stage, perhaps even from childhood? Researchers on the Pittsburgh Youth Study analysed possible links between a series of risk factors and the likelihood of being convicted of homicide (Farrington and Loeber, 2011a, 2011b; Farrington, Loeber and Berg, 2012). Of the total sample size of 1,517 boys, 37 were convicted of homicide over the 22-year period studied. Loeber *et al.* (2005) found that the principal motives recorded in 33 of these homicides were: retaliation/dispute, 40 per cent; robbery, 23 per cent; a drug deal 'gone bad', 17 per cent; gang-related activity, 10 per cent; with 3 per cent unknown.

The best predictions came from an integrated homicide risk score, a composite of several variables. There were seven items in this final list: (a) other/conspiracy conviction (i.e. having planned an offence jointly with someone else); (b) a history of suspension from school; (c) self-reported weapon-carrying; (d) prior arrest for simple assault; (e) a positive attitude to delinquency; (f) a bad neighbourhood; and (g) born to a young mother. As the number of risk factors increased, so did the rate of homicide; so that amongst the highest-risk group, with five, six or all seven of these factors, 19 per cent were convicted of homicide. These are remarkable findings, given that predictions were being made from childhood variables to a homicide conviction up to 22 years later.

Nevertheless, some caution is in order. First, the Pittsburgh study found there was 'significant predictability but also a high false-positive rate' (Farrington and Loeber, 2011a, p. 64). Of 290 boys judged to be 'the worst' on the basis of risk factors, only 8 per cent went on to kill someone; in other words 92 per cent did not. There was a false-negative rate of 38 per cent (those who would be expected not to commit homicide but who did so); and 87 per cent were false-positives (predicted to commit homicide but did not). (An explanation of these terms is given in Chapter 18.) Second, other studies have yielded very different findings from these. Dobash *et al.* (2007) analysed the criminal histories and developmental problems of 786 convicted male homicide offenders from the *Murder in Britain* database. The majority (67 per cent) were late-onset offenders, and had more in common with a group whose first offence was a homicide, in the absence of any prior criminal history, than with an early-onset group who had had troubled childhoods and other familiar risk factors.

Overall, despite what we might expect intuitively, there does not appear to be anything that decisively marks out those who will go on to kill. It seems likely that the situational factors and interactional dynamics considered earlier play a part in such catastrophic events. But they may be more likely to result in a homicide if one or both of the parties also has a high number of the kinds of risk factors identified in the Pittsburgh study.

These findings potentially raise difficulties for a task that has been extensively developed within forensic psychology, that of *offender profiling*. One of the core assumptions underlining this task is that there is some consistency over time in the patterning of serious offences (such as homicides) committed by individuals. Crabbé, Decoene and Vertommen (2008) have reviewed evidence indicating that this may apply to some features of offences but not others. This is an issue we will probe in more depth in Chapter 13.

The Pittsburgh Youth Study is notable for the very thorough effort made within it to discern which factors during development are associated with going on to commit homicide as an adult. A number of studies have focused specifically on homicides committed by younger offenders (those aged below 18). While the rate of homicide by youths is comparatively low, it gives rise to understandable concern when individuals commit such serious acts at an early stage of their lives.

Heide (2003) reviewed the extensive literature on this area, finding that it consisted mainly of small-sample descriptive or clinical case studies of youths aged 12–17. These offer the advantage of in-depth analysis of motivations for offences of this type. The corresponding disadvantage, though, is that they cannot really form a basis for drawing generalisable conclusions, as it remains unclear how representative any case may be of the patterns likely to be found in others. There were a few group-comparison studies and examples of attempts to develop typologies. Heide (2003) suggested that the 'typical' juvenile homicide offender was male, was not doing well in school, was from a dysfunctional family where he had been exposed to violence, was likely to have been arrested for other crimes, and had abused drugs and alcohol; but was unlikely to be psychotic or to have learning difficulties. Such a profile, however, is not unlike one we might find in many who commit repeated offences but not necessarily homicide, and it has proved difficult to find distinguishing features of young people who kill. However, in a comparative study, Zagar *et al.* (2009) tracked the records of 26 youths convicted of homicide over an 11-year period (8 years before and 3 years after the offence), together with a further group of 101 homicidal youths from previous studies. They compared this combined sample of 127 (age range 10–17) with a matched group of 127 'nonviolent delinquents', and found that the former were significantly more likely to show poorer executive functioning, to demonstrate lower social maturity, to have been allotted special educational services, and to have carried weapons.

In a larger-scale study in England and Wales, Rodway *et al.* (2011) collected details of the backgrounds and characteristics of 363 young people aged below 18 who had committed a homicide in the period 1996–2004. As with adults, the majority (91 per cent) were male and three-quarters (74 per cent) were white. Methods of killing included using a sharp instrument (40 per cent), hitting or kicking (25 per cent), or using a blunt instrument (14 per cent); only a small fraction involved a firearm (3 per cent). Comprehensive reports were available for 165 of this group. Amongst them, 48 per cent had a history of drug abuse and 24 per cent of alcohol abuse. A large proportion (73 per cent) had had discipline problems in school and 49 per cent had been excluded; 20 per cent were diagnosed with mental disorders, and although the largest single category amongst these was 'conduct disorder', there was considerable variety amongst the presentations. Rodway *et al.* reported that 35 victims (13 per cent of the total) were family members; there were 11 homicides of parents. Overall, the group was described as showing a great deal of heterogeneity, with a range of family problems, altercations and fights thought to have precipitated the killing.

Apart from the preponderance of males, in some respects this pattern differs markedly from that found in other US studies, where for the period 1980–2008 the average rate of homicide committed by youths aged 14–17 years was far higher than in many other countries, at 15 per 100,000 (Cooper and Smith, 2011). Across all ages, a much larger proportion of both victims and perpetrators were African-American (for victims, in a ratio of 6:1; for perpetrators, almost 8:1). These ratios have fluctuated considerably over time, but show a net downward trend. Amongst black male teenagers, the homicide offending rate rose to an astonishing 246.9 per 100,000 in 1993 (the rate for 18–24-year-olds was even higher), but had declined to 64.8 per 100,000 by 2008. Paralleling adult homicides, many offences involved the use of a firearm, but these numbers too varied markedly over time: in 1993, there were over 3,500 homicides by 14–17-year-olds using a gun, whereas by 2008 that number had fallen to approximately 1,200 (Cooper and Smith, 2011).

Homicide within families

Many research studies have focused on killings by or of close relatives. *Matricide, patricide* and *parricide* are respectively killing one's mother, father, or either (or both) of one's parents. Other terms include *mariticide* (a wife killing her husband), *uxoricide* (a husband killing his wife), *sororicide, fratricide* and *siblicide* (respectively, killing one's sister or brother, or either or both of them), *filicide* (killing one's child, usually after infancy but can refer to any age), *infanticide* (killing a child, usually below the age of one year, though this differs across jurisdictions), *neonaticide* (killing a newborn within 24 hours of the birth), *fœticide* (the unlawful killing of an unborn child), and *familicide* (killing an entire family, or several of its members). There is no firm consensus on the definition of some of these terms, and most of them are rarely used in everyday discussions – we would more often talk of, for example, 'child murder' – but they are used in legal documents and in research.

There are separate studies of most of these permutations of perpetrator and victim, although once again the majority are either statistically based descriptive studies – for example, reporting demographic data or trends over time – or clinical case reports. For explanatory purposes, this leaves a crucial gap where it would be useful to have more systematic information on motives and other factors.

Parricide

Looking first at parricides, we should note that research literature in this area poses methodological problems: there are often different kinds of overlaps in study samples. For example, single-victim and multiple-victim homicides, and killings of natural parents or step-parents, are sometimes separated but at other times lumped together. Completed homicides may be combined with attempted homicides; and data on males and females may be merged. Few studies include any detailed information on motives, perhaps because many aspects of offences remained confidential.

In overviews of the relevant literature, Hillbrand, Alexandre, Young and Spitz (1999) and Palermo (2010) noted that parricide constituted 2 per cent of all homicides; that it involved more male than female perpetrators (ratio 15:1); that killings by younger offenders were more often of fathers than of mothers (ratio 2:1), but that the reverse was true for adult offenders. In contrast to the general pattern of homicides, very few parricides are committed by black offenders. Many earlier studies focused on parricides that were committed in order to end prolonged periods of parental abuse, and this appears to be the most common contributing factor, but types and patterns of abuse have rarely been analysed in depth. The precipitating factor in a parricidal event often appeared to be a sudden change in the relationship between the child and his or her parent. There were smaller proportions in which the principal factor was severe mental illness, though for older parricidal offenders this appeared to play a more crucial role; Hillbrand and Cipriano (2007) report that parents are victims in 20–30 per cent of the homicides committed by those with psychotic illnesses. Combining a set of 237 cases from previous studies, Hillbrand *et al.* (1999) found that there was evidence of mental disorder in 79 per cent, but for several reasons (such as the diagnoses having been made after the event) they considered that this might be an overestimate. In most cases, there had been a long period of conflict between the offender and victim leading up to the crime, and the fatal assault itself happened in an outburst of explosive anger. Malmquist (2010, p. 77) considered that many parricides were in part 'a protest against continuing humiliation' and described a case of an adolescent driving away after having shot his parent, repeating thankfully to himself 'Free at last'. In some patricides, there is evidence of alcohol-dependent fathers and passive mothers; whereas in matricides, a pattern of sexual enmeshment with mothers has often been found, alongside distant and passive fathers.

Heide and Petee (2007) studied a large sample of 5,781 parricides, committed over a 24-year period (1976–1999) by 5,558 offenders. They extracted information from a database we have encountered before, the FBI's *Supplementary Homicide Reports* (SHR). The discrepancy between numbers of victims and offenders is explained by the fact that 8 per cent of the offenders had multiple victims. The mean age of those who committed patricide was 25, and of those who committed matricide slightly older, at 30; but 25 per cent of the former and 17 per cent of the latter were aged under 18. The majority of the offences (patricide, 81 per cent; matricide, 76 per cent) were thought to originate from family arguments, though not about money or property. Heide and Frei (2010) undertook a similar exercise focusing on matricide in the USA, and in addition surveyed a total of 40 case studies from 13 other countries. They noted that, in the USA, of those who killed their mothers, one in six of adults and one in five of juveniles were female.

On the basis of her extensive research and psycho-legal work in this area, Heide (2013) has forwarded a typology which has received fairly consistent support. Amongst children who kill their parents, she identified four major patterns: (a) severely abused children who kill to end the abuse; (b) children with severe mental illness; (c) a group she calls 'dangerously antisocial' children; and (d) a group whose underlying anger was fuelled by alcohol or drugs.

Eldercide

The age above which the killing of adults is classed as *eldercide* is 60 in some studies and 65 in others. Bachman and Meloy (2008) analysed details of such homicides recorded in the FBI SHR for the period 1976–2004, and found that the largest identifiable portion of those for victims under age 65 resulted from conflicts or arguments (39 per cent). For those aged 65 or over, 35 per cent of homicides were associated with another crime (such as a robbery). Even so, for the majority of victims aged 65 or over, the offender was either a family member (35 per cent) or otherwise known to the victim (38 per cent). Krienert and Walsh (2010) examined data on 828 homicides recorded in the USA's National Incident-Based Reporting System (NIBRS) for the six-year period 2000–2005, and also made some comparisons with the trends in the SHR. Fitting the near-ubiquitous pattern, most victims and offenders were male. Most assailants were not youths but showed a wide spread of ages, with a mean of 46 years. However, the age distribution of female and male eldercides differed slightly: female victims were generally older, with a corresponding difference for the perpetrators (a higher proportion over age 45). Victims' acquaintances formed the largest proportion of offenders (31.6 per cent), followed by spouses (26.9 per cent), children (17.3 per cent), or other family members (11.6 per cent), with only 12 per cent being killed by strangers. More of the older females were killed by spouses, while more of the older males were killed by acquaintances. Thus only a proportion of these deaths can be classed as family violence as such, though altogether still more than half of the killings are by family members (55.8 per cent). These patterns were broadly similar to those found in the SHR database, though the latter showed fewer family victims and more who were strangers.

As can be seen, then, not all killings of older adults are intrafamilial, and a proportion of them occur in the course of an acquisitive offence (*felony eldercide*, killing of an older adult committed in the course of a felony). During the period since the mid-1990s the number of these has slowly risen in the United States, while other types of homicide have been falling. This is thought to be a function of the 'aging population': the changing demographic composition of many countries, in which the proportion of the population aged over 65 has been growing. Thus felony eldercide might be best understood in terms of Routine Activity Theory (see Chapter 4), as it is related to the numbers of older adults living alone in a community who are available as targets for property crime (Roberts and Willits, 2011).

Filicide

The reverse situation – murder of children by their parents – is considerably more common than parricide. Amongst family homicides, it is the second most frequent after killing of spouses or partners. The World

Health Organization (Krug *et al.*, 2002) estimated that in the year 2000 there were 57,000 child victims of homicide worldwide. The most common cause of death was head injury. For the United Kingdom in the year 2012–2013, Jütte, Bentley, Miller and Jetha (2014) report that although the rate had declined by almost 30 per cent since the early 1980s, there were still 69 child homicides a year.

'For many, the murder of a child by his or her own parent is an unfathomable act' (Pitt and Bale, 1995, p. 375). Few would dissent from this statement, yet Pitt and Bale (1995) suggest that infanticide has existed since the earliest recorded era of human history. For example, child sacrifice was practised in many societies; and some societies had laws permitting parents to dispose of children, or allowing them to be buried (alive) with their parents when the latter died. But there are large variations in such laws, both between societies and over time.

Notwithstanding our revulsion at the idea of killing a child, as Brookman and Nolan (2006) note, in terms of the likelihood of becoming a homicide victim, the first year of life is the riskiest. Children of 12 months or under have the highest victimisation rate of any age-group. In 2012–2013, the rate of homicide for children aged under one year in England and Wales was 30 per million, whereas the rate for the population as a whole was 9.7 per million (Jütte *et al.*, 2014). In the United States from 1980 to 2008, the child homicide rate per 100,000 was consistently highest for those less than one year old, and progressively lower for succeeding year-groups (Cooper and Smith, 2011).

Several authors have reviewed different segments of research on the killing of children (Bourget, Grace and Whitehurst, 2007; Friedman, Horwitz and Resnick, 2005; Porter and Gavin, 2010; Stanton and Simpson, 2002). While there is much variation, there are also patterns within this, associated with different sets of perpetrators and types of motive. Although there is no legal category of neonaticide – it is subsumed under infanticide – there are characteristic features that differentiate neonaticide from infanticide and from filicides of older children. Studies in several countries show that most neonaticides are committed by mothers; indeed, unlike every other form of homicide, this is the only category where the majority of perpetrators are female rather than male. One situation in which this occurs is fairly straightforward. Often, the mother is the only person who knows of the birth: she may have concealed it, and may even have denied being pregnant. For a variety of possible reasons, the child is unwanted, and is disposed of quickly after birth. Disposal may be by simple abandonment, but in many cases the newborn is suffocated, drowned, strangled or stabbed. It is widely thought that some neonaticides are never discovered, and the total number cannot be known with any certainty; there could be a substantial 'hidden figure' for this type of crime. As the age of the victim increases, so the proportion of filicides committed by men steadily rises also.

Neonaticide and infanticide

Neonaticide is predominantly committed by women aged 25 years or less, and sometimes in their mid or even early teens. They are not usually in a partner relationship, and have rarely committed offences before. They are often in very difficult personal circumstances, typically including poverty or abusive relationships.

In a study of 40 female offenders in the USA, all were thought to have had something to gain from killing the child, primarily 'removal of burden' (Beyer, Mack and Shelton, 2008, p. 528). Most were not considered to have had mental health problems, though a sizeable minority (25 per cent) were. In a **cluster analysis** study of 110 offenders in Italy, Camperio Ciani and Fontanesi (2012) found a 'consistent profile' for those who had committed neonaticide, distinct from that for infanticide and filicide, which had more features in common. They too found that neonaticide was committed by younger, economically poorer mothers, who had tried to kill their offspring non-violently, who had usually concealed the body, and who had never attempted suicide. Those who had killed older children had more often used violent methods, and a high proportion had had mental health problems. Camperio Ciani and Fontanesi (2012) proposed that neonaticide was distinct from other infanticides and could be explained in evolutionary terms: it was an 'adaptive reproductive disinvestment', in which the mother realised that the child's life was non-viable, as she lacked resources to support the child, and she therefore postponed child-rearing to a time when it could be more successful. By contrast, infanticide and filicide were, in the view of these authors, 'improper functioning of adaptation' that required explanation in other terms.

Brookman and Nolan (2006) analysed all 298 recorded case of infanticide in England and Wales in the period 1995–2002. They noted that neonaticide is particularly likely to remain undiscovered, but that there could also be a similar problem of under-recording of *other* killings of infants. The question arises from uncertainties over the status of sudden infant death syndrome (SIDS), in which a cause of death cannot be established, and a broader category of 'sudden unexplained deaths in infancy' (SUDI). They cited a range of estimates of the numbers of cases in which what was diagnosed as SIDS could actually have been infanticide, suggesting 10 per cent as a 'conservative' figure in this regard.

There are thought to be several main kinds of motive for the killing of children, and several authors have suggested ways of classifying the factors that give rise to it (Porter and Gavin, 2010; Stanton and Simpson, 2002). The majority are variations of a scheme first put forward by Resnick (1969), who examined 131 cases and proposed a fivefold typology with the following categories:

» *Altruistic filicide* Filicide committed to relieve the child's real or perceived suffering due to serious illness or anticipated harm.

» *Acutely psychotic* Filicide committed because the mother has experienced an episode of severe mental illness including delusions.

» *Unwanted child* Filicide committed because the mother did not want the pregnancy, leading her to conceal or deny both the pregnancy and then the existence of the child, and because she cannot accept the child – this is most frequently seen in neonaticide.

» *Accidental* There was violent abuse of the child, and although death was not an intended outcome, the child died as a result.

» *Revenge or retaliation* In reaction to earlier events, the perpetrator is seeking to damage someone else – usually a former partner, but sometimes another relative.

There are other, rarer motives, but the above list covers the majority of cases dealt with as homicide by courts. It does not, however, include child killing that is based on beliefs about the relative value placed on baby girls and boys; that is linked to the problems of selective abortion and fœticide, where the numbers are on such a scale that in some countries (e.g. India) they have shown through in the gender ratio of the population as a whole (Jha *et al.*, 2011).

Putkonen *et al.* (2011) undertook more detailed analysis of the motives of 75 women and 45 men in two countries, Austria and Finland, who had killed their children. They found that the perpetrators had been beset with a wide range of difficult and stressful circumstances and personal problems, from poverty and isolation to physical illnesses and relational conflict. Some were motivated by fear of abandonment by a partner, whereas others considered themselves already failures as parents. There were also some for whom the killing of the child was part of an extended suicide.

Some filicides are the result of serious mental disorders in the perpetrator or perpetrators. Krischer, Stone, Sevecke and Steinmeyer (2007) assessed 57 women detained in a psychiatric hospital in New York State. They found schizophrenia to be the commonest diagnosis, followed by a range of severe depressive disorders. In a review of other studies, Bourget, Grace and Whitehurst (2007) found depressive and psychotic disorders to be frequent, but also found a high proportion of personality disorders both in mothers and in fathers who had committed filicide. Mothers, who were more often paranoid or depressed, were more likely to have killed for 'altruistic' motives: to save the child from something thought to be worse. Fathers were more likely to kill older children; more often killed boys; used greater violence; and more often killed in retaliation or in fatal abusive assaults.

Many countries have specific legal provisions demarcating infanticide from the killing of other children or older victims. Malmquist (2013) collated details of the relevant statutes in 50 countries, drawing attention to their absence in the United States and noting the considerable disparities that arise in how cases are dealt with there. Porter and Gavin (2010), in contrast, discuss findings that in their view call into question the appropriateness of having a separate legal category of infanticide. They cite evidence of the extreme unlikelihood of a woman not knowing she is pregnant, implying that in some cases such claims are implausible and may not be genuine. This is in stark contrast to the view of Stanton and Simpson (2002), who considered that denial of pregnancy may be so powerful as to result in shock when the mother goes into labour, leading to a dissociative state in which she then kills the child. Jenkins, Millar and Robins (2011) summarised what was known about the prevalence of 'denial of pregnancy', which is on average 1 in 475 at 20 weeks, dropping to 1 in 2,500 at full term. While such rates are low, they are similar to those of some other birth complications, and far more frequent than neonaticide.

Homicide by a partner

The commonest form of homicide within families or other close relationships is the killing of partners (Liem and Roberts, 2009). Mostly this entails the killing of women by men, but the converse also happens, and homicides occur too in same-sex partnerships. Although homicide is the least likely outcome of partner violence (Barnett, Miller-Perrin and Perrin, 2011), it is obviously the most serious; and as it is often found to be the final act in a history of violent abuse, such an outcome is potentially foreseeable and preventable. We will discuss it briefly here, turning to the broader problem of intimate partner violence in Chapter 9.

Stöckl *et al.* (2013) reported a **systematic review** of 118 studies, conducted across 66 countries, of the prevalence of *intimate partner homicide* (IPH). They also incorporated data from official statistics of recorded crime, analysing a total of 492,340 homicides. For total fatalities, the familiar pattern was found: a majority of homicide victims (80 per cent) were male. Turning to partner homicides, however, the figures reversed. Globally, one in seven homicide victims (13.5 per cent) was killed by an intimate partner. Across all countries, an average of 38.6 per cent of female homicides was committed by an intimate partner, whereas the corresponding figure amongst males was 6.3 per cent. There were large variations between continental regions, with the biggest gender differential emerging in South-east Asia, where partners committed 58.75 per cent of female but only 0.87 per cent of male homicides. By contrast, in two Latin American countries, Brazil and Panama, the figures were almost equal.

For high-income countries, which included most of Europe, Israel, the United States, Canada, Australia, New Zealand and Japan, the proportions of women and of men killed by partners averaged 41.2 per cent and 6.3 per cent respectively, a ratio of 6.5:1. However, this was a conservative estimate, as cases with some missing data were classed as non-partner homicides. When analysis was confined to known cases, the ratio was higher at 7.3:1. In sum, 'women's main risk of homicide is from an intimate partner' (Stöckl *et al.*, 2013, p. 863). These authors noted that for many countries no data were available, and some existing data may have been unreliable. This is a major drawback, given strong evidence that the dynamics of partner homicide differ markedly from the more numerous male–male homicides.

Partner homicide can be defined in different ways, but in England and Wales it is taken to include lethal assaults by both current and former partners. In fact the category covers a wide range of people, and the Office for National Statistics (2014, p. 13) notes that 'partner/ex-partner' includes 'the subcategories spouse, cohabiting partner, boyfriend/girlfriend, ex-spouse/ex-cohabiting partner/ex-boyfriend/ex-girlfriend, adulterous relationship, lover's spouse or emotional rival'. Combining data across the three years 2010–2011, 2011–2012 and 2012–2013, the ONS report also notes that, as we might expect, almost all female victims of partner homicide are killed by a male suspect.

However, that also held for male victims, because of cases in which men were killed by emotional rivals.

Motives for partner homicide

There can be numerous motives for IPH, and attempts have been made to classify them. Studies examining this topic have generally adopted one of two strategies. Some have drawn on relatively small samples, but have counterbalanced this by collecting extensive in-depth data; others have considered larger samples, but a more limited range of data. In a detailed and searching study of 31 men who killed their female partners, Adams (2007) concluded that there were no clear markers that differentiated these men in advance from others who did not go on to commit homicide. However, most did come from families where fathers had been violent. In most cases there was also – as we saw earlier with reference to homicide generally – a pattern of accumulating hostility in their interactions with the women they later killed. Adams suggested that this group of men included four 'types', though there were sizeable overlaps between them (i.e. some men fitted two of the categories):

- The majority, 71 per cent, showed extreme jealousy and were preoccupied with suspicions of their partners; 65 per cent of this group claimed they had killed in a state of 'jealous rage'.
- The second largest category (61 per cent) consisted of men who habitually abused alcohol or other drugs, or both. These men had been more frequently and more severely abusive than others towards their female partners prior to the homicide itself.
- A third, smaller group was materially motivated. This does not mean simply that they stood to profit financially but rather that there had been some conflict over money, property or other possessions; unlike other groups, these men showed no evident signs of jealousy.
- A final, very small group consisted of men who were *both* homicidal *and* suicidal, a pattern we will examine more fully below. These men were often depressed or experienced other severe mental health problems, and they also tended to be heavy abusers of alcohol.

Drawing on a qualitative study employing in-depth interviews with 15 men in a maximum security prison in Israel, Elisha, Idisis, Timor and Addad (2010) describe all the cases as complex and arising from a mixture of factors, with no single theory explaining all of the patterns observed. The majority of these men reported emotional difficulties in their own backgrounds and development. Nine of them saw themselves as having been the 'victim' of the woman they eventually killed, through (for example) her unfaithful, abandoning, or insubordinate behaviour; hence the woman (the real victim) had 'brought it upon herself'. In their personal narratives of the events leading to the homicide, three stories emerged, leading Elisha *et al.* to suggest a tripartite division of motives:

- One story was that of the *betrayed husband*, usually arising in a couple who had lived settled lives for some time and had had children together, but where the woman met someone else; the dominant feeling was not sexual jealousy but loss of family.
- A second story was that of the *abandoned obsessive lover*, from men who had killed partners who were planning to leave them; this was often preceded or followed by a period of stalking, harassment and threats, and some men were thought to have features of borderline personality disorder.
- The third story was that of the *tyrant*, whose actions worsened over a long period of conflict and a struggle for power; the killing often followed a period of estrangement and acrimony, and was a final effort to gain supremacy over the woman. Some of these men were thought to show features of narcissistic or antisocial personality disorder.

A theme running consistently through all the narratives was that of *control*; but also, alongside it, *dependency*. In contrast to other studies where men who had killed their partners proclaimed that they had loved the victim, Elisha *et al.* (2010) found that their

7

participants often had ambivalent or negative feelings, in which love was mixed with anger and hatred.

Dobash and Dobash (2011) reported a study of cognitions of 104 men from the *Murder in Britain* study (briefly described earlier) who had been convicted of murdering a female partner. They employed a method of documentary content analysis, extracting information from reports by a variety of professional staff in the prison case files of these men. They found a mixture of beliefs, ranging from absolute denial that the murder had even happened, through acknowledgement of the event but denial of responsibility, and blaming the victim (two forms of neutralisation), through other types of rationalisation and justification, to genuine remorse. Many men were described as having difficulties in managing close relationships, as showing rigid attitudes concerning male authority and control over women, and showing evidence of possessiveness and jealousy. The majority of men (59 per cent) had a history of previous violence towards the woman they had killed; many had also been abusive in earlier relationships. An even higher figure was found by Campbell *et al.* (2003) in a study of risk factors for partner femicide, involving 220 cases from 11 American cities, which were compared with a sample of 343 women who had been subject to other forms of partner abuse at some time in the previous two years. Here, 79 per cent of murdered women had been previously abused by the man who killed them; and in 73 per cent of cases, there had been threats to kill. A heightened risk of lethal violence was associated with perpetrators having lower educational levels, less stable employment, more substance and alcohol abuse, one or more previous arrests for violence, and readier access to firearms. This study also highlighted some relational dynamics that were strong risk factors, for example where women had separated themselves from highly controlling men.

Thomas, Dichter and Matejkowski (2011) compared 71 men who had murdered intimate partners with 291 who had killed non-intimates (other family members, acquaintances or strangers). They found large differences in motives between the two groups. The former committed the offence alone, due to emotional concerns, more often in a state of rage, and rarely motivated by money. There were indications that perpetrators of IPH had 'a higher stake in conformity' (p. 304), as they more often had stable jobs and were married, but they were also more likely to have mental health problems. Offences by the latter group were more often linked to other criminality and more often involved an accomplice.

For both sexes, there are some cases in which homicide occurs as a way of enforcing the chilling phrase 'If *I* can't have you, no one can', which expresses a level of jealousy, possessiveness, or entitlement so intense as to lead to extreme violence. Hannawa, Spitzberg, Wiering and Teranishi (2006) developed a scale for measuring the strength of such territorial beliefs, which at their strongest produce an individual who regards another person as 'belonging' to him or her in much the same way as personal property. In the majority of cases such beliefs are held by men in relation to women, and are often culturally endorsed to such an extent that – in some places at some times – killing may even have been legally sanctioned.

The predominance of sexual jealousy amongst the motives for partner homicide has led to the formulation of a *male sexual proprietariness theory* (Daly and Wilson, 1988). This suggests that, in many societies, men historically have, in effect, been given 'ownership' of women for reproductive purposes. This had evolutionary value, but resulted in 'double standards' whereby the infidelity of women can be more severely punished than the infidelity of men and can even be seen as a mitigating factor when husbands kill their wives. At the centre of such an attitude is a belief whereby men view female partners as their property, whom they are entitled to control. Suspicious or jealous reactions are only part of a broader system of coercion, of which violence was traditionally a legitimised part. In some instances, however, women's defensive reactions to this experience may lead to retaliatory violence, and eventually to a reverse situation in which women kill their male partners.

As noted earlier, then, women sometimes kill their male partners. A large amount of research suggests that a primary motive for this is as a response to male violence or threats of violence: in other words, in self-defence. Felson and Messner (1998) found that incidents in which women killed their husbands were more likely to involve 'victim precipitation' than incidents in which men killed their wives. Belknap *et al.* (2012) analysed the findings of 117 cases investigated by Domestic Violence Fatality Review Committees (DVFRCs) in Denver, Colorado. Only a few women appeared to exhibit, and to have acted from, the sense of ownership or sexual jealousy that has been found in many homicides by male partners or ex-partners. In many more cases, as Campbell *et al.* (2003) found, women had been victimised by their male partners and felt trapped in those relationships. In a review of 35 studies, a history of battering was the strongest risk factor for IPH to emerge (Campbell *et al.*, 2003). Such patterns parallel the generally higher levels of almost all kinds of violence amongst males.

Serran and Firestone (2004) evaluated the male proprietariness and female defensiveness theories as explanations of male and female homicidal acts respectively. Studies they reviewed support the hypothesis that a sense of proprietary power is an important influence that drives partner homicide on the part of some males. Many attempts to kill a female following her infidelity or defiance of the man's wishes stem from this belief. However, we should of course keep in mind that the overwhelming majority of men who become estranged from their partners do not go on to kill them; other factors are likely to be involved in offences of this gravity. Serran and Firestone (p. 5) quote statistics for Canada to the effect that 'the number of wives divorced in a single year is 55 times greater than the number of wives murdered by their partners over a 19-year period'. By contrast, the evidence for female defensive violence in abusive relationships is relatively strong, and it was in this context that the 'battered woman syndrome' was first described. Most studies suggest that there are few differences between women who kill and those who do not; they suggest rather that there is a higher level of violence shown by the male partners of the former. Roberts (1996) found that women who committed partner homicide were more likely to have been sexually assaulted when a child, to have had drugs problems, to have made suicide attempts through a drugs overdose, and to have been repeatedly assaulted and threatened with death by their partners.

Homicide by a same-sex partner

Homicide also occurs amongst same-sex couples, and Mize and Shackelford (2008) compared IPH in heterosexual, gay and lesbian relationships, focusing particularly on the level of brutality involved in the killings. Drawing on evolutionary theory, this research was designed to test the hypotheses that there would be higher levels of brutality in homicides committed within homosexual as compared to heterosexual relationships, and in ones committed by males as compared to females. The authors accessed the FBI's SHR database for the period 1976–2001, analysing a total of 51,007 cases of partner homicide. Amongst them, 959 (1.8 per cent) of the victims were gay men and 133 (0.3 per cent) were lesbians. The homicide rate was highest in male homosexual relationships (63 per million) and lowest in lesbian relationships (9 per million), with heterosexual relationships between the two (21 per million). Methods of killing were classified by the authors as entailing higher or lower levels of brutality ('very brutal' versus 'less brutal'). The former including stabbing and beating to death; the latter shooting and asphyxiation (suffocation, drowning or strangulation). Overall, 65 per cent of the homicides involved shooting. As hypothesised, when gay men killed their partners, the level of brutality was higher than when heterosexual men killed theirs; the same held for gay women as compared to heterosexual women. Contrary to predictions, however, a higher proportion of women than men used more brutal methods of killing; but this fits with evidence outlined earlier which showed that women more often killed in self-defence, resorting to knives as the most readily available weapons in most households. The authors acknowledged that there could be other factors at work, such as the availability of guns, which may have been an important factor influencing whether or not homicides occurred at all (an issue we examine in Chapter 8).

Homicide followed by suicide

Some of those who kill a close relative then go on to kill themselves, and this is particularly likely when they have killed more than one other family member. The most frequent pattern is one in which a man kills his female intimate partner, and then commits suicide; though sometimes the first victim is a son or daughter (filicide–suicide: Friedman *et al.*, 2005). Harper and Voigt (2007, p. 306) suggest that, 'whereas women are less likely than men to take their own lives after killing an intimate partner, they are more apt to commit suicide after killing their children, except in the case of newborn infants' (a pattern noted above). Some researchers restrict the definition of homicide–suicide to cases where the latter occurs within 24 hours of the former, though others have included cases with a gap of up to 30 days between them (Harper and Voigt, 2007). Murder followed by suicide is very difficult to study closely, given that the perpetrators are not directly available for forensic investigation or research after the event. However, some suicide attempts fail, and there is often other evidence from beforehand that can be analysed to provide indications of the factors at work in producing such horrific outcomes.

Notwithstanding the obstacles, there have been many studies of this sequence of events. Flynn and others (2009) studied a series of 203 incidents of homicide–suicide in England and Wales over a nine-year period (1996–2005). Liem and Roberts (2009) analysed homicides in the Netherlands to test for differences between those that were or were not followed by a self-destructive act (i.e. actual or attempted suicide), comparing 44 of the former with 279 of the latter. Banks, Crandall, Sklar and Bauer (2008) compared IPH with murder–suicide in the state of New Mexico; while Barber *et al.* (2008) reported a similar study in four American states and several other counties. Of 1,503 homicides recorded in the US National Violent Death Reporting System (NVDRS), Barber *et al.* found that just under 5 per cent were followed by the suicide of the perpetrator, and just over 1 per cent by a suicide attempt.

There have been several reviews based on examining rates and patterns of homicide–suicide in different parts of the world. Large, Smith and Neilssen (2009) surveyed 49 studies which together described a total of 64 samples from 17 countries (plus Greenland, which though autonomous is a sovereign part of Denmark), cumulatively including 110,800 homicides, of which 8 per cent had been followed by suicide. Prevalence rates (per 100,000) differed by a factor of 55 (a single far higher figure from Greenland was excluded as an outlier). Large discrepancies in the numbers of events studied, and data-collection periods of varying lengths and at widely dispersed points between 1900 and 2005, make it difficult to draw any general conclusions regarding possible causes of the variations. There have been several attempts to develop typologies of homicide–suicide; and, collating information from nine countries, Liem (2010) used relationship type as a means of classification (according to whether suicide is preceded by killing of the partner, of a child, of an entire family, or of outsiders). Liem *et al.* (2011) made further international comparisons. Panczak *et al.* (2013) conducted a systematic review and located 27 studies from eight countries (Australia, Canada, England and Wales, Finland, Netherlands, South Africa, Switzerland, USA), leading them to conclude that homicide–suicide is a 'distinct entity' – that is, it has features that are not explicable purely in terms of a combination of elements of homicide and elements of suicide. There are specific dynamics and motives that lead to the combination of actions that it entails. Their study found a very high correlation (+0.81) between numbers of homicide–suicides and the rate of civilian gun ownership.

Many of the studies subsumed in these reviews focus on what might be called 'external' features of homicide–suicide, as contrasted with homicide or suicide alone. These variables include the gender and ages of perpetrators and victims; methods of killing the victim and then the perpetrator himself or herself; the numbers of victims; and their relationships to the perpetrator. There are fewer sources of information on motives, or on circumstances prior to the events themselves, other than the suggestion that a proportion of perpetrators are experiencing severe depression and that the killings are often triggered by separation or rejection, or by some other sharp loss such as that of a job or other aspect of status. To obtain more information about possible motives, some studies have analysed reports prepared by coroners conducting inquests into deaths.

In a study based on analysis of coroners' reports in Tasmania, Haines, Williams and Lester (2010) compared murder–suicide with suicides. They found a tendency for higher levels of anger and hostility, and of previous violence, in the former, and also evidence of interpersonal conflict, crisis and loss, but these differences were not statistically significant. Those who committed homicide–suicide were more likely to have been in employment and to have used firearms, but in most other respects there were no features that differentiated homicide–suicide from suicide. Friedman *et al.* (2005) examined coroner's office files in 30 cases of filicide–suicide in Ohio, which involved the deaths of 51 children. In most cases the motive appeared to be 'altruistic', in that the perpetrator believed he or she was saving the child from a worse fate (such as death from a serious illness), though in a quarter of those cases such beliefs were delusional. There were signs of serious mental health problems (depression or psychosis) in 80 per cent of cases, but few of the perpetrators had previous hospital admissions or had made suicide attempts.

Several studies have found that those who kill another family member and then themselves are more likely than those who commit only homicide to have been experiencing a mental health problem, most commonly depression. Based on a study of 341 men accused of attempted or completed IPH in the Netherlands, Liem and Roberts (2009, p. 344) noted evidence that such an outcome was likelier to occur where there had been *symbiosis* or 'far-reaching interdependency' within the partner relationship. When threatened with its loss, the perpetrator felt the need to destroy both his partner and himself. The same authors also suggest that some male perpetrators of homicide–suicide may manifest self-love at a level that is pathological: a highly fragile state accompanied by a lack of **empathy**, resulting in what Liem and Roberts called a state of 'narcissistic rage' during which the killing takes place. The occurrence of homicide–suicide might then be an indicator of the perceived strength of an emotional bond. In a study in Japan, Sakuta (1995) found a preponderance of filicide–suicide and attributed this to the strength of parent–child relationship, considered to be more powerful in Japanese culture than in Western nations (where the spousal or lovers' relationship is assumed to be the strongest emotional connection).

Harper and Voigt (2007) developed an integrated theory of homicide–suicide events, endorsing the view that it is a phenomenon with characteristics distinct from those of either homicide or suicide alone. This was based on a research review and their own analysis of 42 cases that occurred in New Orleans in the period 1989–2001. The underlying causal factor was always some form of conflict, but they suggest that this had to be understood within a framework of 'conflict intensity structures'. That in turn draws on a model of the 'social geometry' of violent conflict forwarded by Black (2004), whereby violence is often used for what is mistakenly believed to be a moralistic purpose, to right a perceived wrong. Harper and Voigt delineate several routes along which such conflict amplifies to produce this scale of violence. One major influence is the intensity of the relationship between the perpetrator and the victim or victims, which predicts the degree of hostile emotion that arises within the partnership and eventually precipitates lethal violence. A second key factor is personal and social *strain*, as conceptualised by Agnew (1992, 2006a, 2007; which we discussed in Chapter 3), whereby many needs – money, sex, status, or independence – may be blocked. The third main element is power dominance, which may already have been presenting as abuse, but at its extremity may be expressed in the aforementioned self-aggrandising 'If *I* can't have you ...' mantra. In most homicide–suicides, many (or all) of these processes may be at work. That, as Harper and Voigt recognise, makes the theory difficult to evaluate in an area that is already very difficult to comprehend.

In a revision of this model, Gregory (2012) considered that Harper and Voigt (2007) underestimated the importance of 'hegemonic masculinity' as a principal contributory factor. Gregory undertook an analysis of all 30 homicide–suicide cases (including 5 of familicide) that had occurred in Yorkshire and Humberside over a 15-year period (1993–2007). All perpetrators were male, and 32 of the 37 victims were female. Gregory suggested that male proprietoriness had played a significant part in these offences and that the resolve to commit suicide preceded the formation of homicidal intent. Thus for a majority of perpetrators, 'the performance of masculinity has become bound up with his ability to be in full charge of his partner' (2012, p. 142). Violence 'escalates towards homicide', according to Gregory, when there is a sense that such control has been lost. In cases of family annihilation, the perpetrator's anger in killing his children was directed at his partner or ex-partner. In most of these cases there had been a history of domestic abuse, a steady rise in aggression, and a major threat to the offender's status in relationships, work, or both.

Homicide recidivism

The majority of homicides involve a single victim only, and official data and follow-up studies indicate that the likelihood of repeating such an act is very low. The Homicide Index developed in England and Wales showed that in 2012–2013 there were three convictions for homicide of individuals who had had a conviction of this kind before. Over the ten-year period from 2002, 43 people who had a previous homicide conviction were convicted of killing again (ONS, 2014). In Finland, Eronen, Hakola and Tiihonen (1996) found a rate for homicide recidivism over thirteen years of 2.2 per cent; factors most strongly associated with its recurrence were alcohol problems and a diagnosis of personality disorder. Roberts, Zgoba and Shahidullah (2007) reported post-release data on a random sample of 336 homicide perpetrators in the American state of New Jersey. Several had committed further offences, although none had committed another murder; however, the follow-up period here was only five years. Regarding the small proportions who do kill again, Bjørkly and Waage (2005) reviewed the available literature on *recidivistic single-victim homicide*, finding only eleven relevant studies and only three that examined the phenomenon specifically. Prevalence rates were typically in the range 1.0–3.5 per cent. Clearly, any repeat of a homicide offence is an extremely serious development. Its low frequency points towards the rarity of the circumstances in which homicides take place. However, there certainly are cases of people who take more than one life, and they give rise to some of the most notorious crimes and the greatest levels of public alarm.

No relevant data are available for those who commit multiple homicides, different forms of which we discuss in the next chapter. As we have seen, a large proportion of those who commit familicide or mass homicide also commit suicide. Like serial murderers, if they are arrested and convicted they are unlikely ever to be released, and in some countries they are likely to be executed. In the United Kingdom, almost all of those given 'whole life tariffs' have committed more than one homicide (see Chapter 16).

Chapter summary

- This chapter focused on homicides that result in the death of a single victim, in the majority of cases being carried out by a single perpetrator. This is by far the most frequent form of homicide. The law focuses on investigating motives in order to establish whether the *mens rea* for murder was present, but lethal events are also often a product of interactional exchanges, relational dynamics, spatial and structural factors, and, farther back in time, each participant's developmental processes and patterns. There was more detailed consideration of homicide within families, killing of partners, and homicide followed by suicide.
- It has proved difficult to find any features that decisively mark out those who will go on to kill, even amongst people who commit other kinds of violent offences. Situational factors and interactional dynamics may play a crucial part in such catastrophic events. A homicide may be more likely if either the victim or the perpetrator has a high number of the kinds of risk factors identified in longitudinal research.
- A brief review of information on what is known about levels of recidivism following single-victim homicide shows that it is very low: most people who commit this type of offence do not do so again.

7

Further reading

Despite its seriousness, there are surprisingly few serious texts on the subject of homicide, though there are numerous sensational treatments. The following books are recommended as sources firmly based on what is known from the study of homicide from criminological and psychological perspectives.

- Fiona Brookman (2005). *Understanding Homicide* (London: Sage Publications). This is one of only a few books that provide an overview of the study of homicide, addressing general issues, differing explanations, motivations, and the particular patterns that homicide takes.
- Terance D. Miethe and Wendy C. Regoeczi (2004). *Rethinking Homicide: Exploring the Structure and Process Underlying Deadly Situations* (Cambridge: Cambridge University Press). Examines the roles of situations and processes leading up to homicides.
- David Adams (2007). *Why Do They Kill? Men Who Murder Their Intimate Partners* (Nashville, TN: Vanderbilt University Press). This is a valuable source, offering an extended focus on intimate partner homicide.
- Joan Swart and Lee Mellor (eds) (2016). *Homicide: A Forensic Psychology Casebook* (Boca Raton, FL: CRC Press/Taylor & Francis). This very useful book contains chapters on most of the types of homicide likely to be seen in the course of forensic psychology practice.

Multiple Homicide

The crimes that have the potential to cause the most widespread public alarm are those in which more than one person is killed, either together in a massacre (mass killing), or in succession but with features that suggest that the same person is responsible for each one (serial killing). The motives for such crimes at first seem incomprehensible, and some may remain beyond understanding as the perpetrators go on to kill themselves. Nevertheless, some offer explanations for their conduct before they begin, and others have been arrested and have given accounts of their motivations afterwards. This chapter reviews what has been learned from the assessment of those who commit these offences and from indirect evidence collected from the study of crime events themselves.

Chapter objectives

- To describe the range of violent crimes involving multiple victims and crimes that involve more than one perpetrator, and the different patterns they take.
- To review what is known about the factors that contribute to the occurrence of such events, including what has been learned about motives, focusing on familicide, mass killing and serial murder.
- More briefly, to consider some possible contributions of psychology in understanding large-scale violence in political, ethnic or religious contexts, manifesting as terrorism or genocide.

All homicides can be said to create multiple victims, in the sense that relatives of the deceased are also caused significant and enduring distress of several kinds. A small proportion of homicides, however, involve the *killing* of more than one person.

Multiple homicide takes a number of forms; and the possibility of it happening is an understandable source of far-reaching concern, and sometimes outright terror, in any community. Alongside those reactions there is also a kind of morbid fascination, fed by a steady stream of crime novels, films and television series, which often depict how such individuals are eventually caught in a way that bears little resemblance to actual events. (Perhaps it is this, more than anything else, that has created a misleading image of what most forensic psychologists do for a living.) The reality of the crimes, however, is often extremely grisly in itself and can pose extraordinary challenges on a number of levels, without any need for creative embellishment.

Multiple homicides are often divided into two main types, *mass* and *serial* (Meloy and Felthous, 2004):

- *Mass murders* usually consists of single events in which several people are killed either simultaneously or in a prolonged and continuous violent outburst. Dietz (1986) suggested that use of this term should be confined to incidents in which all of the deaths occurred within a 24-hour period. The victims may be from the offender's family (*familicide*), or complete strangers, or a mixture of the two. Whereas most events of this kind involve a number of murders in a single episode at a single place, in some events the offender moves between places over a period of several hours; this is generally referred to as a *spree murder*.
- In *serial murder*, by contrast, the killings, usually of one victim at a time, are spread out over a longer period, potentially many years. Some are localised, while others are carried out over a large area.

As Fox and Levin (2012, pp. 19, 20) have commented, it is best not to worry too much over exactly how *mass*, *spree* and *serial murder* are defined, as there are some crimes that fit all three definitions.

Multiple homicides differ from single-victim homicides in ways other than the number of victims. Evidence suggests that they are far more often premeditated, sometimes meticulously; and they are usually driven by markedly different motives. To achieve the desired results, mass killers most often use firearms, and they are far more likely than serial killers to commit suicide afterwards, as the final act, and what the perpetrator perhaps considers the culmination, of the murderous sequence. In serial homicide, by contrast, methods of killing more commonly involve direct physical contact, employing knives, blunt instruments, or ligatures; there are also cases, though much rarer, of the serial use of poison. Some types of serial killing are preceded by acts of sadism and torture, and some perpetrators retain 'souvenirs' of their victims or of the crime location. This implies that often the process of killing has become an objective in itself, rather than being the means of eliminating the victim. But there are exceptions to this also, such as John Allen Muhammad and Lee Malvo, the 'Beltway snipers', who over three weeks in October 2002 shot from long range a series of ten people in Maryland and Washington DC. Serial killers may evade detection for lengthy periods, and some have been known to send messages to the police or the press, appearing to relish playing a game of cat-and-mouse. In other cases they show signs of relief when eventually caught.

Familicide

One form of mass homicide is *familicide*, sometimes called *family annihilation*, the killing an entire family or several of its members. While it involves the deaths of a number of people, it is often considered separately from other mass killings in which most or all of the victims are non-relatives. What is usually called 'mass murder' or 'massacre' mainly involves strangers, though some victims may be known to the perpetrator. That pattern of homicide will be considered separately below, as the motives often differ from those linked to familicide.

Both intrafamilial and extrafamilial massacres are very rare events, although the former occur slightly more often than the latter in most countries where information has been collected. Yardley, Wilson and Lynes (2014) developed a taxonomy of male British family annihilators over the period 1980–2012. They found 71 cases in which parents deliberately set out to kill their children. Some then went on to kill the other parent, or themselves, or both. In 59 of these cases the perpetrators were men. While the number of these events is small relative to other forms of homicide, it appears to have risen in the UK in the period since 1980. The source of information in this study, accessed through the *Nexis* database, was newspaper reports of the events, and their accuracy and completeness may be questionable. Just over half (55 per cent) of the perpetrators were in their thirties; most (71 per cent) were employed, and came from a wide range of occupational groups; after killing their relatives, 81 per cent committed suicide or attempted to do so. Amongst these, the majority (77.5 per cent) of completed suicides occurred immediately after the killings. Where children were killed, 96.6 per cent were progeny of the perpetrator, and only 3.4 per cent were step-children. Family break-up was imminent or was threatened preceding 66 per cent of events; in a further 17 per cent there were financial problems.

Yardley *et al.* (2014, p. 137) suggest that family annihilation is a 'distinct category of murder' and proposed four subgroups for classifying these men, which in order of prominence they called *self-righteous*, *disappointed*, *anomic* and *paranoid*, acknowledging that there was some 'seepage' between them. Those in the first and largest group (56 per cent) blamed their partners for problems in the family. They had a rigid concept of an ideal family, and breakdown of this unit was seen as a catastrophic failure, unacceptable to the man's 'domineering, masculine identity'; some of the man's communications had dramatic and narcissistic elements. The *disappointed* group (16 per cent) shared some of these features, but thought that the family had let them down in some fundamental way; as a result, it had lost its function for them, and could be dispensed with totally and permanently. For those in the *anomic* group (14 per cent), having a family was closely linked to their own economic status and social standing, and was also a symbol of achievement: when that was threatened by their own prospective financial ruin, they feared a form of reputational death, with familicide the only escape. Members of the fourth, *paranoid* group (14 per cent) perceive a major external threat, imagined or actual, that is undermining their role as protector of their children, such as a suspected alliance between an estranged partner and a social institution such as a childcare agencies.

Liem, Levin, Holland and Fox (2013) undertook a similar task in the United States, analysing two sets of data: the widely used FBI *Supplementary Homicide Reports* (SHR), supplemented by newspaper reports of familicide, which contained more detail about the relationships between victims and those who killed them. Covering the nine-year period from June 2000 to June 2009, they found a total of 629 cases, but focused attention on a subset of 207 (an average of almost two per month) that met a 'narrow definition' of familicide, meaning that the victims included an estranged partner and at least one child. The vast majority (96 per cent) were committed by males and most (73 per cent) involved use of firearms. In 74 per cent of cases where there was information on motives, news reports cited problems between partners as the precipitating factor in homicides; in 39 per cent the main problems were thought to be financial, while in 11 per cent there were disputes over child custody. Child victims were the biological offspring of perpetrators in 76 per cent of cases. Homicides were followed by suicides in 64 per cent of cases.

Liem and Reichelmann (2014) sought to take this a stage further by analysing motives in more depth. They applied cluster analysis, a method of identifying subgroups within a larger sample, to a set of 238 familicides, using similar data sources to those in the study just described; but they also included examples in which individuals killed their parents (parricide) and one or more of their siblings whom they perceived to be siding with the parent who was dominating or oppressing them (as they saw it). Again, most killings (94 per cent) were carried out by men, and (as in other US studies) mainly involved firearms; 70 per cent showed indications of premeditation and planning; and 57 per cent were followed by suicide or attempted suicide. Four types of familicide emerged from the analysis, labelled: (a) *despondent husbands*; (b) *spousal revenge*; (c) *extended parricides*; and (d) *diffuse conflict*. The first category (46 per cent) reflects a far higher proportion of these killings that were a result of financial problems than in the Yardley *et al.* (2014) UK sample (though money problems coexisted with other marital difficulties). This group also showed the highest proportion of evidence of premeditation (92 per cent), and all of its members committed suicide. The second and fourth categories (17 per cent and 24 per cent) were more often associated with previous partner violence, but spousal revenge was never followed by suicide. The third and smallest group (13 per cent) included the killing of parents and siblings, as mentioned above. The fourth group was more mixed, but also included a very high proportion of cases in which there was a history of domestic abuse, and the highest proportion in which there had been a restraining order.

Massacres

The less frequent, but in many people's minds more frightening, form of mass killing is one targeted partially, or sometimes entirely, at strangers. While those who commit these atrocities often have specific victims in mind, after having killed those individuals they often continue their attacks on other people selected seemingly at random, a pattern Meloy *et al.* (2001; Meloy and Felthous, 2004) called *bifurcated*. They used this term to refer to adolescents who first killed family members and then moved on to attack people at school; although only two of their cases fitted this pattern. However Hickey (2013) lists seventeen examples of such bifurcated mass homicides in the United States in the period 1927–2011; these were mainly committed by adults. Most showed the 'private to public' pattern, killing first relatives and then strangers, but some involved attacks in two or more public locations. Most episodes begin with shootings targeted at preselected individuals, followed by a period of more sporadic, random firing. The sense that victims were simply 'in the wrong place at the wrong time' causes this form of homicide to be among the most feared. By its nature, if many victims are to be killed, this crime for the most part involves weapons that can be used at a distance (such as firearms or explosives). However, there are instances when attacks have involved arson, as in the 1990 fire in the *Happy Land* club in New York, which killed 87 people; where a toxic substance has been released, as in the sarin gas attack on Tokyo underground trains in 1995, which killed 13 people; or where numerous stabbings have been carried out in rapid sequence, as in the April 2014 attack at a house party in Calgary, Alberta, in which 5 people died.

There is a historically documented phenomenon of sudden, unexplained killing rampages known as *amok*. Such rampages were recorded in India, Malaysia and other countries between the 16th and early 20th centuries (Kon, 1994). The person who went on such a rampage was often said to have been depressed beforehand, and after a frenzied attack on others had complete amnesia for the event. This was traditionally explained in terms of spirit possession or mental illness, but later came to be seen as a product of a set of cultural norms that prohibited direct personal confrontations and placed stringent controls on the expression of aggression. The latter interpretations of unexpressed anger and stifled aggression are consistent with what is known about the kinds of multiple homicides that have been reported in many other countries over recent decades. Perpetrators are often described as having previously been passive, dejected and alienated; and as 'loner' males who have accumulated grievances, become embittered, and formed a belief that they need to 'get even' with society. Sometimes such individuals have been described as highly narcissistic, having a 'superman' complex, and being bent on an act of cathartic self-assertion. Palermo (1997) considered this similar to the drug-induced *berserk* state of Norse warriors of medieval times, and suggested that it could explain killings carried out by individuals who were consumed by extreme levels of hatred and who were in a state of vengeful rage as a result.

Mass killings fitting this pattern have taken place in public venues such as restaurants, shops or cinemas, in the street, in workplaces, schools and university campuses. As already noted, they are often referred to as *rampages*. Böckler, Seeger, Sitzer and Heitmeyer (2013) distinguish them from genocide and terrorism in that there is a greater focus on personal thoughts and feelings that have perhaps become fixations, as opposed to political or religious factors. They are also distinct from multiple gangland killings and drive-by shootings, which often have several victims but are generally rooted in economic rivalries. Böckler and his colleagues divide rampages into three types: *'classic' rampages*, usually committed by adults in a public place; *workplace violence*, usually arising from a grievance against employers or workmates; and *school shootings*, most of which are committed by younger people. The vast majority of offenders in all three types are male.

These events cause the level of devastation that they do because they are typically committed using assault weapons (semi-automatic pistols, rifles or shotguns which can fire at high speed and have a large-capacity magazine). In some cases explosives or arson have been used; and in a small number of cases, as just noted, there have been multiple stabbings or mass poisoning. To fire on people from the tower of the University of Texas at Austin in August 1966, Charles Whitman armed himself with two shotguns, three rifles, two pistols and a revolver, together with a large supply of ammunition for each weapon, and a formidable array of other equipment that would enable him to sustain a lengthy siege. Having already killed his wife and his mother, he killed a further 13 people in the ensuing massacre, and wounded 32 more.

It now seems clear that an offence on this scale is primarily predatory and requires considerable forethought. The psychological state of the offender is very different from that of someone who kills on impulse following provocation or escalation of an interpersonal conflict. The perpetrator may still be exceedingly angry or agitated, but the process differs from spontaneous reactive aggression in having been rationalised. Where individuals have made statements concerning their intentions, they appear to believe that their actions are justified. In some cases their fury has been directed against women, as in the murder by Mark Lépine of 14 female students at the École Polytechnique, Montreal, in 1989; or the murderous attack launched by George Hennard on a restaurant in the town of Killeen, Texas, in October 1991, when he killed 23 people and wounded 19 others. Firing on diners, Hennard shouted words of vengeance against women whom he felt had maligned him, imagining that he was teaching them a lesson. In other cases, the attacker has an overwhelming vendetta against virtually everyone. The video-recorded messages of Seung-Hui Cho, who killed 32 people and wounded 17 others at Virginia Polytechnic in April 2007, set out specific reasons why he believed he had been wronged, asserting that he had been 'forced into a corner' and that people had brought it on themselves (Hickey, 2013).

Homicides of this type have been called *autogenic massacres*, on the basis that they are driven by 'highly personal agendas arising from the perpetrator's own specific social situation and psychopathologies' (Mullen, 2004, p. 313). Analysis indicates that they are most often committed by 'low status males' with a troubled history, who not long before the massacre have experienced some personal insult of a kind that they find intolerable (Harrison and Bowers, 2010). Most perpetrators are men in their thirties and forties. There have been several instances of this in the UK, including the attacks by Michael Ryan in the Berkshire village of Hungerford in August 1987; by Thomas Hamilton in Dunblane, Perthshire, in March 1996; and by Derrick Bird in Cumbria in June 2010. Mullen (2004) has reported a case series of five individuals who carried out mass homicides in Australia, and while the details varied in several respects, the perpetrators showed some striking features in common. All were male, aged under 40, and unemployed or in casual employment; all were socially isolated, had been bullied or were solitary in childhood; all had a history of fascination with guns. Most had no prior histories of offending or of contact with mental health services. All had been depressed prior to the killings, and they also had persecutory ideas, though in most cases neither of these features was at a clinically diagnosable level (see Chapter 11). Mullen (2004) considered that they displayed rigid beliefs, suspiciousness and self-righteousness; and that they experienced resentment and ruminations, engaged in fantasy, and showed evidence of grandiosity and narcissism. In carrying out their acts, they mostly followed a 'script' they had obtained from elsewhere, usually from what they knew about previous mass killings. Similar features were found in other studies (e.g. Meloy *et al.*, 2001; Meloy and Felthous, 2004), although there was often a higher rate of recorded mental disorder. Some perpetrators have been described as manifesting a 'warrior mentality' or a kind of self-image that has been called that of a 'pseudo-commando', a compensatory identity that permits angry and alienated individuals to take lethal vengeance against those whom they believe have thwarted or humiliated them (Knoll, 2010a, 2010b).

Fox and DeLateur (2014) have exposed and debunked some of what they call the 'myths and misconceptions' that are associated with mass homicides. They analysed a series of 672 such assaults in the United States in the period 1976–2011, in each of which four or more people were killed. That is an average of about 20 massacres per year, approximating to one every 2½ weeks or so. Contrary to a widely held belief, in the USA their number has not been rising across that period but has showed a fluctuating pattern.

While the perpetrators are often acting out of a sense of fury against those whom they kill, these crimes are not committed on impulse but are carefully planned, sometimes many months in advance, and the killers often appear perfectly calm and methodical during the event itself. Nor are victims killed completely indiscriminately; while that may occur for part of the time, there is often a targeting strategy linked to themes of revenge and power. Most weapons are obtained legally, and the majority of perpetrators had displayed no problems that would have disqualified them from purchasing guns.

Mass killings in schools

As noted above, these acts may be carried out in a wide range of locations, but the impact is particularly disturbing when the target is a school and the victims are children and their teachers – perhaps even more so when the perpetrators, too, are of school age. Given the near-defencelessness of such locations, they have often been the focus of attacks. The United States has by far the highest rate of these events. The Academy for Critical Incident Analysis at John Jay College of Justice in New York (2012; McCarthy, 2012) developed a database of 294 massacres between 1764 and 2009, which had caused 672 deaths in schools across 38 countries. They then compared the number of these massacres during the period 2000–2010, and found that the USA, with a population of 308 million, had 27 such attacks – only one fewer than 36 other countries together, with a combined population of 3.8 billion. The majority of massacres in the USA (85 per cent) were carried out by a single perpetrator; and while the mean age was 23, half of the sample were aged between 13 and 20, 85 per cent had a history of being bullied, and 71 per cent committed suicide afterwards. Most (95 per cent) carried at least two weapons.

Mass homicides in schools are not a recent phenomenon. The highest death toll arose in the Bath School disaster in Michigan in May 1927, when 38 children and 6 adults died after Andrew Kehoe, a local farmer who was treasurer of the school board, exploded home-made bombs containing a mixture of dynamite and the incendiary chemical pyrotol. More often, though, such attacks have involved firearms. They have been committed in primary (elementary) schools (for example, at Sandy Hook in Newtown, Connecticut, in December 2012), in secondary schools (Columbine High School, Denver, in April 1999), and on college campuses (Virginia Tech massacre, in April 2007). Elsewhere, other weapons have been used, as in March 2010 when Zheng Minsheng stabbed 13 children, 8 of whom died, at an infant school in Nanping, China.

Böckler, Seeger, Sitzer and Heitmeyer (2013) developed an international database of 120 school rampages in 24 countries. They suggest that, in contrast to the position in the USA, the number has slowly increased over the period 1957 to 2011, particularly since the 1990s. The numbers of dead and injured also appear to have risen. Their sources, however, were news reports, and they acknowledge the questionable reliability of these reports. Among the perpetrators, 76 per cent were aged 12–21, and 97 per cent were male.

Both psychological and numerous other factors have been identified as possibly contributing to mass homicides in schools. As these events often involve the suicide of the perpetrator (or perpetrators), there are few cases in which individuals can be assessed afterwards. However, some do survive, and there is usually intense investigation of their lives even if they do not. Several have communicated their reasons for their actions before carrying them out. Some recorded their thoughts leading up to the event, or posted their ideas on websites. Others left suicide messages, and a few despatched 'manifestos' setting out why they had decided to commit the offences. Dutton, White and Fogarty (2013) analysed the diaries and blogs of four mass killers (including three school shooters) and suggested that their behaviour was driven by a combination of extreme paranoia with 'malignant narcissism', giving rise to seething hatred. Langman (2009a, 2009b, 2013) has reported an analysis of 35 case histories of school shooters, mainly from the USA but a smaller number from Canada, Germany, Finland and Brazil. Unlike those who commit other mass killings, most (75 per cent) were aged less than 20, and the youngest (Andrew Golden) was just 11. Langman stresses that school massacres are not a single phenomenon and that there is considerable variability among them. He suggests that those who commit them can be divided into three main types, defined as *psychotic*, *traumatised* or *psychopathic*. Those in the first and largest group, *psychotic*, show a number of marked symptoms of schizophrenia or schizotypal personality disorder, have delusions or hallucinations, are socially eccentric, and usually are also anxious and depressed. Langman's second type, *traumatised*, have experienced physical, sexual or emotional abuse (or any combination), and have parents with substance-abuse problems and criminal records, with disrupted families often living in squalor; perpetrators show a range of trauma symptoms linked to earlier victimisation. The third group, *psychopathic*, are marked by features such as grandiosity, callousness and lack of guilt; they reject rules and morality; and several are also sadistic. Some of the 35 appeared to fit one of these categories fairly well, whereas others did so more tentatively.

Other researchers have emphasised situational and cultural influences that create conditions in which such extreme events may be more likely to occur. They occur in communities where a school plays a dominant role in individuals' lives and where other sources of social validation are limited; and where there is a strong status hierarchy within adolescent groups, often reinforced by the reactions of parents. There can be intensive competition within adolescent society, which has profound effects on individuals' self-evaluations: 'American teenagers are ruthless arbiters of one another's social worth' (Newman, 2013, p. 76). There is often evidence of extensive bullying, and a culture that emphasises masculinity and associated values in young males, who are by far the most numerous perpetrators of school mass homicides. Within teenage culture a cultural script can emerge that attaches importance to attractiveness, popularity, athletic prowess, and particular patterns of dress and social demeanour. Some who are on the margins of social groups, or excluded from them, may acquire an aversive attitude to the school society, an attitude that through rumination and fantasy gradually mounts into hostility and then rage. In an integrative approach, Newman *et al.* (2004) listed ten factors widely invoked to explain these patterns: mental disorder; sudden loss of control (where after earlier insults, the person 'snapped'); family dysfunction; bullying; peer support (sometimes others have known the events were about to happen, and gave encouragement, or were even forewarned to stay away); community disruption; a culture of violence (engendering a belief that revenge is justified); media violence; gun availability; and copycat effects. Newman and her colleagues proposed a model containing five 'necessary but not sufficient' factors. These are characteristics they considered must be present for the event to occur, though none of them in itself is enough to make it happen – and even then, note that these offences are almost exclusively committed by males. The five factors are:

- that the shooter perceives himself as an outsider from the social groups that he thinks are important
- that he suffers from psychosocial problems that magnify the effect of this feeling of being excluded or ostracised
- that there are available 'cultural scripts' for redressing this problem through violence, especially as that relates to notions of masculinity
- that there is a failure of monitoring systems that would identify a troubled youth and provide support or intervention
- that there is ready access to guns.

Newman *et al.* tested their model against three datasets which contained information about a total of 78 school shootings. They concluded that in 20 of 25 cases in their dataset, the perpetrator had been attacking the adolescent social hierarchy (many victims were members of high-status groups), and in the remainder the perpetrator was attacking the school's institutional structure (most victims were teachers). Across the three datasets, a high proportion of the boys who had engaged in the school shootings manifested the above features, lending support to the theory, though as expected it could not account for the full range of cases. Newman *et al.* (2004) were at pains to point out that their list of variables could not be used to construct a profile of *prospective* perpetrators, as many offending youths show only some of these features.

The higher rate of these types of crimes in the United States is often attributed to the number of guns in circulation in that country and to their ready accessibility, but it is also a function of attitudes towards them which have deep roots in American society and culture. Almost always in the wake of any such incidents, an agonised public debate concerning this is reinvigorated. The general points that often arise within it are considered in the next 'Where do you stand?' box. The debate also occurs in relation to the use of guns in other types of crimes that are far more frequent than school massacres.

WHERE DO YOU STAND?

Homicide, firearms and gun control

In England and Wales in 2014–2015, there were 26,370 offences involving knives or other sharp implements, and 4,862 offences involving firearms other than air weapons (Office for National Statistics, 2015). These figures represent only a small proportion of total police recorded crime (6 per cent and 0.2 per cent respectively) and both had shown large drops over the preceding 10-year period.

Many assaults and homicides do not involve use of weapons. But where they *are* used, weapons of almost any kind are likely to lead to more severe injury than hands or fists alone – though use of the feet can be worse (Brennan, Moore and Shepherd, 2006). What is less clear is whether the *availability* of weapons makes violent crime more likely.

The relationship between violence and weapon use is complex. For example, people who decide to attack someone might first arm themselves. Here the use of a weapon could be seen as part of the aggression sequence. However, there are many other cases where 'the decision to carry a weapon and the use of a weapon cannot be reduced to the motivations associated with aggression' (Brennan and Moore, 2009, p. 217). We need to understand *why* a knife or gun was kept at hand.

Regarding possession of knives, following a steep rise in fatal attacks on young people in London in 2007–2008, there was mounting concern over an 'epidemic' of knife-carrying (Wood, 2010). Although studies both in the UK (Palasinski, 2013) and in Australia (Brown and Sutton, 2007) found that significant proportions of young people often carried knives, survey and interview data suggested they did so mainly for protective and self-image purposes, rather than with aggressive intent. This lends support to the stance of Brennan and Moore (2009).

Far greater controversy arises, however, in relation to firearms. There are recurrent and very bitter debates on this issue. They centre on the number of gun-related deaths, the availability of firearms, and the issue of gun control; most notably in the USA, which has the world's highest number of guns in private ownership.

The Graduate Institute of International and Development Studies in Geneva produces an annual report on the problem of weapon use (the *Small Arms Survey*). Its 2007 report provided statistics on 'civilian firearms arsenals' across 178 countries, rank ordered by the numbers of firearms per 100 people. For comparison, here are the top five, followed by a selection of the other figures:

USA	88.8	Northern Ireland	21.9
Yemen	54.8	Australia	15.0
Switzerland	45.7	South Africa	12.7
Finland	45.3	Brazil	8.0
Serbia	37.8	England and Wales	6.2
Canada	30.8	Scotland	5.5
Germany	30.3	India	4.2
New Zealand	22.6		

While several countries have high rates of gun-related homicides, the USA's is well above that of comparable high-income countries (though over the period 1993–2011 it fell by 39 per cent: Planty and Truman, 2013). As we saw earlier, it also has quite frequent multiple killings, almost all carried out using firearms – often using semi-automatic weapons, which can be purchased legally and with few obstacles in many states. This has led to the question: is the easy availability of these weapons a contributory factor in the homicide/massacre rate?

These issues have a high political and media profile. Key players in the dispute include the major political parties, a very influential 'gun lobby' pressure group, the National Rifle Association (founded in 1871), and the more recently formed Brady Campaign to Prevent Gun Violence (begun in 1974). Part of the background to this debate is the Second Amendment to the American constitution (dated 1791), concerning the 'right to bear arms'. Some people interpret that to mean that the Amendment bestows such a right on individual citizens. Other people, however,

8

insist that it refers to citizens' duty, in particular circumstances, to form or to join a militia for the protection of the people from the central government (Spitzer, 2012).

Supporters of 'gun rights' argue that 'guns make society safer'. In 1982 the town of Kennesaw, Georgia, passed a local law making it mandatory for residents to own a gun, though certain exceptions were allowed. It was claimed that this law had reduced the number of burglaries in the town, and some data suggested that that was the case. However, the data used to support this proved to be highly selective. A ten-year time-series analysis of burglary rates in Kennesaw before and after the enactment of the new law found no such effect (McDowall, Wiersema and Loftin, 1989). A larger-scale survey analysing national US data on handguns and burglary found no support for the suggestion that gun ownership deterred house burglary. On the contrary, the rate of burglary increased when guns were more prevalent, and indeed there was evidence that guns provided an inducement to burglary (Cook and Ludwig, 2002).

The accumulated data concerning firearms and violence lend more support to the contention that their availability is a factor more likely to increase gun-related injuries, homicides and suicides than to prevent them. In a compelling 'tale of two cities', Sloan *et al.* (1988) compared the US city of Seattle and the Canadian city of Vancouver, which have different laws on the ownership of firearms. While the two cities had quite similar rates of assault and aggravated assault, rates in Seattle were slightly higher. However, the rate of assault using guns was 7.0 times higher in Seattle, and the rate of handgun homicide was 4.8 times higher.

Reviews since then have confirmed an association between rates of gun ownership and rates of suicide, homicide and accidental injury (Anglemeyer, Horvath and Rutherford, 2014; Hepburn and Hemenway, 2004; Miller, Hemenway and Azrael, 2007; Stroebe, 2013). In a survey comparing 27 countries, Bangalore and Messerli (2013) found that the number of guns per capita in a country was a direct and significant predictor of firearm-related deaths. This relationship was independent of the rate of mental illness, which is often perceived as a cause of rampages and other incidents but which was not significantly correlated with firearm deaths. There is, however, an inverse association between the numbers of laws controlling firearms and levels of gun-related homicides and suicides (Lee et al., 2017).

What then are we to make of countries such as Switzerland with large numbers of guns in private ownership that do not have high homicide rates? Does this mean that the availability of guns is not a factor? Killias and Markwalder (2012) suggested that the extent to which firearms are used in homicide is a function not simply of the numbers of guns in a country but also of fundamental beliefs concerning them. In Switzerland they are issued following military service, and are kept under lock and key to be used only in a national crisis, rather than as a routine way of achieving personal protection.

But when guns are easily in people's hands, the impact on them can be perceptible. Bartholow, Anderson, Carnagey and Benjamin (2005) conducted an experiment in which they compared two groups: those who hunted regularly and were familiar with guns, and others with no gun experience. They found that amongst both groups, thoughts about guns had a 'priming effect', increasing the levels of participants' aggressive thoughts, and that this increase was linked to aggressive behaviour in a competitive situation.

In an analysis of 677 incidents in Philadelphia in the period 2003–2006 in which guns were used in assaults, Branas *et al.* (2009) found that possession of guns did not protect citizens from being shot. Although there were instances in which people had been able to use guns defensively, individuals in possession of a gun were 4.46 times more likely to be shot in an assault than those who did not have a gun, and 4.23 times more likely to be killed.

This finding is reinforced by research on what are called 'Stand your ground' laws, which allow citizens to use lethal force in self-defence. These laws have been introduced in some American states. Humphreys, Gasparrini and Wiebe (2017) evaluated their effect on rates of homicide generally, and on gun-related homicide, examining rates over 16 years (1999–2014), covering the period before and after the change in law. Homicide rates in Florida, which adopted the laws on 1st October, 2005, were compared with those in four other states (New York, New Jersey, Ohio and Virginia) that did not adopt them, and with suicide rates by firearm in Florida itself. In the phase prior to the change in law homicide rates in Florida were stable but showed a slight downward trend. Over the total study period, there was no evidence of change in either total homicide rates or firearm-related homicides in the other states, nor in the rate of suicides in Florida. However, the rate of gun-related homicide in Florida showed an 'abrupt and sustained' increase of 31.6 per cent in the phase following the legal change, and that for homicide in general showed a 24.4 per cent increase. This is strong evidence that permitting citizens to defend themselves with firearms resulted in larger numbers of them being killed.

Where do you stand on this issue?

1 Does the availability of guns make violence, including homicide, more likely?

2 Where guns are freely available, should they be controlled more tightly? Or should controls on them be loosened, to enable citizens to protect themselves?

3 You have just been appointed a government minister with a remit to develop a new set of laws governing gun ownership. What rules will you include within these laws?

Serial murder

As one expert suggests, the public (and probably professionals too) have a complex and contradictory reaction to crimes of this type. While we are 'enthralled by the serial killer', at the same time we are 'also afraid of him ... simultaneously fascinated and repelled' (Miller, 2014a, pp. 3, 4). The extent of violence in some serial murders horrifies us and also evokes primal fears at the thought of each victim's agonising fate. Although most serial murderers have killed fewer than ten victims (Hickey, 2013), a proportion kill many more. The majority are caught, but some evade detection over periods of many years. The identities of others have never been established: there are series of cases that remain unsolved.

Serial murder is defined by Fox and Levin (2012, p. 30) as 'a string of four or more homicides committed by one or a few perpetrators that spans a period of days, weeks, months or even years' (an earlier FBI definition used a cut-off point of two homicides). Fox and Levin assembled details of a total of 614 individuals who, alone or in partnership, had committed serial murders in the USA at some time in the years since 1900. While calculating an exact number of victims is impossible, they estimate that these offenders were collectively responsible for 3,700 homicides. But they suggest that the real figure may be higher, as some murders committed by the same person are not recognised as such, a problem that has been called *linkage blindness* (Egger, 1984).

Examination of their database showed that 93 per cent of serial killers were male; 65 per cent were white; the largest single group (42 per cent) embarked on their killing careers in their twenties, and the second largest (31 per cent) in their thirties. Just under 70 per cent confined their crimes to a local area, with the remainder killing on a regional (22.8 per cent) or national (9 per cent) basis, and a small number operating internationally. Fox and Levin also document that in the USA such crimes have changed in frequency across successive decades, showing a low rate prior to the 1970s, rising steeply to a peak in the 1980s, and with a gradual decline since then. The explanation for this might lie in changes in recording practices and forensic techniques, which have influenced the police's ability to establish connections between crimes; but it also parallels the trends for violent crime overall. Fox and Levin (2012) argued that some earlier suggestions to the effect that as many as 5,000 murders per year were the work of serial killers were almost certainly erroneous, and suggestions that there were hundreds of serial killers at large in the USA were wildly exaggerated. (They suggested that this might have been done to strengthen a case for increased funding of the FBI.) It is worth noting that there have been criticisms of the FBI method of classifying multiple homicides.

Borrowing medical terminology, Reid (2017) called for a 'new nosology' to be developed, and forwarded proposals accordingly.

Serial homicide has been recorded in many countries of the world and – as with violent crimes in general – the majority of perpetrators are male. Unlike single-victim homicide, however, most victims of serial killing are female (Kraemer, Lord and Heilbrun, 2004). A large proportion of these offences have a sexual motive, and while this can obviously be regarded as a form of sex crime, it is not legally classified as such in England and Wales. It does share some features of other types of sexual crimes we will discuss in Chapter 9, but also takes various forms and may be driven by a different combination of motives (Miller, 2014b).

As suggested earlier, the objective in serial homicide is often the act of killing itself, and in most cases the motives are psychological rather than economic. In sadistic murder, for example, the offender obtains excitement and pleasure from inflicting suffering or from observing the suffering of the victim, or both. Serial murders often produce more victims than mass murders do, but they are killed consecutively, with a latency or 'cooling off' period in between. The length of the latter can vary markedly, from a few days to a number of years. For example, Gary Ridgway (the 'Green River Killer') is known to have killed 49 women, and confessed to killing over 20 more, in the American states of Washington and California over the years 1982–1998. However, the majority (42) were killed in a much shorter period, 1982–1984, often with only a few days between them. Dennis Rader (the 'Bind, Torture, Kill' or BTK Killer, a name he gave himself) committed ten homicides in the years 1974–1991, after some of which he sent letters to the police and to newspapers. That was followed by a 14-year gap before he resumed sending letters again, which led to his capture and conviction. Ted Kaczynski (the 'Unabomber'), who carried out 16 attacks between 1978 and 1995, desisted from his activities at one stage for a period of six years (1987–1993).

Kraemer, Lord and Heilbrun (2004) compared a set of 170 serial-homicide offenders with a control group of 195 single-homicide offenders. The latter group were perhaps somewhat unusual in containing a high proportion of individuals who had been involved with someone else in joint killings (the number of victims was 133). Single-homicide offenders more often had initial contact with the victim, killed him or her, and disposed of the body all at the same location. For serial offenders, these three locations tended to be different. Principal intentions also differed: single offenders more often committed 'emotion-based' crimes against paramours and acquaintances; serial offenders more often committed sexual killings of strangers.

Classification of serial killing

There have been numerous attempts to find a viable and potentially useful way to classify serial homicides. Some are based on analysing measurable features of the crime scene, whereas others focus on analysis of motives. Any system based on the former almost always fails, as there are typically some sequences of murders that fit more than one category. A similar problem arises with motives, however: here too many offences are influenced by multiple factors and defy neat classification. Miller (2014a) reviewed a total of four such classificatory frameworks and suggested a generic, integrated account with four broad categories: *sexually sadistic*, *delusional*, *custodial* and *utilitarian* killers.

The first group consists of *sexual sadists* who kill for the excitement of sex itself, intensified by the accompanying feelings of domination and control the offender obtains from inflicting pain. Andrei Chikatilo (the 'Butcher of Rostov') committed 53 murders in the period 1978–1990 across a wide area of what are now the Russian Federation, Ukraine and Uzbekistan. His victims included 21 boys, 14 girls and 18 women; the youngest was aged 7 and the oldest 45, but the majority were in their teens and twenties. These were very brutal crimes as a result of Chikatilo's reported pattern of eviscerating his victims before or after death in order to obtain sexual gratification. In the years 1974–1978, Ted (Theodore) Bundy killed at least 30 females, ranging in age from 12 to 26, across several American states. He was suspected of many other murders in addition. Sometimes he entered victims' bedrooms while they were asleep and bludgeoned them to death. On other occasions he used his good looks and charm to lure victims from apparently safe places, often in view of many other people, and once out of sight forced his victims into his car, before abducting and killing them.

A second group consists of individuals who are acting on *delusional* or *paranoid beliefs*. They may feel themselves to have been given a 'mission' to clear the world of a specific class of persons – usually a group they perceive as of low social status, such as sex workers. Peter Sutcliffe (the 'Yorkshire Ripper') fits into this category. He killed 13 women and attempted to kill 7 others, in the north of England in the period 1975–1979; most of his victims worked as prostitutes, though a few did not. He mutilated some of the corpses afterwards. Several psychiatrists testified at his trial that he suffered from paranoid schizophrenia, but he was found guilty of murder and sentenced to life imprisonment. Subsequently, he was transferred to a high security hospital and later still he was placed on a whole life tariff (see Chapter 16). Between 1982 and 1997, Ahmad Suradji killed 42 women near the Indonesian city of Medan. He was a sorcerer who reportedly believed that he could gain healing power by drinking the saliva of his victims, whom he buried up to their waists and then strangled. They were then completely buried, with their heads facing towards his house, which he believed gave him further power. While a belief in forces of magic may be culturally normative in many parts of the world, it does not usually include the idea of killing others so that power can be obtained from them, and the latter amounts to a delusional state. Ahmad Suradji was found guilty of murder and executed by firing squad in 2008.

A third category includes what are called '*custodial*' *killers*. These are individuals whose professional relationship with others is outwardly a responsible and caring one, but who in fact have an underlying motive wholly at odds with that role. As a result of their professional positions, these individuals have succeeded in gaining the trust of others, to such an extent that in some cases they were able to continue offending even after a third party had become suspicious. Examples in the UK are the general practitioner Harold Shipman, who was convicted of murdering 15 of his patients but was strongly suspected of having killed 215 more; and the nurse Beverley Allitt, who was found guilty of the murder of 4 children, the attempted murder of 3 others, and causing grievous bodily harm to a further 6. There may be a power motive within this, insofar as the perpetrator is able to exercise, quite literally, 'life or death' control over the victim. In Harold Shipman's case, there appears in relation to his final victim to have been an additional motive of financial gain. Beverley Allitt was diagnosed with a rare mental disorder, *Münchausen's syndrome by proxy*, in which an individual causes illness in someone else in order to gain attention. Note however, that the status of this disorder is controversial (Mart, 2004).

Miller's fourth group consists of those whose motives are partly *utilitarian*. In these homicides, there are material gains to be made, though this motive could be mixed with other motives of a different kind, such as anger or revenge. This category includes professional *contract killers* ('hit men'), who are functionaries of organised criminal gangs or who operate on a freelance basis for money (see Chapter 10). Here too, however, a sense of power may be an influence.

The largest proportion of serial homicides belongs in the first of the above categories and contains not only a major sexual element but one that is also connected to sadism, in which the killer obtains pleasure from witnessing another person's pain (or inducing it, or both). Some researchers consider this to be the prominent motivation in these offences (Myers, 2004; Myers, Husted, Safarik and O'Toole, 2006). Prior to the first homicide, the offender engages in fantasy concerning the possibility of it, and a series of influences and events combine to instil a sense that he (almost all are males) can act out such fantasies. The combination of this with an absorbing urge for power and control over another is a highly dangerous one, and some of the most appalling cases of serial murder, whether heterosexual or homosexual, have incorporated these elements. Having committed one homicide, a cycle begins whereby the urge to repeat the act may grow until it becomes intolerable. In the case of Ted Bundy the period between these acts was comparatively short (30 victims in a three-year period, sometimes with multiple killings in a single day), whereas for other killers it has been longer or more variable.

The victims of serial homicide are almost always exclusively strangers, and this facilitates a process whereby some perpetrators are able to inflict excruciating pain on their victims and act towards them in other ways that signify objectification and dehumanisation. In some cases the brutality and deviance extends further, to acts of torture, **necrophilia**, or cannibalism. Several patterns of action found amongst serial murderers illustrate extremes of human behaviour in their bizarreness and gruesomeness. Alongside the macabre killing of two women and the suspected murder of a number of others in the period 1954–1957 in rural Wisconsin, Ed Gein also unearthed remains from a local cemetery. He dismembered bodies from both sources, fashioned bones into household items, and made lampshades from human skin. It emerged that he had made a mask from an actual face and a vest from a woman's torso. He would dance outside his home at night wearing both. He is described as having had a psychosexually very intricate relationship with his mother, reportedly a devoutly religious, rigid and domineering woman, who compelled him to live an isolated life. Characters in several horror films, including *Psycho*, *The Texas Chainsaw Massacre* and *The Silence of the Lambs*, are reputedly based on Ed Gein.

Jeffrey Dahmer claimed 17 victims, all male, in the period 1978–1991. His killings changed form over time. By the latter stages he had developed a *modus operandi* in which he lured victims to his apartment, often having offered them money for sex. Homosexual acts might then take place, after which he drugged and then strangled most of his victims. He masturbated over their bodies and then dismembered them, photographing them at various stages, and preserved parts of their bodies. He later committed necrophilia and cannibalism, and made household items out of body parts. He drilled holes in two of his victims' skulls while they were still alive, introducing a corrosive chemical, hydrochloric (muriatic) acid, into their brains in an effort to create compliant, zombie-like persons whom he could keep under his control and accessible for sexual purposes. When police entered his home after one near-victim escaped, they found a severed human head and two hearts in the refrigerator. Other human remains were found in a freezer and in a large tank of acid. Dahmer told police he had eaten the hearts, livers and portions of the muscles of several victims. He was described as having collected animal bones when a young boy and having been intensely interested in dissection. His social ineptness and reclusiveness led Silver, Ferrari and Leong (2002) to contend that he suffered from Asperger's syndrome, a type of developmental disorder considered to be part of the 'autistic spectrum'. Jeffrey Dahmer had taken to heavy drinking from an early age. Neither of his parents was available to him emotionally; their marriage was riven with conflict, and when he was in his late teens they parted acrimoniously. There appeared to be a compulsive element to his murderous behaviour. Although some expert witnesses diagnosed him with borderline personality disorder, the court decided he was sane and found him guilty.

There is a strand within Jeffrey Dahmer's case similar to one found in that of Dennis Nilsen, who killed 15 young men in the period 1978–1983 in London. He too met his victims in local pubs and took them back to his lodgings. There, after strangling them, he washed their bodies and made sketches of them (Masters, 1985), often keeping the bodies with him even as they began to decompose. Parallels have been drawn between these two cases in terms of the absence or loss of other relationships in the perpetrators' lives, their social isolation and extreme loneliness starting from childhood, and their engagement in deviant fantasy leading to an urge to secure complete control over their victims (Martens and Palermo, 2005; Palermo, 2008).

Factors involved in sexual homicide

How is it possible to explain a pattern in which an individual can obtain sexual gratification from inflicting abominable pain on another person and then proceeding to kill her or him? We will discuss other kinds of sexual violence separately in the next chapter, but it is worth focusing briefly here on some of the elements that contribute to sexual murder. While those who commit this type of homicide are routinely referred to as 'monsters', 'beasts' and so on, their actions are in fact extreme manifestations of processes that occur in many individuals:

- *Classical conditioning model* An early theory of sexually deviant behaviour, propounded by McGuire, Carlisle and Young (1964), applied the behavioural concept of conditioning. In this context individuals reinforce a type of sexual interest by repeatedly masturbating to imagery associated with it. Surveys have suggested that many men have erotic fantasies that incorporate themes of sexual power and aggressiveness (Crépault and Couture, 1980). MacCulloch, Snowden, Wood and Mills (1983) investigated this in relation to sadism, and, based on their work with a series of 16 patients detained in a secure hospital, illuminated the process whereby elaborate fantasies influenced their likelihood of committing violent sexual offences. Sexually sadistic fantasies can become established at a comparatively young age, from early adolescence onwards (Johnson and Becker, 1997). There is a consensus that engagement in sadistic fantasy is a core mechanism in the creation of an individual capable of sexual homicide, in the absence of counterbalancing inhibitory mechanisms such as prosocial relationships (in which individuals act for the benefit of each other) or moral controls (Chan and Heide, 2009).
- *Motivational model* Burgess *et al.* (1986) took this a stage further by examining how such fantasies become a prime preoccupation for some men. For that to occur there is likely to have been some other form of developmental failure, one result of which is often social isolation. The fantasy life then takes on greater salience, replacing ordinary social relationships, and gradually acquiring compulsive force. This continued cognitive processing reaches a stage where, in an individual who because of other developmental experiences feels no reason to inhibit such cravings, the urge to act on them becomes irresistible.
- *Trauma control model* Hickey (2013) refers to developmental processes through which individuals may acquire the capacity to commit serial murder. The personal histories of many of those who commit serial sexual homicides show a series of destabilising events, which Hickey (2013) call *traumatisations*. These might include an unstable early life, the loss of parents, witnessing violence, direct maltreatment, and in some cases brain injury. While similar things happen to many individuals, amongst some they contribute to an inability to cope with certain kinds of stress. Rejection, isolation, absence of support and a lack of skills in solving problems in constructive ways produces a person with a strong sense of 'inadequacy, self-doubt, and worthlessness' (2013, p. 137). To manage such pervasive feelings, the individual reverts to *dissociation* as a coping strategy. This can induce *compartmentalisation*, enabling the individual to maintain more conventional relationships, whilst inwardly continuing to experience profound negative feelings. The oscillation between these two personal worlds may be the mechanism that accounts for the cyclical nature of serial homicides, with violent incidents separated by interludes of 'cooling off'.
- *Integrative paraphilic model* Purcell and Arrigo (2006) proposed a model of what they have labelled 'lust murder', which combines aspects of the three models just described. This focuses on the emergence of sexual sadism as one form of paraphilia, a pattern of atypical sexual arousal and ongoing deviant interest (see Chapter 11), in this case of an extreme type. As a result of the developmental factors specified in the other models – failures of learning and traumatisation – and via the process of orgasmic conditioning to violent sexual imagery, the individual recurrently employs the latter as a form of self-soothing or compensatory mechanism when faced with emotional stress. However, this cycle steadily increases in amplitude, suggest Purcell and Arrigo, until 'when violent erotic imagery no longer sates the person's sexual appetite, behavioral manifestations follow' (p. 57) – manifestations that include sadistic sexual violence.

It is sometimes claimed – as news reports highlight whenever the suggestion emerges – that spectacular crimes of this type are influenced by the viewing preferences and habits of those who commit them. That is, they are said to have watched violent films or other images, sometimes repeatedly, prior to committing the offence. This is a key part of the recurring debate about the impact of media violence on aggression. Helfgott (2008, pp. 379–384) compiled a list of no fewer than 44 examples in which there is anecdotal evidence of a 'copycat' effect on serious violent crimes. The alleged influences cover a wide range and include novels such as *The Catcher in the Rye*, which is thought to have influenced Mark David Chapman, who shot and killed John Lennon. More often video games such as *Grand Theft Auto* or films such as *A Clockwork Orange*, *Robocop II*, *Child's Play 3* and *The Matrix* are implicated as preoccupying the minds of individuals who mentally rehearsed scenes from them and subsequently acted them out. A few films, such as *The Matrix* and perhaps most notoriously *Natural Born Killers*, have each been linked to several murders. In some cases juries have been shown the films in court, in trials arising from a homicide thought to have been influenced by viewing such films.

Miller (2014a, p. 9) suggests that serial killers 'have been around for as long as people have lived in aggregated societies'. A frequently cited example is that of the medieval French nobleman, Gilles de Rais (1405–1440), who, after retiring from a successful career as a soldier (during which he was a key ally of Joan of Arc), is alleged to have tortured and murdered a large number of children (200, and perhaps even more) at his chateau not far from Nantes. There are disputes over whether or not these events took place, but it is thought that a person of his social rank may have been in a position to act with impunity in a way not possible for most citizens. Walker (2001), on the other hand, doubts the likelihood that in the remoter past there would have been any such problem as serial murder. He suggests that in small-scale societies, it would almost certainly have been impossible for the identity of any person carrying out such acts to remain unknown. While willingness to kill might have been valued in conflicts with outgroups, no one who displayed regular severe violence towards members of the ingroup would have been tolerated. Examples of decisive action against 'overly violent men and bullies' have been reported in present-day hunter-gatherer societies (Fry, 2011, p. 237). Serial crime as we know it today is very likely a relatively recent phenomenon: a function of the opportunities that arise from the spatial dispersal and social anonymity of mass societies with low levels of informal control.

Multiple perpetrators

Multiple homicide, of course, usually refers to numbers of *victims*. But there are also homicides that are committed by multiple *perpetrators*. When two or more individuals have cooperated to commit deadly assaults, the results have been some of the most notorious crimes in recent history – particularly when there is a sexual element and the perpetrators were sexual partners, and even more so if the victims were children. Within the large database of serial homicides compiled by Fox and Levin (2012), they identified 56 partnerships or 'serial killer teams', of which 71.4 per cent were all-male combinations, 5.4 per cent comprised females only, and 23.3 per cent were mixed-sex.

Gurian (2013) reviewed possible explanations of homicide by mixed-sex partners, in which the offences are committed by a combination of at least one man and one woman, usually sexual partners, acting together as accomplices. Gurian reviewed a series of 34 documented cases of partnered co-offenders, from a number of countries, comprising a total of 111 individuals (63 males, 48 females) who had each committed at least two homicides during the period 1900–2006. Infamous examples in the USA include Bonnie Parker and Clyde Barrow ('Bonnie and Clyde') in the 1930s and the 'Manson family' in the 1960s; and two duos in the UK, Ian Brady and Myra Hindley (the 'Moors Murderers') in the 1960s, and Fred and Rosemary West, in the 1980s. It is usually taken for granted that the male is the principal culprit in these partnerships, and that may often be correct. However, cases such as that of Paul Bernardo and Karla Homolka, who killed three young women in Ontario in the early 1990s (including the latter's younger sister), suggest that it is not always accurate. In that case, videotape evidence that Karla Homolka had played an active part in the rape and murder of victims became available only after she had already made a 'plea bargain' with prosecutors, on the basis that she would testify against her partner.

Potential explanations of what happens in these relationships include the suggestion that they are a result of sensation-seeking, and that both parties excite each other into doing things that neither of them would have done alone. Another possibility is that of *hybristophilia*, a term referring to a type of paraphilia in response to a person who does outrageous or dangerous things. (Note that this is not classed as a mental disorder as such.) This is also suggested to explain the reported admiration of many women for serial murderers such as Ted Bundy, who whilst in prison is said to have received hundreds of amorous letters from women, many containing propositions of marriage. A third possibility is the psychiatric syndrome known as *folie à deux*, in which two individuals (or three, in *folie à trois*, and so on) experience a commingling of fantasies or delusional states. In this case, the participating individuals are each likely to have been at risk of mental disorder prior to entering into the relationship. Another, though perhaps more prosaic, explanation is in terms of the social psychology of obedience and influence by authority or other powerful figures, processes to which many people may be susceptible and which may be at work in many offending peer-groups involved in other types of crimes.

Individuals who embark on a joint enterprise of serial killing are each likely to have come from a disturbed background and may manifest many of the features associated with repeated involvement in violence. But co-action with another person could weaken or remove some of the inhibitions that might otherwise have operated. That could apply to both male and female members of homicidal partnerships. As Gurian (2013) suggests, not enough is known about offending by women to evaluate the motivations at play in such relationships.

It is very difficult to choose between the various options that have been offered to account for this rare form of offending. It is also plausible, given the diversity of patterns it takes, that each of the aforementioned processes explains some of the instances of it.

Terrorism

In the final sections of this chapter we move from the study of multiple homicide at the personal, familial or local level, to types of multiple killing that take very different patterns and stem from different sets of motives. We discuss each of these only briefly, however, as forensic psychologists are unlikely to encounter many perpetrators of these types of offences. In any case, they are rarely apprehended and there are few certainties regarding them.

Acts identified as *terrorism* have in common a motive of inducing extreme fear in civilian or non-combatant populations, usually with the intention of pressuring governments in the pursuit of a political, ideological or religious objective, or some fusion of these. The immediate means of accomplishing this is to cause death or injury by making indiscriminate attacks or by threatening to make them. The currently dominant form of terrorism involves attempting to maximise these effects by attacking places where people are going about their routine everyday business. The targets are not military installations or government buildings, but shopping centres, markets, performance venues, buses, trains, or busy streets. The sense that lethal violence could happen anywhere at any moment is part of the message conveyed, to instil and spread fear as widely as possible. To the extent that terror attacks heighten individuals' awareness of their own possibly imminent death, they also appear to increase prejudice against 'outgroups' (Das *et al.*, 2009).

The *Global Terrorism Index* is an annually produced report comparing rates of terrorist incidents in 163 countries. During 2015, there were 29,376 deaths caused by terrorism, a reduction of 10 per cent compared to the year before. The five countries most badly affected were Iraq, Afghanistan, Nigeria, Pakistan and Syria, together accounting for 72 per cent of all deaths from terrorism. However, the 34 countries of the OECD (Organisation for Economic Co-operation and Development, the world's wealthiest countries) experienced a 650 per cent increase in such deaths from 2014 to 2015, making it the worst year since 2001, when the 9/11 attacks occurred. In those events, four passenger aircraft were hijacked; two were flown into the towers of the World Trade Center in New York, one into the Pentagon building in Arlington, Virginia, and a fourth crashed in Pennsylvania. Yet notwithstanding the massive public concern over terrorist incidents that has arisen in OECD countries, more than 90 per cent of terrorist attacks occurred in countries that were engaged in violent conflicts.

Terrorism is an issue that sparks vociferous debate between individuals, in the news media, amongst politicians and between academic experts. As with many concepts discussed in this book, there is no consensus definition of the term. Krueger and Malečková (2003) noted that there were over 100 definitions. Martin (2016) reviewed a range of attempts to define it, but noted that none of them is universally accepted. It has become conventional to apply the term to certain groups which – in recent years, and especially since the attacks of September 2001 in the United States – have committed atrocities in Europe, the Middle East, North Africa and elsewhere. Acts of terrorism today are closely associated with groups often described as 'fanatical'. Thus terrorism is almost universally viewed as without moral justification and is condemned as a crime (Stevens, 2005). However, some legitimate governments that publicly take that stance have themselves directly used, or indirectly sponsored, terrorist activity, thereby compromising their position on these points.

Over recent decades, terrorist attacks have been perpetrated by a wide variety of groups and for numerous causes. Examining the proclaimed justifications issued by different terrorism groups, O'Boyle (2002) classified them under six headings: the revolutionary left; radical ecological; national liberation; religious Christian right; secular right fascist or race-hate groups; and Islamic extremism. Each group sought to base its rationale on a different combination of moral, religious and political principles.

Considerable effort has been expended in trying to identify features of individuals who might be associated with involvement in terrorism. An initial assumption that those who carry it out come from economically deprived families has been contradicted by research. Studies suggest, in fact, that they are more likely to come from slightly better-off backgrounds and to have above-average levels of education. Another keenly debated question has been whether those who carry out such acts are mentally disturbed, especially if their involvement has led to self-destruction. Sheehan (2014) notes that in 2013 there were 384 suicide attacks in 18 countries, causing 3,743 deaths. Even if individuals see themselves as being at war, the chosen course of deliberately killing non-combatants and then oneself seems to signify grossly distorted beliefs, and possibly a deranged state of mind.

There are differences of opinion over whether suicide-terrorism is indicative of mental disorder. Some authors suggest that in the contexts in which it occurs it is not fundamentally irrational (Kacou, 2013), while others consider that perpetrators of suicide-terrorism show features in common with perpetrators of other cases of massacres followed by suicide (Lankford, 2010; Lankford and Hakim, 2011). A review of the limited evidence on this issue suggests that some elements of suicidality may be present in a minority of perpetrators, but that more in-depth studies are needed of those who are intercepted before committing suicide attacks, as well as 'psychological autopsies' of those who die (Sheehan, 2014). More generally, there is no clear evidence that the rate of mental disorder is higher amongst those involved in terrorist acts than in any other group (Ruby, 2002). In that respect, the practice of employing risk assessment methods that have been developed for use with patients in forensic mental health services has been called into question (Dernevik *et al.*, 2009). Monahan (2012) expressed doubt as to whether *any* instrument designed to predict the risk of terrorism can be prospectively validated in the same way that this can be done for instruments designed to predict the risk of common violence.

Forensic psychologists have been involved in the assessment of individuals who have been arrested for, or convicted of, terror-related offences. In the United

Kingdom, the statutes governing this are the Terrorism Act 2000 and the Counter-Terrorism and Security Act 2015. In 2003, the UK government introduced a counter-terrorism strategy for public safety with four strands: PREVENT, PREPARE, PROTECT, and PURSUE. This policy was continued, although in a revised format from 2011 onwards. The first strand is focused on identification of individuals who may be at risk of being drawn into an affiliation with terrorist ideology, and who may go a step further and become adherents of a terrorist organisation, a process known as *radicalisation*. While most referrals for assessment under PREVENT occur in schools, social services, health clinics or other community settings, there is evidence from a survey of 15 countries that radicalisation may occur in some cases to people who are serving prison sentences for other types of crime (Neumann, 2010). Several models have been proposed as to how the process occurs (King and Taylor, 2011). The commonalities between them are thought to be threefold: the relative deprivation of the community to which the individual belongs; personal crisis and a search for identity; and certain personality vulnerabilities. However, there are inconsistencies in the evidence pertaining to each of these.

Given the levels of concern regarding radicalisation, attempts have been made to find a means of identifying individuals who may be potentially at risk of becoming radicalised and who may then go on to commit terrorist offences. One such 'consultative tool' is the VERA 2 (*Violent Extremism Risk Assessment*) protocol described by Pressman and Flockton (2012), which contains 31 items concerned with beliefs, attitudes, intentions, capability, training, commitment and other aspects of the individual. However, apart from a small-scale case study by Beardsley and Beech (2013), there is a lack of validating evidence. The UK Ministry of Justice devised its own approach to assessing these risks, entitled the *Extremism Risk Guidance* (ERG-20; Lloyd and Dean, 2015). However, the use of this measure has proved to be controversial due to the absence of published evaluative data, and the approach has been subject to considerable criticism (Qureshi, 2016; Royal College of Psychiatrists, 2016).

Over recent years, the extremist terrorists most likely to commit attacks in European countries have been members of 'terror networks', with whom they are connected via the internet (Dalgaard-Nielsen, 2010; Sageman, 2004). Such networks may undertake recruitment and training and may also provide strategic direction. A major focus of the work of the security services is on monitoring those networks and communications. It remains markedly more difficult to predict the behaviour of those who operate in isolation, who have been called lone-actor (or sometimes 'lone wolf') terrorists, about whom considerably less is known (Pantucci, Ellis and Chaplais, 2015).

Genocide

During the 20th century, by far the largest numbers of deaths committed in any manner that is now formally classified as crime took the form known as **genocide**. Apart from war, but sometimes carried out as part of it, episodes of genocide are the most appalling events in history, and have resulted in enormous numbers of casualties. The 20th century witnessed some of the most horrific acts of this kind, with total numbers of deaths estimated at over 100 million (Jones, 2017; Totten and Parsons, 2009).

Genocide has occurred in many locations throughout the world; and on the basis of historical accounts, incidents that appear to fit the description have occurred over many centuries. Naimark (2017) outlines different forms it has taken, both in the ancient world and in other historical and cultural contexts since then. Naimark's account includes massacres of indigenous groups that occurred during the course of European settlement and colonialism in different parts of the world, resulting in the obliteration of some peoples in the Americas, Africa and Australia.

During the last century, genocidal acts were often systematically planned to decimate or exterminate an entire group of people. Examples include Ottoman Turkey and the killing of one million Armenians in 1915; the *Holodomor*, the enforced starvation under Josef Stalin of between five and seven million people in the Ukraine in the early 1930s; the massacre of an estimated half a million members of the Indonesian Communist Party in 1965–1966; the torture and murder of nearly two million people by the Khmer Rouge in Cambodia in the 1970s; and the massacre of an estimated 800,000 Tutsi in Rwanda over a period of less than four months in 1994 (Totten and Parsons, 2009). Most notorious of all, the *Holocaust* in Nazi Germany entailed the carefully planned, industrial-scale murder of six million Jews in gas chambers and by other methods, and the murder of several hundred thousand Slavs, Roma, people with disabilities and other derided and despised groups.

The term 'genocide' as used today owes its origins to the work of Raphael Lemkin (1900–1959), a Polish and Jewish lawyer who challenged the contradiction whereby one person killing another could be charged with murder, while those who authorised or conducted the eradication of an entire group were not classed as having committed a crime. Lemkin campaigned for many years to have this rectified, both before and after his flight from Poland to the United States to escape persecution. After World War II he called for it to be denounced by the United Nations (Power, 2013).

Lemkin's work culminated in the establishment in 1948 of the UN *Convention on the Prevention and Punishment of the Crime of Genocide*. This defines genocide as actions carried out with the intention of destroying, in whole or in part, a national, ethnic, racial or religious group by killing members of that group, by causing serious bodily or mental harm to them, by deliberately inflicting conditions of life designed to bring about the group's destruction, by imposing measures to prevent births within the group, or by forcibly transferring children to another group. Essentially, these are all different methods of seeking the annihilation or extermination of a community of people. The *mens rea* component of this definition – intent to destroy – if seemingly straightforward, has been a matter of close legal analysis (Ambos, 2009). For example, the ruthless commercial exploitation of the Congo in the period 1880–1920 by King Leopold II of Belgium is thought to have led to ten million deaths, but is not usually regarded as a genocide (Hochschild, 1998).

Genocides occur in particular historical circumstances, often, although not always, where there have been long-standing or recurring conflicts between two or more groups, with mutual perceptions of distrust, fear and threat. In these contexts ambitious leaders, whether in pursuit of an ideology or simply to consolidate their power, may incite or take advantage of mounting tension in order to escalate suspicion and hatred to an incendiary point at which mass violence comes to seem not only permissible but necessary.

Staub (1989, 1999, 2000) developed a theory of the causes of genocide, combining historical, political, cultural, situational and psychological factors. Staub employed the word 'evil', but defined it not as a supernatural force or as a defect of human character, but rather as a specific type of act: the deliberate destruction of human beings. What can lead to people launching such drastic violence against each other? Staub (1989, p. 18) notes that: 'The most terrible human capacity is that of profoundly devaluing others who are merely different.' Precursors of mass violence usually include difficult life conditions on the part of the eventual perpetrators, who perceive the eventual victims as partly or wholly responsible for their predicament, and as threats not only to their welfare but also to their self-esteem. Manipulative leaders can exploit this to intensify the devaluation of the perceived outgroup. Under further pressures, and bolstered by propaganda and often by what nowadays would be called 'fake news', tensions continue to rise and there is an 'inculcation of fear' (Dutton, Boyanowsky and Bond, 2005), with the outgroup progressively presented as a threat to the very existence of the perpetrators. Some flashpoint event may be used as a pretext for calls to take action against the outgroup. Staub describes a 'continuum of destruction' that can then ensue, with genocide as its ultimate form. Other contributing conditions include a populace who have lived in conditions of acceptance of authority, and the rise of antisocial persons to positions of power within the society.

Contemplating the horror that genocidal events entail, it remains difficult to grasp how they can have occurred, and to accept possibly the most horrifying aspects of them:

that those who carry them out are often 'ordinary people' who would be unlikely to be violent in other circumstances. Waller (2006) reviewed extensive historical material which indicated that many perpetrators of the most astonishing cruelty were not individuals who could be diagnosed as sadists or psychopaths, but simply people who, through a series of psychological processes operating in particular circumstances, came to believe that they had no choice other than to annihilate members of another group – even if, prior to that time, some of them had been neighbours. Drawing together studies on conformity, beliefs, socialisation, group cohesion, ethnocentrism, deindividuation and dehumanisation, Waller developed a model that combined these processes and showed how people can be persuaded into roles in which their thinking can be transformed to a point at which they are prepared to inflict the most horrendous violence.

Chapter summary

- The chapter examined various forms of multiple homicide, recognising that this is an extremely difficult area to investigate as those who perpetrate such crimes often end by killing themselves, or are unable to explain their own actions.
- Such killings have taken several forms, including familicide (family annihilation), massacres and spree killings, school rampages and serial homicide.
- Combining evidence from statements made by perpetrators in advance, from analysis of what is known about individuals' movements, and from a small number of cases in which offenders have discussed their motives, it has been possible to discover patterns of resentment and hostility building up over extended periods prior to the occurrence of mass killings, or associated with fluctuations in rates of crime by serial murderers. Several models of those processes have been forwarded, but for understandable reasons are difficult to test. The available evidence does not, unfortunately, allow the drawing of any clear conclusions with regard to causal relationships.
- Some types of large-scale multiple killings, terrorism and genocide arise from complex combinations of motives. In order to understand these motives, the events need to be placed in a wider historical and political context. Psychological research has helped to elucidate the mental states, beliefs and social-influence processes that make such atrocities possible.

Further reading

As with single-victim homicide, there are many sensationalised accounts of these events, and more sober, evidence-based studies are fewer than for other types of crime, for reasons discussed in the text. The following can, however, be recommended:

- James Alan Fox and Jack Levin (2015), *Extreme Killing: Understanding Serial and Mass Murder*, 3rd edition (Thousand Oaks, CA: Sage Publications). This is an extensively researched book covering numerous issues within this area in a relatively concise volume. Also Ronald M. Holmes and Stephen T. Holmes (2010), *Serial Murder*, 3rd edition (Thousand Oaks, CA: Sage Publications). This focuses mainly on serial killing, but touches on mass killing in less depth.
- On serial homicide, key sources are Eric W. Hickey (2013), *Serial Murderers and Their Victims*, 7th edition (Belmont, CA: Wadsworth Publishing), which includes many brief accounts of the perpetrators; and the books by Richard N. Kocsis (2008), *Serial Murder and the Psychology of Violent Crimes* (Totowa, NJ: Humana Press), and

Catherine Purcell and Bruce A. Arrigo (2006), *The Psychology of Lust Murder: Paraphilia, Sexual Killing and Serial Homicide* (Amsterdam: Academic Press).

» On multiple killings in schools, see Peter Langman (2009), *Why Kids Kill: Inside the Minds of School Shooters* (New York, NY: Palgrave Macmillan); and Katherine S. Newman, Cybelle Fox, David J. Harding, Jal Mehta and Wendy Roth (2004), *Rampage: The Social Roots of School Shootings* (New York, NY: Basic Books). The edited book by Nils Böckler, Thorsten Seeger, Peter Sitzer and Wilhelm Heitmeyer (2013), *School Shootings: International Research, Case Studies and Concepts for Prevention* (New York, NY: Springer) contains chapters by many of the leading experts in the field. These are all thoughtful and in-depth analyses of the factors that appear to give rise to these extremely disturbing events. As its title suggests, the book by Donald G. Dutton (2007), *The Psychology of Genocide, Massacres, and Extreme Violence: Why 'Normal' People Come to Commit Atrocities* (Westport, CT: Praeger Security International), makes links between several types of extreme violence involving multiple homicides.

» For a wide-ranging volume on terrorism, see Gary Martin (2016), *Understanding Terrorism: Challenges, Perspectives, and Issues*, 5th edition (Thousand Oaks, CA: Sage Publications).

» For a relatively brief but broad-ranging historical outline of genocide, Norman M. Naimark (2017), *Genocide: A World History* (New York, NY: Oxford University Press), provides a valuable overview. For more depth on many other dimensions of genocide, see Adam Jones (2017), *Genocide: A Comprehensive Introduction*, 3rd edition (Abingdon: Routledge).

» For examination of the psychological factors in genocide, see the books by Ervin Staub (1989), *The Roots of Evil: The Origins of Genocide and Other Group Violence* (New York, NY: Plenum Press); and James Waller (2002), *Becoming Evil: How Ordinary People Commit Genocide and Mass Killing* (Oxford: Oxford University Press).

» A gruesome but informative comparison of the worst mass killings in history has been compiled by Matthew White (2011), *Atrocitology: Humanity's 100 Deadliest Achievements* (Edinburgh: Canongate).

Sexual Offences and Partner Assault

This chapter describes and discusses forms of aggression and violence that are sexually motivated or that contain a sexual element, or that occur in the context of close personal relationships. The largest part of the chapter focuses on the problem of sexual offending against adults and against children, outlining the different patterns of such offending and the factors associated with it. The second major area covered in the chapter is that of violence within close relationships, focusing particularly on domestic abuse or intimate partner violence. A third, briefer section of the chapter discusses the offences of stalking and harassment. In each of these areas, where possible we consider the relationships between multiple levels of explanation, from individuals to the social and cultural context in which those individuals develop.

Chapter objectives

- To gain an understanding of the psychological and other factors that influence specific forms of violence and associated serious offences. These offences include:
  - sexual offending
  - domestic abuse or intimate partner violence
  - sexual harassment and stalking.

Violent offences can result from a range of motives, which sometimes appear to be of a relatively simple and fairly obvious nature. That applies particularly to offences that are *reactive*, the result of expressive or emotional aggression: a person who is provoked or threatened responds almost automatically. In other situations, motives may be wholly *instrumental*: individuals plan to use violence, or are prepared to use violence, to achieve other ends. In many more cases, however, there is a complex mix of these two patterns.

This chapter will focus on serious crimes that entail some form of aggression towards or disregard for others, and in which the offences committed take a number of particular forms, usually combining reactive and instrumental aggression. In the course of the chapter we will focus on a succession of offence categories, including: rape, sexual assault and related offences against adults and children; domestic or intimate partner violence; and harassment and stalking.

Sexual offences

Sexual offences have been a major focus of practice and of research in forensic psychology. Forensic psychologists are extensively involved in the assessment and treatment of individuals who have committed crimes of this type, and have devised a range of methods for working with such individuals. The shape of current responses to many aspects of this type of offending, including the approaches to managing those who have committed such offences, has been significantly influenced by models of sexual offending developed within psychology, and by practical applications derived from those models. These include a number of widely used psychological and risk assessment tools, intervention programmes and management procedures. Use of these now forms part of the work done in police investigations, in prisons, in the community, in youth justice and in forensic mental health settings.

The general term 'sexual offence' covers a wide spectrum of crimes, presently defined (in England and Wales) in the Sexual Offences Act 2003, which drew together provisions of a number of earlier statutes dating back over a lengthy period. The 2003 Act clarified a range of issues, abolished some offences, and also created a number of new ones. The offences covered by that Act include rape and other forms of sexual assault; sexual activity with a child, and other sexual offences against children; meeting a child under 16 following sexual grooming; abuses of trust that involve sexual activity; taking indecent photographs of children; abuse of children through prostitution and pornography; exploitation of prostitution; trafficking for sexual purposes; and administering a substance to a person without her or his consent, with the intention of overpowering that person in order to be able to have sex with her or him. The Act also covers several other types of aberrant behaviour, such as indecent exposure, voyeurism, intercourse with an animal, and sexual penetration of a corpse.

Sexual offences generally constitute only a small proportion of recorded crime incidents: for example, in most years they form just 1 per cent of the total number of offences recorded by police in England and Wales. Given their nature, however, they are a regular focus of media attention, and the type of harm involved gives rise to considerable public concern. As with other areas of antisocial behaviour, the level of concern might be because of an overestimation of how often such offences occur. Concern might also reflect a stereotypical picture of who commits such offences: that of a depraved and insatiable predatory male. While such individuals do exist, they are comparatively rare; yet the stigmatising language often used in news media makes them appear something other than human. Sexual offences may be committed by individuals from any background, and a majority occur between people who are known to one another. A report by the Ministry of Justice, the Home Office and the Office for National Statistics (2013) divides sexual offences into two major categories: the 'most serious', which includes rape, attempted rape and sexual assault; and 'other sexual offences', which includes sexual activity with minors (excluding rape and sexual assaults), exposure, voyeurism and other offences. In the 'most serious' offences, averaged across a three-year period, over 90 per cent of victims knew the perpetrator. In 56 per cent of cases the perpetrator was a current or former partner; in 31 per cent an acquaintance; and a stranger in just 10 per cent. For the lesser offences, by contrast, the offender was a stranger in 52 per cent of cases.

There is a tendency for *all* sexual offending to be considered serious in comparison with other kinds of crime. That might be because it 'corrupts what in other contexts should be the most intimate and tender of human encounters' (Miller, 2014c, p. 68). Therefore, more or less any form of sexual offending gives rise to a sense of revulsion. By crossing a line into this kind of offence, those who break such basic rules of conduct are often seen as total outsiders. In reality, however, there is a wide *range* of seriousness within the varied mix of offences listed earlier. We saw in Chapter 6 that there have been several attempts to gauge seriousness of crimes in general; there have also been attempts to measure the seriousness of sexual offending. Two examples are given in the 'Focus on ...' box on page 171.

The majority of perpetrators of sexual offences are male, and the majority of victims are female. Nevertheless, the reverse can and does occur (Peterson, Voller, Polusny and Murdoch, 2011), as do same-sex victim–offender combinations: homosexual assaults are committed by both males and females. The detection and therefore the study of serious sexual crimes are bedevilled by a major problem of under-reporting. Across three 'sweeps' of the Crime Survey for England and Wales between 2007 and 2012, only 15 per cent of female victims of a serious sexual offence informed the police; 57 per cent told someone other than the police, and 28 per cent told no one (Ministry of Justice, Home Office and Office for National Statistics, 2013). In some countries, reporting sexual victimisation can carry a heavy price for the victim, who may be assumed to have provoked it. Thus the 'true' rate of sexual offending, in the sense of the number of times one person's action towards another could be formally defined as unlawful if it came to light, is more difficult to estimate than for many other types of crime.

FOCUS ON ...

Measuring the seriousness of sexual offending

Aylwin *et al.* (2000), focusing on sexual assaults committed by adolescents, developed a set of *Offence Severity Codes* denoting six levels of gradually increasing seriousness. The levels describe features of behaviour in the offence and are not an attempt to assess the extent of impact on the victim.

Aylwin and his colleagues used these codes to assess the offence patterns of a group of 434 adult and 121 young offenders convicted of sexual offences. In their findings, 10 per cent of the former and 7 per cent of the latter had committed crimes of the most 'severe invasiveness'. Unexpectedly, a significantly larger number of younger offenders than of adult offenders committed offences at severity level 5.

COPINE and SAP scales

The *Combating Paedophile Information Networks in Europe* (COPINE) scale was developed for the specific purpose of classifying illicit sexual images of children disseminated via the internet (Taylor, Holland and Quayle, 2001). There are ten levels. The lowest score classifies images that are non-erotic and non-sexualised, such as pictures of children in their underwear that might have been used in advertising. Median scores refer to photographs of children who have been made to pose sexually. The highest items refer to depictions of actual assaults or sadistic or bestial acts.

The Sentencing Advisory Panel (SAP) scale contains five categories, roughly paralleling those in the COPINE scale, but making fewer differentiations in the middle range (Beech *et al.*, 2008).

FBI Depravity Standard

Focusing specifically on a range of 'the worst of crimes' in the FBI's *Crime Classification Manual*, Welner (2013) developed a scale for assessing the amount of depravity involved in a crime. This was designed for classifying crimes that contained elements considered 'heinous, atrocious and cruel'. It extrapolated from the established concept of aggravating factors, with the objective of constructing a *Depravity Standard* that can be used in sentencing perpetrators.

The scale contains 25 items, each referring to an action or an intent on the part of the offender that would worsen or prolong a victim's suffering, would cause permanent damage or disfigurement, or would be inflicted on a victim who was already helpless. Some of the forms of depravity identified were associated with the presence of one or more forms of mental disorder.

9

Severity level	Offence behaviour
1	Victim fondled (clothed); victim fondled offender (clothed); victim voyeured without knowledge; obscene phone calls.
2	Victim fondled (clothes off)- includes digital penetration, masturbation; victim fondled offender (clothes off)- includes digital penetration, masturbation; victim incited to fondle other victim(s) (clothes off); victim exposed to (exhibitionism); frotteurism.
3	Victim performed oral sex upon; victim made to perform oral sex on offender; victim incited to perform oral sex on other victims; simulated intercourse.
4	Vaginal intercourse performed on victim or actively attempted.
5	Victim sodomised or actively attempted; victim gang raped.
6	Offense of particular brutality. Offense of severity levels 2 to 5 with added dimension of severe degradation/humiliation; weapon used in the course of assault; use of forced confinement; force employed was much more than required for victim compliance.

Source: reprinted from International Journal of Law and Psychiatry, 23(2), Aylwin, A. S., Clelland, S. R., Kirkby, L., Reddon, J. R., Studer, L. H. & Johnston, J., Sexual Offense Severity and Victim Gender Preference: A Comparison of Adolescent and Adult Sex Offenders, p. 117. Copyright © 2000, with permission from Elsevier. DOI: https://doi.org/10.1016/S0160-2527(99)00038-2

For an estimate of the quantity of sexual aggression that goes unreported, a review article by Krahé, Tomaszewska, Kuyper and Vanwesenbeeck (2014) is informative. This article collates the findings from 113 studies conducted as part of the Youth Sexual Aggression and Victimization (Y-SAV) project, in which 27 countries of the European Union participated. Data were obtained from surveys of males and females, focused both on victimisation and on perpetration, within the age range 12–25. Interpretation is hampered by some differences of definition: in some countries data were restricted to the use of physical force, while in others 'sexual aggression' was defined more widely to include behaviours such as harassment. Even so, the range of figures gives a clear indication that officially recorded rates of sexual offences are likely to be considerable underestimations of the true rates. The *lifetime prevalence rates* (see Chapter 2) of female sexual victimisation (excluding sexual abuse before age 12) varied from 9 per cent to 83 per cent, while the corresponding range for males was from 2 per cent to 66 per cent. The lifetime prevalence rates of engaging in sexual aggression ranged from 0 per cent to 80 per cent for males and from 0.8 per cent to 40 per cent for females.

Some of the stages through which a probably large number of actual offences is attenuated into a far lower number of reported crimes, and a still lower number of convictions, are illustrated in Figure 9.1. Taking the mid-point of the offence estimates on the left – and assuming that these figures are close to correct – that gives a rate of conviction for sexual offences in general of 1 in 84, and for rape of 1 in 72. Similar patterns of attrition between the numbers of reported rapes and the numbers of those convicted can be found in several European countries (Turquet *et al.*, 2011). Thus most people who offend sexually are not brought to justice. This may also mean that those who are, and the still smaller fraction of those who then participate in psychological research, may not be representative of the far larger number who commit such acts.

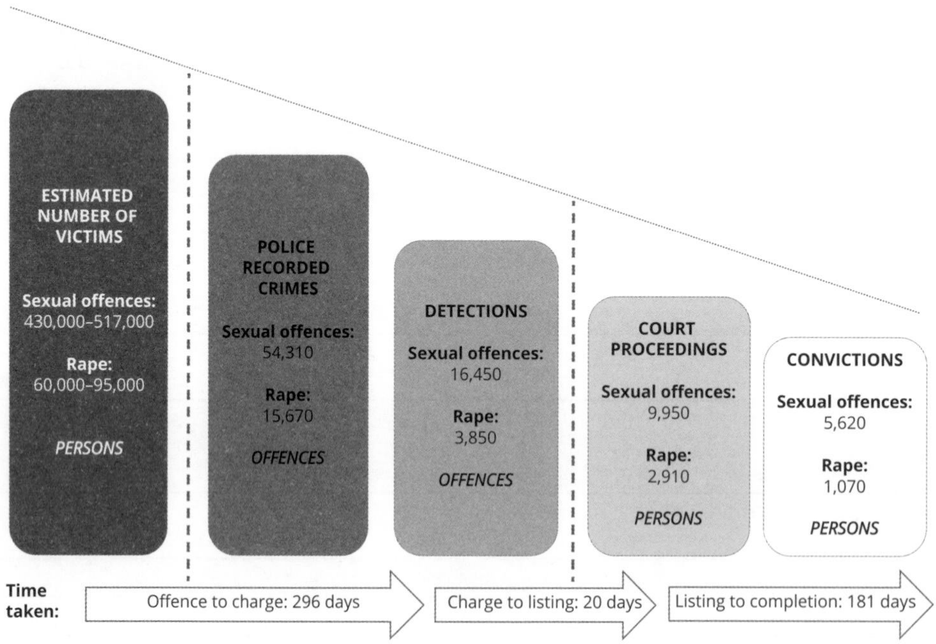
ESTIMATED NUMBER OF VICTIMS
Sexual offences: 430,000–517,000
Rape: 60,000–95,000
PERSONS
POLICE RECORDED CRIMES
Sexual offences: 54,310
Rape: 15,670
OFFENCES
DETECTIONS
Sexual offences: 16,450
Rape: 3,850
OFFENCES
COURT PROCEEDINGS
Sexual offences: 9,950
Rape: 2,910
PERSONS
CONVICTIONS
Sexual offences: 5,620
Rape: 1,070
PERSONS
Time taken:
Offence to charge: 296 days
Charge to listing: 20 days
Listing to completion: 181 days

Figure 9.1

Flow of sexual offence cases through the criminal justice system in England and Wales, showing attrition at each stage. The figures for persons, offences and time intervals are averages over a three-year period (2009/10, 2010/11 and 2011/12). Note that the figure is not to scale.

Source: adapted from Ministry of Justice, Home Office & Office for National Statistics (2013). © Crown copyright, licensed under the Open Government Licence v3.0: http://www.nationalarchives.gov.uk/doc/open-government-licence/version/3

Between 2000 and 2016 the number of offenders in England and Wales imprisoned for sexual offences rose steadily. By March 2016 the total stood at 13,114 male and 120 female prisoners (Allen and Dempsey, 2016). As a proportion of the prison population, this was a rise from 9 per cent to 15 per cent. Over most of that period, the numbers given Community Orders rather than custodial sentences grew even faster, from under 200 in 2005 to almost 2,000 in 2011. Amongst those sentenced for sexual offences in 2011, 83.7 per cent had no previous cautions or convictions for this type of offence (for rape, the figure was higher, at 86.4 per cent), while 3.4 per cent had previously been found guilty of five or more such crimes.

As illustrated by the coverage of the Sexual Offences Act 2003 (described earlier), sexual offending takes a wide variety of forms. Many influences are at work in its occurrence. In what follows, offences are grouped into two broad categories, as there are separate strands of research on each: sexual offences against adults and sexual offences against children. Sexual offences are also often divided into 'contact' and 'non-contact' categories. The former refers to all offences that involve direct physical activity against a victim (rape, indecent assault, incest, or frotteurism). The latter includes indecent exposure and exhibitionism, voyeurism, making obscene phone calls (telephone scatologia), and internet-based offending.

Sexual offences against adults

Apart from sexual homicide – which is not itself a legal classification, as types of homicide and motives for it are not usually codified in statutes – the most serious kinds of sexual offence are those of rape and other kinds of penetration. In some jurisdictions, 'rape' is defined generally as sexual intercourse without consent. Under the Sexual Offences Act 2003 of England and Wales, a man or boy (*A*) commits an offence of rape if he intentionally penetrates the vagina, anus or mouth of another person (*B*) with his penis, where that person has not consented to the penetration, and where *A* does not reasonably believe that *B* has consented. 'Assault by penetration' is a separate offence, and applies where the penetration is of a sexual nature and is done with a part of the body or anything else. The offence of 'sexual assault' makes the same provisions as for rape or penetration (intention, absence of consent) with reference to touching another person sexually. Rape and penetration can lead to life imprisonment; assault to a sentence of up to ten years.

There are large variations between countries in recorded rates of rape. The United Nations Office on Drugs and Crime (UNODC, 2013) collated statistics on the rate of rape from 130 countries. According to these data, the five countries with the highest rates per 100,000 population in 2012 were: Sweden (66.5), Jamaica (34.1), Guyana (33.8), Bolivia (33.0) and Panama (31.2). Those with the lowest rates were Azerbaijan, Bahrain, Palestine and Syria (all 0.2 per 100,000), Armenia and Montenegro (both 0.5) and Indonesia (0.7). The corresponding figure for the United States was 26.6. Notwithstanding the figure mentioned earlier, which shows that sexual offences constitute only a small fraction of all crimes, the cumulative proportion of the population who are victims of rape can be remarkably high. Survey data from the 2011 National Intimate Partner and Sexual Violence Survey in the United States showed that an estimated 19.3 per cent of women and 1.7 per cent of men have been raped during their lifetimes (Breiding *et al.*, 2014). The UNODC does not provide separate data for the three United Kingdom jurisdictions but, using a different metric, for serious sexual offences in England and Wales the average 12-month prevalence rate in the years 2009–2012 was 2.5 per cent of females and 0.4 per cent of males (Ministry of Justice, Home Office and Office for National Statistics, 2013).

Given the reasons for not reporting sexual crimes, however, it is unclear how much these data can tell us about the underlying patterns of such offences in different places. There are many influences on reported crime rates, and since we cannot be confident that the figures are genuinely comparable, their relationship to actual crime events is highly questionable. They do point towards large differences between societies, and other information suggests that such differences are meaningful and reflect 'real' variations. But the high rate for Sweden, for example, is partly a function of recording practices, in which each crime incident is counted separately, a procedure known as 'expansive' offence counts (von Hofer, 2000). In some other European countries, one offender raping the same victim several times would be recorded as one offence (Aebi *et al.*, 2014). Sweden's high rate is also believed to be a consequence of an acknowledged greater level of gender equality, which has led to lower fear about reporting. Using the *Gender Inequality Index* – a United Nations measure of the social position of women as an indicator of human development – Sweden emerges as one of the most highly ranked countries. Thus the underlying rate of rape in Sweden may not really be higher than that of other countries, as the UNODC figures imply; on the contrary, Sweden might in fact be a safer country than many others that have apparently lower rates of rape.

The figures quoted above are from official (police) records or from victim reports. Some research has also been done using reports of (male) perpetrators. The *UN Multi-country Cross-sectional Study on Men and Violence* surveyed 10,178 men from nine samples across six Asian countries – Bangladesh, China, Cambodia, Indonesia, Papua New Guinea and Sri Lanka – mainly to investigate rates of non-partner rape (Jewkes *et al.*, 2013). Again there was wide variation in reported rates, with the highest at 26.6 per cent in Papua New Guinea. Rates of intimate partner rape were higher than for non-partner rape in all countries. Almost 50 per cent of the men who reported having raped someone had first done so while a teenager, and 16 per cent said they had raped four or more women. These data indicate the likely large scale of the difference between recorded and unreported sexual crimes.

Patterns of rape

Rape occurs in several sets of circumstances and different factors may be operating within each. What Miller (2014c) calls 'forcible rape' is the closest to a broad definition of illegal coercive penetrative assault. This is what most people understand as 'rape', and most of what we know about rape is based on information about this form. However, in some countries there is also a category of offence called 'statutory rape', which involves penetrative sexual contact between an individual over the age of legal consent and a victim legally defined as not capable of consenting to sexual activity. This could be a child below the age of legal consent, or a person with intellectual disabilities. 'Date rape' and 'marital rape' (or 'spousal rape') occur in the context of the named relationships. The latter was not made illegal in England and Wales until the advent of the Criminal Justice and Public Order Act 1994. Until that moment, therefore, there was a presumption in law that husbands did not require consent for sexual intercourse with their wives. In the USA, the process of criminalising marital rape across all states extended over an 18-year period, from 1976 (Nebraska) to 1993 (North Carolina and Oklahoma). Even following those legal changes, marital rape was not consistently dealt with as seriously as rape outside marriage (Bennice and Resick, 2003). According to the United Nations, as of 2011 there were still no laws explicitly criminalising marital rape in 127 countries (Turquet *et al.*, 2011).

'Multiple rape' occurs when a victim is raped by more than one aggressor; in most cases where this occurs there are two or three perpetrators – incidents involving larger numbers are far less common (Chambers, Horvath and Kelly, 2010). In 30 (9 per cent) of 348 rape cases studied by Groth and Birnbaum (1979) there was more than one assailant. Most (24 cases) involved two co-offenders, but five cases involved three attackers, and one case involved four. Hazelwood (2009) reserved the term 'gang rape' for offences involving three or more perpetrators. Porter and Alison (2006) retrieved information from law reports and other sources on a series of 223 group rapes from 11 countries (the majority from the USA and UK). These involved a total of 739 offenders, and 22 per cent resulted in the death of the victim; almost of the latter were in the USA. A small number of cases also involved multiple (2 or 3) victims.

Rape in warfare is a widely documented mass crime, sometimes resulting in enormous numbers of victims (Rittner and Roth, 2012). There is evidence of such offences going back several thousand years (Vikman, 2005a, 2005b). While rape in warfare has often been thought to result from conquering armies of sexually deprived males rampaging out of control, in modern times it has been described as a weapon of war, deliberately used to spread terror in a population, and even as a form of genocide. In the conflict in Bosnia-Herzegovina in the 1990s, for example, there is evidence that, amongst many other atrocities, Bosnian women were detained in 'rape camps' and forced to give birth to a child who was then considered Serbian (Boose, 2002).

Given the many sensitive and controversial aspects surrounding how it is regarded and dealt with, debates concerning rape can become highly polarised. In some societies female victims are often seen as having *caused* the offence, and as having disgraced their families. In such cases the victims may be publicly shamed and vilified, sometimes even being excluded from their communities (Parrot and Cummings, 2006). We might expect that this would occur only in societies in which the legal status of women is compromised (Turquet *et al.*, 2011), but evidence suggests that it can also happen in societies in which, at least superficially, males and females are recognised as equals (van der Bruggen and Grubb, 2014). Stereotypical beliefs and what are called 'rape myths', discussed later in this chapter, can even influence the deliberations of juries (Dinos, Burrowes, Hammond and Cunliffe, 2015).

Rape typologies

The legal definition of the offence of rape is fairly precise in defining the *actus reus* that constitutes the crime. However, the patterns in which rape occurs and the motivations underlying it show considerable variation. Though obviously a sexual crime, rape can be committed for non-sexual motives, and these can also arise in different combinations. A major, often disputed issue in relation to rape is the relative balance of sexual and other motives in driving the offence. Assessing which factors are operating on a case-by-case basis can be a pivotal element in providing appropriate intervention to reduce the likelihood of the offence being repeated. Given that rape involves enforced sexual penetration, it might seem to follow that it has its roots in sexual deviation, and understandably, sexual deviation is often thought to be the central if not the sole factor in its aetiology. Lohr, Adams and Davis (1997) examined the possibility that rape may be a type of paraphilia. This refers to the experience of being sexually aroused by, and obtaining gratification from, atypical objects or situations. Note that paraphilia in itself is not necessarily either pathological or criminal. However, in some cases it may cause distress to the individual or to others and may be classed as a mental disorder (see Chapter 11), and in some cases may also result in causing harm to others. Lohr *et al.* considered that a propensity to rape may be similar to this, resulting from the *classical conditioning* of rape as a sexual preference. In a study using *penile plethysmography* (see Chapter 18), Lohr *et al.* found that some men became more aroused to scenes involving sexual coercion, and did not inhibit their arousal. Classical conditioning is thought to be a key mechanism in developing a pattern of deviant arousal in individuals, and other research on rape has shown that it plays a part in some offence patterns (Barbaree, Marshall and Lanthier, 1979, Baxter, Barbaree and Marshall, 1986).

9

However, research carried out in the 1970s led to recognition that non-sexual factors often played a major role in precipitating behaviour that is then channelled into sexual aggression. The discovery that rape can result from a range and indeed a mixture of motives has led to the development of several typologies of rape motivation (Robertiello and Terry, 2007). Based on an initial study of 133 rapists and 92 victims, and a fuller set of interviews with 500 rape perpetrators, Groth and his colleagues (Groth, Burgess and Holstrom, 1977; Groth and Birnbaum, 1979) concluded that rape was a result of three types of motive, working in varying combinations: power, anger and sexuality. Sexuality almost always plays a part, but the relative balance between that and the other factors varies markedly. On this basis Groth and Birnbaum delineated three main types of rapists according to the motives that predominate in each:

» *Power-driven rape* 'Power-driven rape' is divided into two types. In 'power-assertive rape', the offender's intention is to secure enough power over the victim to be able to compel her or him to have sex, or to impose on the victim whatever he desires: the offender's objective is to attain that feeling of power. The level of force used will be limited to what is necessary to achieve this. As part of the rape the offender also wants to believe that the victim too was aroused and excited by the act, as this would validate his sense of masculinity. In 'power-reassurance rape', the act serves a compensatory function for other feelings of inadequacy in the individual's life. In 'anger-excitation' rape on the other hand, there is a fusion of aggression and sexuality, and perpetrators of this kind of offence obtain direct gratification from the victim's suffering; aggression is itself 'eroticised'.

- *Anger-driven rape* In some other rapes, 'it is very apparent that sexuality becomes a means of expressing and discharging pent-up feelings of anger and rage' (Groth and Birnbaum, 1979, p. 13). In such 'anger-driven rapes', the focus of the offender's fury might be the victim alone, but often she or he is a substitute for, or symbol of, someone else. In 'anger-retaliatory rape', the perpetrator has a strong need to take revenge against a specific individual or in some cases against women in general, as a result of feeling that they are responsible for difficulties in his life. Victims are chosen at random and assaults may last for a long period.
- *Sadistic rape* Although similar in some ways to 'anger-excitation' rapes, assaults of this type are likely to be planned and premeditated, not spontaneous or opportunistic. Here, sexual satisfaction is gained primarily through inflicting severe suffering and degradation on the victim. These offenders thus cause more physical harm than other types of rapist, and offences are more likely to result in homicide.

Groth and Birnbaum (1979) estimated that the proportions of the three principal types of rape among the offenders they assessed was: power rape, 55 per cent; anger rape, 40 per cent; and sadistic rape, 5 per cent. Given the biases that can arise from studying incarcerated samples, however, the authors suggest that most rapes probably belong in the 'power' category. Robertiello and Terry (2007) suggest that most marital and acquaintance rapes conform to that pattern.

This taxonomy was adapted by the FBI and applied to rape and sexual assault cases in its *Crime Classification Manual* (Douglas, Burgess, Burgess and Ressler, 2013; see also Burgess and Hazelwood, 2009). It was further developed to cover 14 main types of rape, encompassing no fewer than 45 subtypes. The taxonomy was also extended to other patterns, such as 'criminal enterprise rape' (where the assault is committed for material gain), 'felony rape' (where it is committed in the course of another serious crime), and 'abduction rape' in which a victim is forcibly taken from one place to another, kept there for a lengthy period (sometimes months or even years), and repeatedly raped. Several of these were subdivided according to the age range of the victims. There are other subgroups, too, consisting of 'opportunistic' and 'gang' rapists. Each has a different primary motive and distinct 'style of attack'.

This partition of motives is based on analyses of interviews, or of file-based accounts, and has been criticised on the grounds that there is a lack of independent validation of the categories so derived. Another classification system was developed at the Massachusetts Treatment Center (MTC), a large secure facility specialising in work with sex offenders (Knight and Prentky, 1990). This relied more on the use of psychometric assessments, and has undergone a number of revisions, leading to a typology (MTC:R3) which delineates five main types of rapist, as shown in Figure 9.2.

Barbaree *et al.* (1994) analysed data on a series of 60 referrals to the Warkworth Sexual Behaviour Clinic in Ontario and found some support for the MTC model. It worked for the majority of the sample, but the authors left 20 potential participants out of their study because they did not fit any of the MTC categories. In an Australian study, McCabe and Wauchope (2005) analysed two sets of files (130 police files and 50 court transcripts) in terms of a series of 42 variables, and also found general support for the MTC typology. However, they suggested that the types could be further subdivided, and even then there were some 'outliers'.

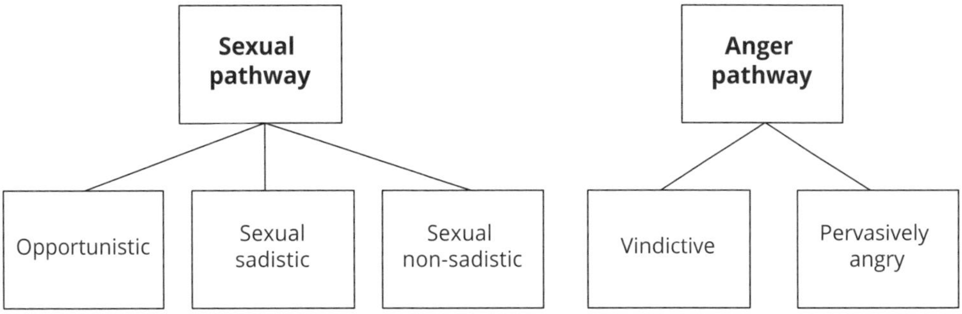
Sexual pathway
Anger pathway
Opportunistic
Sexual sadistic
Sexual non-sadistic
Vindictive
Pervasively angry

Figure 9.2
Typology of rape motives used as a basis for identifying subgroups of rapists, drawing on the Massachusetts Treatment Center (MTC) model.

Source: Figure 14.1 The offender types in the MTC: R3 as described by Knight and Prentky (1990). From Reid, S., Wilson, N. J. & Boer, D. P. (2011). Risk, Needs, and Responsivity Principles in Action: Tailoring Rapist's Treatment to Rapist Typologies. In D. P. Boer, R. Eher, L. A. Craig, M. H. Miner & F. Pfäfflin (eds.), International Perspectives on the Assessment and Treatment of Sexual Offenders: Theory, Practice, and Research. pp. 287–297. Chichester: Wiley-Blackwell. Copyright © 2011 John Wiley & Sons Ltd.

9

While the typological approach captures some important distinctions between different patterns of rape motives and behaviour, no single model has emerged as entirely satisfactory and (so far) there have always been cases that do not fit the proposed frameworks. Nevertheless, Reid, Wilson and Boer (2011) considered it important to recognise the variation in rape motivations as a key step in deciding on the most appropriate treatment approaches. Keep in mind, however, that as the samples on which these typologies are based mostly consist of male perpetrators of rape against adult female victims – which is by far the commonest pattern – the research findings cannot be extrapolated to other offender–victim combinations.

It is a mistake, however, to associate rape exclusively with some form of individual psychopathology. The view that rape is committed by a small minority of highly deviant males is at odds with what is known about the patterning of this offence. The UK data cited earlier, and similar statistics from many other countries, indicate that the majority of rapes are committed by people known to the victim. This suggests that factors other than sexually deviant interests are at work in precipitating sexual violence, and numerous findings accord with that suggestion. Several risk factors have been found to be associated with rape and other serious sexual assaults, and we will consider them in a later section of this chapter.

Sexual offences against children

Although maltreatment of children – whether consisting of physical, emotional, or sexual abuse, or of neglect – has probably occurred throughout history, it was largely hidden or ignored until the late 19th century. According to a report by the National Society for the Prevention of Cruelty to Children (NSPCC; Radford *et al.*, 2011), there have been three waves of 'discovery' of the problem of child maltreatment since then. The specific offence of child sexual abuse was rarely reported, indeed scarcely acknowledged until only a few decades ago. The scale of the problem began to be revealed following the first methodical investigations published in the 1980s (Olafson, Corwin and Summit, 1993). Over the last few decades, the rate of reporting of many kinds of sexual offences has risen steadily. In recent years, a number of retrospective investigations have been launched in several countries on the basis of emerging evidence of extensive abuse of children by members of religious orders and clergy. In response to other revelations, police forces in the United Kingdom have launched major operations such as the Yewtree Inquiry, begun in 2012 following a series of allegations about the media celebrity Jimmy Savile. Thus what was once a concealed and disowned activity has been subjected more recently to more careful scrutiny. It seems likely that even now the full extent of child sexual abuse is not fully understood.

A preliminary question that arises in this area is that of what society formally defines as the dividing line between childhood and adulthood (the age of *majority*), and the related issue of when a developing individual is believed to be capable of understanding and agreeing to sexual activity (the age of *consent*). The first does not vary greatly between countries. By contrast, as we will see in Chapter 16, the age of *criminal responsibility* – the age at which a developing individual is considered capable of deciding whether or not to commit what society regards as a crime – varies widely across the world. Similarly, as the 'Focus on ...' box illustrates, the age of consent also varies markedly.

FOCUS ON ...

The age of consent

Like the age of criminal responsibility, the age of consent also varies from one country to another (Waites, 2005). For example, it is:

- 13 in Spain and Japan
- 14 in Austria, Bangladesh, China, Germany, Hungary, Italy, Serbia and Portugal
- 15 in Croatia, Denmark, France, Poland, Romania and Sweden
- 16 in most states of Australia, in Belgium, Canada, Netherlands, New Zealand, Norway, Malaysia, Russia, the United Kingdom, and many other countries
- 16–18 in the different states of the USA
- 17 in South Australia, Tasmania and Ireland
- 18 in India and Turkey
- 21 in Bahrain.

There is no age of consent in Saudi Arabia: all sex outside marriage is illegal, but there is no minimum age set for marriage. Some countries have complex rules rather than a simple age limit, for example designating different ages at which different sexual activities may be permissible, or taking into account the age difference or nature of the relationship between those involved.

The age of consent has been adjusted both upwards and downwards in different countries over time. In the jurisdictions of United Kingdom, it has changed several times. From the 13th century to the 19th century in England it was set at 12, but in England, Wales and Ireland the Offences Against the Person Act 1875 increased it to 13. Subsequently, under the Criminal Law Amendment Act 1885, it was increased to its present level of 16 (Waites, 2005).

The effects of sexual abuse during childhood, especially if it occurs on repeated occasions, can be lifelong, and may be manifested in a wide range of adjustment and emotional problems. Maniglio (2009) amalgamated findings from a series of 14 systematic reviews published between 1995 and 2008, encompassing results from 587 studies involving over 270,000 participants. There was evidence of raised rates of a wide variety of difficulties amongst victims of sexual abuse. They ranged from behavioural and sexual problems to substance misuse and other psychological and emotional disturbances. The latter included depression, anxiety, post-traumatic stress symptoms, self-harm and risk of suicide, amongst others. Having been a victim of child sexual abuse (CSA) was also associated with later risk of sexual **revictimisation** in adulthood. Thus child sexual abuse has been linked to an extensive sequelae of behavioural and emotional problems of varying levels of seriousness.

Finkelhor and Browne (1985) proposed possible 'traumagenic dynamics' – mechanisms that can explain the injurious impact of CSA. They identified four such processes: inappropriate sexualisation; betrayal of trust; the experience of disempowerment; and stigmatisation. The ensuing problems are markedly worse when individuals have been maltreated in multiple ways, a pattern Finkelhor, Ormrod and Turner (2007, 2009) called 'poly-victimisation'. In a random community survey of 1,467 children aged 2–17 (the Developmental Victimization Survey), information was requested on 33 different types of victim experiences. Those aged over 10 responded for themselves; for younger ones, a caregiver gave replies. For 18 per cent of the sample who had been victimised in four or more different ways, that cumulative experience was the strongest predictor of their level of trauma symptoms.

However, in many of the reviews collated by Maniglio (2009) the quality of studies was very variable and often poor. Furthermore, there was evidence to suggest that other factors – including family dysfunction, conflict, neglect and other types of child abuse (physical and emotional) – were also often associated with a history of sexual abuse, and may have played a larger part in causing later problems than the sexual abuse in and of itself. The latter conclusion, and the suggestion that the impact of sexual abuse *per se* on later development of problems may sometimes have been overestimated, has led to some bitter controversies, as briefly discussed in the 'Where do you stand?' box.

WHERE DO YOU STAND?

Child sexual abuse controversies

There is no doubt that being a victim of sexual abuse in childhood can cause major psychological harm to individuals, but the impact may be more variable than is commonly thought. Research into this, and the conclusions drawn from that research, has been highly controversial in a number of respects. One is the role of sexual abuse as compared to other factors in the causation of later adjustment problems. Another is the exceedingly divisive and rancorous issue of whether it is possible for children to forget or to repress their memories of having been sexually victimised, and then to recall them later in life.

Following the publication of a review by Rind, Tromovitch and Bauserman (1998), the first of these debates became extremely heated in the United States, to the extent that their article was not only widely criticised but, after a campaign of lobbying, was ultimately condemned by the US Senate. On the basis of their review, Rind *et al.* had concluded that some victims of child sexual abuse (CSA) were not as badly damaged by it as is sometimes assumed, and showed only mild adjustment problems in adult life; and that in many cases their later problems were caused by dysfunctional family environments rather than by CSA itself. There was a considerable media and political outcry against these conclusions and the authors' professional standing was called into question. However, an examination of the criticisms by the American Association for the Advancement of Science indicated that the contents of the paper had been misrepresented by many of its critics, and that there was no reason to doubt the methodology the authors had employed (Rind, Tromovitch and Bauserman, 2000).

This specific dispute arose in the midst of an even more acrimonious debate concerning what for a time were called 'recovered memories' of childhood abuse. During the 1970s and 1980s, there were increasing numbers of cases in the USA in which adult clients in therapy claimed that they had been sexually abused in childhood, some by parents or other relatives, and some by staff of children's homes where they had been resident. Such abuse undoubtedly occurs, and it is true that much of it remains concealed, but in these cases it was claimed that the children had forgotten or repressed their memories of the abuse – in effect, they had amnesia for the events, and had only recovered those memories through the process of psychotherapy. Many thousands of relatives and care staff were sued or prosecuted on the basis of these claims, and some were convicted and sentenced to lengthy terms of imprisonment. Many children made allegations against their parents or others that were later shown to be unfounded.

Based on studies of memory functioning, of children's testimony and on evidence concerning the processes of psychological therapy, Loftus (1993, 1997), Brandon, Boakes, Glaser and Green (1998) and other researchers suggested that there was no scientific basis for the claim that such 'memories' could be 'recovered'. What were described by some therapists as recollections of traumatic events (sexual abuse during childhood) that had initially been hidden from conscious awareness were instead 'false memories' that had been generated or implanted through interactions between therapy client 'victims' and their therapists.

Where do you stand on these issues?

1 Do you consider that child sexual abuse must always be extremely harmful, independently of other possible causes of emotional disturbance?

2 Do you find it credible that memories of childhood abuse could be influenced by interactions with therapists in adulthood?

Two meta-analyses by Pereda, Guilera, Forns and Gómez-Benito (2009a, 2009b) have brought together the findings of research on the epidemiology of sexual abuse of children. On the basis of 65 studies from 22 countries, Pereda *et al.* concluded that on average almost 1 in 5 women (19.7 per cent) and almost 1 in 13 men (7.9 per cent) had experienced sexual abuse before reaching the age of 18. Not surprisingly, there are large variations in these figures, and given the taboos and the levels of secrecy and of shame surrounding these types of offences many of them may be underestimates.

Despite the publicly feared image of the marauding sexual predator, stereotypically classed as an unrestrained paedophile, crimes involving such individuals are in fact statistically infrequent. The intense media attention they receive when they do occur probably plays a large part in exaggerated perceptions of their likelihood (an illustration of the *availability heuristic*: Stalans, 1993). Most sexual abuse of children takes place within families, and most such abuse is carried out by close relatives, including parents, or by other acquaintances of the victim. Table 9.1 illustrates the distribution of perpetrators of child sex abuse in terms of their relationship to victims. This is based on analysis of a large database of almost 1.3 million cases in Australia (Richards, 2011), but similar patterns can be found in many countries and the figures are similar to those found in England and Wales.

Child sexual abuse and Finkelhor's 'preconditions' model

Given the vulnerability of children and the value that all societies profess to place on keeping children safe, the finding that sizeable numbers of adults sexually assault and abuse them may seem difficult to understand. The process through which sexual

Relationship	Proportion of abusers (%)
Male relative other than father or stepfather	30.2
Family friend	16.3
Acquaintance or neighbour	15.6
Known person (not in other categories)	15.3
Father or stepfather	13.5
Stranger	11.1
Female relative other than mother or stepmother	0.9
Mother or stepmother	0.8

Table 9.1 Distribution of relationships of child abusers to child victims in Australia. Sample size: 1,294,000.

Source: based on Australian Bureau of Statistics data. From Australian Bureau of Statistics, 2006, Personal Safety Survey, cat. no. 4906.0, viewed 07 October 2017, http://www.abs.gov.au/AUSSTATS/abs@.nsf/DetailsPage/4906.02005%20(Reissue)?OpenDocument Copyright © Commonwealth of Australia 2006, licensed under https://creativecommons.org/licenses/by/2.5/au

offending against children occurs has been the subject of considerable investigation.

In a highly influential statement of the factors that operate to make it possible, the sociologist David Finkelhor (1984) suggested that certain 'preconditions' have to be met. For an adult to abuse a child sexually, the following four processes had to occur; that is, they are considered necessary:

- *Motivation to abuse a child* The adult needs to have an interest in, or urge towards, sexual activity with a child. This in itself has several components, and Finkelhor and Araji (1986) provided an expanded analysis of them. They suggest that for adults to carry out abusive acts certain features are likely present, though not all will be found in every individual. The principal features are:
  - *Deviant arousal* Individuals experience sexual excitement and attraction to children, which if persistent and exclusive may be symptomatic of *paedophilia* (discussed more fully below and in Chapter 11). This may be due to early learning or conditioning, but its origins remain unclear.
  - *Emotional congruence* Some potential abusers describe a sense of closeness between themselves and children. That is, apart from a feeling of sexual arousal in itself, they also have an emotional need for connection with children or feel an affinity with them.
  - *Blockage* For some individuals, there may have been a failure to form satisfactory sexual partnerships or to achieve emotional intimacy with adults, due to factors such as fragile self-esteem, social anxiety, or a lack of interactional skills for establishing close relationships. (As Ward and Hudson (2001) have pointed out in a critique, this concept and that of emotional congruence overlap somewhat and are difficult to distinguish.)
- *Overcome internal inhibitions* Given the strong feelings of protectiveness most adults have towards children, for any such adult to abuse a child the inhibitions against doing so would have to be weakened. Some individuals may have generally poor impulse controls; more often, though, the state of disinhibition is a temporary one, induced by other influences such as alcohol intake or pornography use. Individuals may turn to such behaviours when they are under some form of emotional strain; and an individual's inability to cope appropriately with such strain may have precursors through events in his or her own earlier history. Individuals may also develop and deploy specific cognitions through which they convince themselves that it is permissible to act on their urges; in some cases, those may be part of a system of *implicit beliefs* about children's sexuality, another point we will discuss later. Such disinhibitory influences appear in most cases of CSA, but are especially marked amongst perpetrators who show a sexual preference for children.
- *Overcome external inhibitions* Given the severe social disapproval of anything that harms children, the individual also has to negate or to circumvent the force of that disapproval. Some ways of doing so may derive from situational and opportunistic factors, such as the absence or weakness of other caregivers who would otherwise protect the child. In other cases, efforts may be made, and sometimes planned in advance, to be with the child when other adults or siblings are not. If the abuse is to be repeated, and if the offender is not to be caught, the offence must not be discovered; therefore efforts are made to ensure concealment, or in other ways to manipulate the environment so that the abuse can continue in secret.
- *Overcome the child's resistance* Finally, children themselves do not want to be abused, so other steps are taken to engage the child's compliance. A child's insecurity, lack of knowledge or understanding, and willingness to trust adults are all factors that the perpetrator may exploit to obtain power over the child and to create conditions in which the abuse can occur. This may be accomplished through manipulation and 'grooming' over an extended period. ('Grooming' refers to a process whereby an offender gradually builds an emotional connection with a child in order to gain her or his trust.) In some cases, however, the child's resistance

may be overcome using direct coercion or threats, which may also be used to preserve secrecy and so avoid discovery.

When certain features are present over time, perpetrators can be classified as having a form of mental disorder, **paedophilia**. This is defined as a type of paraphilia (as described above) entailing a persistent sexual interest in and preference for prepubescent children. A related type of paraphilic pattern, *hebephilia*, is defined as a sexual interest in children who are pubescent but not yet sexually mature. However, less is known regarding this, and it is not separately defined as a mental disorder (Stephens and Seto, 2016).

These disorders have been approached from both medical (Hughes, 2007) and psychological (Seto, 2009) perspectives. It is essential to note that 'paedophilia is not synonymous with sexual offending against children' (Seto, 2009, p. 403). In incest offences, for example, there may be disturbed family dynamics that divert an adult's sexual focus from a partner onto a child. Thus it does not follow that an individual who has sexually abused a child is necessarily a paedophile: on average, only 40–50 per cent of those who carry out such acts meet the clinical criteria for paedophilia (Seto, 2009); Grubin (1998) provided an estimate lower than this, of 25 to 40 per cent. Also, it is important to note that sexual attraction to children is not in itself a crime, and that some individuals experience such urges but do not engage in sexual activity with children. In Chapter 11 we will return to this issue when we discuss its mental health aspects.

Child pornography and internet sexual offending

A large fraction of what are called 'non-contact' sexual offences entail the use of child pornographic materials to obtain sexual gratification. This pattern has emerged and developed in tandem with the expanding availability of indecent images of children, and with the use of the internet as a means of conveying and accessing pornography (Sheldon and Howitt, 2007). Pornography of course existed before the arrival of the internet: according to data collected for the US General Social Survey, across the years 1973–2010, an average of 30.8 per cent of adult males said they had viewed a pornographic film in the previous 12 months (Wright, 2013). But a large volume of pornographic material of many types is now available via the internet, and evidence suggests it is viewed by many people. In an online survey in the USA, 75 per cent of men and 42 per cent of women indicated that they had intentionally viewed or downloaded pornographic material; 21 per cent of men and 17 per cent of women said they had done so while at work (Albright, 2008, 2009).

While the transmission of adult erotic images is not illegal in the UK (provided it is not of an 'extreme' nature), the production and uploading of sexual images of children is. The creation of such images often directly involves sexual abuse of a child and thus constitutes an offence in itself. In England and Wales, viewing or downloading images of this kind is an offence under the Sexual Offences Act 2003. Some individuals arrested for such crimes have been found to hold many thousands of these images on their personal computers. In a study by Webb, Craissati and Keen (2007), a mean of 16,698 images was found, though the distribution was very skewed, with a median of 317 and a maximum of 920,000.

There has been a debate over whether this material should be called 'child pornography', as much of it directly involves non-consenting, abusive, violent and therefore criminal activity. That is, it consists predominantly of actual recordings of children being sexually assaulted. A separate proportion reportedly consists of 'pseudo-pornography' or 'pseudo-pictures' in which images are created in other ways, for example by superimposing an image of a child onto a sexualised picture of an adult (Taylor, Holland and Quayle, 2001).

Beech, Elliott, Birgden and Findlater (2008) examined the different ways in which the internet had been used for purposes linked to child sexual abuse. These include the production and dissemination of abusive images for personal or commercial reasons (or both); the creation or maintenance of online networks of those with paedophilic interests; and movement from non-contact to contact offending, including communicating with children as possible targets of future indecent assaults. Elliott and Beech (2009) proposed a typology of internet offenders with four categories: (a) periodically prurient offenders, who act impulsively or out of curiosity, do not have a specific sexual interest in children, but do have a broad interest in pornography; (b) fantasy-only offenders, who are sexually interested in children but have no history of contact offending; (c) direct victimisation offenders, who engage in both online and contact offending; and (d) commercial exploitation offenders, who are mainly seeking financial profit and are not themselves pursuing sexually deviant interests. It is unclear what proportions of offenders could be said to fit into each of these groups.

Given the solitary and secretive nature of internet offending, and its presumed anonymity, it has been widely speculated that those who engage in it may show some kinds of emotional or 'socio-affective' difficulties, or 'intimacy deficits', leading to depression or loneliness. In addition, some studies found online offenders to be less generally antisocial than those who have actually molested children; while the latter show more indicators of psychopathic traits, and more evidence of substance-abuse problems. Similar findings were obtained by Webb, Craissati and Keen (2007) in samples of offenders on probation in London, and by Magaletta, Faust, Bickart and McLearen (2014) amongst male prisoner samples in the United States.

There have now been several reviews of studies that compare internet-based with contact sex offenders. Babchishin, Hanson and Hermann (2011) and Henshaw, Ogloff and Clough (2015) both covered this field. Offenders who accessed child pornography online were mainly Caucasian, tended to be younger, and were less likely to be married. They were 'higher functioning' with respect to education and employment, and less likely to have criminal histories or substance-abuse problems. Lower proportions of this group had endured physical or sexual abuse in childhood than was the case for offline offenders, but for both groups the proportions were higher than in normative samples. Online offenders showed higher levels of emotional loneliness, under-assertiveness and passivity, and lower self-esteem. They also showed a greater capacity for empathy with their victims, but alongside indices of higher sexual deviance and investment in sexual fantasy. These differences did not emerge consistently from all analyses, but are indicative of the two populations being distinct in some basic ways.

There has been understandable alarm at the prospect that some offenders use internet chatrooms to establish a connection with a child, concealing their own age, and then cultivating the relationship with the aim of making face-to-face contact with the child later for sexual purposes. Following the establishment in 2006 of a specialised police command in the UK, the Child Exploitation and Online Protection Centre (later absorbed into the National Crime Agency), there were a number of prosecutions and convictions for this type of crime, and the agency claimed that it had also disrupted a large number of image-sharing networks. Kloess, Beech and Harkins (2014) reported that of over 2,300 allegations received by the agency in 2010, 64 per cent related to online grooming. They described a model of *cybersexploitation* through which such grooming proceeds, and the strategies used by offenders to secure a child's compliance with their requests.

However, it has also been argued that the nature of these offences has been erroneously described. Wolak, Finkelhor, Mitchell and Ybarra (2008) suggest that in the majority of such cases, the offences are better understood not as stemming from predatory urges but as a form of statutory rape. That is, while the people who commit such offences are seeking a sexual relationship with an adolescent, very few of those interviewed in a series of surveys by Wolak *et al.* (2008) pretended they were teenagers themselves, and most of the eventual victims knew that they had been conversing online with an adult. Internet offenders were rarely paedophiless and rarely violent. In a study of 51 chatroom sex offenders, 90 per cent of whom had been arrested as a result of undercover 'sting' operations, Briggs, Simon and Simonsen (2011) suggested that their behaviour was less often a function of sexual deviance or criminal intent and more often of 'social isolation, dysphoric moods, and increased social isolation due to increasing involvement in the internet community' (p. 87). While this still presents a serious problem, Wolak *et al.* (2008) argued that the pattern

9

is less 'archetypically frightening' than the media-manufactured image of the scheming and deceptive paedophile offender.

They suggested that a different approach to prevention is needed with respect to the kinds of messages given to children and adolescents about the risks of internet use, an approach that involves more emphasis on education, relationship awareness and avoidance strategies.

Escalation

Viewing pornographic images, becoming sexually aroused and masturbating to them can reinforce sexually deviant preoccupations (Quayle, Vaughan and Taylor, 2009). Based on a meta-analysis of 22 studies, there is also evidence of a significant association between use of pornography and measures of verbal and physical sexual aggression (Wright, Tokunaga and Kraus, 2016). An obvious question that follows is whether anyone engaging in such behaviour is then likely to go on to commit contact sexual offences. As we saw earlier, available evidence suggests that only a small proportion are likely to follow such a path, and those are individuals who would probably have done so anyway, either because they experience stronger deviant urges or because they have broader antisocial tendencies. Seto and Eke (2005) studied the offending pathways of child pornography users over time. Of the 201 offenders in their sample, 4 per cent went on to commit a contact offence. Whether or not individuals offended again was most closely associated with whether they had previous convictions (which 56 per cent of this sample did have). Those who committed both non-contact and contact offences had the highest rates of sexual and of any other kind of reoffending. Similarly, in a Swiss study of 231 men charged with consumption of illegal pornographic material, Endrass et al. (2009) found that just 3 per cent committed a subsequent violent or sexual offence over a six-year follow-up.

Houtepen, Sijtsema and Bogaerts (2014) reviewed evidence on the specific question of which factors are associated with the transition from internet to contact sexual offending. They found that such factors fell into three areas. First, the most prominent factor was that which is frequently seen in higher-risk groups, namely a general antisocial tendency manifested in a history of several types of offending. Other features were often present also, including low empathy, poor inhibitory control and cognitive distortions concerning children. Second, individuals more likely to commit child sexual abuse spent more time on the internet and had larger collections of pornographic materials, including more explicitly abusive images. Spending prolonged periods on the internet increased the likelihood of establishing contact with other child pornography users and becoming part of a network sharing images and reinforcing sexually deviant interests. The third set of factors included the individual's offline or everyday lifestyle and potential access to child victims, though these were usually extrafamilial.

A particularly thorough meta-analysis of 30 study samples by Babchishin, Hanson and VanZuylen (2015) is also relevant to this question, as the authors reported an extensive comparison between individuals who offend online only (child pornography offenders, or CPOs), those who engage in contact offending only (sexual offenders against children, or SOCs), and those who had committed both (mixed group). The differences between the first two groups were similar to those found in the reviews by Babchishin *et al.* (2011) and Henshaw *et al.* (2015), discussed earlier. There were significant differences between all of the groups in paired comparisons. The mixed group showed higher levels of sexual interest in children than either of the other two groups, and a level of other antisocial features akin to the SOC group and higher than the CPO group. The authors suggested that the patterning of offences could be explained in terms of Routine Activity Theory (see Chapter 4), as SOCs had greater direct access to children, whereas CPOs had greater access to the internet. The mixed group had access to both. The CPOs had more lifestyle and psychological barriers to offending against children, including higher levels of empathy and lower levels of cognitive distortions.

These results are linked to the broader question of whether there is a general progression in seriousness of sexual offending across various other types. For example, do those who commit non-contact offences such as indecent exposure (exhibitionism) proceed at a later stage to commit contact offences such as indecent assault? Some researchers have sought to address this. McNally and Fremouw (2014) reviewed 12 studies, published between 1983 and 2008, which examined temporal links between exhibitionism and other kinds of sexual offences, over an average follow-up period of over five years. Six of the studies used a correlational design (testing for associations between different types of offence) and six examined recidivism rates (comparing rates for those who had shown different patterns of prior offending). Despite a number of methodological problems, it was concluded that certain trends were identifiable. Approximately 25 per cent of exhibitionistic offenders later committed some further kind of sexual offence. The proportion who went on to commit contact offences ranged from 0.9 to 16.2 per cent; those who had committed a contact sexual offence prior to an incident of indecent exposure had higher rates of escalation to further contact sexual offending. The familiar finding that those who escalated to more serious offending had other features of a general antisocial tendency also emerged in these studies.

Specialisation, versatility and crossover

People who commit sexual offences are often perceived as being a distinct group. Is that impression accurate? This raises a fundamental question: do those who commit such offences also break the law in other ways, or do they mainly or solely commit offences of a sexual nature? A related question is whether *within* sexual offending there are narrower forms of concentration on one type of offence as compared to another. Thus there are two levels at which patterns of offence 'specialisation' have been studied, and numerous research studies have been carried out in efforts to answer these questions.

As with rape, there have been attempts to develop typologies of those who sexually abuse children, and these are linked to the question of whether or not some offenders 'specialise'. Wortley and Smallbone (2014) investigated dimensions along which patterns of offending vary, using a 'criminal careers' approach. This was based on whether or not individuals were first offenders or had prior convictions for sexual offences ('limited' as compared to 'persistent' careers) and on whether or not they also had convictions for non-sexual offences ('specialised' as compared to 'versatile' offending patterns). Amongst a sample of 362 convicted offenders in Queensland, Australia, four groups were then identified: 'limited-versatile', 41 per cent of the sample; 'limited-specialised', 36.4 per cent; 'persistent-versatile', 17.8 per cent; and 'persistent-specialised', 4.8 per cent. Self-report data on aspects of offending were available for 177 of the participants. These suggested that the four subgroups were distinct in several ways, differing significantly on a number of self-reported variables concerned with problematic characteristics. The two largest groups, both 'limited', were on average older at the time of their first conviction, and were more likely to live with the child they abused. Neither of these groups was thought to require specialised sex offender treatment. The third group, 'persistent-versatile', began offending earlier, and had larger numbers of victims. The fourth group, 'persistent-specialised', though the smallest (less than 5 per cent of the sample), had the largest number of sexual victims, more of these being outside the family, and could be described as the highest-risk group. Findings paralleling these were obtained by Harris, Mazerolle and Knight (2009) in a study of 374 men at the Massachusetts Treatment Center. 'Versatile' offenders showed more indicators of a wider antisocial tendency; and rapists bore a greater resemblance to those classified as 'versatile' than to child molesters, with just 11.8 per cent of them having committed rape only. More child molesters than rapists specialised in sexual offences: 42.6 per cent could be classed as 'specialists' in having committed that offence only. 'Specialists' showed higher levels of sexual deviance.

One of the earliest studies of specialisation *within* sexual offending was reported by Abel *et al.* (1988), who conducted in-depth interviews with 561 men diagnosed with one or more forms of paraphilia, seen during the period 1977–1985 in two community-based psychiatric clinics in the USA. The study included a large proportion of men who had committed sexual assaults, and others who had committed offences such as exhibitionism or making obscene telephone calls, or who reported other forms of paraphilic behaviour including voyeurism, frottage, fetishism or bestiality. Participants who had committed assaults were classified according to their victims' gender and age range, and the offenders' relationship to them. Just 10 per cent of the sample had a single paraphilia diagnosis. More than 50 per cent were diagnosed with 2–4 forms of paraphilia, with the remainder having 5–10 forms. While half of the sample had targeted only one age-group (child, adolescent, or adult), 31 per cent had targeted two age-groups, and 11 per cent all three. The majority had selected either male or female victims, but 20 per cent had targeted both; 23 per cent had victims both inside and outside their families.

In later research, efforts have been made to arrive at more precise definitions of the degree to which patterns of offending are 'specialised' or 'versatile'. These terms have been defined in different ways and a variety of proposals have been made about how to measure the key variables. Lussier and Cale (2013, p. 447) define *specialisation* as 'the tendency to limit offending to one particular form of crime'. Thus an individual may be defined as 'specialist' if he or she commits the same type of offence on successive occasions. *Versatility*, also called 'generalist' offending, is defined as 'the number of different crimes committed'.

There are several ways of measuring these patterns:

» *Percentage* The simplest measure is to class someone as 'specialising' when a certain proportion of his or her criminal record consists of one type of offence (e.g. >50 per cent, >75 per cent). This is sometimes called the 'specialisation threshold'. There is no agreed rule regarding the cut-off for this and it therefore remains somewhat arbitrary, but 50 per cent is common.

» *Diversity index* The probability that any two offences drawn randomly from someone's record belong to different offence categories (Miethe, Olson and Mitchell, 2006).

» *Transitional probability* The likelihood of repeating the same type of offence in successive time periods or 'arrest cycles' in a person's criminal history.

» *Forward Specialisation Coefficient* (FSC) A measure computed from the difference between observed and expected frequencies of particular types of offence over time.

The term **crossover** is generally used to refer to a pattern of sexual offending in which individuals commit offences against victims in two or more of the principal categories defined according to gender, age-group and the nature of the relationship (intrafamilial or extrafamilial).

To investigate these patterns, several studies have analysed criminal histories and repeat convictions of sex offender samples. Soothill, Francis, Sanderson and Ackerley (2000) studied a sample of 6,097 men who had been convicted of four different kinds of offences in England and Wales. They examined offence patterns of this group over a 32-year period – from 1963, when the Offenders Index was begun, to 1994. The four offences were: indecent assault against a female; indecent assault against a male; unlawful sexual intercourse with a girl aged under 16; and indecency between males. (Although homosexuality was decriminalised in England and Wales in 1967, the last category of offence remained on statute until the Sexual Offences Act 2003.) The principal finding was 'remarkably clear-cut' evidence of specialisation, with members of all groups being most likely, when reconvicted of another sex offence, to be reconvicted of the same kind of offence as before. But there was also evidence of versatility within one of the groups: those who had committed indecent assault against males. That group also had elevated rates of new convictions: for indecent assault on a female; for gross indecency with a child; and for buggery (in legal terms, anal rape) or attempted buggery.

In an American study, Heil, Ahlmeyer and Simons (2003) undertook a comparison between a group of 223 prisoners and 226 parolees (all with convictions for sexual offences). This study found more extensive evidence of crossover between different offence and victim types. That may be partly attributable to the employment of a polygraph assessment, which amongst the prisoner group dramatically increased the amount of offending to which they admitted;

and also to their participation in a fairly intense treatment programme that emphasised disclosure and openness. Only 11 per cent of prisoners admitted to just one type of victim; for the remainder, there were high proportions of crossover in relation to both age and relationship, but the rate of crossover for gender was lower. Different results emerged in an Australian study by Sim and Proeve (2010) of victim categories across three successive offence transitions. Here, victim choices tended to be stable in both the gender and relationship domains (i.e. there was more evidence of specialisation), but were more varied in relation to age-group.

Within a total population of 38,000 prisoners, Miethe, Olson and Mitchell (2006) undertook some comparisons between 10,000 men convicted of sexual offences and other groups who had been convicted of violence, property and public order offences. Amongst the sex offenders, only 5 per cent of those convicted of sexual crimes had committed that kind of offence and no other. The study also found a subgroup who were classed as 'versatile specialists'. Though sounding oxymoronic, this defined a number of offenders who committed 'sprees' of one type of offence and then, after a gap, embarked on an episode of committing another type of offence.

Cann, Friendship and Gozna (2007) found that a quarter (24.5 per cent) of their sample of 1,345 discharged prisoners showed some form of crossover with reference to age, gender, or relationship to victim. However, the proportions showing two types of crossover were relatively low and only seven individuals (0.05 per cent) showed crossovers in all three categories. Thus the majority of the study group could be described as 'specialised'. These findings and others, such as those of Harris *et al.* (2009) cited earlier, raise a broader question concerning the aetiology of sexual offending. One view is that it forms only a part of a wider pattern of antisocial behaviour characterised by involvement in a variety of criminal acts; another is that it has specific and unique features involving separate causal processes, such as conditioning. The likelihood is that both accounts have some substance, and that they describe different subgroups and separate pathways, with the more specialised sex offenders manifesting higher levels of sexual deviance.

Most of these studies preceded the rise of internet-based sexual offending. However, Howard, Barnett and Mann (2014) analysed patterns of this alongside other forms of sexual offending amongst a large sample of repeat male offenders (n=14,804) in England and Wales. Four initial offence groups were defined: contact child offences; contact adult offences; use of indecent images; and offences linked to paraphilia. The groups were also combined to produce aggregates of contact versus non-contact offences, and child versus non-child offences. Specialisation was measured by examining the ratio of proven reoffending to the expected rate for different kinds of offence. Specialisation was highest for indecent image offences; men who committed those also had a far lower rate of reoffending of any other type than those in the rest of the groups. There was a weaker tendency towards specialisation amongst paraphilia offenders; but no evidence of it in contact offenders, who also were more often reconvicted of non-sexual offences. The strongest tendency towards involvement in a range of offence types was amongst adult contact offenders, supporting the view that their offences may be a manifestation of a broader antisocial tendency.

We might anticipate that those who show a crossover pattern (especially of multiple kinds) are likely to be assessed as representing a higher risk. This was found in some studies (Cann, Friendship and Gozna, 2007), but not in others (Sim and Proeve, 2010). However, the sample size in the former is considerably larger and should be allotted greater weight. As the authors of some of these studies make clear, it is necessary to keep in mind the disadvantage of relying on official records, which typically underestimate the numbers of offences that individuals have actually committed. Some researchers, however, used interviews and self-report data, and supplemented those with procedures to test the veracity of information. For example, Abel *et al.* (1988) repeated their interviews until answers to questions were consistent; and Heil *et al.* (2003) assessed participants and accompanied this with a polygraph. A further difficulty is that studies used different methods of counting offences – including arrest rates, charges, court appearances ('sentencing occasions'), or convictions. Thus direct comparisons across studies are not always meaningful.

Despite these limitations, there are some discernible patterns of variation within sexual offending. Some researchers in criminology have nevertheless insisted that sexual offending can be understood using general models applicable to all *other* types of crime, and that the inclusion of specifically sexual risk factors adds very little. A study of imprisoned sex offenders by Lussier, Proulx and LeBlanc (2005) led them to suggest that 'specificity in developmental antecedents is modest at best' (p. 270). They considered that both sexual and other types of offending are 'all different manifestations of the general deviance syndrome that can manifest itself differently across time and situations'. They also noted that 'chronic offenders commit more than their share of sexual aggression' (p. 271). In a larger sample and using different measures, however, the same research group found some support for what they called a 'sexual deviance' as opposed to a 'general deviance' syndrome (Lussier, LeClerc, Cale and Proulx, 2007). Sexual recidivists showed evidence both of antisocial tendencies and of hypersexuality (frequent experience of high levels of libido or sexual urges) through the course of development.

In summary, it is possible to find examples of both specialist and generalist trends, and also of varying permutations of the two. A majority of individuals show an exclusive sexual predilection towards child or adult victims; while a proportion feel sexual attraction to both, or may offend opportunistically when their preferred target is not accessible. The firmest evidence of specialisation is amongst internet offenders. Amongst contact offenders, the most common type of crossover is with respect to victim age. While most offenders are solely heterosexual or homosexual in orientation, others may assault both females and males. Some individuals may offend only against family members, while others target strangers. Given these variations, it is unlikely that all of the possibilities can be explained by a single unifying theory.

Risk factors for sexual offending

Massive opprobrium is directed against those who commit sexual offences, judging at least by how they are portrayed in the media (Harper and Hogue, 2015). However, there is no basis for widely held stereotypes to the effect that offenders are in some basic way *different* from those who have not engaged in such acts (Richards, 2011). Joyal, Beaulieu-Plante and de Chantérac (2014) reviewed 23 studies, with a combined sample of 1,756 participants (including non-offending comparison samples), that investigated the neuropsychology of sexual offending. Given the objectives of their review, the number of available studies was not large, and conclusions proved difficult to draw. The first main finding was that sex offenders are a very heterogeneous group. Second, on average, these offenders showed some cognitive impairments compared to the general population, but there was no specific pattern within these. Those who had offended against adults had similar neuropsychological profiles to non-offenders, whereas those who had offended against children had lower scores on some cognitive measures. The studies that were located supported few conclusions beyond these.

The 'risk factors' approach does not rely on the expectation that individuals belong in discrete categories but tests the proposition that combinations of different variables are associated with more frequent or more serious sexual offending. Researchers have expended significant efforts in trying to identify these variables. In the course of that search, a long list of possibilities has been considered. Results have gradually eliminated some and downplayed the likely role of others. As new findings emerge, the pattern of the best-supported factors has gradually evolved. There have been several major reviews of the research on this (e.g. Hanson and Bussière, 1998; Hanson and Morton-Bourgon, 2005, 2009; Helmus, Hanson, Babchishin and Mann, 2013; Knight and Thornton, 2007).

Drawing the results of these and other reviews together, Mann, Hanson and Thornton (2010) allotted hypothesised risk factors into four categories: those that were 'empirically supported'; others that were 'promising'; some that were 'unsupported', but with interesting exceptions; and those with 'little or no relationship' to sexual recidivism. To be placed in the first category, a variable had to show a specified minimum effect size obtained from at least three studies. Factors should also be 'psychologically meaningful' – that is, they should describe individual propensities, defined as 'enduring characteristics that lead to predictable expressions of thoughts, feelings or behaviour' (p. 194), through interactions with the environment. For example, aggressive offenders are not aggressive all the time, but are more likely than others to respond aggressively to events they interpret in certain ways. Thornton (2013) provides a list of the best-supported risk factors under four main headings or 'domains': *sexual interests* (sexual preoccupation and offence-related sexual interests); *distorted attitudes*; *aspects of relational style*; and *problems in self-management*. Some factors are specifically, perhaps uniquely, associated with sexual aggression. Others co-occur with the factors that are associated with offending in general. A proportion intersect with those that are associated with violent offending; and, as we saw in Chapter 6, the latter two sets (relational style and skills, and self-management problems) also overlap to a considerable degree. In what follows we focus mainly on the first set of such factors (sexual interests and preoccupations).

Alongside other developments, the examination of risk factors has led to the construction of specially designed instruments for risk assessment, prediction of recidivism, and management of those who have been convicted of sexual offences. There is now a sizeable number of these instruments in circulation, and several have been extensively researched. We will consider them in Chapter 18, when we discuss forensic assessment with an explicit focus on the question of risk.

Sexual preoccupation and offence-related sexual interests

There are two interrelated aspects of the sexual interest component of risk. One is *sexual preoccupation*, an 'abnormally intense interest in sex that dominates psychological functioning' (Mann *et al.*, 2010, p. 198), in which engagement in sexual activity is often impersonal. The other is *sexually deviant interests*, a preference for gaining satisfaction from non-consenting sex. Clegg and Fremouw (2009) identified two versions of the latter, 'strong' and 'weak'. In the strong version, it is held that rapists have an 'absolute preference' for coercive over consensual sex. In the weak version, it is thought that rapists are more aroused than others by enforced sex. Clegg and Fremouw (2009) reviewed 19 studies of the phallometric assessment of rapists and child molesters (this method is described in Chapter 18), to test the strength of the association between arousal and different kinds of sexual stimuli. No studies were found that directly supported the 'strong' version of the preference hypothesis, but there was tentative support for the 'weak' version – that is, higher arousal than non-sex offenders, but not an exclusive proclivity.

In a meta-analysis of 82 studies with a cumulative sample size of 29,450 offenders, Hanson and Morton-Bourgon (2005) found that deviant sexual interest, which refers to 'enduring attractions to sexual acts that are illegal (e.g. sex with children, rape) or highly unusual (e.g. fetishism, autoerotic asphyxia)' (p. 1154), was one of the two strongest predictors of sexual recidivism. While those who commit sexual offences do not necessarily have deviant interests, the risk of reoffending is much higher when they do. The other key predictor was antisocial orientation and lifestyle instability, though this was more highly correlated with violent and general recidivism than with sexual recidivism. This factor has been associated with several types of criminal activity, so it is not a distinguishing feature of sexual offending.

These patterns are corroborated by evidence concerning adolescent males who commit sexual offences. Are the same predictors that are associated with general offending also applicable to those who commit sexual offences, during the critical phase of adolescence when patterns of delinquency emerge? In a large-scale review of this area encompassing 59 studies, Seto and Lalumière (2010) concluded that some additional variables were needed to understand adolescent sexual offending. The two strongest predictors of involvement in it were atypical sexual interests (which includes sexual arousal response to children or to coercive sexual acts) and having been a victim of child sexual abuse. Both of these showed moderate-to-large effect sizes (Cohen's *d* of 0.67 and 0.62 respectively). Some factors found with general delinquency were negatively correlated with sex offending: for example, having antisocial associates, substance misuse and antisocial attitudes.

Notwithstanding the importance of deviant sexual preference as a risk factor, some researchers have voiced doubt about the usefulness of focusing on that as a target of change in sex offender treatment (Marshall and Fernandez, 2003).

Abuse history

There is evidence that those who commit sexual offences are more likely than those who commit other types of crimes to have been victimised sexually themselves. Jesperson, Lalumière and Seto (2009) conducted two interrelated meta-analyses. One focused on 17 studies which had compared rates of child sexual abuse in adult sex offenders and non-sex offenders. The other focused on 15 studies which had compared those who had sexually offended against adults with those who had sexually offended against children. In each case they compared abuse history variables across three domains: sexual abuse; physical abuse; and emotional abuse and neglect.

There was a significantly higher rate of sexual abuse history amongst sex offenders than amongst non-sex offenders, with an odds ratio of 3.36; that is, sex offenders were 3.36 times more likely to have been victims of sexual abuse than non-sex offenders; but there was no significant difference in histories of physical abuse. Those who had sexually offended against adults had a significantly lower prevalence of sexual abuse history than those who had offended against children, with an odds ratio of 0.51; but they had a higher rate of physical abuse history, with an odds ratio of 1.43. While the number of studies used to make some of the comparisons was fairly small, the authors were able to eliminate publication bias as a factor in their results. They concluded that the results provided support for the hypothesis that those who have been sexually abused themselves are more likely to become sexual abusers. Babchishin, Hanson and VanZuylen (2015) found that those who had committed sexual abuse against children had higher rates of both sexual and physical abuse histories than internet sex offenders. In their review of sexually abusive adolescents, Seto and Lalumière (2010) found that a history of sexual victimisation was the second strongest predictor of sexual offending by adolescent males, after atypical sexual interests. In a British study of 700 adolescents who had perpetrated abuse, there was documented evidence that they had previously been victims in 31 per cent of cases, and allegations or strong indications in a further 19 per cent (Hackett, Masson, Balfe and Phillips, 2013). Amongst the 24 girls included in their sample, the corresponding figures were 37 per cent and 32 per cent, higher proportions than for boys.

Two other points concerning this area are worth keeping in mind. First, there is evidence that adults may under-report childhood abuse. Two studies compared records of abuse from contemporaneous records during childhood with individuals' reports based on in-depth interviews 20 years later. In both cases, a large proportion of those who were known to have been abused physically (40 per cent; Widom and Shepard, 1996) or sexually (36 per cent of women and 84 per cent of men; Widom and Morris, 1997) did not report this as adults. Second, there is no direct or linear causal relationship between victimisation and abusiveness. That is, child sexual abuse does not make it inevitable that the victim will in due course become an abuser. Equally, some individuals who commit sexual offences have never been victimised. This is a probabilistic relationship, influenced also by many other factors that act in combination.

Attitudes

A number of attitudinal and cognitive variables have been investigated for their possible associations with sexual offending. Some patterns have emerged from research on this, despite the challenges of studying it. For example, it is notoriously difficult to assess factors such as attitudes, given the potential guardedness of participants when asked questions pertaining to sexual coercion or aggression. It is difficult to design measures that do not suffer from a major weakness of *transparency*, such that respondents can easily see what is being assessed. In most areas of assessment transparency would be seen as advantageous (*face validity*), but if respondents are being assessed in relation to a trait or attitude that they know is sensitive or subject to social disapproval, they may be forewarned and respond defensively, withholding or misrepresenting their real thoughts or opinions.

Helmus, Hanson, Babchishin and Mann (2013) reported a meta-analysis of 45 studies of attitudes hypothesised to be linked to sexual recidivism. The studies were published in the period 1986–2012, and had a combined sample size of 13,782 participants. Study samples were followed up for an average of 5.6 years and the overall sexual recidivism rate was 9.2 per cent. Attitudes had been measured at one of two points in time, either before or after participation in treatment. While it was expected that the former would supply more accurate predictions, and there was a difference in accordance with that, it was statistically non-significant. Overall, Helmus and her colleagues found that some attitudes were predictive of sexual recidivism, though the effect size for the association was small (a Cohen's *d* of 0.22). These were attitudes that condoned or justified sexual offending, although Helmus *et al.* noted that many of them remain very 'poorly defined' (p. 47). The effects showed more strongly for child molestation, on which there were more studies, than for rape. Helmus *et al.* identified a small number of attitude scales which they classed as 'empirically validated', in that in each case there were three or more studies supporting their usefulness. Thus there are some attitudes that are associated with sexual reoffending.

A disturbing aspect of these findings is that attitudes potentially supportive of rape are apparently not uncommon, and when assessed in terms of personality functioning, males expressing such views have generally been found to be within the 'normal' range in other respects. This was found some years ago by Petty and Dawson (1989), who reviewed literature and reported their own results, which showed that a sizeable minority of US male college students had stated that they would be prepared to use force in sexual encounters if they could be assured of not being caught. On a personality inventory, the subgroup of men expressing such views the most strongly were within one standard deviation of the mean of the student population as a whole. In a meta-analysis of 29 studies, Murnen and Kohlman (2007) found that attitudes supportive of rape or other sexual assault were held by higher proportions of those who participated regularly in sports. There is evidence of an association between *hypermasculinity* – a cluster of attitudes in which violence, dominance and sexual conquest are perceived as manly – and acceptance of 'rape myths' (Gage, 2008; see below). College students who held these attitudes were more likely to engage in dating aggression and sexual coercion (Forbes, Adams-Curtos, Pakalka and White, 2006). Alleyne, Gannon, Ó Ciardha and Wood (2014) found that as many as 66 per cent of a sample of university students 'did not emphatically reject' some sexual interest in multiple-perpetrator rape. Beliefs perhaps not overtly supportive of, but not convincingly dismissive of, sexual aggression appear to be internalised by a sizeable proportion of the male population. This is not linked to any traits usually considered abnormal, but appears to be tacitly endorsed within the surrounding culture.

In the survey of males from six Asian countries reported by Jewkes *et al.* (2013), which was described earlier, respondents were asked the main reasons why they had committed rape. This was done as a component of individual interviews, but these specific data were collected using a series of statements with four-point Likert scales. The commonest reasons endorsed were 'sexual entitlement' (73.3 per cent), 'seeking entertainment' (58.7 per cent), and 'as a form of punishment' (37.9 per cent). Broader factors thought to be operating were poverty, previous victimisation, images of masculinity emphasising sexual prowess, male dominance, low empathy, and alcohol misuse. Although the methodology here was

9

relatively simple, clinical research employing in-depth interviews and more elaborate psychometrics has generated similar patterns of results.

Cognitions

Attitudes are usually defined as having *affective, behavioural* and *cognitive* components. The last of these has been a particular focus of research on sexual offending. As that research has progressed, there has been a gradual change of emphasis in terms of the types of cognitive variables that are thought to be related to sexual offending.

Cognitive distortion, a concept adapted from cognitive therapy, refers to irrational or ill-founded statements individuals make to themselves, which sustain states of mind or patterns of behaviour. While these statements might secure certain goals for those individuals, they are in other ways maladaptive. Abel, Becker and Cunningham-Rathner (1984) described seven examples of such distortions which were verbalised by men who had sexually molested children, and developed a scale for assessing them (Abel *et al.*, 1989). The examples were these men's ideas that:

1. 'A child who does not physically resist advances really wants to have sex.'
2. 'Having sex with a child is a good way for the child to learn about sex.'
3. 'Children do not tell others about this because they want it to continue.'
4. 'In the future society will realise that sex between children and adults is all right.'
5. 'An adult who only touches a child's genitals is not really being sexual, so no harm is done.'
6. 'When a child asks an adult about sex, this means that the child wants to see the adult's genitals or to have sex.'
7. 'A parent's relationship with a son or daughter is enhanced by having sex with him or her.'

Statements of these kinds by child molesters sometimes emerge as retrospective justifications – rationalisations ('excuses') for behaviour – in a manner akin to the techniques of neutralisation we encountered in Chapter 5. They may also be used to deflect or to nullify reasons for *not* doing something, and there is evidence that cognitive distortions are associated with denial and minimisation (Nunes and Jung, 2012). Thus interest in these distortions was driven by the hypothesis that they may play a part in facilitating and maintaining offending behaviour. This provided the rationale for making them a target of change, and sessions focusing on cognition have been a standard feature of many treatment programmes.

However, attempts to assess such cognitions have not produced consistent results in differentiating child molesters from other groups (Ward, Hudson, Johnston and Marshall, 1997), and so have not securely established the aetiological significance of distortions (Gannon and Polaschek, 2006). Indeed, Maruna and Mann (2006) cast doubt on the value of addressing distorted thinking in treatment programmes, and the concept of 'cognitive distortion' has since been criticised as 'unacceptably fuzzy' (Helmus *et al.*, 2013, p. 35).

Some researchers have investigated whether distortions in thinking may be traceable to a more deeply embedded plane of cognition, at the level of *implicit theories* (Polascheck and and Gannon, 2004; Polaschek and Ward, 2002; Ward, 2000; Ward and Keenan, 1999). These are cognitive structures that operate at an automatic level, outside conscious awareness, and which affect how individuals process information from the social world. With reference to sexual offending, several researchers have suggested that implicit theories may be a critical influence on how potential perpetrators view others, in ways that can facilitate and even (in their minds) justify their offending. Several such beliefs have been hypothesised, and we paraphrase them as follows (these refer to rape, but parallel ideas arise in relation to molesting children):

- *Women as unknowable* Women are fundamentally different from men. It is impossible to grasp how their minds work; encounters with them are sure to be adversarial.

- *Women as sexual objects* Men's sexual needs dominate everything, and women want sex even when they don't know it; their body language is a better clue than what they say.
- *Entitlement* Men have a right to sex, and to impose it on women. Essentially, men's needs should be met and women's place is to let that happen.
- *Male sex drive is uncontrollable* Men's arousal builds up and beyond a certain point cannot be contained. It is then difficult for them or a woman to halt the process.
- *Dangerous world* The world is a hostile and threatening place, and people will exploit you if you let them, so you must look after your own interests.

In a study of 37 rapists, Polaschek and Gannon (2004) found that almost all endorsed the first three of the implicit theories above, though a smaller proportion endorsed the last two. Collectively, these ideas have close similarities to what were originally called **rape myths**, an idea introduced in a renowned cultural and historical examination of rape by Brownmiller (1975) and first employed in research on sexual offending by Burt (1980). This term denotes a cluster of erroneous beliefs to the effect that (for example) in most cases rape victims are promiscuous, or in most cases women only accuse men of rape when they are trying to get back at someone they are angry with. In a random sample of 598 adults from the general population, Burt that found that these beliefs were predicted by an acceptance of interpersonal violence and of traditional gender stereotypes, and by an expectation of gender relations being adversarial. Here again, however, as found in studies of attitudes, some non-sexual offenders, and some non-offenders, also appeared to subscribe to potentially offence-related beliefs.

Theories of sexual offending

Sexual offending consists of a wide assortment of behaviours, both in the nature of the acts committed and in their levels of seriousness. The variability within sexual offending makes the production of robust theories a challenging task. A sound theory in this area has to account for a perplexing variety of phenomena. Numerous theories have been forwarded, with large variations in their span of applicability.

Ward and Hudson (1998; see also Ward, Polaschek and Beech, 2006) proposed a *meta-theoretical framework* for classifying the theories that have appeared, organising them into three levels:

- *Level I: Comprehensive and multifactorial theories* These combine a number of discrete variables and are likely to focus on distal or long-term causes, such as family dysfunction or poor parenting. An example is Finkelhor's 'preconditions' model of child sexual abuse (discussed earlier).
- *Level II: Single-factor theories* These have been developed to explain the occurrence of specific phenomena within sexual offending, drawing on specific factors such as self-regulation problems, or empathy or intimacy deficits. These theories, too, tend to consider mainly distal causes.
- *Level III: Micro-level or offence process theories* Theories at this level focus on more proximal causes: factors in the situation immediately prior to the onset of offending. An example is the concept of the 'offence chain' process, a sequence of nine steps through which individuals travel before molesting a child (Ward, Louden, Hudson and Marshall, 1995).

From a long list of possibilities, therefore, we focus on just one theory which represents probably the most wide-ranging explanatory model of sexual offending published to date: the 'Integrated Theory of Sexual Offending'.

Integrated Theory of Sexual Offending

The *Integrated Theory of Sexual Offending* (hereafter, the ITSO) was forwarded by Ward and Beech (2006, 2008; Ward, Fisher and Beech, 2016). In their initial paper, Ward and Beech (2006) first sought to establish that the ITSO possesses what they considered were the seven attributes of a good scientific theory: empirical adequacy; internal coherence; external consistency; unifying power; heuristic value in generating hypotheses; explanatory depth; and simplicity.

They also regarded it as important that a theory in any specific domain be connected with broader conceptualisations of human behaviour. The ITSO synthesises variables from a wide array of domains, including evolution and genetics, brain development, the physical and cultural environment, individual circumstances, social learning and the resultant ongoing pattern of neuropsychological and cognitive functioning. These are harnessed together to help explain the emergence of mental states or clinical symptoms associated with sexual offending.

The ITSO assimilates elements from other theories, including an earlier 'Pathways' model of sexual offending (Ward and Siegert, 2002). This held that there were four discrete routes to sexual offending: via intimacy and social skills deficits; via antisocial cognitions; via distorted sexual 'scripts' and cognitions; or via emotional dysregulation. To these four trajectories Middleton, Elliot, Mandeville-Norden and Beech (2006) proposed adding a fifth, 'multiple dysfunctional mechanisms' (p. 594), which combined ingredients of the other four. The integrated theory embraces all of these combinations, and the pathways through which they are thought to interact, as shown in Figure 9.3.

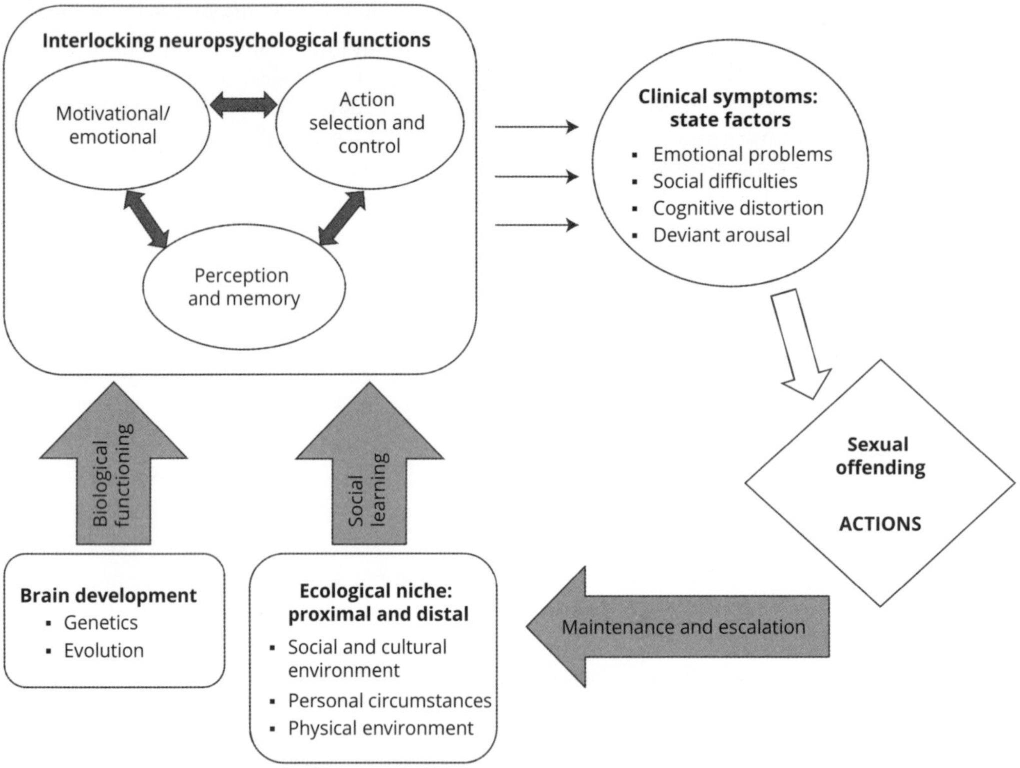
Interlocking neuropsychological functions
Motivational/ emotional
Action selection and control
Perception and memory
Clinical symptoms: state factors
Emotional problems
Social difficulties
Cognitive distortion
Deviant arousal
Sexual offending
ACTIONS
Biological functioning
Social learning
Brain development
Genetics
Evolution
Ecological niche: proximal and distal
Social and cultural environment
Personal circumstances
Physical environment
Maintenance and escalation

Figure 9.3
Integrated Theory of Sexual Offending (ITSO) of Ward and Beech.

Source: reprinted from Aggression and Violent Behavior, 11 (1), Ward, T. & Beech, A., An integrated theory of sexual offending, p. 51. Copyright 2006, with permission from Elsevier. DOI: https://doi.org/10.1016/j.avb.2005.05.002

Ward, Fisher and Beech (2016) were not trying to dispense with the 'risk factors' approach, but to incorporate it within what they consider a more formal theoretical framework. In the ITSO, there are four broad categories of '**stable dynamic risk factors**' (Thornton, 2002), or domains of problematic psychological functioning (Ward and Siegert, 2002). Using slightly different terminology, they are shown as the clinical symptoms or 'state factors' in the top right of Figure 9.3, and are:

» *emotional problems*, deficits in control and self-management, negative moods, impulsivity

- *social difficulties*, emotional loneliness, low self-esteem, attachment problems, victim stance
- *cognitive distortion*, offence-supportive cognitions, dysfunctional **schemas**, implicit theories
- *deviant arousal* and sexual interests, preferences and fantasy, including paraphilias.

In interaction with proximal experiences and events, the above may cause the emergence of acute risk states. Ward and Beech (2006, p. 47) proposed that 'combinations of these vulnerabilities may result in illegal sexual behaviours under certain circumstances'. The broader configuration of the ITSO shows the major pathways (depicted as the larger arrows) through which combinations of biological (evolutionary, genetic) and ecological and environmental factors shape an individual's neuropsychological functioning (top left of Figure 9.3) and the three interlocking systems that compose it – *motivational/emotional, perception and mem*ory and *action selection and control.*

Findings indicate that various forms of emotional dysregulation can contribute to the development and maintenance of some patterns of offending. However, while the ITSO provides a valuable framework for synthesising a broad spectrum of variables, when addressing the detailed processes, specific combinations of which make offending more likely, there is still an inevitable lack of precision. For example, emotional dysregulation can itself take a number of forms. The variable of 'negative emotionality', included in Ward *et al.*'s *emotional problems* category, has emerged (as we saw in in Chapter 5) in several longitudinal studies of the onset, establishment and escalation of delinquency and other antisocial behaviours (e.g. DeLisi and Vaughan, 2014; Lahey and Waldman, 2005; Pulkkinen, Kyyra and Kokko, 2009). Difficulties in managing or channelling negative emotion, and what Ward *et al.* (2016, p. 7) call 'emotional competency deficits' are implicated in several forms of rule violation, including delinquent acts. Interview-based research with high-frequency adult offenders has found that inability or unwillingness to address personal problems is accompanied by marked negative feelings (dysphoria). This often results in an accumulation of difficulties, to a point where coping mechanisms fail and a new offence occurs (Zamble and Quinsey, 1997). For those with some of the other features specified in the ITSO, that is likely to be a sexual offence.

The advantages of the ITSO, Ward *et al.* contend, are its breadth and depth, and that it fuses together more contributory factors than any other model. Its major limitation, which besets all theories in this area, arises from what philosophers of science call the **underdetermination of theory**. This describes a situation in which the available evidence is compatible with a number of different theoretical formulations, with no means of choosing between them. When addressing a problem as complex as sexual offending, it is very difficult to devise a theory that is sufficiently refined that it could be tested alongside competing explanations, using empirical data to decide which one had greater explanatory power. For example, Smallbone and Cale (2015) have forwarded a theory with many similarities to the ITSO, though with a different emphasis as it places sexual offending within the perspective of 'developmental life-course' criminology. But of necessity, many of the same psychological variables are included in both theories.

Sexual offence recidivism

A question in the mind of anyone who works with those convicted of sexual offences has been expressed very simply by one of the field's leading researchers (Hanson, 2000): 'Will they do it again?' There have been numerous statistical analyses, follow-up evaluations and reviews with a bearing on this question. The general finding is that recidivism rates for this group are on average lower than for people convicted of other types of offences. This picture emerges from both UK and international data.

Looking first at short-term reconviction rates, the Ministry of Justice (2017a) in England and Wales publishes 12-month 'proven reoffending' data in its *Quarterly Bulletins*. For adults, the average one-year rate across all offences for those convicted of any offence in the 12 months to March 2015 was 24.3 per cent; while for those who had received custodial sentences it was 44.7 per cent. For those whose index offence was sexual, the one-year reoffending rate was 13.0 per cent. This compares with a figure of 42.2 per cent for those whose index offence was theft. The follow-up figures include all types of reoffence. Data are not given on the proportion that were new sexual offences, but as we saw earlier most offenders are 'generalists' who also break the criminal law in other ways.

Turning to longer-term studies, Cann, Falshaw and Friendship (2004) reported a 21-year follow-up of all 419 adult male sex offenders released from English prisons in 1979. At the end of the period, 24.6 per cent had been reconvicted of a sexual offence, 21.7 per cent of a violent offence, and 63.8 per cent of any offence. In a later study, amongst a large cohort of 3,027 released sex offenders, Wakeling, Beech and Freemantle (2013) found a two-year sexual offence recidivism rate of 1.7 per cent, a sexual plus violent reconviction rate of 4.4 per cent, and a general reconviction rate of 12 per cent. Concerning younger sexual offenders in the UK, Hargreaves and Francis (2014) conducted a long-term analysis of reconvictions for a period of up to 35 years. Using a specific form of analysis, they determined that those convicted of sex offences return to a risk level commensurate with that for those who have never been so convicted after a period of 17 years.

In the United States, Langan, Schmitt and Durose (2003) reported an analysis of recidivism rates of 9,691 male sex offenders released from prison in 1994. These men had served an average of 3.5 years in prison. At three years post-release, members of the study sample were four times more likely to be rearrested for a sexual crime than other released prisoners (a population of over a quarter of a million). Their rearrest rate for this was 5.3 per cent, as compared with 1.3 per cent for other prisoners; their sexual reconviction rate was 3.5 per cent. Their rearrest rate for any offence was 43 per cent, compared to 68 per cent for other prisoners. Of the new sexual offences 40 per cent occurred within the first 12 months after release.

Harris and Hanson (2004) compared data from ten follow-up studies (seven Canadian, two American and one British). Follow-up periods ranged from 2 to 23 years. Overall recidivism rates were as follows: after 5 years, 14 per cent; 10 years, 20 per cent; and 15 years, 24 per cent. They found that while recidivism rates for rapists and child molesters were broadly similar, within the latter group extrafamilial offenders against boy victims had the highest rates (35 per cent after 15 years), while incest offenders had the lowest rates (13 per cent after 15 years). Similar patterns were found in a 15-year follow-up of 2,474 offenders released from prisons in New Zealand (Vess and Skelton, 2010). In contrast to the prevalent image of those who commit these types of crimes, 'most sexual offenders do not re-offend sexually over time' (Harris and Hanson, 2004, p. 11).

In a meta-analysis of a set of 100 study samples with a combined total of 28,757 participants, Hanson and Morton-Bourgon (2009) found a mean observed sexual recidivism rate of 11.5 per cent over an average 70-month follow-up. In 50 of those studies where sexual or violent recidivism was measured, its rate was 19.5 per cent; in the 65 studies where any recidivism was recorded, its rate was 33.2 per cent. In a later study, Hanson, Harris, Helmus and Thornton (2014) reported survival analyses over a 20-year follow-up period. This entailed monitoring the proportions of groups remaining offence-free as time progressed. Their study aggregated data on 7,740 offenders from 21 samples. Cases were classified as 'low', 'moderate', or 'high' risk using the *Static-99R*, a widely used risk-assessment instrument. Respective sexual recidivism rates, after an average follow-up period of 8.2 years, were these: low risk, 2.9 per cent; moderate risk, 8.5 per cent; and high risk, 24.2 per cent. If individuals remained offence-free for the first five years, their recidivism rates for ensuing years were significantly reduced, a finding obtained even with high-risk offenders.

However, based on evidence that some of those who offend sexually subsequently admit to larger numbers of offences than those of which they are convicted, it may be that official records underestimate the 'true' recidivism rate. Groth, Longo and McFadin (1982) invited 83 convicted rapists and 54 convicted child molesters from two different institutions in the United States to complete an anonymous and confidential questionnaire which asked them about their history of sexual assaults, regardless of whether or not these had ever been detected. In the rape group, the average number of known offences was 2.8, whereas the members of that group admitted to an average of a further 5.2 undetected rapes. Corresponding figures for the child-molester group were 1.7 and 4.7. Thus the ratio of undetected to recorded offences ranged from 1.8:1 to 2.7:1. Overall, given the distribution of results, it appeared that there was a portion of offenders who could be described as 'prolific' in their offence histories. For a small minority of the group, omitted from the averages quoted above, it was far higher: 7 per cent admitted to more than 50 undetected offences each.

An even larger discrepancy between different sources of reoffending data was found by Falshaw, Friendship and Bates (2003). They reported a follow-up study of 173 offenders who attended a community-based treatment programme in England. They compared official reconviction rates from the Offenders Index with other markers. The latter included a measure of 'sexual reoffending', defined as committing another illegal sexual act whether or not it led to arrest, and 'sexual recidivism', defined as offence-related behaviour with a sexual motivation, even if legal. Offenders' average period 'at risk' (that is, the period during which they could have committed a new offence) varied widely, from two to nearly six years, with an average of just under four years. The recidivism rate counted by these other methods was 5.3 times the officially recorded rate. However, the status of the measure of recidivism used here is unclear, as it is defined in the report as including legal acts that might *indicate* risk. With all sources combined, the average recidivism rate was 21 per cent after just slightly less than four years.

Given the nature of sexual offending, it is usually thought possible that anyone who commits a sexual offence then poses a potentially lifelong risk of reoffending. While the highest probability of reoffending is within the first five years after release, the risk of reconviction does not follow the same shape as that of the age–crime curve for offending in general, so individuals may continue to be at risk of further offending for long periods. However, the introduction of registration, monitoring and notification procedures is likely to have reduced the likelihood of sexual offences or offence-related risk behaviours remaining unreported. Moreover, the probability of committing further sexual offences reduces with increasing age (Craig, 2008; Harris and Hanson, 2004). This may be a function of the decline in libido that occurs as age advances (Barbaree, Blanchard and Langton, 2003), or it may be related to other changes in individuals' lives.

Intimate partner violence

Non-sexual abuse of one family member by another has at different times been known by several names, including *family violence*, *domestic abuse* (DA), *domestic violence* (DV), *intimate partner violence* (IPV), *spousal assault*, *partner abuse*, or *battering*. The broadest term, *family violence*, can refer to conflicts or abuse between generations. Various terms are often used interchangeably, although in some respects they may refer to slightly different patterns depending on whether there is a single victim (usually a spouse or partner) or multiple victims (other family members, such as children or older parents).

The term 'violence' in its narrow sense refers specifically to physical assaults, but it is also often used more broadly to refer to other aspects of domination of one partner by the other within a close relationship, and may thus include sexual, emotional, financial and other forms of coercion and control. The term 'abuse' has been used to include all forms of behaviour in which one individual causes harm to, or violates the rights of, another. For the purpose of recording by police in England and Wales, for example, domestic abuse incidents are currently defined as 'any incidence of threatening behaviour, violence or abuse (psychological, physical, sexual, financial or emotional) between adults, aged 16 and over, who are or have been intimate partners or family members, regardless of gender or sexuality' (Office for National Statistics, 2016d, p. 8).

Until not very long ago, public discussion of domestic violence was virtually non-existent. The problem was almost entirely concealed in the privacy of family homes. Given long-standing social attitudes, it seemed to be either taken for granted or ignored. Groves and Thomas (2014) described how the 'naming' of domestic abuse had to precede any attempt to define it. For these and other reasons, there are strong indications that the frequency of DA/IPV is still markedly underestimated in official statistics: 'It is known that only a small proportion of domestic abuse incidents are reported to the police' (Office for National Statistics, 2016d, p. 8). Often, therefore, this remains in many senses a 'hidden' type of crime.

Prevalence

Statistics from the Crime Survey for England and Wales (CSEW) show that during the year ending March 2015 the police recorded 943,628 incidents of domestic abuse (Office for National Statistics, 2016d). During 2014–2015, 8.2 per cent of women and 4.0 per cent of men reported having been victims of domestic abuse on one occasion or more, while 5.8 per cent of women and 2.6 per cent of men reported having been victims of non-sexual partner abuse. The corresponding figures for long-term experience of victimisation amongst those aged 16–59 were: for any domestic abuse, 27.1 per cent for women and 13.2 per cent for men; and for non-sexual partner abuse, 20.7 per cent for women and 8.6 per cent for men. For the year 2014–2015, domestic-abuse crimes formed 10 per cent of all recorded crime, and a third of all recorded assaults that resulted in injury (HM Inspector of Constabulary, 2015). The largest single group of victims of domestic abuse were women in the age range 20–34.

In addition to direct assaults, other types of offences are considered by police officers to be *linked* to domestic abuse. One-third of offences of 'violence against the person' fell into this category, and these include, for example, threat or possession with intent to commit criminal damage (31 per cent), public order offences (23 per cent), perverting the course of justice (18 per cent), and criminal damage to a dwelling (14 per cent) or to a vehicle (3 per cent). The percentages in brackets are the proportions of *all* offences of that type that were classed by police as related to domestic abuse.

There are surprisingly wide variations in the officially recorded prevalence rates of DA/IPV across different countries and world regions, but it is difficult to tell to what extent they may reflect differential rates of reporting and recording practices rather than differences in actual underlying ('true') rates. Alhabib, Nur and Jones (2010) collated results from a total of 134 studies on the prevalence of domestic violence (physical, sexual or emotional) against women from 50 countries across all major world regions, published in the period 1995–2006. They found considerable variation in prevalence rates, ranging from 1.9 per cent to 70 per cent – with both of those extremes occurring within a single country (the United States). Esquivel-Santoveña and Dixon (2012) sought to establish a true rate of IPV against women and against men by collating data from 11 surveys, conducted mainly in the USA but with others in Mexico, Ukraine and South Africa. However, inconsistencies in the methodology of the surveys that were found precluded the drawing of any clear conclusions. In a review of over 200 studies from 83 countries outside the USA and industrialised Anglophone countries, Esquivel-Santoveña, Lambert and Hamel (2013) found generally higher rates of both partner violence and psychological abuse than in the USA and UK. There were very large variations in IPV prevalence, but they were not correlated with the Human Development Index, used worldwide as a composite measure of health, education, income and living standards.

In Europe, surveys of violence against women have been conducted by the European Union Agency for Fundamental Rights (FRA), across all 28 EU member countries (FRA, 2014b). This found an average reported rate, for either physical or sexual violence by a partner since the age of 15, of 22 per cent. The lowest rate of 13 per cent was in Austria, Croatia, Poland, Slovenia and Spain, while the highest at 32 per cent was in Denmark and Latvia. The corresponding figure for the UK was 29 per cent. Several regional and global surveys have been conducted, under the auspices of international bodies such as the World Health Organization (WHO; 2013) and other composite agencies of the United Nations (UN; García-Moreno *et al.*, 2013; Stöckl *et al.*, 2013). These have found relatively lower rates in the high-income countries of the European region and Japan (23.2 per cent and 24.6 per cent respectively), but higher rates for the African, Eastern Mediterranean and South-east Asian regions (36.6 per cent, 37.0 per cent and 37.7 per cent respectively).

A portion of IPV is fatal, and it has been reported that approximately 14 per cent of homicides occur in partner relationships (39 per cent of killings of women and 6 per cent of killings of men). Corradi and Stöckl (2014) analysed patterns of intimate partner homicide in ten European countries, including the UK. Over the period 2000–2011, there were 2,559 female and 5,530 male homicides in the UK, of which respectively 1,076 (42.0 per cent) and 306 (5.5 per cent) were committed by intimate partners. While overall there are more male victims of homicide, most are killed by other men outside the context of close relationships, whereas a large fraction of female victims are killed by male partners.

Partner violence is not confined to heterosexual relationships: it also occurs in both male and female same-sex couples. Many of the correlates of abuse in same-sex couples parallel those found in heterosexual relationships (Bartholomew, Regan, Oram and White, 2008), but there is some evidence that the overall level of violence is higher (Badenes-Ribera *et al.*, 2015); and differences have also been reported, for example, in patterns of jealousy (Barelds and Dijkstra, 2005).

Nor is the problem of partner violence solely 'domestic' – that is, occurring only in couples who cohabit the same household. It also arises in other intimate relationships. Straus (2008) summarised data from the International Dating Violence Study, a survey involving a total of 13,601 participants in 32 countries. Focusing on respondents within this sample who had been in a relationship for at least one month, Straus (2008) found a mean reported rate of assault within their relationships during the previous 12 months of 31.2 per cent, with a range from 16.6 per cent in Portugal to 77.1 per cent in Iran. Data from studies of this type have given rise to a number of issues that are frequently debated in the study of IPV. They include the questions of directionality and gender symmetry, the role of reactivity, and whether or not there are unique risk factors operating in partner violence that are not found for violence in general:

» *Directionality* A first question concerns the relative proportions of partner abuse that are committed by males against females, by females against males, or in same-sex couples. This raises frequently disputed issues. For example, from the feminist perspective, part of the explanation of domestic abuse is considered to derive from patriarchal power structures (male dominance). On that basis, the violence by males against female partners would be expected to be more common, and police and victim survey statistics suggest that that is indeed the case. However, other survey data concerning the scale of the difference are more variable. A comprehensive review integrating 48 studies provided more support for the bidirectionality perspective (Langhinrichsen-Rohling, Misra, Selwyn and Rohling, 2012). Thus there is acknowledged to be 'bidirectionality': there are perpetrators in both genders.

» *Gender symmetry* A second, related question is whether there is gender 'symmetry': that is, do men assault women and women assault men at similar rates, or is the former more prevalent? That the number and proportion of assaults committed by males is higher would accord with the general picture regarding crime as a whole, and violent and sexual offences in particular, including homicides. Some researchers, however, have contended that symmetry (or even 'mutuality') is the more customary pattern, but that this is unrecognised, or even denied, by other workers in the field (Straus, 2010, 2014). One interpretation is that violence by men towards women is more frequent at all levels of seriousness, and that while the difference may be marginal at the lowest levels of aggression (sometimes called 'ordinary' or 'situational' partner violence), it becomes far larger with increasing levels of seriousness; and in relation to grievous harm and to murder or manslaughter, the difference is very pronounced. An alternative interpretation is that there is symmetry at most levels of severity, other than in a small proportion of cases where there is 'extreme' violence that is driven by 'clinical' factors (meaning mental disorders in perpetrators).

- *Reactivity* A third dispute that emerges from this research is the extent to which female violence towards males is reactive – that is, that it is not initiated by women but is more typically a defensive response against male aggression. Evidence indicates that while this may be true in a proportion of cases, there is also some violence that is clearly instigated by females and not solely in response to assaults by males.
- *Gender and risk factors* There are also disagreements over whether the risk factors for intimate partner violence differ from those for violence in general. Some researchers say they do not. In a study of 2,124 prisoners convicted of partner violence, Felson and Lane (2010) found no features specific to IPV. There was a slightly higher rate of child sexual abuse and of alcohol misuse amongst IPV perpetrators, but otherwise they were 'like other violent offenders'. Similar findings were obtained by Bates, Graham-Kevan and Archer (2014) in a survey of 1,104 UK university students. Other authors, however, suggest that there are distinct influences at work in IPV. On the basis of a study of 1,306 women in South Africa, Jewkes, Levin and Penn-Kekana (2002) reported that in addition to the factors involved in other types of violence there were further influences on IPV, notably the relative status of women in society, conservative ideas about their social position, and the perceived acceptability of using violence as a means of exercising male authority in relationships. This depended at the individual level on the extent to which men absorbed 'normative' ideologies of male superiority over females. These studies illustrate the polarisation of views concerning the origins of IPV, and the extent to which gender power differences play a role.

Notwithstanding these disputes, it is universally accepted that IPV can have a number of serious consequences in terms of the health of victims. The WHO prevalence research (García-Moreno *et al.*, 2013) documents a range of sequelae for women, and studies show these include increased rates of depression and other mental health problems (Devries *et al.*, 2011), and elevated suicide risk (McLaughlin, O'Carroll and O'Connor, 2012), and an increased likelihood of having an abortion or of giving birth to a low-weight baby. IPV also has a significant impact on children who witness it (and who may be used instrumentally by some men against female partners: Beeble, Bybee and Sullivan, 2007). Effects include elevated risks of behaviour problems and of deficits in cognitive and social functioning. But there is also considerable variability in the effects of exposure to IPV, influenced by a number of other factors (Hungerford, Wait, Fritz and Clements, 2012).

Several typologies or attempts at classification have been forwarded regarding IPV. Possibly the simplest, which parallels one we have encountered before in discussion of sexual offending, involves dividing perpetrators into 'generalists', who have also committed other types of violent offences, as compared with 'specialists', who have not (Herrero, Torres, Fernández-Suárez and Rodríquez-Díaz, 2016; Huss and Ralston, 2008). Other approaches have identified varying levels of criminality and psychopathology linked to lethal violence (Dixon, Hamilton-Giachristis and Browne, 2008). One of the most widely used classifications was devised by Johnson (2008), who argued that the large discrepancies in estimates of the prevalence of domestic abuse (in the United States) can be understood only by realising that the figures that are available often refer to different forms of IPV. Johnson combined individual and relational features, according to the level to which violence was used as a means of control. This enabled him to distinguish four patterns of conflict, each of them characterised by particular features of the dynamics within couples, varying according to levels of violence and motives of control:

- *Intimate terrorism* This refers to the exclusive exercise of power by one partner, using a wide variety of means, including violence and also economic control, and the use of children to coerce the other partner, who is abused, subjugated, and isolated.

- *Violent resistance* One partner is dominant, violent and controlling. The other is violent and fights back, but is not controlling.
- *Situational couple violence* Neither partner is trying to control the relationship, but there are many incidents of conflict in which violence can be situationally provoked, for a mixture of reasons. (This is thought to be the most common type of couple violence.)
- *Violent mutuality* In a small minority of couples, individuals are repeatedly aggressive towards each other and engage in mutual combat in efforts to achieve control.

Some researchers have evaluated whether the use of typologies is helpful and whether 'batterers' do indeed fall into different categories (Huss and Ralston, 2008). Using cluster analysis, Huss and Ralston (2008) found some separate groups, but there were also some similarities between these. To date, cluster analysis has not been applied to investigating the differences identified by Johnson.

Explaining domestic abuse and partner violence

As we found with sexual offending, many factors play a contributory role in the occurrence of domestic abuse, and research investigations have found large numbers of variables associated with it. Ali and Naylor (2013a, 2013b) have reviewed the major categories of factors – biological, psychological, feminist, social and ecological – that have been found to play a part in the occurrence and patterning of IPV and the principal theories that have been offered to account for how they operate. Based on a household survey carried out in both urban and rural locations in ten countries, Abramsky *et al.* (2011) found that, despite sizeable variations in prevalence, there were some consistent associations between domestic violence towards women and a number of risk and protective factors. The risk factors included alcohol abuse, cohabitation status, younger age, attitudes supportive of spouse abuse, sexual partners outside the relationship, prior child abuse and exposure to DA. The protective factors included secondary education, high socioeconomic status and legally registered marriage. However, there is no straightforward link between multiple deprivation and rates of domestic violence – even when investigated in a single area, such as the city of São Paulo, Brazil (Kiss *et al.*, 2012).

In a review of 17 carefully selected studies published in the period 2000–2010, VanderEnde, Yount, Dynes and Sibley (2012) examined associations between DA and a number of community-level variables, such as indicators of social disorganisation, neighbourhood cohesion, socioeconomic status, levels of other forms of violence, and norms for behaviour between males and females. Levels of DA/IPV were not uniformly a direct function of concentrated disadvantage. While a relationship of that kind was reliably found in some large cities, it failed to emerge in other settings. In some societies, widespread acceptance of partner mistreatment, amongst both perpetrators and victims, appears to be a stronger influencing factor than poverty and associated hardships. The WHO has issued 'a call to action' for all nation-states to address the specific and endemic problem of violence against women as a vital aspect of ongoing global development (García-Moreno *et al.*, 2015).

At present, however, there is no satisfactory unified account regarding how potential contributory factors interconnect (Bell and Naugle, 2008; Dixon and Graham-Kevan, 2011). No single, comprehensive explanatory model of the causation of DA/IPV has attracted consensus support. What does seem clear is that in order to encompass the breadth of influences that appear to be directly or indirectly involved, several sets of factors, operating on different levels, need to be included in an integrative framework. A potentially useful way of conceptualising this is in terms of an 'ecological model' of the type forwarded by Heise (1998; see also Beyer, Wallis and Hamberger, 2015), as shown in Figure 9.4. This suggests that if we are to understand partner violence, we need to incorporate variables from four levels. Looking at Figure 9.4, we can consider the operating variables, moving from the right to the left of the overlapping ellipses:

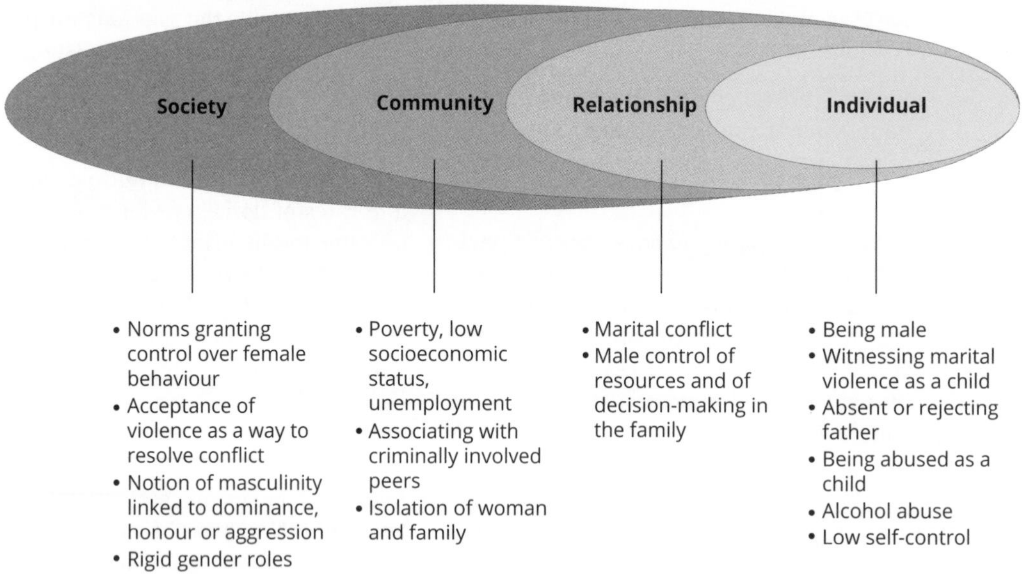
Society
Community
Relationship
Individual
• Norms granting control over female behaviour
• Acceptance of violence as a way to resolve conflict
• Notion of masculinity linked to dominance, honour or aggression
• Rigid gender roles
• Poverty, low socioeconomic status, unemployment
• Associating with criminally involved peers
• Isolation of woman and family
• Marital conflict
• Male control of resources and of decision-making in the family
• Being male
• Witnessing marital violence as a child
• Absent or rejecting father
• Being abused as a child
• Alcohol abuse
• Low self-control

Figure 9.4
An ecological model of intimate partner violence (IPV).

Source: adapted from Heise, L. L. (1998). Violence Against Women: An Integrated, Ecological Framework. Violence Against Women, 4 (3), 262–290, SAGE. DOI: https://doi.org/10.1177/1077801298004003002. Ideas additionally taken from Beyer, Wallis & Hamberger (2015).

» *Individual* Factors often associated with a higher risk of perpetrating IPV include being male, having witnessed marital violence as a child, having had an absent or rejecting father in early life, having been abused as a child, alcohol abuse, and low self-control. Although perpetrators show considerable heterogeneity (Dixon and Browne, 2003; Dixon and Graham-Kevan, 2011), several key variables, such as impulsivity or features of anger, often emerge from assessments (Birkley and Eckhardt, 2015; Eckhardt, Samper and Murphy, 2008; Norlander and Eckhardt, 2005).

» *Relationship* There are different patterns of dynamics within relationships, which may be egalitarian or may be marked by the exercise of power by one partner over another (Straus, 2008). Marital conflict more commonly results in male control of resources and of decision-making in the family. Violence may be triggered by specific events and situations in the course of the relationship (Wilkinson and Hamerschlag, 2005).

» *Community* The community surrounding the couple may be characterised by features often associated with higher levels of family stress and dysfunction (Beyer, Wallis and Hamberger, 2015; VanderEnde *et al.*, 2012). These include poverty, low socioeconomic status and unemployment, often resulting in the isolation of women and families. Adult males and females often spend large portions of time in segregated same-sex groups, which is thought likely to reinforce entrenched beliefs, perhaps more so if groups are composed of criminally involved peers.

» *Society* Many societies have rigid gender roles and norms that institute male control over female behaviour; and some accept violence as a way to resolve relational conflict. There is a widespread notion of masculinity linked to dominance, honour or aggression. The cultural norms within the society as a whole may permit or even instil dominance and inequity between females and males, with associated links to rates of relationship violence (Yodanis, 2004).

Responding to partner violence

In a historical review of provision for victims of partner violence, beginning in an era where such violence was often unrecognised, Barner and Carney (2011) described the emergence of legislation designed to address the problem of spousal abuse in the United States. They recounted the origins of the first women's refuges. There are now reportedly over 1,200 such shelters in the United Kingdom alone, the first having been established in 1972 (Corradi and Stöckl, 2014). From that period onwards, there has been steadily widening recognition of the extent of IPV as a major social problem, resulting in a series of changes in the law, in policing and in victims' services. The Vienna-based organisation WAVE (Women Against Violence Europe), housed by the Austrian Women's Shelter Network, has produced a series of reports on aspects of the provision of support services in 46 countries. Stelmaszek and Fisher (2012) and Logar and the WAVE Team (2016) provided a Europe-wide, country-by-country summary of what services are available. Across the 46 European countries surveyed, with a combined population of 831 million people, there are 2,937 women's centres. The majority (92 per cent) of these centres are in the 28 European Union member countries, while many other countries have only very limited provision.

These services have been largely self-organised by women victims of domestic assault, sometimes with help from volunteer agencies or health departments. Several types of public-service response have also been made in efforts to address domestic abuse. The principal patterns of action taken have included arrest of alleged perpetrators, obviously with the aim of proceeding to charges and prosecution. Due to case attrition, however, which occurs for a number of reasons – including insufficient evidence, and victim retraction and withdrawal – that process is often cut short. A number of other police or multi-agency community responses have been developed, most linked to women's refuges and other sources of support, and some mandated through court procedures (such as Protection or Restraining Orders).

Finally, there is a wide spectrum of psychologically based treatment or intervention programmes focused either on the perpetrator of violence and abuse or on the couple as a unit (Bowen, 2011). We will discuss some of these approaches and what is known about their effectiveness in Chapter 19.

Harassment and stalking

Harassment, whereby a person engages in repeated conduct that causes another person alarm or distress, may take place in a variety of contexts, but has been most extensively studied in work and educational environments, and in racial and other group conflicts. Because of the discrepancy in perceptions between perpetrators and victims, instances of harassment are often disputed. Possibly its most frequent form and the one we consider in most detail here, *sexual harassment*, has been 'defined psychologically as unwanted gender-based comments and behaviors that the targeted person appraises as offensive, that exceeds his/her available coping resources, and/or that threatens his/her well-being' (Buchanan and Harrell, 2011, p. 8). This has been found to be extremely widespread, with a survey of 16 European countries finding that between 40 per cent and 50 per cent of women experience some form of unwanted sexual attention at some point during their lifetime (European Commission, 1998). *Stalking* has similarities to harassment – which may also be part of it – but is a more specific pattern of behaviours in which an individual repeatedly seeks contact with another person who does not desire such contact.

By comparison with many other types of offence, harassment and stalking have been criminalised only quite recently in the UK and other countries. American states brought in laws for this purpose from 1990 onwards, with other countries doing so through the 1990s and 2000s. The relevant statutes in England and Wales include the Protection from Harassment Act 1997, which made it illegal to pursue a form of conduct that amounts to harassment of another. This did not formally ban stalking, but the Protection of Freedoms Act 2012 added a section (2A) to the 1997 Act, specifically to define the offences of *Stalking* and of *Stalking involving fear of violence or serious alarm and distress.* This made it against the law to contact, or to attempt to contact, someone who does not want such contact; to monitor his or her

9

activity, either directly or through internet, email or other electronic communication; or to watch or to spy on a person, or to loiter in any private or public place to be able to do so. The Sex Discrimination Act 1975 had made it unlawful to discriminate against someone on the grounds of gender. However, it did not specifically outlaw sexual harassment; that only occurred following an Amendment introduced in 2008, which required employers to protect employees from harassment by third parties.

During the year 2015–2016, 155,444 incidents of harassment and 4,155 cases of stalking were recorded by police in England and Wales. In the majority of cases, victims were female – for harassment preponderantly so, but for stalking in a ratio generally estimated at 3:1. As with the other types of crime discussed in this chapter, it is likely that numerous incidents of harassment remain unreported. Some evidence suggests that in the case of stalking, incidents may be reported but not acted upon unless they reach a quite serious level. A United States National Victimization Survey found that, over a 12-month period, 5.1 million women and 2.4 million men were victims of stalking. The estimated lifetime prevalence of stalking victimisation was 5.7 per cent for men and 15.2 per cent for women (6.5 million male and 18.3 million female victims: Breiding *et al.*, 2014). In trying to explain the 'dark figure' (hidden figure, see Chapter 2) of stalking in the United States, Brady and Nobles (2015) studied patterns of seeking and receiving help in relation to stalking in Houston, Texas. Over an eight-year period, Houston Police Department received a total of 3,756 calls requesting such help, but only 66 resulted in stalking incident reports, and there were only 12 arrests. No explanation could be found for this, but part of it appeared to be that the 'threshold' for defining stalking as a crime was set too high.

Sexual harassment

Sexual harassment can have a range of consequences for victims, usually considered in two main categories. The first is its impact on work or educational careers, as some element of those may often have been the levers that perpetrators used to manipulate victims (Willness, Steel and Lee, 2007). There may be effects on job satisfaction and on productivity; and, as opportunities for promotion are withheld or blocked, victims may withdraw from organisations in which they would otherwise have stayed. The second is its impact on personal well-being and health. These may include anxiety, stress, depression and other psychological reactions. If the harassment is prolonged or includes actual assault, the consequences may be similar to those found amongst victims of any other form of sexual assault.

Pina, Gannon and Saunders (2009) reviewed research on perpetrators of sexual harassment and on attempts to explain their behaviour. While we might expect harassment to be abuse of power by someone higher in an organisational hierarchy over someone lower in that hierarchy, that is not always the case. Since it appears to occur in a very wide range of workplaces, there are no clear social or demographic characteristics of perpetrators. Several scales have been developed for possible identification of those with a proclivity to harass, but only one, the *Likelihood to Sexually Harass Scale* (LSH), has been well validated (Pina and Gannon, 2012). It has, however, proved difficult to isolate any clear pattern of personality features amongst those who harass, and an understanding of this behaviour requires the application of the model of person–situation interactions that we have described in other chapters of this book.

Pina and Gannon (2012) appraised several theories that have been forwarded in attempts to explain harassment. They include *Sociocultural Theory*, a variant of Feminist Theory that views harassment as an extension of male dominance. This, however, fails to account for the fact that most men do not engage in sexual harassment, and that the trend towards convergence of gender roles in recent decades has not led to a reduction in the frequency of sexual harassment. *Organisational Theory* attributes greater explanatory potential to features of power relations and atmosphere within workplaces and other environments. *Sex-role Spillover Theory* suggests that individuals bring with them to their workplaces wider beliefs or attitudes related to gender stereotypes, such as the view that women should not rise to powerful positions, and that this results in conflict and in making use of opportunities to harass. *Natural/biological theories* view harassment as an extension of mating strategies programmed through human evolution, whereby males, held to be more innately sexually aggressive, use harassment to increase their access to the maximum number of females. In addition to these, there is a *four-factor theory* which combines features of the previous models, and which sets out a series of preconditions for harassment which parallel those stated in Finkelhor's theory of child sexual abuse, described earlier in this chapter.

Willness *et al.* (2007) reported a meta-analysis of 41 studies of work-based sexual harassment, with an aggregate study sample of 68,343 participants. This indicated that the strongest predictor of sexual harassment was *organisational climate*, meaning the extent of tolerance within a company or institution for people acting in sexually exploitative ways, and whether or not there were formal guidelines naming objectionable behaviour and making it possible for those affected to file grievances. A second key variable was *job gender context*, the extent to which occupational work roles were defined along traditional 'gendered' lines.

Harassing behaviours can be placed along a continuum that includes verbal and non-verbal components. As noted in a study of sexual harassment on a college campus, 'situational characteristics and individual differences of perceivers affect interpretations of social-sexual behavior' (Stockdale, Vaux and Cashin, 1995, p. 471). Harassment may begin with repeated glances or compliments, which at first might not be unwelcome. But these may progress to inappropriate staring, increasing over-familiarity, intrusiveness, use of innuendo, unwanted touching, sexual manipulation, intimidation and coercion. Victims may be vulnerable in some respect, and that may be a reason why they are targeted.

Pina and Gannon (2012) reviewed evidence concerning the antecedents and consequences of sexual harassment and developed a model of how variables interact. Antecedents include the overall gender ratio within an organisation, but more specifically the ratio at different levels or grades. Permissive attitudes or adverse relationships may allow perpetrators to create patterns of dominance and submissiveness. Individuals who exploit such opportunities show high scores on the LSH scale and may also show features in common with other sex offenders, such as endorsement of 'rape myths' or sexual hostility, alongside poor perspective-taking ability and authoritarian attitudes (Begany and Milburn, 2002).

Stalking

There is a stereotypical image of stalking: that the main victims are celebrities who, as a result of their media exposure, become a fixation for someone with severe mental health problems. Such cases do occur; and the introduction of the first laws against stalking, in California in 1990, followed on the murder of a young actress, Rebecca Schaeffer, by a fan who had become first infatuated and then very angry with her (Saunders, 1998). But the two had never previously met. This type of outcome is very uncommon, however: in the majority of cases, stalking arises as an extension or aberration of normal relationship processes.

Stalking was defined by Mullen, Pathé and Purcell (2001, p. 335) as behaviour characterised by repeated intrusions that involve 'unwanted contacts such as following, approaching or surveillance, unwanted telephone calls, e-mails, letters or graffiti'. Today we can also include communications via other social networks: *cyberstalking* has been described as possibly more threatening than physical stalking because the identity of the perpetrator remains concealed (Miller, 2012).

A strategy we have seen applied elsewhere is to establish whether a problem manifests itself in different ways, which suggests that distinct risk or causal factors may be operating. Based on a study of 145 stalkers in Australia (79 per cent male), Mullen, Pathé, Purcell and Stuart (1999) developed a typology that has had a wide influence on other research (e.g. Youngs, Ioannou and Straszewicz, 2013). They divided their study sample into five groups, as follows:

» *Rejected* Individuals who pursue former intimate partners following a break-up, seeking either reconciliation or in some cases revenge. This is described as the most commonly encountered group.

- *Intimacy-seeking* Individuals who probably have unmet emotional needs and who become romantically attached to someone whom they are convinced will eventually reciprocate their feelings, and who persist despite being rebuffed.
- *Incompetent suitor* Socially inept yet often intimidating individuals, who intrude on strangers or others only casually known to them. A given episode may be short-lived, but it may be repeated with different targets, one after another.
- *Resentful* Individuals who pursue a victim to obtain revenge for a perceived or an actual injury, who are motivated by an urge to cause distress to their victims, and who are gratified by the sense of power they obtain from doing so.
- *Predatory* Individuals whose stalking is part of a wider pattern of sexual offending and represents a stage in the process of planning an assault.

Many other typologies have been forwarded. Spitzberg and Cupach (2007) list 24 of them, and both they and Miller (2012) note that similar themes run though nearly all the classifications. These include rejection from relationships; *erotomania* (love obsession); the exercise of power through threat or revenge; and delusional states or other forms of mental disorder.

Spitzberg and Cupach (2007) reported a meta-analysis of 175 studies of stalking. They distinguish it from unwanted pursuit of intimacy, which they termed *obsessive relational intrusion* (ORI). This resembles stalking and clearly must be very aggravating to the recipient, but does not surpass a 'reasonable threshold of fear or threat'. It can, however, develop into stalking. Different sets of studies within their meta-analysis illuminate separate aspects of the problem. While a majority of victims (60–80 per cent) were women, the proportion of male victims was markedly higher than for harassment. Across both genders, most victims (79 per cent) were acquainted with the person who stalked them. Where duration of stalking was recorded, it was found to continue for an average of 22 months. In 82 studies that analysed whether stalking led to violence, 32 per cent of stalking cases involved physical and 12 per cent involved sexual violence.

As with harassment, behaviours that gradually take shape as stalking can initially be hard to distinguish from activities that occur in normal close relationships. The stalker and victim may previously have shared an intimate or romantic attachment. There is a continuum of behaviours, from repeatedly sending messages or gifts, via intently watching someone or shadowing their movements, to intimidation, threats and violence. Rather than develop a typology of individuals, the objective of some research has been to classify stalking behaviours.

Spitzberg and Cupach (2014) identified a set of eight clusters of actions that they considered to be distinct features of stalking. They are: (a) *hyper-intimacy*, or subjecting someone to intense and often highly demonstrative levels of attention; (b) *mediated contacts*, meaning very frequent messaging or other cyber activity; (c) *interactional contacts*, which consist of arranging to cross paths with, even to ambush, the victim; (d) *surveillance*, which involves keeping close watch on the victim's activities, even by clandestine methods such as spyware; (e) *invasion*, whether by gaining illegal access to personal information or by breaking into the victim's home; (f) *harassment and intimidation*, involving acts such as making threats, being insulting, or spreading rumours; (g) *coercion and threat*, issuing explicit statements or demands linked to menacing consequences; and (h) *aggression and violence*, which may include assault, property damage, or, in the most extreme cases, killing the victim and even relatives.

Of the studies in Spitzberg and Cupach's (2007) review, 24 reported evidence on *motives* for stalking. A series of 124 motives was compiled, which the authors assigned to four major categories as follows:

- *Intimacy* These included rage at abandonment, pain of rejection, loss, loneliness, dependency, infatuation, jealousy, love, obsession, seeking reconciliation, sexual desire, or preoccupation. Collectively, these were present in a third of the cases studied.

- *Aggression* These included anger, hostility, retaliation, revenge, projection of blame, possession/control, power, or intimidation. These represented 20–25 per cent of cases.
- *Disability-based motives* These related to drugs or to mental disorder. They represented just over 10 per cent of cases.
- *Task conflict or related issues* These arose, for example, from business, financial or neighbour disputes. These too represented in the region of 10 per cent of cases.

Other cases showed multiple motives, and only a small number remained 'miscellaneous' or 'unclassifiable'.

Clearly, for any victim of stalking, a key concern is that it should stop. Victim surveys suggest that being stalked results in considerable emotional damage (McEwan, Pathé and Ogloff, 2011). Also of key concern is whether stalking is likely to culminate in violence. Assessing this presents a challenging task. Amongst a series of 85 men convicted of stalking, James and Farnham (2003) found that serious violence, including homicide, was more likely to be committed by those *without* previous convictions for assault, and who did not have a problem of substance misuse or a diagnosis of personality disorder. This is quite unlike the links usually found for violence in general. Whether or not threats of violence are associated with actual violence appears to depend on the groups studied. Spitzberg, Cupach and Ciceraro (2010) collated the findings of 21 studies of reports of obsessional relational intrusion (ORI; described earlier) and of stalking amongst US student populations, and the findings of a meta-analysis of 274 studies from several countries that included both victims and perpetrators of stalking (total sample size 331,121). When they analysed the correlation between issuing threats of violence and carrying them out, this was low and non-significant in forensic and clinical study samples, but was 'substantial in magnitude' (p. 278) and statistically significant in general population and college samples; unfortunately the authors do not present statistical outcomes relating to this.

On the basis of several studies, Mullen, McEwan and their colleagues developed the *Stalking Risk Profile* (SRP), an assessment of factors that could be used to predict the path an individual's actions might follow once stalking incidents had been reported (McEwan, Pathé and Ogloff, 2011; Mullen *et al.*, 2006). This assessment involves collecting five kinds of information: on the nature of the relationship between the stalker and the victim; on the stalker's motives; on psychological and social aspects of the stalker, including any mental health problems; on any patterns of vulnerability in the victim; and on the legal and mental health context of the stalking events. This information first allows classification of individuals according to the typology outlined earlier, and can also provide a framework for making judgments of risk. McEwan *et al.* (2016) have reported a validation study of the SRP based on a follow-up of 241 individuals (7.7 per cent female), referred to a forensic mental health clinic as a result of stalking, over an average period of four years. The SRP was moderately successful in predicting levels of stalking recurrence (of either the same or a different victim) for those classified in high-, medium- and low-risk bands. However, the overall predictive accuracy of the profile was low. Results showed some success in its capacity to predict the stalking of new victims, but poor discrimination in terms of predicting new stalking behaviours against existing victims. These findings underline the difficulty of predicting the course of events in this complex form of behaviour.

In a study comparing 479 male with 71 female stalkers in Sweden and Australia, Strand and McEwan (2012) found that similar factors predicted the likelihood of violence in both genders. The rate of violence was slightly but not significantly higher amongst males; and the combination of three factors – existence of a prior intimate relationship, persistent approach behaviour and making threats – was predictive of stalking violence for both sexes.

Explanations of stalking

Several attempts have been made to explain stalking. Given the dysfunctional nature of the behaviour, and that stalkers are often profoundly agitated and unhappy, an obvious step is to attribute it to some form of mental disorder, and it is true that a proportion of those who engage in stalking have been or are subsequently diagnosed with one or other form of such disorder (Kamphuis and Emmelkamp, 2000). Yet that finding in itself does not constitute an explanation, as we then have to explain the origin of the associated disorder, with the additional problem of explaining why it has taken this form with one individual when another with a similar diagnosis does not stalk.

There are five main theoretical accounts that have been offered:

» *Evolutionary theory* Duntley and Buss (2012) have forwarded the view that stalking is a product of human evolution. It presents one strategy amongst others in mate selection, as a means of regaining sexual access to a former partner, or of preventing access by others. The fact that this sometimes succeeds, even if that is rare, shows its usefulness as an adaptive mechanism. Brüne (2003) applies similar concepts in seeking to explain why erotomania, which is associated with some patterns of stalking, is more prevalent in men than in women.

» *Coercive control theory* According to this view, stalking serves the purposes of maintaining surveillance and control over the victim's everyday activities and social environment, and includes making threats and progressively isolating the stalking target (Dutton and Goodman, 2005). As such it has close links to the factors that drive intimate partner violence, and both can be understood in the same context, that of male dominance over females, which is deeply embedded in many cultures.

» *Relational goal pursuit* This model, forwarded by Spitzberg *et al.* (2010), draws on their proposal (discussed earlier) that stalking is an extended version of obsessive relational intrusion. While ORI is usually annoying and troublesome but not inherently threatening, stalking exceeds the boundaries of acceptable behaviour as a result of the self-regulation problems of the perpetrator. Individuals narrow the concept of their relationship goals and focus exclusively on one other person. If they are then rejected, they energetically resist that rejection and experience a strong negative affect as a result, leading to the sequence of behaviours that Spitzberg and Cupach (2014) defined as characteristic of stalking.

» *Attachment theory* This theory is widely adopted as an account of problems in close relationships and emotional regulation in adulthood. It traces the origins of such difficulties to dysfunctional family environments or disrupted emotional links with caregivers during childhood, as a result of which individuals did not develop secure attachments to adult figures and so did not internalise healthy working models of how to relate happily to others. In a study with 2,783 American college students, Patton, Nobles and Fox (2010) found that those who admitted to having stalked someone (5.8 per cent of the sample) showed significantly higher rates of anger-related problems and of anxious, insecure attachment styles than those who did not.

» *Social learning* Fox, Nobles and Akers (2010) reported a self-report survey of stalking in 2,766 American college students, in which they were also asked to provide information about patterns of association with others. Stalking perpetrators, 5.79 per cent of the survey group, were significantly more likely to report having friends who had also stalked, and had more tolerant attitudes towards the behaviour, including use of neutralisations, suggesting that differential association and peer learning may be factors in permitting individuals to act in this way.

At present there is not enough evidence to evaluate the relative strengths of each of these approaches. Davis, Swan and Gambone (2012) outline a possible programme of research that could generate information for testing some of them, or for combining concepts from each theory and formulating a more comprehensive model that was also more firmly evidence-based.

Chapter summary

The chapter has focused on three groups of offences which evidence suggests, despite many changes in recent years, continue to be massively under-reported and under-recorded. One is sexual offending against children and adults, and related types of crime. The second is domestic abuse or violence against intimate partners. The third is harassment and stalking.

Sexual offending takes a wide variety of forms. After considering legal definitions and data on prevalence, the chapter focused on several of its most serious forms. We first discussed approaches to estimating offence seriousness, which in itself is a complex task. We then reviewed what is known concerning the relationship between the different motives that influence rape, and typologies that have been developed for classifying rape.

The chapter then reviewed evidence on the causes of sex offending against children, the 'preconditions' model, and the role of paedophilia (discussed again in Chapter 11). We examined the role of pornography and the emergence of non-contact, internet-based offending, and what is known about the amount of movement between this and contact crime. This was followed by a discussion of the nature and extent of 'crossover' between different categories of victim.

We next summarised the findings from the accumulated evidence on risk factors for sexual offending, and moved from the correlational approach to models of causation. From a wide spectrum of possibilities, we focused on the Integrated Theory of Sexual Offending (ITSO), which combines concepts from a number of earlier approaches. Finally, we reviewed follow-up data on the rate of sexual recidivism, which is generally lower than for most other types of offence.

The second major area covered in the chapter was that of violence between intimate partners (IPV). The chapter considered definitions, reviewed data on prevalence, and examined several disputed issues associated with this type of offence. We considered a number of explanatory factors leading to the presentation of a multi-level 'ecological' model which appears to be the most comprehensive approach to understanding these kinds of offences.

The third area covered was that of sexual harassment and stalking. The former is a relatively common experience for many women, and evidence suggests that there are insufficient protections against it in many organisations. An important aspect of the latter is that it is not something that happens only to people with a highly visible public image, but something that can emerge in other contexts, including the breakdown of, or the desire for, close relationships.

9

Further reading

» There are several edited volumes that address the field of sexual offending or particular aspects of it. The largest and most compendious are expensive but should be accessible in libraries. The most voluminous and up to date are these:

- Amy Phenix and Harry M. Hoberman (eds) (2016). *Sexual Offending: Predisposing Antecedents, Assessments and Management*. New York: Springer.
- Douglas P. Boer (ed.) (2016). *The Wiley Handbook on the Theories, Assessment and Treatment of Sexual Offending*. New York: Wiley-Blackwell. (Three volumes.)

» Slightly less recent, but still weighty and wide-ranging books include:

- D. Richard Laws and William T. O'Donohue (eds) (2008). *Sexual Deviance: Theory, Assessment and Treatment*, 2nd edition. New York: Guilford Press.
- Douglas P. Boer, Reinhard Eher, Leam A. Craig, Michael H. Miner and Friedemann

Pfäfflin (eds) (2011). *International Perspectives on the Assessment and Treatment of Sexual Offenders*. Chichester: Wiley-Blackwell.

- Anthony R. Beech and Leam A. Craig (eds) (2009). *Assessment and Treatment of Sex Offenders*. Chichester: Wiley-Blackwell.

» On partner and other family violence, for a book that also covers sexual abuse inside families, see:

- Ola W. Barnett, Cindy L. Miller-Perrin and Robin D. Perrin (2011). *Family Violence Across the Lifespan: An Introduction*, 3rd edition. Thousand Oaks, CA: Sage Publications.

» Specifically on partner violence, see:

- Nicola Groves and Terry Thomas (2014). *Domestic Violence and Criminal Justice*. Abingdon: Routledge.
- Michael P. Johnson (2008). *A Typology of Domestic Violence: Intimate Terrorism, Violent Resistance, and Situational Couple Violence*. Boston, MA: Northeastern University Press.

Although the book is mainly focused on treatment, there is good background material in:

- Erica Bowen (2011). *The Rehabilitation of Partner-Violent Men*. Chichester: Wiley-Blackwell.

Other Serious Crimes

This chapter considers the role of psychological factors in a variety of serious crimes. We begin with substance-related offences. Many criminal acts occur when individuals are under the influence of alcohol. In a smaller proportion of cases, individuals may be affected by other substances, or may commit offences in order to maintain a drug-using habit. Possession or sales of controlled substances are offences in themselves, and often lead to other crimes including violence. The first section of the chapter explores the nature of these connections.

We then go on to consider several quite different kinds of offences, including robbery, arson and kidnapping. The chapter concludes with an exploration of serious economic crimes, which criminologists often contrast with 'street crimes' as they arise in different contexts and are often disregarded in mainstream discussions. Throughout, we focus on what is known about psychological factors in the offences described, although for some types of offence the extent of that knowledge is very limited.

Chapter objectives

- To survey what is known about psychological factors and processes in substance misuse, and in what ways they are related to crime.
- To examine psychological factors involved in the offences of robbery, arson and kidnapping.
- To consider the role of psychological factors in serious economic crimes.

Alcohol- and substance-related offending

There is evidence that we humans have made use of psychotropic or 'mind-altering' substances since prehistory, and some form of such uses appears in virtually every society on Earth. Today, alcohol, tobacco and caffeine are readily obtainable throughout most of the world. Some communities use other substances, such as *kava*, a type of shrub, the roots of which are brewed on many islands of the Pacific to make a drink that contains several psychoactive ingredients. In the past, indigenous peoples of the Americas extracted *mescaline*, a hallucinogenic drug believed to produce spiritual experiences, from different kinds of cactus. Archaeologists have found that leaves of the *coca* plant, the source of cocaine, were used in Peru up to 10,000 years ago (Dillehay *et al.*, 2010). There is even a claim that the Neolithic revolution, the momentous change from nomadic to settled lifestyles and the development of agriculture, was spurred by a desire not to bake bread but to brew beer (Braidwood *et al.*, 1953).

The list of substances with sedative, stimulant, euphoric or other pleasurable effects is a very long one. Alongside their allure, however, such substances also have a downside. All of them are essentially toxins. They affect not just the brain, which is why they are sought after, but also the kidneys, the liver, the heart and other vital organs. Consumed in sufficient quantities, they can be ruinous to health, and can even prove fatal. They are often the means by which people take their own lives. As a result, most drugs are subject to legal controls. In the United Kingdom, the relevant law is the Misuse of Drugs Act 1971, which divides controlled drugs into three classes (A, B and C) according to their risk of causing harm. The Home Office (2016a) has published a *Controlled Drugs List*, though it is stated to be 'not exhaustive'.

The relevance of this to forensic psychologists is, of course, that substance use is also linked to several forms of crime. We can divide this into three broad categories:

» The possession of controlled substances, even if only for personal use, is an offence in itself. Under the Misuse of Drugs Act 1971, possession can result in a prison sentence of up to two years for a Class C drug, and seven years for a Class A drug, though many cases are dealt with more leniently.

» The manufacture, distribution, sale and trafficking of illegal drugs are more serious offences, which under the Misuse of Drugs Act can lead to life imprisonment. Given the scale of drugs markets, these activities are often associated with other types of serious crime.

» Substance use alters individuals' thinking and feeling (otherwise, why do it?). The resulting behavioural changes often include committing criminal acts. In terms of the sheer numbers of offences, this type of connection is by far the most common.

Apart from possession, the link between substances and crime is not a straightforward causal one and it is not inevitable. Nevertheless, the connection occurs with sufficient regularity for substance misuse to be considered one of the principal risk factors for involvement in crime (and is one of the 'central eight' risk/need factors identified by Bonta and Andrews, 2017).

Investigation of the links between substances and crime has followed different pathways, mainly influenced by the levels of legal control applied to each drug. Given its accessibility, alcohol is often considered separately and is the most intensively researched. It is subject to some restrictions (licensing laws) regarding who can buy or sell it and when. Yet many people drink alcohol in a moderate and problem-free way, and its use is so widespread that often people do not even think of it as a drug. According to the World Health Organization (2011a), however, alcohol is associated with no fewer than 60 different diseases. In 2012 there were 3.3 million deaths globally due to alcohol consumption, and harmful drinking 'ranks among the top five risk factors for disease, disability and death throughout the world' (WHO, 2014, p. 2). The cost of alcoholic beverages can be very low and, given their availability, alcohol is the substance most often associated with offending.

What is called 'substance-related offending' more often refers to use of controlled drugs, sometimes loosely referred to as 'street drugs'. These include cannabis, ecstasy, cocaine, heroin and many other substances prohibited in most countries, often with severe penalties for their use or sale. These drugs can be classified in various ways – for example, as narcotics, hallucinogens and so on – but the terminology in this area is often employed very loosely. More precise definitions are given in the World Health Organization's (1994) *Lexicon of Alcohol and Drug Terms.*

In addition, there is also a sizeable underground market in some prescription medicines, controlled pharmaceuticals which are instead used 'recreationally' for their impact on mood. These include amphetamines (taken for their stimulant effects), barbiturates or benzodiazepines (taken for soothing effects), analgesics (taken for pain-relieving but also calming effects) and hypnotics (sleep inducers).

These patterns have existed for some time. To complicate the picture somewhat, in recent years a novel phenomenon has emerged, in the form of 'new psychoactive substances' (NPSs). The synthetic production of compounds that had similar properties to existing illicit drugs but had not yet been placed under formal control led to the appearance of a succession of what were popularly called 'legal highs', which could be bought via the internet. The most potent of these include drugs that contain synthetic cannabinoids: similar to the chemicals found in the marijuana plant, but made in a laboratory. They include the drug known as K2 or Spice, which is thought to have contributed to rising levels of violence in prisons in 2015–2016. Between 2010 and 2016 in England and Wales, over 500 NPSs were banned using the Misuse of Drugs Act. To impose a 'blanket ban' on further innovations of this type, the Psychoactive Substances Act 2016 was introduced. Nevertheless, some NPSs continue to be widely available.

There are many thousands of compounds that have effects on the human body and on personal experience that are pleasurable in the short term but harmful in the longer term. Which ones are the most often used in ways that cause harm? It has been argued that the threefold classification used in the Misuse of Drugs Act 1971 is not an accurate reflection of harms caused by drugs. That issue has been researched for the UK, producing a set of results discussed in the 'Focus on ...' box below.

FOCUS ON ...

Comparing drug harms

People use a wide range of mind-altering substances to induce pleasant states or to reduce unpleasant ones. These substances have the disadvantage that all of them also have toxic effects; they are all harmful to some extent. When consumed in large amounts or over long periods, they can cause major health problems and cut lives short.

In a report prepared for the Department of Health in London, Jones, Bates *et al*. (2011) presented tables giving detailed information on the types of harm associated with 17 major categories of drugs. These included both those that are legal and regulated (such as alcohol, tobacco and prescription drugs) and those that are wholly prohibited. Most potentially harmful drugs are controlled by law, and attempts have also been made to classify them according to the levels of harm associated with each. Nutt, King, Saulsbury and Blakemore (2007) set out to do this by measuring three types of drug harm: (a) the physical harm caused to the individual; (b) the extent to which people are likely to develop dependence; and (c) the wider effect of the drug on other individuals and on society. Applying this to a series of 20 substances, it was clear that the levels of harm caused by each drug bore only a loose relation to its classification (A, B or C) under the Misuse of Drugs Act 1971.

This analysis attracted some criticism, as one of its outcomes was that heroin was ranked as the UK's most dangerous drug, even though in terms of sheer numbers there are more deaths associated with alcohol and tobacco. Caulkins, Reuter and Coulson (2011, p. 1886) argued that *individual* and *aggregate* levels of harm are 'entirely different concepts' and should not be mingled: and that the harm rankings obtained from each are entirely different and averaging or merging them makes no sense.

By then, Nutt, King and Phillips (2010) had already produced a revised list of harm levels. They did this using a fuller set of 16 criteria, each weighted according to its relative importance as assigned by a committee of experts. Crime was third in the list of categories of social cost, after economic cost and injury cost. The rank ordering of the ten most dangerous substances then became, in descending order: alcohol, heroin, crack cocaine, metamphetamine, cocaine, tobacco, amphetamine, cannabis, GHB and benzodiazepines.

The substances associated with the highest levels of harm were alcohol, heroin and crack cocaine. More detailed analysis showed associations of each substance with crime. Most drugs showed some links of this kind, with the strongest for heroin, alcohol, crack cocaine, cannabis and amphetamines (p. 1563). This may underestimate the role of alcohol, partly as a result of its frequency of use, and partly because some of its various effects are indirect.

Question

In your view, which approach is the more informative: to classify drugs solely in terms of their known risks to health, or to take account of social factors such as the extent of their use?

Humans appear to be the only species that has learned to make deliberate use of the mood-altering capacities of a variety of chemical compounds, which when swallowed, inhaled or injected can produce such a range of keenly coveted effects. Although there are documented cases of animals becoming intoxicated, that has usually occurred by accident in laboratory situations. There seems to be no real basis for the tale that African elephants allow fruits of the *Marula* tree to ferment in order to produce alcohol. It has been estimated that the amount of fruit an adult elephant would need to ingest in order to become inebriated in this way is 400 per cent of its normal dietary intake (Morris, Humphreys and Reynolds, 2006), an unlikely scenario even on feast days.

Alcohol and crime

Although alcohol is a legalised drug in most societies, there are laws governing access to it. Under some circumstances offences can arise in direct violation of those laws, such as driving while intoxicated, public drunkenness, or sales to under-age persons. In addition, information of different kinds and from several sources also shows that alcohol is a risk factor for involvement in numerous other kinds of antisocial conduct and criminal activity, including both acquisitive and violent offending.

Alcohol appears to have a particular role in relation to violence. Such violence includes not only fighting in bars or public places, but also intimate partner violence (Foran and O'Leary, 2008; Langenderfer, 2013; Murphy *et al.*, 2005), sexual assault (Finney, 2003) and homicide (Shaw *et al.*, 2006; Wieczorek, Welte and Abel, 1990). Regarding the last of these, Kuhns, Exum, Clodfelter and Bottia (2014) reported a meta-analysis of 23 studies across nine countries and a cumulative sample of 28,265 homicide offenders. They found that an average of 48 per cent of perpetrators were described as 'under the influence' of alcohol at the time of the offence, and 37 per cent were 'intoxicated' (the effects were more pronounced). (Note that these findings are based on witness reports and not on breath or blood tests.) Similar proportions were found amongst homicide victims (Kuhns *et al.*, 2011). In addition, alcohol is thought to play a part in both the abuse and the neglect of children (Robinson and Hassle, 2001; Wilczynski, 1995). Generally, heavy drinking by parents can have a detrimental effect on children's physical and psychological well-being (Kroll and Taylor, 2003).

Other findings relevant to the alcohol–crime relationship include the following:

- *Violent offences* Arrest records from several countries suggest that a large proportion of violent offences (with a range of 40–66 per cent) are committed when perpetrators are under the influence of alcohol (Graham, Parkes, McAuley and Doi, 2012).
- *Victims' perceptions* A large proportion of victims participating in the Crime Survey for England and Wales (47 per cent in 2014–2015) believed offenders to be under the influence of alcohol at the time of a violent incident (Office for National Statistics, 2016b).
- *Alcohol-related problems* Surveys show that sizeable proportions of convicted adults in prison or on probation have alcohol-related problems. For example, a UK survey found 63 per cent of male and 39 per cent of female sentenced prisoners had engaged in 'hazardous drinking' in the year before being imprisoned (Singleton *et al.*, 1998).
- *Life stresses* In-depth interview studies with persistent offenders reveal a temporal relationship between life stresses, alcohol consumption and criminal recidivism (Zamble and Quinsey, 1997). That is, the offenders' personal narratives typically show close connections between experiencing problems, resorting to drink, and then committing an offence.
- *Interpersonal violence* Self-report diary studies show specific temporal associations between drinking and assaults on intimate partners (e.g. Fals-Stewart, 2003); and a Swedish study with remand prisoners also found alcohol to be a significant trigger of interpersonal violence (Lundholm *et al.*, 2013).
- *Sexual assaults* Reviews of research on links between alcohol and sexual assault suggest that while alcohol may not play a direct causal role in sexual aggression, the timing of its use may be a precipitating factor (Abbey, 2011; Kraanen and Emmelkamp, 2011; Lorenz and Ullman, 2016).
- *General aggression* In a study carried out in a secure mental health unit in Sweden, alcohol was found to be associated with a higher risk of aggression within a 24-hour period of ingestion than other types of drugs (Haggard-Grann, Hallqvist, Långström and Möller, 2006). Thus it is possible that there are some direct neurophysiological effects of alcohol on liability to become aggressive amongst some individuals, though it is difficult to isolate this connection from other factors that may also be involved. Alternatively, the effect may be indirect, via the suppression of behavioural inhibition (self-control) capacities.

» *Mental and emotional functioning* Laboratory and experimental studies in psychopharmacology show that alcohol has various deleterious effects on reasoning, emotional control and decision-making (Exum, 2006; Field *et al.*, 2010). These effects appear to be particularly pronounced following a pattern of binge drinking. In a review, Courtney and Polich (2009) found evidence of deficits in frontal-lobe and working-memory functioning amongst binge as compared to non-binge drinkers, although they noted that there was no consensus definition of exactly what constituted a 'binge'.

Additional evidence comes from a 30-year follow-up study of a New Zealand birth cohort (n=1,265), showing that when other factors have been taken into account, alcohol has particular links with two kinds of offence: impulsive violent assaults; and property damage, vandalism and arson (Boden, Fergusson and Horwood, 2012). Similar results emerged from a study of offence patterns amongst a large representative sample of American prisoners (n=18,016). Homicide, physical assault, sexual assault, robbery and other 'confrontational' offences were more likely to be committed by an intoxicated offender than were other types of crime (Felson and Staff, 2010).

Does alcohol cause violent offending?

Thus there are well established *associations* between alcohol and violent offending, but does alcohol actually *cause* violent crime? One very extensive review concluded that there is indeed an unequivocal causal relationship between alcohol and aggression (Tomlinson, Brown and Hoaken, 2016).

Notwithstanding the sizeable amount of research, however, the mechanisms that mediate the alcohol–crime connection are not fully understood. Ethanol, the active ingredient in alcoholic drinks, has a pharmacological effect largely as a CNS depressant. This makes it seem an unlikely candidate for directly *inducing* violent or other criminal behaviour (Boles and Miotto, 2003), but it is thought it might do so in conjunction with a pre-existing propensity to aggressiveness (Giancola, 2006). Overall, alcohol appears more likely to contribute to violence via one or more of several possible mediating processes:

» *Disinhibition* After drinking, there is a reduced capacity for exercising deliberate, conscious or 'executive' control over impulses. One proposal is that this is due to the 'depletion of cognitive resources' caused by intoxication (Hirsch, Galinksy and Zhong, 2011); although the extent of this disinhibition is a function of the level of consumption, and the effects may be very specific (Montgomery *et al.*, 2012).

» *Narrowing of selective attention* Focusing on a limited range of information, such as perceived threats within a shortened time-span, can produce an effect that has been called 'alcoholic myopia' (Steele and Josephs, 1990; Giancola, Josephs, Parrott and Duke, 2010).

» *Anxiety reduction* Some individuals drink in order to gain social confidence, and when drinking may experience a temporary lowering of anxiety and a temporary lift in self-esteem. However, they may still feel vulnerable to interpersonal risks and threats, and therefore be prone to aggression (McMurran, 2011).

» *Outcome expectancies* Individuals' beliefs about alcohol, and what they anticipate will be its effects, will influence their pattern of drinking, alongside their prior likelihood of being aggressive (McMurran, 2007). Decisions to drink may be a function of these factors (Zhang, Welte and Wieczorek, 2002). In a naturalistic experiment, Bègue *et al.* (2009) compared the effects of alcohol expectancies with actual alcohol consumption, and found that the former, as well as aggressive dispositions, better predicted aggressive behaviour on a specially designed task than disposition alone. Similar results were obtained in a self-report study by Barnwell, Borders and Earleywine (2006). In two larger experiments involving a deceptive retaliation task, Levinson, Giancola and Parrott (2011) found that alcohol increased aggression amongst individuals with permissive or approving beliefs about aggression, but not amongst those who did not hold such beliefs.

Through complex interactions, a range of other individual factors influence the strength of the alcohol–crime relationship. It may be modulated by personality, by attitudes, and possibly by specific constellations of factors such as a hypermasculine or 'macho' orientation that also fosters high alcohol consumption (Graham and West, 2001). This may be particularly likely in a subgroup of the young adult male population (McMurran, Hoyte and Jinks, 2012; de Visser and Smith, 2007), at least in Western economies.

A multiplicity of sociocultural, temporal and situational factors come into operation when people drink alcohol, deriving from the places or events where that occurs, the purposes that alcohol serves, and the contexts in which individuals have learned to consume alcohol (Moore, 2001). The latter are associated in many societies not only with reward and pleasure, but with social ease and enjoyment, high excitement and 'letting go'. Problems of antisocial, criminal and violent behavior are most likely to arise in the context of prolonged or habitual heavy drinking, or of binge drinking, especially where that involves 'pre-loading' – drinking more cheaply at home prior to visiting costly night-time venues (Foster and Ferguson, 2012; Hughes, Anderson, Morleo and Bellis, 2008). The settings in which people drink may also be an important factor, as outlined in Chapter 6.

The availability of cheap alcoholic drinks is thought to be linked to levels of consumption, and thereby to health and public order problems. Concerns over this have influenced some governments towards a policy of *minimal unit pricing* for alcohol. This entails specifying a sale price per unit below which supermarkets and other retail outlets cannot drop. International evidence has shown that minimum pricing reduces overall rates of alcohol consumption (Wagenaar, Salois and Komro, 2009), of violence-related injuries (Matthews, Shepherd and Sivarajasingham, 2006), and of alcohol-related deaths (Zhao *et al.*, 2013). A proposal of this kind was considered by the UK government, but was abandoned. That decision was widely believed to have been a result of intensive behind-the-scenes lobbying by alcohol industry representatives (Gilmore and Daube, 2014; Gornall, 2014). A similar proposal was agreed in Scotland, and despite legal challenges by the Scotch Whisky Association (Woodhouse, 2017) was approved in 2017.

Other substance misuse

Estimated numbers of people using different illicit drugs around the world are set out in the annual reports of the United Nations Office on Drugs and Crime (UNODC). In January 2016 there were 244 drugs under international control. The UNODC (2016) estimated that globally 247 million people had used illicit drugs in the preceding year. Amongst them, 183 million people had used cannabis; 33 million had used opiates; and there was a steady flow of new psychoactive substances. The widespread desire for these drugs has resulted in the growth of a highly profitable world market for them, which in 2012 was estimated as having a value of over US $320 billion. The UNODC report includes maps showing rates of drug use in individual countries and of known drug-trafficking routes. Some aspects of drug trafficking as economic crime are discussed later in this chapter; here we focus on substance misuses at the individual level.

Data from the Crime Survey for England and Wales (Home Office, 2016b) show that the rate of misuse of several substances has been gradually declining in recent years. The rate of reported use of any drug in the preceding 12 months by the 16–24 age-group fell sharply from a high of 31.8 per cent in 1998 to 18 per cent in 2015–2016. Amongst a wider age band, 16–59, it fell more gently, from 12.1 per cent to 8.4 per cent, over the same period. There was a fall in the use of any Class A drug for 16–24-year-olds (8.6 per cent to 6.6 per cent), but the rate for 16–59-year-olds held steady (hovering in the range 3–4 per cent throughout the period). Only a small proportion of these two age-groups, 8 per cent (16–24) and 4 per cent (16–59), said they used a drug every day; 41 per cent (16–24) and 42 per cent (16–59) said they used a drug only once or twice in the entire year. The proportions of the two age-groups reporting use of a new psychoactive substance were 6 per cent (16–24) and 2.7 per cent (16–59). For the three most widely used drugs, cannabis, powder cocaine and ecstasy, those in the age band 16–59 saying they used the drug just once a month or less were 63 per cent, 89 per cent and 93 per cent respectively; thus the majority were only occasional users. There were more male than female users of every type of drug.

There are several forms of drug–crime connections. Goldstein (1985) proposed a taxonomy for the relationship between drug use and violent crime, involving three broad types:

- *Psychopharmacological* The first type describes the behaviour of habitual drug users that may be a result of the action of the substance. While, as with alcohol, there is little evidence of such a direct cause–effect relationship, Goldstein cites examples of individuals who became more vulnerable (having increased irritability and impulsiveness) and out of control during the process of withdrawal from drugs, or when their supplies were running short. These effects may be part of a process where, as with alcohol, drug abuse is also associated with an elevated risk of partner violence, as Moore *et al.* (2008) found in a meta-analysis of 96 studies, although the association was moderated by other factors.

- *Economic-compulsive* The second type consists of crime that arises from a drug-using individual's need to obtain more of the drug, or money to purchase it. A pattern of this kind was documented in two studies, by Parker and Newcombe (1987) and Jarvis and Parker (1989), who investigated how heroin users in England financed their substance use, which was often through acquisitive crime, mainly burglary and shoplifting, and also drug dealing. Of 46 heroin users interviewed in one study, 35 were spending far more than they could earn by legitimate means. After commencing regular heroin use, their rate of convictions had more than doubled.

- *Systemic* The third type refers to the conflicts that erupt between competing gangs in the drug supply chain. Given the sums involved, dealing in drugs is intensely competitive; and since it is outside the law, disputes are resolved by committing other crimes. Direct retaliation is therefore the preferred mode of addressing grievances in this context (Topalli, Wright and Fornango, 2002). Goldstein, Brownstein, Ryan and Bellucci (1988) analysed 414 homicides committed between March and October 1988 in New York City. They found that 52.7 per cent of them were drug-related, and amongst those 39.1 per cent were in the 'systemic' category.

Goldstein's 'tripartite' categorisation proved useful in proposing a framework for drugs research (Brownstein and Crossland, 2003). However, it has also been subjected to some criticisms, mainly on the grounds that there are other connections that it does not cover. Based on detailed interviews with 41 prisoners serving sentences for drug-related offences in the UK, Bennett and Holloway (2009) suggested some refinements. They analysed the connections between ten types of drug (including alcohol) and ten types of crime. They found that 56 per cent of the links could be placed in the 'economic-compulsive' category, and 37 per cent in the 'psychopharmacological' category. The remaining 7 per cent were linked to 'lifestyle'. In large measure, these findings validated Goldstein's typology, but with an added 'lifestyle' category at the individual level.

The drug–crime connection is vividly illustrated by results obtained from the *New English and Welsh Arrestee Drug Abuse Monitoring* (NEW-ADAM) study. Over an eight-year period, Bennett and Holloway (2007) contacted a total sample of 4,645 arrestees in 16 police custody suites. Amongst them, 2,833 tested positive for having used at least one drug. Within this cohort, 75 per cent of males and 81 per cent of females had a pattern of 'multiple drug use', meaning that they used two or more drugs over a 12-month period. Arrestees with that pattern reported twice as many property offences as those who used one drug only (a mean of 229 as compared to 104). There was also a close association between the incidence of crime in individuals' lives and the numbers of *different* drugs used. Those who used just one type had a mean offending rate only slightly higher than those who did not use drugs at all (104 as compared to 93).

However, those who used five different types of drug reported a mean of 195 offences, and those who used eleven different types of drug a mean of 337 offences. When asked if their substance use and crime were connected, 63 per cent replied that they were, and within that group 71 per cent said that that applied to all of their offences.

Bennett, Holloway and Farrington (2008b) adopted a different approach to analysing drug–crime connections, by making a meta-analysis of 30 studies. Each study reported data on one or more of five types of drugs – heroin, crack, cocaine, amphetamines and marijuana – and their relationship with total offending rates, and also with several specific types of offence (e.g. shop theft, property theft, drug supply and prostitution). They also examined the influence of gender and age. Analysis in terms of odds ratios showed that, overall, individuals involved in substance use were 2.8–3.8 times more likely to be involved in offending than others who were not involved. The ratios were highest for crack cocaine (>6), were 3.0–3.5 for heroin, and were approximately 2.5 for powder cocaine. Rates for amphetamines and for marijuana were lower, at 1.8–1.9 and 1.4–1.5 respectively.

However, these associations do not establish a causal path from drugs to crime. Hayhurst *et al.* (2017) reported a meta-analysis of 20 studies in an attempt to identify temporal patterns in the relationship between involvement in substance use and crime. Unfortunately, as all the located studies dealt only with opiates, they did not allow a test of the relationship between cocaine and crime, the drug that had the highest odds ratio in the Bennett *et al.* (2008b) meta-analysis. The average age of onset of offending across the studies was 16.7 years, while the average age of onset of opiate use was 19.6 years – the reverse of what would be expected if substance use *caused* crime. However, across the majority of samples in the studies, there was an increase in rates of theft, burglary and robbery following opiate use. The studies were too heterogeneous for computation of a mean effect size to make sense. Given the methodological weakness of some studies, the authors advised that more research was needed before a clear conclusion could be drawn.

Factors influencing substance use

Analysing trends over time, it emerges consistently that drug use is more prevalent in the teenage and early adult years with a steady decline thereafter, not unlike the pattern of the age–crime curve. Hence the division in Home Office data, cited earlier, into '16–24' and '16–59' age-groups.

Frisher *et al.* (2007) reviewed research on factors that predicted illicit substance use among young people. From a total of 251 relevant studies identified, 78 (62 quantitative and 16 qualitative) were analysed in detail. Risk factors were separated into four main categories: 'personal/biological', including evidence on the influence of genes, gender, ethnicity, mental disorder and variables such as sensation-seeking; 'personal/behavioural', including educational variables, conduct, delinquency, tobacco/alcohol use, attitudes and rebelliousness; 'relationship variables', including family bonds, parental controls and peer-group membership; and 'structural factors', including socioeconomic status, neighbourhood variables and drug availability.

The strongest and also the most consistent associations to emerge were for family variables. Patterns of family interaction, parental discipline and monitoring emerged as significant, and there was very limited evidence that such links were due to genetic factors. Having problems at school, such as poor attendance and truancy, predicted substance use. Peer influence also played a role, as did permissive attitudes towards drug use and drug availability. For many other variables, findings were contradictory.

Gateway hypothesis

The question has often been posed as to whether there is a kind of 'natural progression' in the order in which people become regular drug users, such that trying 'soft drugs' will be an inevitable route into using 'hard drugs'.

These terms are fairly arbitrary and difficult to define, but generally refer to drugs carrying lower versus higher risks of **addiction**. Sources differ with respect to which substances they place in each category. Sometimes alcohol and tobacco are described as 'gateway drugs', sometimes cannabis. The *Opium Law* in the Netherlands formally codifies 'soft drugs' as including cannabis, sleeping pills and sedatives, and 'hard drugs' as heroin, cocaine, amphetamine, ecstasy and gamma-hydroxybutyric acid (GHB), widely labelled as the 'date-rape drug'.

Research on this question to date has not produced a definitive answer. In essence, the *gateway hypothesis* is a causal one, in one version specifying that nicotine use affects the brain (probably via dopamine systems) in such a way as to make it more likely that an individual will go on to use cocaine (Kandel and Kandel, 2015). Competing ideas include the possibilities that (a) individuals who use cannabis are more likely to be exposed to opportunities to try other drugs (the *social environment hypothesis*), or that (b) those who become cannabis users have characteristics that incline them towards interest in other drugs in any case (the *common liability hypothesis*). Studies generally find that the majority of those who use soft drugs (however defined) do not move on to hard drugs, and the bulk of evidence seems more compatible with the common liability hypothesis.

Once a pattern of substance misuse has become established, it is often a predictor of later involvement in crime, though that is usually a function of other factors in addition. Dowden and Brown (2002) reported a meta-analysis of 45 studies, yielding 116 effect-size estimates of the relationship between substance-abuse factors (including alcohol) and recidivism. Almost 60 per cent of the studies entailed follow-up periods of two years or more, with an aggregate sample size of 44,498. There was a small but significant association between substance use and general recidivism, with the largest effect size for combined alcohol and drug misuse. Drug abuse and alcohol abuse were each significantly associated with future violent recidivism. For women offenders, the strongest predictor of recidivism was having had a parent who abused substances, though that finding was based on just six study samples.

Substance use and dependence

Substance use may become so firmly ingrained in people's lives that they find it extremely difficult to escape from, and some never succeed in doing so. When drinking or taking a drug becomes a feature of every day, and preoccupies someone to an extent that it dominates other activities, he or she may experience steadily worsening problems in relationships, work and health. If substance use continues to damage the person's functioning despite repeated attempts to control it, he or she would be regarded as suffering from a *substance-use disorder* or *addiction*. Under the systems of psychiatric diagnosis we will discuss in Chapter 11, these are classified as mental disorders.

'Substance-use disorders' are defined in psychiatric terms as the chronic and relapsing use of alcohol or another drug to an extent that it causes significant impairment of functioning and distress to the individual users or those around them. Such disorders may be 'mild', 'moderate' or 'severe'. The term 'addiction' is reserved for the severe end of this spectrum, characterised by recurrent, compulsive and damaging use of a substance, which is resistant to efforts to stop it. Kraanen, Scholing and Emmelkamp (2012) assessed 237 offenders attending a forensic psychiatry outpatient clinic in Amsterdam. They found that 27.3 per cent met criteria for alcohol-use disorder, 20.3 per cent for cannabis-use disorder, and 5.3 per cent for cocaine-use disorder. At the time of their offences, across the whole group 30 per cent were intoxicated in some way. Amongst those who had committed violent offences, the proportion was larger, at 48.5 per cent; for partner violence, 25 per cent; for sexual offences, 17.4 per cent; and for other offences, 21 per cent.

From a medical point of view, addiction is defined in simple terms as a 'brain disease', though of course the processes underlying that may far from simple. It 'involves the chronic pharmacological actions of substances in the brain' (Nutt and Nestor, 2013, p. 1). The Brain Disease Model of Addiction (BDMA) centres on the premise that the central mechanism in dependence and addiction is a *biological* one: an effect of the substance on the operation of brain cells. Features of dependence, craving and loss of self-control, with all their consequences, flow from this altered state. This is a direct result of the action of a drug on brain chemistry within particular neural structures (Volkow, Koob and McLellan, 2016). The BDMA has been lauded as counteracting a long history in which those who develop addictions have been denigrated and stigmatised on the presumption that they were somehow morally deficient or lacked enough willpower to control their problem.

Brain changes occur following introduction of any psychotropic substance, and over time, if a substance continues to be used, the brain adapts to those changes ('drug-induced neuroplasticity': Volkow *et al.*, 2016). While the BDMA may appear to be a convincing account, the mechanisms underlying addiction are still keenly debated. However, the purely neurological approach cannot account for all the phenomena of addiction. First, in the long term, chronic addiction is the exception rather than the rule: follow-up research shows that the majority of those labelled as 'addicts' recover from substance misuse. Second, there are also behavioural addictions that do not involve any psychoactive substance – they include gambling, binge eating, sex, and even exercise. Third, the results that support the BDMA are over-reliant on animal models and studies, and it is unclear how reliably some evidence can be applied to humans. Fourth, the brain changes said to be pivotal in addiction also occur in other forms of learning and change, and like those are reversible. Overall, the preponderance of evidence calls the BDMA into question as too simplistic (Hall, Carter and Forline, 2015; Lewis, 2015, 2017; Satel and Lilienfeld, 2014).

A fuller understanding of habitual substance abuse involves a number of different mechanisms that converge and result in entry to a highly dependent, addicted state. They include instrumental and conditioned learning, the role of rational choice at early stages, and modulation of mood and emotion over time through use of the drug. West and Brown (2013) have formulated a model integrating these features and processes, as illustrated in Figure 10.1. The model also takes account of individual differences in

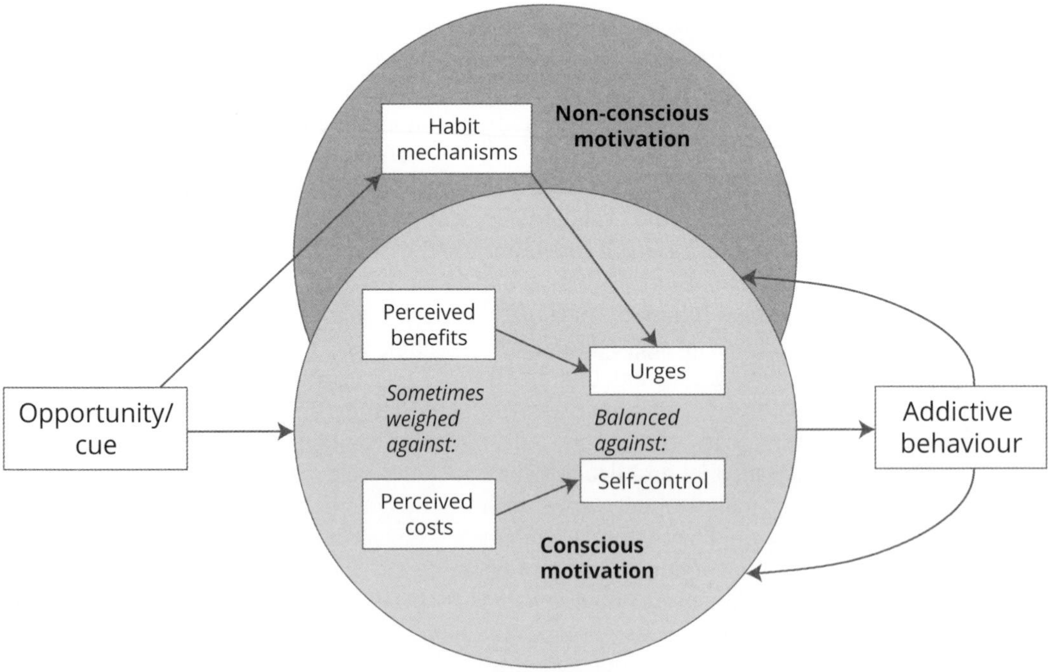
Habit
mechanisms
Non-conscious
motivation
Perceived
benefits
Urges
Opportunity/
cue
Sometimes
weighed
against:
Balanced
against:
Addictive
behaviour
Self-control
Perceived
costs
Conscious
motivation

Figure 10.1
An integrative model of addiction. The model incorporates elements of choice, self-control and automatic processes (habit mechanisms).

Source: Figure 7.4 A simplified diagram of a Choice Theory of addiction with self-control, and instrumental learning added. From West, R. & Brown, J. (2013). Theory of Addiction. 2nd edition. Chichester, UK: Wiley-Blackwell. This edition first published 2013, © 2013 by John Wiley & Sons, Ltd. First edition published 2009, © 2009 Robert West.

impulsivity, self-control and other factors which may make individuals more susceptible to repeated substance use, alongside environmental factors.

As West and Brown (2013) point out, addiction is a social construct. There is no fixed or objective definition of addiction. Nor, at present, is there a consensus on which of the numerous theoretical accounts of addiction is best supported by the evidence. Becoming a habitual substance user is a gradual process and a function of multiple factors on several levels.

Robbery

In terms of motive, *robbery* is primarily an acquisitive crime, but given its nature it is usually seen as a violent one. It is a form of theft in which money or goods are taken by force or with the threat of force. In England and Wales, 'robbery' is defined in Section 8(1) of the Theft Act 1968 as comprising those two elements (theft and force). Ashworth (2015) characterises the legal definition of robbery as unusual when compared to other offences. For example, in the Offences Against the Person Act 1861, 'assault' is divided into different types both by the nature of a crime and by its seriousness, each of them classified in separate sections of the statute. In robbery the amount of force or the severity of a threat can vary widely, but all are included within the same offence definition.

As described by Ashworth (2015), with reference to how the law operates and which sentences are imposed, there are five gradations of robbery. The principal factor that influences its seriousness (and therefore the severity of the penalty) is the level of harm or threat employed in the offence. An offence will be judged as more serious if there is evidence of advanced planning, if offenders wore disguises, if they acted in a group, and in relation to an individual who played a lead role:

» *Level 1* Usually street robberies ('mugging'). These involve the theft of purses, bags or other valuables.

» *Level 2* Generally robberies of small businesses, and usually entailing the use of a weapon.

» *Level 3* Robberies involving the use of significant force or in which serious injury occurred.

» *Level 4* Violent personal robberies in someone's home.

» *Level 5* Commercial robberies that have been professionally planned and where firearms are likely to have been carried and perhaps used (which would probably mean that other types of offences had been committed in addition).

If a robbery is thwarted, under Section 8(2) of the Theft Act 1968 the perpetrator can be charged with *assault with intent to rob*. This is not regarded in law as a lesser offence than robbery: the two crimes can be punished by the same terms of imprisonment.

In the period between March 2006 and March 2016, the number of robberies recorded in England and Wales fell by 48 per cent, and the number involving firearms by 62 per cent (Office for National Statistics, 2017). Of the 28,859 offences involving a knife or other sharp instrument recorded in the year ending March 2016, 36 per cent were robberies; they also accounted for 18 per cent of the offences in which a firearm was used. The downward slope of the trend for robbery is encouraging, but has to be set against the more dismal finding that for 2015–2016 the highest one-year proven reoffending rate was for robbery by juveniles at 44.2 per cent (Ministry of Justice, 2017a).

On a global scale, in the majority of cases the risk of becoming involved in street robbery has to be understood against a background of economic deprivation and poverty, as differentials in income and material wealth magnify in some countries. Like other acquisitive and violent crimes, robbery is often associated with disorganised neighbourhoods and rapid urban growth. (The comparative rates discussed in Chapter 2 reflect this.) However, robbery also occurs in more prosperous societies. Here it is often associated with substance misuse, which creates a need for money to sustain the habit, and some research discussed earlier has examined those connections. For other individuals, street crime may be driven by a wish to have ready access to 'fast cash' in order to maintain a 'partying' lifestyle (Jacobs and Wright, 1999; Wright, Brookman and Bennett, 2006).

In contrast, it may also be associated with homelessness amongst youth. Heerde, Hemphill and Scholes-Balog (2014) undertook a review of 29 studies of physically violent behaviour experienced by or committed by homeless young people in the age range 12–24. In a few studies that examined this, their rate of robbery was higher than that for the general population; and there was an association between the length of time for which the person had been homeless and the event of mugging someone, though the effect sizes for these links were fairly small. On the other hand, members of this group were themselves often attacked and robbed, and were in several respects a highly vulnerable group.

Patterns and motives in robbery

The offence of robbery is sometimes seen as providing a prototypical example of a crime based on rational calculation, fitting the model of the 'reasoning criminal' as outlined in Chapter 4. The would-be robber is likely to choose 'targets' on the basis of estimating the balance of likely gains (the value of items to be obtained) as compared to the effort and the potential risks involved (of encountering resistance, of being caught, or of committing a more serious crime than planned), according to research (Bennett and Brookman, 2010).

Research on decision-making processes amongst those who commit armed robbery shows that in a proportion of cases they do take these factors into account, but this may be more likely when the target is a commercial premises (Level 5 robbery), such as a building society or betting shop, than in street robbery. For example, based on case-file analysis and interviews with 88 men convicted of armed robbery in London, Morrison and O'Donnell (1994) discovered that the offenders had carried out detailed planning prior to their offences. One indicator of this was that once they had reached the place they intended to rob, in a large proportion of cases they handed a written note to a member of staff demanding money. Similarly, in a series of interviews with 86 armed robbers (14 of them female) in St Louis, Missouri, carried out with a 'live' sample actively engaged in such crimes, Wright and Decker (1997) found that considerable thought was given to the location, timing and targeting of robberies. In terms of their crime histories, this was a highly accomplished group: 71 per cent admitted to ten or more robberies, and 36 per cent to fifty or more. These offenders made general decisions to embark on robbery as a means of acquiring money. They could earn very little in law-abiding jobs and preferred the freedom of not being in employment. As a criminal choice, robbery required less effort than burglary. Most of Wright and Decker's participants had consciously deliberated on this, taking a number of factors into account. But there were also occasions when they acted quickly on opportunities that suddenly appeared. All of this needs to be seen, however, in the setting of a hard-edged street culture, itself part of a broader context of disadvantaged neighbourhoods and dysfunctional personal backgrounds (Jacobs and Wright, 1999).

In street robberies, including those that are linked to substance use, the repeated need for additional money shows a cyclical pattern according to when the amount of it in someone's possession becomes depleted and eventually runs out. This cycle is represented in Figure 10.2. Even at the outset individuals are in a state of 'bounded rationality' – that is, their thinking is focused on a narrow range of issues, detached from their broader context. As the moment of the offence approaches, desperation steadily rises. Gradually, the range of an individual's potential targets widens and the preparedness to take greater risks increases. These offences may then entail almost no forethought at all. The individual reaches a point at which any chance will be acted on, with little planning preceding it. Topalli and Wright (2014) mapped out this pattern of the changing motivational state and gradually shifting priorities. They characterised this as a transition from a state of 'alert opportunism' to one of 'motivated opportunism'. In the former, there is a maximal range of choices for action, but only what appears to be a very good crime opportunity will be taken. In the latter, the range of possible actions is minimal and almost any target will do.

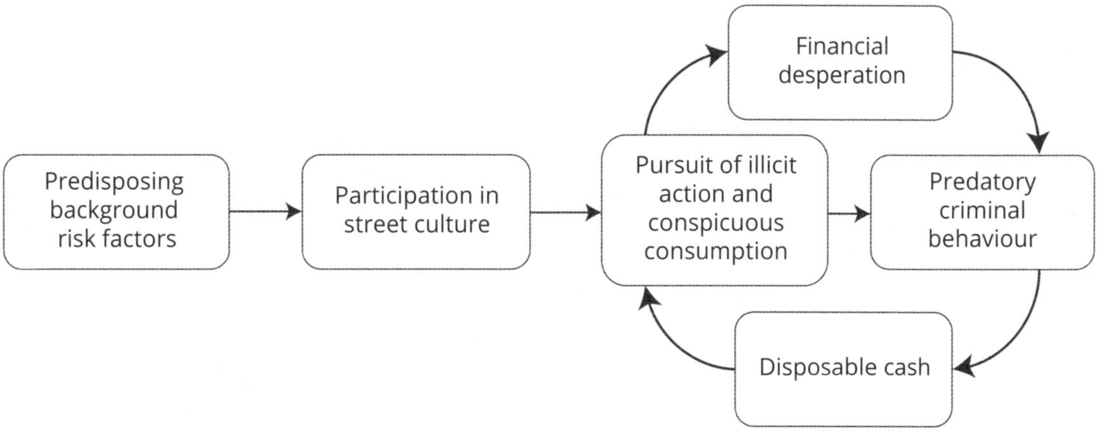
Financial desperation
Predisposing background risk factors
Participation in street culture
Pursuit of illicit action and conspicuous consumption
Predatory criminal behaviour
Disposable cash

Figure 10.2
The aetiological cycle of predatory crime.

Source: Figure 3.1 The etiological cycle of predatory criminality. From Topalli, V. & Wright, R. (2014). Affect and the dynamic foreground of predatory street crime: Desperation, anger, and fear. In J. L. van Gelder, H. Elffers, D. Reynald & D. S. Nagin (eds.), Affect and Cognition in Criminal Decision Making. p. 44. Abingdon, Oxon: Routledge. Copyright © 2014 Routledge. Reproduced by permission of Taylor & Francis Books UK.

By this time the individual is in a state of 'psychosocial encapsulation' in which he or she becomes fixated on relieving what is by then 'visceral' distress.

Working with a group of 76 offenders convicted of robbery in the Netherlands, Lindegaard, Bernasco, Jacques and Zevenbergen (2014) charted fluctuations in their experiences of different emotions (fear, anger and shame) before, during and after an offence. They suggested that a clearer picture of this state of flux and how individuals manage it may be an important component in understanding the nature of the offence.

Thus although the motives for robbery are fundamentally economic, it seems unlikely that Rational Crime Theory alone can provide an adequate explanation of these offences. Research has shown that motivational and emotional states also play crucial parts in the onset of offending, and they help to explain the cyclical pattern just mentioned. In addition, it is important to recognise that the cultural context of many robberies is that of the street in which many people are pursuing a hedonistic lifestyle, and one that involves not just conspicuous consumption but also high status derived from appearing to live effortlessly. Thus 'the motivation to offend arises out of shared values rather than personal utilities' (Bennett and Brookman, 2010, p. 280), or some combination of the two.

In Chapter 7 we discussed the work of Luckenbill (1977), who studied interaction sequences that led up to some crimes of homicide. Luckenbill (1981) later suggested that there are also patterns of exchange that occur in the course of robberies. He analysed 261 cases out of 732 reported in one year in a city in Texas (179 completed, 82 attempts). To commit a robbery, it is necessary to get close to the intended target. In one-third of cases that was achieved through a surprise attack: the offender lurked unseen and then rushed on the victim. In the remainder, the offender 'established co-presence' by acting as a person normally would in the situation – for example, in a car park, pretending to be looking for their car. Having got close, the assailant then took steps to control the situation, ensuring the victim's **compliance** by the use or threat of force. What happened next was dependent on several factors, including whether or not the victim could just be commanded to hand items over (wallet, car keys) or was needed to take action (unlock a door) and whether or not he or she resisted. The victim's level of resistance might depend on moment-by-moment perceptions of the offender's demeanour, or the proximity of help. The technique of the street robber is to gain control of the micro-interactional situation, imposing his (or her) momentum upon the victim. In the words of Wright and Decker (1997, p. 66), the assailant must create 'the illusion of impending death' in the mind of the victim. Thus repeat offenders have acquired skills for maximising the likelihood of success in an offence, including techniques for instilling and managing fear and of intimidating and controlling victims.

Deakin, Smithson, Spencer and Medina-Ariza (2007) investigated the *modus operandi* of 20 offenders convicted of street robbery in Manchester. The offenders described having operated in groups, using distraction as a ploy in overwhelming victims. In other respects their methods were similar to those outlined by Luckenbill, including 'blitz' attacks or subtle manoeuvrings into close range. Selection of victims involved careful analysis and judgment, though there were favoured target groups: these included students; people using cash machines; men out looking for prostitutes; and other offenders known to have committed robbery, who might be carrying the proceeds from their own offences.

Extortion

Extortion has some similarities with robbery, in that it also involves the securing of money, goods or services from someone, or perhaps gaining control over them, through coercion. But it differs in that rather than entailing the immediate threat of assault, it involves the instillation of fear over time. This can happen on an individual level, but more often develops as part of a network of organised criminal activity. It can become widespread in areas where there is an active criminal 'underworld' of gangs engaged in 'racketeering'. That can vary in scale from urban neighbourhoods, such as the parts of London dominated by the notorious Kray twins in the 1960s, to entire regions of a country, as illustrated by the operations of the Sicilian Mafia across several generations (Hobbs, 2010a). It particularly thrives in many parts of the world with socioeconomic systems in which 'the state is weak and where agents of the state do not have a monopoly over the means of violence' (Hobbs, 2010a, p. 726).

Blackmail is a specific form of extortion centred on extracting money, goods or services from someone by using a threat to disclose damaging or incriminating information about that person to a third party unless he or she complies.

Carjacking

Most car theft consists of gaining entry to a vehicle when it is parked and empty, usually by breaking a door handle or a window, and taking and driving it away without the owner's consent. In *carjacking* the vehicle is occupied, and the offender employs a ruse to persuade the driver out of the car, then forcibly ejects or threatens any other occupants and steals the car. Between 1993 and 2003 there were on average 38,000 carjacking incidents per year in the United States (Bureau of Justice Statistics, 2004). Most offences (68 per cent) occurred at night; 74 per cent of offenders were armed; and 56 per cent had committed the offence more than once. According to US government warnings, 'common attack plans' included bumping a victim's car from behind, then seizing it when he or she got out of the vehicle; flashing lights to convince drivers to pull over, thinking that their car had a problem; staging an apparent accident and flagging drivers down; and following drivers home and stealing their car as they left it (Bureau of Diplomatic Security, 2002).

Topalli, Jacques and Wright (2015) have argued that successful completion of carjacking involves certain types of expertise. There are two sets of skills. The first is perceptual, in identifying suitable vehicles and victims (one of their respondents describing a suitable target car as 'heroin on four wheels', p. 22). The second is procedural, in enacting the offence successfully. While this must take some time to learn, it is perhaps an exaggeration to call it 'expertise', a word perhaps better reserved for the safecracking and other 'craft crime' skills that were in use during what Hobbs (2010b) called the 'golden age' of armed robbers in the UK, between 1960 and 1980.

Home invasion

Home invasion shares some features with burglary, but has more similarities to robbery; or, as Douglas, Burgess, Burgess and Ressler (2013) suggest, with carjacking.

House burglars mostly work alone, and break into dwellings during daytime when the buildings are likely to be unoccupied.

The last thing most burglars want is to encounter a resident, and the majority try hard to avoid it. By contrast, in home invasion perpetrators work as a group, more often at night, are often armed, and expect residents to be at home as that will better serve their plans. This is a highly confrontational offence that involves controlling victims and ransacking houses, sometimes stealing valuables and forcing victims to disclose their PIN for bank cards or the code for a safe if they have one. Victims may also be forced to hand over their car keys, with the invaders then stealing their cars also. Home invasions often result in serious injury and trauma; some involve rape and even murder. This offence is commoner in the United States and some other countries than in the UK. It is not usually classified as a separate type of offence, although some American states have legislated to make it so.

Arson

Arson is a form of criminal damage, an act of crime that involves intentionally setting fire to property. Targets of such offences can include anything flammable, but the commonest are cars, houses, garages, shops, less often schools and other public or commercial buildings, and occasionally also open areas such as fields and woodlands. Given the unpredictability of fire, what someone intends as a limited event may go far beyond anything anticipated. *Happy Land*, an unlicensed nightclub in the Bronx, New York, was the target of an arson attack in 1990. Julio González, estranged from his girlfriend who worked there and angry with a doorman who had barred him from entering, poured petrol at the only exit from the club and set it alight, an action that led to the deaths of 87 people.

In England and Wales, arson is legally defined in Section 1(3) of the Criminal Damage Act 1971. As the title of that Act implies, it covers any offence in which without lawful excuse someone destroys or damages another person's property, either with the intention of doing so or having been reckless as to whether the action could have that outcome. Where the damage is done or was intended to be done by fire, the offence 'will be charged as arson'. If found guilty of that offence, the offender may be liable to life imprisonment. These offences are classified differently in Scotland, where there are separate common law offences of 'wilful fire-raising' and of 'culpable and reckless fire-raising'.

Doley, Dickens and Gannon (2016) discuss issues of terminology in this area. They suggest that the term 'firesetting' be used, and define this as 'any problematic act of setting fire to property, including the natural environment, outside accepted social and cultural boundaries' (p. 1). This is distinct from the lighting of fires for conventional purposes, such as campfires, bonfires, waste disposal, or burning candles.

Prevalence of arson

While it may seem surprising given the conspicuousness of fires, statistics on firesetting are thought to be quite unreliable. That is partly because some fires that have been deliberately set burn out harmlessly, and partly because some incidents of this type are not recorded as arson. For example, if a car is stolen and later found burnt out, the offence is likely to be recorded as vehicle theft.

The Home Office publishes statistics on the number of fire incidents recorded annually in England. During the year to the end of March 2016, fire and rescue services attended 528,700 fire-related incidents; there were also 214,100 false alarms (Home Office, 2016c). Of the 162,000 fires attended, 73,400, or 45 per cent of the total, were thought to have been started deliberately, while 55 per cent were accidental. These proportions had remained the same over the previous few years. Over a ten-year period up to 2013, numbers of deliberately set fires fell by 76 per cent (Arson Prevention Forum, 2014). However, there was then an increase in 'primary fires' – more serious fires that harm people or damage property – which totalled 19,300 in 2015–2016 (Home Office, 2016c). There were 303 fire-related fatalities in that year. The Arson Prevention Forum suggests that, on average, 25 per cent of fire deaths are deliberate, and analysis of trends over the period 2009-2014 found that 45 per cent of those were suicides.

Many acts of deliberate firesetting are carried out by young people. Research suggests that an interest in starting fires, or a tendency actually to start fires, first develops in childhood, and that a surprisingly large proportion of children and adolescents have purposefully set a fire at some stage. For example, a large epidemiological study with 43,093 participants aged 18 or over in the United States showed a lifetime prevalence for firesetting of 1 per cent (Vaughn *et al.*, 2010). By contrast, in a representative community sample of 4,595 adolescents aged 12–17, the prevalence of self-reported firesetting was 6.3 per cent (8.4 per cent for boys and 4.2 per cent for girls: Chen, Arria and Anthony, 2003). Rates of involvement in firesetting are lower than for other forms of delinquency, yet statistics from several countries show that a large proportion of fires are set by youths, and a disturbing proportion by children aged under 10 (Lambie and Randell, 2011).

Why would young children engage in a behaviour that potentially puts them at great risk, even more so than many other things they do? One explanation that has been offered is that to many children in Western societies, fire is seen as something exciting and entertaining, perhaps even fascinating, because they do not have the opportunities that children in some other cultures have, for learning from a young age to use fire as a tool. Fessler (2006) examined this from an anthropological perspective, conducting an informal survey of his colleagues who carried out ethnographic work in 19 different cultures. In most of those societies, children began interacting with fire from an early age, regarded it almost entirely in utilitarian terms, rarely played with it, and did not think of it as having entertainment value. While Fessler proposes that this illustrates the working of an evolutionary mechanism, the patterns he describes and their contrast with technological societies seem more easily explained as a function of social learning.

Risk factors and motives

What is known about firesetting from a psychological point of view? Alongside the cultural differences just outlined, there are also pronounced individual differences, with some individuals apparently drawn to starting fires, while others are very wary of them.

Research has revealed a number of factors in the backgrounds and developmental experiences of children and adolescents in the former group. Lambie and Randell (2011) reviewed 15 studies of factors associated with firesetting behaviour. Boys are two to three times more likely than girls to set fires. There is often evidence of family dysfunction and parental stress, though these are often more closely associated with repeating the behaviour than with its first occurrence. There is also an association with maltreatment, including physical and sexual abuse. This was supported in a brief review of seven studies by Burnett and Omar (2014). A proportion of young people who set fires also experience mental health problems, including depression, conduct disorder and attention deficit hyperactivity disorder (ADHD). In comparison with non-firesetters, those who set fires also showed higher levels of aggression generally, as well as higher levels of hostility and lower levels of self-regulation.

Many of these factors, however, are often found to be associated with other forms of antisocial behaviour. Some research suggests that those who set fires may show extreme levels of other types of aggression, and of substance misuse, but to date the only variable that emerges as uniquely associated with firesetting tendencies is 'fire interest'. This refers to a persistent curiosity about and attraction to fire, and while findings on this are not wholly consistent, those exhibiting higher levels of such interest are more likely to be involved in multiple incidents of setting fires. This may be crucial for understanding the pathways of those who continue such behaviour into adulthood, but those connections for the moment remain poorly understood.

In any case, not all firesetting is carried out by this particularly troubled group; deliberate setting of fires can occur for a variety of reasons, and more so amongst adults, where additional factors are likely to be operating alongside those that affect children (Del Bove and MacKay, 2011). Initial attempts to develop a typology of firesetting based this on an analysis of assumed motives, but this gradually evolved to take account of individual offender characteristics (Doley, 2003). Studies suggest that motives fall into a number of major categories. As with other areas discussed in this chapter, there are often several frameworks to choose from in classifying offences of a particular type into subgroups, and they often overlap in their coverage.

For arson as a criminal offence, the principal motives have been grouped as follows:

- *Acquisitive/economic* Burning down a property so that its owner can claim insurance on it, or in other cases to destroy a rival business; or arson for personal gain.
- *Instrumental* To cover up another crime; or to kill someone and conceal evidence of having done so (fire-associated homicide: Davies and Mouzos, 2007).
- *Vandalism* For excitement, sensation-seeking, or tension relief.
- *Emotional reasons* To express anger; as a way of seeking attention; or as an act of suicide (self-immolation). A specific subcategory here may be as an act of revenge following an interpersonal conflict (Barnoux and Gannon, 2014).
- *Mental disorder* Research has shown links between firesetting and several diagnosed psychiatric disorders, including psychotic and delusional states, and substance-use (especially alcohol-use) disorder. On the other hand, *pyromania* is relatively rare (Tyler and Gannon, 2012). There is no evidence that any specific disorder causes firesetting, but such problems may increase the risk of firesetting in particular circumstances (McEwan and Ducat, 2016).

Theories of firesetting

Clearly, many factors play a part in firesetting; firesetting can stem from a variety of motives; and the individuals who perpetrate firesetting are a heterogeneous group. It is unlikely that any single factor would be sufficient on its own to provide an explanation. Gannon (2016) reviews a number of 'single factor' theories, and it may be that each accounts for one aspect of the problem. However, in efforts to understand arson or firesetting more fully, three separate theoretical approaches have appeared. As each draws on multiple variables, they present multifactorial theories.

Functional analysis

Jackson, Hope and Glass (1987) developed a behavioural model for understanding patterns of recidivist arson. Essentially, individuals who commit arson are likely to come from origins where they have been disadvantaged in some key ways. They are experiencing significant dissatisfaction in life, but are not effective through conventional channels in accomplishing personal goals. Vicarious experience of the power of fire encourages an expectation that setting a fire could bring about a major change in the individual's life. At some point when negative emotions accumulate, a trigger event leads the individual to set a fire in an attempt to redress the situation. All of this is couched in functional analysis of the changing contingencies of reinforcement over time.

Dynamic-behaviour theory

Fineman (1995) proposed a social-psychological theory which also draws on behavioural models but places greater emphasis on individual differences than in the functional-analytic approach. It also incorporates an account of the process whereby feelings and cognitions converge in a sequence that increases firesetting risk. Common features of that sequence that are likely to occur in all firesetters are identified, and this is then followed by analysis of how different potential motives may influence the particular route this sequence follows.

Multi-Trajectory Theory of Adult Firesetting

Gannon, Ó Ciardha, Doley and Alleyne (2012) developed a more comprehensive account, the Multi-Trajectory Theory of Adult Firesetting (M-TTAF), which builds on features of the previous two models but assimilates a still broader range of variables, and also follows through to a stage of action where the individual desists from firesetting. Developmental and contextual factors are examined which explain how individuals may have developed psychological vulnerabilities that in a specific combination might increase the risk of firesetting. These include inappropriate fire interest, offence-supportive attitudes, difficulties in emotional self-regulation, and problems in communication. Taking into account different motives and different possible triggers, the theory maps out possible diverse, but convergent routes (trajectories) into firesetting. Two qualitative, interview-based studies, respectively of 23 firesetters diagnosed with mental disorders (16 males, 7 females: Tyler *et al.*, 2014), and of 38 imprisoned adult male firesetters (Barnoux, Gannon and Ó Ciardha, 2015), found support for the M-TTAF in analysis of the 'offence chain' that unfolded as different factors influenced their development and their experiences before and after they committed their offences.

Kidnapping and abduction

Under common law in the countries where it prevails, it is an offence to infringe the liberty of another person by taking him or her captive, by force or deception, without that person's consent and without lawful justification. This is the essence of *kidnapping*, in which a person is 'taken away'; but there is also a related offence of *false imprisonment*, which involves depriving another person of liberty by unlawfully confining them. Thus one offence as it were 'compels movement', while the other restricts it (Law Commission, 2014). There are laws applying to some specific forms of kidnap. For example, the Child Abduction Act 1984 in England, Wales, and Scotland makes it an offence to take or to send a child out of the UK without appropriate consent; and the Modern Slavery Act 2015 defines offences of *slavery*, *servitude*, *forced* or *compulsory labour* and *human trafficking*.

As Wright (2009) notes, kidnapping has a history going back several thousand years; there have been times when entire populations have been kidnapped (he gives as examples the biblical account of the deportation of the Hebrew people from Judah to Bablyon in the 6th century BCE; and that there were sieges of cities in 17th-century Europe that were only lifted on payment of ransom). The criminal offence of kidnapping in the modern era can consist of several different types of acts, ranging from abduction of children by estranged parents, to people trafficking, hostage-taking, or hijacking of an aircraft. As definitions of these acts are not always set out in formal statutes, the boundaries of 'kidnapping' are not precisely defined. The contexts within which people carry out offences of this kind show considerable variety, and different forms of it overlap with one another. The result is a state of what Noor-Mohamed (2014) has called 'definitional ambiguity'. Several attempts have been made to classify ways in which kidnapping occurs. While the number of cases of kidnapping in the UK and in most parts of Europe seem relatively low – though we cannot be sure, as the offence is not always recorded separately – there are regions of the world where it is far more frequent.

In the year ending March 2016, there were in total 2,998 reported offences of kidnapping in England and Wales. That was fairly similar to the figure for the year 2002–2003 (3,198), but in ensuing years the numbers declined, reaching their lowest in 2012–2013 (1,388) but then rising again. Soothill, Francis and Ackerley (2007) analysed data on convictions for kidnapping in England and Wales in the period 1979–2001, finding a total of 7,042 for men and 545 for women. Approximately half of those convicted had also committed other types of offence, and nearly 60 per cent had convictions for violence. However, the proportion convicted of a second kidnapping offence was very low: 3.9 per cent of men and 2.6 per cent of women. There is no evidence of 'specialisation' in this type of crime.

Concannon (2013) generated a set of 43 variables for comparing some key features of kidnaps. These included characteristics of the victim, the offender, the abduction site, the *modus operandi* in the offence, and the outcome. Examining a series of 100 kidnaps, she and her colleagues were able to classify them under seven main headings:

» *Domestic* This refers to kidnap in the context of previously close relationships that have broken down. In one type, one partner (usually male) takes the other (usually female) by force and keeps her in a place of his choosing. In a second type, a court has assigned custody of a child to one parent and the other abducts the child; this situation is made more complex if the parents are citizens of different countries.

» *Predatory* These are usually sexually motivated crimes that result in assaults on the victim. Note that this category is divided into two types according to whether the victim is an adult or a child, as each has some different features and a different course. While most victims survive, in the cases analysed a proportion were murdered.

» *Profit* In these cases the main objective is financial gain through demanding a ransom. While this is often a form of organised crime, Wright (2009) notes that there has been a growing overlap between this and demands for money in politically motivated kidnaps – a form of fund-raising, usually for terrorist groups.

» *Revenge* In this type, kidnap is used as a means of retaliation, either directly against someone whom the offender sees as having wronged him or her, or indirectly against someone associated with that person whose kidnap will cause her or him distress. Most people subject to this kind of kidnap do not survive.

» *Political* Kidnappings in this category are themselves very varied: they may be committed to publicise a cause or an issue, to pressure a government to release prisoners from the kidnapper's group, to instil fear, or to make a government appear unable to protect its own people. The majority of victims of political kidnap are killed by those who have taken them.

» *Staged* In these incidents, no real kidnap has taken place. In some cases the offender has faked the event, usually to cover up another crime (such as that they have actually killed the victim). In other cases the victim and offender are cooperating with each other for fraudulent purposes.

Noor-Mohamed (2013) reviews other attempts to develop a typology of kidnapping, including one developed by the United Nations Office on Drugs and Crime, and offers a new scheme with 19 separate categories. These are in two major groups. One is abduction of a child or an adult, usually stemming from family conflict, individual psychopathology (paedophilia, baby-snatching), kidnap for marriage (which still exists in some cultures), or 'pseudo-therapeutic' kidnapping, whereby someone is recaptured from a cult. The other main group is kidnap for political or economic purposes, for example for propaganda, for prisoner exchange, or to extract concessions; or for ransom, for debt collection, or for people trafficking for labour (modern slavery) or for sexual exploitation.

Turner (1998) proposed the use of a 'classificatory device' for kidnap, using two dimensions to reflect the relative strength of motives related to politics or to material gains (or neither, or both). The rationale for attempting to classify these acts is to produce an understanding of differences in motivation, as those will influence the direction and course of events, and therefore the response that law enforcement agencies should make. An understanding of kidnappers' or hostage-takers' intentions is a vital piece of information for investigation, and where it becomes part of the process, for negotiating the release of victims. Turner applied this framework to analysis of some notorious kidnapping incidents to illustrate how one could interpret changes in motivations over time. (Such changes are not unusual.)

Attempts have also been made to classify offences of child abduction. Plass (1998) devised a typology with eight categories, differing in three ways. The first was whether or not the parent whose child had been taken knew where the child was; the second, whether the child was being kept by someone in a place, or had been taken by someone to a place, where the child should not be; and the third, whether or not the perpetrator had legal custody of the child (which does not exclude the possibility of isolating a child where it should not be). This approach also allows construction of a scale of seriousness, which can inform the responses authorities should make to the situation. This takes account, for example, of the effect of the episode on the child and the nature of the situation. A child taken to an unknown location by someone who has no custody rights is a very different event from a child being confined in a known location by someone who does have custody rights. Examining a series of 104 cases of children in a project database (NISMART, the US National Incidence Studies of Missing, Abducted, Runaway and Thrownaway Children), Plass found that this system could be used successfully to predict several features of case progression and outcomes.

Tiger kidnapping

Tiger kidnapping refers to a type of hostage-taking in which an individual is compelled to do something because the kidnap victims are close relatives who are kept under threat of harm unless he or she follows the perpetrators' orders. An example is the 2004 kidnapping at gunpoint of family members of two senior employees of the Northern Bank, Belfast, as a result of which on the next working day the two officials organised the theft of £26 million from the bank, after which their family members were released. Offences of this kind were given the name 'tiger kidnapping' because carrying them out requires that the offenders watch routines for a period before striking.

Hijacking and piracy

Hijacking is a highly ambitious and often very dramatic type of offence, which involves the forceful commandeering of a form of transport such as a truck, a ship, or an aircraft. In some cases the objective of such an act is not kidnapping in itself, though that may happen as a by-product of the seizure. For example, where trucks are involved, the purpose may be either robbery or in some cases to procure the vehicle in order to commit another crime: drivers may be ejected immediately or may be held for a short while. Very rarely, ships have been the target, as occurred in 1985 when the Italian cruise liner *Achille Lauro* was hijacked by four members of the Palestinian Liberation Front. This had political objectives, and therefore differed from *piracy*, which is almost always carried out for financial gain. Between 2005 and 2012 there were numerous incidents of piracy in the Indian Ocean off the coast of Somalia, and piracy continues in other parts of the world.

In aerial hijacks there can be several different motives. Holden (1986) analysed a series of 326 hijacks, which occurred between 1953 and 1982, and distinguished two main types. The first focused on transportation: the hijacker ordered that the plane be diverted somewhere other than its planned destination, for example to allow the hijacker to claim asylum. The second had the objective of monetary gain: the hijacker demanded a ransom to ensure the safe return of passengers and crew. Other investigators later added a third major category, political hijackings.

Miller (2007) carried out a cluster analysis of 27 features of 139 hijacks from the period 1993–2003. His objective was to map out possible patterns within them, rather than to classify them by motive. Four clusters emerged:

- The first was unprepared hijackings, usually carried out by a single perpetrator who was often unarmed but had sometimes made an improvised weapon, and who for personal reasons wants a flight diverted to another destination. Incidents of this type generally did not last long, and were often resolved without injury or death; and hijackers rarely achieved their aims.
- The second was politically motivated hijacking, usually carried out by members of a terrorist group, though just over half were committed by individuals acting alone. They were more likely to be armed, and were more often successful in achieving their goals; even so, the proportion who managed this was just 36.8 per cent.
- The third type of hijacking always involved a group, mostly armed, and generally not politically motivated but seeking to divert the plane for other purposes. These incidents were more protracted and one-fifth of them resulted in the death of passengers or crew members.
- The final cluster consisted of hijackings of international flights by solo perpetrators demanding that the plane divert to a new destination. Two-thirds succeeded in this aim, but all of these hijackers were then arrested or gave themselves up. There were no deaths in incidents of this type.

Aircraft hijackings have occurred for many years, but were particularly frequent throughout the 1970s and 1980s. Overall, hijacking was not very effective in achieving its protagonists' aims. There is some evidence of a 'contagion' effect, whereby successful hijacks are quickly followed by others; most, however, are not successful (Dugan, LaFree and Piquero, 2005; Holden, 1986). Due to heightened levels of security at airports, the rate of aerial hijacks has declined since the terror attacks on New York City in September 2001.

Serious acquisitive or economic crime

The crimes we have discussed in the last few chapters are the ones most likely to be the focus of the everyday work of forensic psychologists. Research and practice concerning such crimes are central to the field. There are other types of serious crimes, however, which have acquisitive or economic objectives, and which although they do not involve direct aggression can nevertheless result in serious harm to individuals or communities. To complete this chapter, we turn to serious crimes of this type. We discuss them under several subheadings, but it is best to bear in mind that there are no exact dividing lines between them.

The misappropriation of resources that legally belong to another person is not limited to the forms of property crime we know as pickpocketing, shoplifting, car theft or house burglary. Several types of acquisitive crime are usually placed under the heading 'economic crime'. They include tax evasion; fraudulent claims for insurance payments, work-related expenses, social security, housing, disability or other benefits; deceptive advertising; marketing of counterfeit designer products; overcharging of business costs; short-delivery of goods (fulfilling an order but with some portion of it missing); and many variations on these themes. All the indicators are that these are fairly widespread practices. At an individual level, the amounts gained and lost might not be large, though in some cases they may be. But when such crimes are repeated many times, or coordinated by organised criminal groups, the sums accrued overall can be immense. Further, when carried out in the corporate sector, they typically attain much higher values in terms of money or other assets.

Legitimate businesses suffer extensively from the fraudulent activities of outsiders or of their own employees. The professional financial services company PricewaterhouseCoopers (PWC) has published a series of reports on the volume of commercial crime. For its 2007 report, contact was made, and interviews conducted, with staff in 5,428 firms in 40 countries. The results showed that more than 43 per cent of companies reported suffering at least one significant economic crime during the year, and for over 80 per cent economic crime had caused significant damage to their business. The average value of frauds was the equivalent of US $2.4 million (reaching a total of US $1.3 trillion over the firms surveyed). The report concluded that 'no industry is immune' from such activity (PricewaterhouseCoopers, 2007, p. 7). The loss of funding and the 'level of collateral damage' was in proportion to the level of seniority of the perpetrator. That is, the higher an individual had risen in an organisation, the more command he or she had over segments of its finances. A later report, based on 3,877 responses from 78 countries, revealed a 30 per cent increase in fraud and a 13 per cent increase in cybercrime between 2009 and 2010 (PricewaterhouseCoopers, 2011). More than half (56 per cent) of the most serious frauds were described as having been 'an inside job', and many companies had no strategy in place for dealing with cybercrime.

There is a striking comparison that arises here, and it underlines some of the issues we discussed in Chapter 2 concerning conventional definitions of crime. The overall financial cost of economic crime is many times larger than that attributable to what in the public mind is conventionally labelled 'the crime problem'. Reiman and Leighton (2013) carried out a methodical comparison between the two. For the year 2010, the total sum of money stolen in all reported property crime in the United States amounted to US $15.7 billion. Reiman and Leighton set this alongside the costs of all kinds of financial crime including computer- and internet-related fraud, consumer fraud, credit-card and cheque fraud, embezzlement and pilferage, insurance fraud, theft of securities, and a variety of other types of comparable offence. Under each heading, a range of values was found, sometimes with very large differences between lowest and highest estimates.

In each case, Reiman and Leighton used the most conservative figure available. The total they arrived at was US $610 billion, nearly 40 times more than the quantity of money stolen in 'ordinary' crimes.

White-collar crime

When reporting his seminal studies on what he called 'white-collar crime', the criminologist Edwin Sutherland (1983, p. 7) defined it as 'crime committed by a person of respectability and high social status in the course of his occupation'.

Sutherland considered that the 'differential association' process (discussed in Chapter 4) was a sufficiently powerful mechanism to explain the phenomenon, and that personality factors had little relevance in understanding it. The mechanism can be approached using the methods of social psychology in understanding group interactions and how they influence commonly held attitudes. Thus, in studying attitudes to paying tax and to tax evasion in small businesses (in the hairdressing and beauty sector), Ashby and Webley (2008) suggested that the beliefs people held regarding these issues were a function of their occupational group membership and the 'taxpaying culture'. Other researchers, however, have incorporated individual differences into a more broad-based theory. This has focused, amongst other aspects, on the process of *moral disengagement* whereby some individuals are prepared to initiate and to perpetuate corruption within a business organisation (Moore, 2008). But there is still relatively little psychological research on this form of offending, and what there is has concentrated mainly (though not exclusively) on the highest income levels of the financial spectrum.

The term 'economic crime' is now generally used to refer to the expropriation of money through various fraudulent methods. Naylor (2003) developed a typology of 'profit-driven' crimes and divided them into three subgroups:

» *Predatory offences*, which include robberies and other ordinary acquisitive crimes, involve the illegal redistribution of existing wealth, and are committed by individuals or occasionally gangs.

» *Market-based offences*, such as tax evasion and other subverting of regulations, involve the illegal earning of new income, and are usually committed by organised crime groups.

» *Commercial offences* involve the illegal redistribution of legally earned income, and are usually committed by corporations.

Given the primarily economic perspective adopted by Naylor, comments on 'the nature of the offender' in the three types of cases remain very generalist and speculative.

Superficially, these forms of crime appear quite different from what are variously classed as 'ordinary', 'conventional', 'traditional' or 'street' crimes. The difference may derive from the impersonal and anonymous nature of money itself, and the advantages this offers with respect to crime opportunities, a point emphasised by Engdahl (2008) in an analysis of these crimes. However, Engdahl supplemented this with some motivational analysis, acknowledging that 'many cases of economic crime can be traced back to personal problems not shared with or communicated to others for fear of losing face or position' (2008, p. 163). A case study illustrating this is given in Engdahl's paper. Committing crimes as a function of individual problems sounds not unlike the process that operates in many street-level offences. Moreover, in an exceptionally long-term, 35-year follow-up of offenders identified as middle class, Soothill, Humphreys and Francis (2012) found that these offenders had been reconvicted of a wide range of offence types. Having once embarked on crime, their records subsequently were not dissimilar to those found amongst offenders lower down the socioeconomic ladder.

Nevertheless, there have been several attempts to search for potentially distinctive psychological characteristics of people found guilty of market-based or commercial crimes (adopting Naylor's classification). Some authors have offered mainly anecdotal descriptions of intensely ambitious, perhaps narcissistic individuals, who acquire a sense of omnipotence and begin to believe they are above the law. Alongside such descriptions, however, a contrasting vignette is one of a struggling individual who resorts to fraud to solve mounting financial problems – perhaps accompanied by, and probably worsened by, and possibly even caused by, alcohol problems. Feeley (2006) typified the commercial environment as likely to foster 'ultra-competitiveness' in some individuals, thereby bringing out tendencies to seek dominance, to take risks, or to ignore rules. Such an environment is compounded by the problem that the boundaries between adroit business practice and law-breaking are not always clear (deliberately so, some might argue). Furthermore, because society has an ambivalent attitude towards white-collar crime, perceiving it as distinct from volume crime, perpetrators can 'maintain a non-criminal self-concept' (Dhami, 2007, p. 58). In interviews with 14 males serving prison sentences for fraud or deception whilst holding senior positions in their employing organisations, Dhami (2007) found that the majority believed they had been harshly treated by the courts, but were held in esteem by prison staff. Most believed that they had done no harm to society and that their actions were not real crimes. To this extent, they employed one of the techniques of *neutralisation*, denial of injury (see Chapter 5).

Other researchers have reported more formal group comparisons. Collins and Schmidt (1993) compared a cohort of 365 prisoners, convicted of white-collar crimes, from across 23 US prisons with a non-offending sample of 344 'employed in white-collar positions of authority' (1993, p. 297). These participants were asked to complete a number of questionnaires to assess personality factors and aspects of attitudes to work. Of numerous differences found between the two groups, the largest were on subscales assessing conscientiousness, possession of a sense of responsibility, and adherence to social norms. In a study in Germany, however, Blickle, Schlegel, Fassbender and Klein (2006) found white-collar offenders to be more conscientious than a comparison sample, though they did emerge as having lower self-control, lower integrity, and higher levels of hedonism and narcissism. Terpstra, Rozell and Robinson (1993) asked a sample of 201 business studies students how they would respond in a series of vignettes depicting opportunities to engage in unethical business activity (insider-trading). Those who believed that they would assent to such opportunities were more likely to be young and male. They were significantly more competitive, and had an external locus of control – that is, they were more likely to be influenced by situational factors, as opposed to being internally self-regulating.

Using a qualitative approach, Alalehto (2003) interviewed a series of 128 Swedish businessmen and asked them to nominate, in confidence, an associate whom they knew well and to describe that person's work behaviour and attitudes. The interview focused on aspects that these 'informants' thought were linked to a tendency to engage in fraudulent acts. On the basis of this, several identifiable types of individual emerged as more likely to engage in such acts. Given the indirect third-party informant-based method of data collection, it is difficult to draw firm conclusions from these findings. However, alongside the psychometric studies described in the preceding paragraph, such results suggest that individual differences do play a role in the likelihood of becoming involved in fraud and similar activities. Alalehto (2003) described how Sutherland and others precluded examining individual differences for reasons similar to those we noted in Chapter 3: from a fear that to talk in psychological terms amounts to the imputation of pathology or sickness.

Also using qualitative methodology, but with a quite different participant sample, Willott and Griffin (1999) analysed a series of semi-structured discussions on crime and money with nine groups of men on probation or in prison in the UK. All participants had been convicted of economic crimes and were described as 'working class', so all of them came from 'blue-collar' rather than white-collar occupational groups. Using grounded theory and discourse analysis, the conversations thus recorded were first separated into 'chunks', then condensed into a hierarchy of themes, of which five were classed as superordinate. These revolved around a metaphor of economic crime as a 'lifeboat', resorting to which had been justified by participants on several grounds. The groups considered that politicians and others managing the state and the system were the biggest criminals, and the inequities of the economy and of criminal justice appeared to make them feel that no guilt attached to their own offences. The accounts the men gave 'serve to justify and even valorise economic crime by constructing it as an unavoidable necessity for survival and therefore not a crime at all' (1999, p. 451). Casting themselves in traditional male roles as breadwinners, Willott and Griffin's respondents felt that other means of making a living were closed to them. They were clearly living with marked 'financial strain', which Martire (2010) has argued is a factor that needs to be more fully integrated into forensic psychologists' perceptions of our roles, to place greater emphasis on advocacy. Whatever our views of their predicament, it seems clear that the beliefs of these men perform a neutralising function. As we saw earlier and will see again below, this cognitive process has been found as a contributory factor in several different types of offence.

Ragatz and Fremouw (2010) undertook a review of 16 studies of white-collar crime, including several that addressed psychological aspects. Unfortunately, they found no consistent definition of white-collar crime across these studies, and several were marred by fairly weak methodology; amongst other limitations, they did not analyse samples separately by gender. Overall, although there were some trends in the findings, this review suggested that few clear conclusions could be drawn from existing research and that more robust studies are needed. In a subsequent study, however, Ragatz, Fremouw and Baker (2012) compared three groups of male prisoners – 39 'white-collar only' offenders, a 'white-collar versatile' group of 88 offenders who had also committed other crimes, and 86 non-white-collar offenders. While the first of these groups had lower lifestyle criminality scores, they showed higher psychopathy scores. Both white-collar groups had higher rates of alcohol consumption than the non-white-collar group. The 'versatile' group showed higher levels of criminal thinking than the two other groups, and higher scores on 'Machiavellian egocentricity' than the non-white-collar group.

There could of course be additional variables at work, not explored in these studies. Recall the claim of Gottfredson and Hirschi (1990) that low self-control is the central variable in all crime. Piquero, Exum and Simpson (2005) have suggested that in relation to white-collar crime the *reverse* may apply. Success in a business career is difficult without the capacity to be highly controlled and to delay gratification. At the extreme end, a need or 'desire for control' could itself be a risk factor in that environment. Piquero and her colleagues presented business executives and Masters of Business Administration (MBA) students with vignettes depicting opportunities to commit fraud. Willingness to do so proved to be a function of several variables, but at the individual level an urge to be in control was a significant predictor of choosing criminal options. In later studies, Piquero, Schoepfer and Langton (2010) and Schoepfer, Piquero and Langton (2014) found that whereas low self-control predicted greater willingness to commit shop theft, desire for control predicted greater willingness to shred documents related to a problematic business account. These findings should be interpreted cautiously, however, as although the participants rated the scenarios as highly realistic, they were addressing a *hypothetical* situation and had not themselves been convicted of white-collar crimes. Also, while in two studies the participants worked in the corporate sector or were taking business classes, in the third the sample consisted of undergraduate students.

Drawing this together, is it possible to develop a preliminary model of the factors that influence large-scale fraud and other types of serious economic crime? Are they the same as those found amongst individuals near the bottom of the wealth and income scale? Offences of this kind are often seen as basically rational: the motive is taken to be obvious (acquisitiveness, whether from 'greed or need'), and it is assumed that perpetrators consciously weigh up the benefits and costs (as classical criminology predicts they should). That is very likely to be partly true in many cases. Even within criminology, however, this approach has little direct evidence to support it in this simple form; and there is also evidence that contradicts it (Minkes and Minkes, 2010). Other factors are likely to include 'opportunity structures' – in other words, the circumstances in which people may be able to make financial gains – and these are probably also influenced by the differential association process outlined by Sutherland. Readiness to offend may be a result of moral disengagement; or it may be linked to attitudes and beliefs conducive to or supportive of fraud, such as the views that 'Everyone else is doing it', 'It isn't really a crime', 'It's necessary for survival' and 'There are other people doing far worse things', as well as additional neutralisation techniques. Finally, for crimes to be repeated over an extended period, individual differences in some aspects of personality may play a part. These include variations in conscientiousness and perhaps also in conceitedness and narcissism.

Corporate crime

Individuals may commit economic crimes purely for personal gain, as for example in *embezzlement*, in which case the employing company itself may be the victim. But in other cases such crimes may be committed for the benefit of the corporation; and on occasion such crimes are committed by what are in other ways legitimate and long-established businesses, and sometimes even well-known names. This type of law-breaking is collectively called 'corporate crime', and in monetary terms the scale of such crime is believed to exceed the total proceeds of street crime by a very large margin.

The focus of Sutherland's studies was on the operations of 70 of the largest US corporations in the areas of manufacturing, mining and public utilities during the first half of the last century. He found that these companies had an average of 14 decisions made against them by federal or state courts or by trade commissions. Some decisions covered multiple counts of illegitimate activity. Violations included restraint of trade (subverting competition laws); misrepresentation in advertising; unfair labour practices; and infringement of patents, trademarks or copyright. When the first edition of Sutherland's book *White Collar Crime* appeared in 1949, his publishers, fearful of libel action, and his university employers, fearful of losing sponsors, pressured him to remove identifying information concerning the companies he had studied (Geis and Goff, 1983). The full 'uncut' version of the book, with these details restored, did not appear until 1983.

There have been numerous scandals since that time bearing out the suggestion of many criminologists that corporate crimes are endemic within the financial system (e.g. Minkes, 2010; Robinson and Murphy, 2009). Sometimes they are traceable to slack or even non-existent internal oversight, as in the 1995 collapse of the British bank Barings, which followed the activities of a 'rogue trader' who notched up mammoth losses on the Singapore stock market. In other cases they are carefully planned by a small group, as in the Guinness scandal of 1987, in which four businessmen attempted to manipulate share prices in order to create conditions for a company takeover. In yet other instances, however, they are a result of systematic action involving multiple players, as in the collusion that was exposed in 2012 between Barclays and several other banks to manipulate the London Interbank Offered Rate (LIBOR). This is an interest rate that forms the basis of US $350 trillion worth of trading in financial 'derivatives' markets. The illicit rate-fixing had been happening over two decades, but only came to light in 2012 in what became known as the Libor scandal. Individual frauds can result in the loss of jaw-dropping sums of money, amongst the largest being the cases of the US companies Enron and WorldCom, which collapsed in 2001 and 2002 with losses of US $65 billion and US $104 billion respectively. Minkes (2010) provides details on a number of the most infamous corporate frauds of recent decades. However, later events suggest that these were only forerunners of much worse practices. The financial crisis which overtook many of the world's major economies in 2007–2008 did not have its origins solely in cavalier investment decisions, or in government regulatory laxity. There were also major elements of criminality underlying it, including investment, tax and mortgage fraud. Many types of risk were known but deliberately concealed, as mapped out by Barak (2012). These were part of a toxic mixture that also included major forms of mismanagement and miscalculation (Nelken, 2012). Thus economic crime is sometimes conducted on a scale far beyond that of the individual white-collar offender.

Using data collected by the World Bank, the Tax Justice Network (2011), an international research and advocacy organisation based in London, calculated that for 2010, the total amount of money lost to governments through tax evasion across 145 countries, representing 98.2 per cent of the world's Gross Domestic Product (GDP), was a remarkable US $3.13 trillion, equivalent to 5.1 per cent of the global GDP. The highest loss of potential tax revenue for a single country was in the USA, at US $337 billion; in a somewhat ignoble 'top ten table' for this, the UK came ninth, with a loss of US $109 billion. The same group later reported that overall a minimum of US $21 trillion and possibly as much as US $32 trillion has been diverted to 'offshore tax havens' (Tax Justice Network, 2012). Zucman (2015) estimated that wealthy individuals and multinational companies have in the region of US $7.6 trillion in hidden bank accounts or under the names of 'shell' companies in countries where those services are offered. While such companies – which do not conduct any 'real' business but are simply names for the holding of funds – are not in themselves illegal, it is known that they have often been used as vehicles for concealing financial assets and for tax evasion. Overall, as a drain on the world's national budgets, what is known as the 'shadow economy' outstrips 'ordinary' crime by a fairly colossal margin. It seems paradoxical, then, that these enormous figures are not a cause of greater concern.

One reason for this may lie in the widely discrepant amounts of attention that news media give to different kinds of law-breaking activity. This can be illustrated in relation to tax fraud and benefit fraud respectively. The UK's National Fraud Authority (2013) reported that in 2012 the total quantity of money lost as a result of 'identified fraud' was £15.5 billion, to which should be added a further £36.5 billion of 'hidden' fraud (total: £52 billion). Within that sum, the totals lost to tax fraud and benefit fraud were £14 billion and £1.2 billion respectively.

The latter, however, is the subject of many more news reports than the former. In an online survey of a UK representative sample (n=1,085), conducted in 2012 by the polling agency *YouGov* for the Trades Union Congress (TUC, 2013), respondents thought that 27 per cent of welfare payments were claimed fraudulently. Government figures showed that the actual proportion was 0.7 per cent. The finding can be placed in the wider context of the nature of public discourse surrounding social security payments in the UK, where there is a 'National Benefit Fraud Hotline' – a telephone number that members of the public can call if they suspect someone of making fraudulent welfare claims. In 2009–2010, over 250,000 calls were made to that number. Lundström (2013) compared the discussion of social security in five national newspapers in Britain with coverage of the same subject in four comparable newspapers in Sweden, and also analysed comments on related internet blogs. Very contrasting patterns of meaning emerged from the two settings. In Sweden the problem of social security fraud is perceived by the media as closely linked to concerns about the aggregate level of benefit fraud. The discussion is somewhat removed from the political sphere and the tone of writing is neutral. Although they do occur, there are few stories about individual cases. In the UK, in contrast, the debate is highly charged and politicised, and much more publicity is given to individual cases, with stories that give names and other personal details, and draw parallels with other types of crime in a way that generally calls into question the 'deservingness of recipients' (2013, p. 637). Differences such as this might partly explain why social security fraud provokes such anathema in Britain. As a number of authors have commented, there appear to be different rules applied to crimes committed in 'the streets' as opposed to those committed in 'the suites'. Levi (2009) has suggested reasons why there are no reactions of 'moral panic' surrounding white-collar crime, primarily deriving from the very different way public discussion of it is managed and perceived.

While financial offences do not cause direct physical injury, they can nevertheless be extremely damaging. Clearly, tax evasion deprives the public exchequer of resources that would otherwise be available for public purposes in health, education or other areas. Large-scale fraud, embezzlement, illegal trading in financial markets and related activities can create many victims, costing them their livelihoods through loss of jobs, earnings, savings or pensions, and indirectly, for example through reduced dividends or increased premiums. In addition to the economic hardship caused, there is likely to be accompanying emotional harm to such victims, which may have serious long-term impacts including deterioration in health. Boyd (2006) conducted a postal survey of 550 investors in a mortgage company in British Columbia, Canada, which collapsed due to fraud with total losses of $300 million (Canadian). Most of the investors had been dependent on the proceeds as a means of funding their retirement. More than half of those who had lost upwards of $50,000 described 'extreme or major harm' to their emotional well-being and security; and 20–30 per cent reported damage to their marriages, their friendships and their physical health, with effects similar to or worse than being a victim of a violent crime. In addition to the monetary losses involved, therefore, crimes committed for financial motives can have many less obvious but nevertheless serious consequences. The next 'Focus on...' box describes an infamous example of the crime of fraud.

FOCUS ON ...

Serious fraud: Ponzi schemes

Although Charles Ponzi (1881–1949) did not in fact invent the method of fraud that bears his name, his use of it and the scale of his activity caused a sensation that has linked his name to it ever since.

Ponzi was born in Italy, and moved to the United States in 1903. After a succession of low-paid jobs and failed business ventures, and having served a number of prison sentences, he hit upon a scheme for persuading people to invest money in a company he had set up. He paid *initial* investors using money he gained from *later* investors, thereby creating an impression that large profits could be made very fast. In fact, none of the money he took was invested elsewhere.

Imagine it is the start of the 20th century. You want to contact someone but there is no internet and there are few telephones. Your only option is to send a letter, but you know the people to whom you are writing cannot afford to buy stamps to reply. You therefore also send them a stamped envelope addressed to yourself (an SAE). Now imagine that the person lives in another country – at that time, as now, there were large movements of population around the globe. Not having the local stamps, you cannot send an SAE. But from 1906 onwards, when the International Postal Union was established, it became possible to send an 'international reply coupon' (IRC). This enables the person to reply to you without having to buy the local stamps. They can do this provided their country has signed up to this agreement, and by this time many countries have.

Ponzi noticed that stamps cost less in Italy than in the USA, and saw that there was an opportunity for money to be made – or so it *appeared*. The IRCs that were received were worth more than the cost of the stamps needed to reply. By selling the difference as an investment, Ponzi led people to believe that they could gain from future sales. In effect, he persuaded people that there was a possibility of making profit from this price difference. Essentially, he sold an idea of making good returns if you invested in his company: a company that was setting out to reap those profits. Indeed, he offered very high and speedy rates of return: 50 per cent after only 45 days.

In reality, achieving that was next to impossible. What Ponzi actually did was to pay earlier investors with the money invested by later ones. That created an initial impression of success – but no money was being generated by actual business investment. Over a period of several months in 1920, the number of people who bought shares in his business grew astonishingly fast. Ponzi, meanwhile, pocketed the excess income generated from all the people who had invested because they believed this scheme would work. It is thought that he gained a very large sum in 1920, equivalent to many millions of dollars today. He bought a mansion and lived an opulent lifestyle.

This type of fraud carries Charles Ponzi's name mainly because of the notoriety he gained from using it. There have been other similar schemes. Fast forward 100 years, and the most spectacular to date – said to be the largest fraud in history – was carried out by Bernard ('Bernie') Madoff, based in New York City, between 1991 and 2008.

The effects of these schemes were devastating for the many people who lost money as a result. Some investors could withstand the losses, but in many other instances the sums were people's entire life savings. Bernie Madoff had employed several close relatives in the business and one of his sons committed suicide. In June 2009, Madoff was sentenced to 150 years' imprisonment.

There are other serious types of large-scale fraud including pyramid schemes and matrix schemes. Very little is known about the psychology of those who perpetrate such crimes, but some studies pertaining to this are summarised in the main text.

In the most serious kinds of corporate crime, those who engage intentionally in actions that they know are likely to cause harm may have features more often associated with the very high-risk offenders described in the research literature on *psychopathy*. This concept will be examined more fully in Chapter 11, in its most widely used form as a description of a type of severe mental disorder associated with persistent antisocial behaviour. While this can only be speculative at present, several researchers have considered that the term 'psychopathic' may be applicable to the behaviour of some organisations and some individuals within them. Babiak, Neumann and Hare (2010) reported a study in which they administered the *Psychopathy Checklist* (PCL:R), the principal measure of the construct, to 203 managers and executives from seven corporations. They also obtained information from what are called '360° assessments', a management development tool in which individuals request feedback from those with different perspectives on them inside an organisation. Although the mean psychopathy score was lower than that for a community sample, the distribution was such that the corporate sample contained more individuals with high scores (including eight with PCL:R scores of 30 or more – the cut-off in defining psychopathy). Those emerging as higher on some features of psychopathy were rated by their colleagues as having a more charismatic interpersonal style, but as showing lower responsibility and as being poorer 'team players'.

Pardue, Robinson and Arrigo (2013a, 2013b) suggested that the concept of psychopathy may potentially contribute an important element to the understanding of corporate crime. Reviewing the major theories used to account for conventional crime, they noted that when applied to offences of this type there are some quite large explanatory gaps. They examined several incidents of high levels of harm caused by the oil, car and financial industries (e.g. explosions at British Petroleum (BP) facilities in Texas in 2005 and in the Gulf of Mexico in 2010; the concealment of vehicle faults by Toyota Motor Corporation, which in due course led to the recall of 11 million cars and vans; and the part played by banks such as Citigroup and Goldman Sachs in the 2008 financial crisis). They examined some of the features of psychopathy as specified by Hare (1996), whose description is widely used, and suggested that some of those features are associated with success in a competitive business environment. While recognising the challenge posed by applying an individual-level construct to an organisation, they considered that corporations as entities manifest some features of psychopathy and that 'corporate behaviour corresponds with several psychopathic traits'.

Organised crime

You may have noticed a recurring lament of this book that many terms have no agreed definitions. Unfortunately the same is true here, as the meaning of 'organised crime' is also rather loose. Generally, it refers to cooperation between individuals to commit offences, usually for profit, and likely to require planning, although whether or not there is overall coordination from any central source varies between contexts. As Levi (2012, p. 601) states, 'there is a conceptual problem of judging when a "network" begins and ends'. The extent to which this involves members of what is commonly called the criminal 'underworld' also varies, given that often some of those involved also have legitimate employment that affords them opportunities to commit crimes (von Lampe, 2016).

The kinds of offences that require active collaboration and that spawn the formation of criminal networks are usually ones likely to produce significant monetary gain. They include trafficking in drugs or people, smuggling to avoid taxes or import duties, identity theft and fraud relating to credit or debit cards, kidnapping for ransom, and the illegal dumping of toxic waste, amongst many others (Levi, 2012). To these could be added money-laundering, which often occurs at the intersection between lawful and unlawful activities (Hicks, 2010), and which was estimated to have amounted to US $1.6 trillion, or 2.7 per cent of global GDP, in 2009; a portion of it used to finance terrorism (HM Treasury and the Home Office, 2015). Some of these practices depend on internal corruption within official agencies, for example where a bank employee or executive is in a position to use existing accounts to disguise sources of money or the real identities of payees. Some forms of trafficking depend on illegal transfers of this kind, while others are done through the creation of 'front companies' (Hicks, 2010). Given the risks involved, including the severe penalties if apprehended and in some cases the attentions of potentially violent competitors, it seems likely that the rewards from these endeavours must be high.

Modes of organisation vary considerably. The family-based hierarchies and ritual codes of honour thought to characterise the Sicilian and American Mafia and other crime syndicates, as depicted in films such as *The Godfather*, do not appear to be typical of most organised crime. However, in some contexts there is a high level of structure. Levitt and Venkatesh (2000) studied the operation of a drug gang in an almost exclusively black neighbourhood in a large American city. There was a fairly formal hierarchy and allocation of roles (leader, runner, treasurer, enforcer and 'foot soldiers' who provided the points of sale for the drugs at street level). In some respects the group's organisation was not unlike that found in law-abiding businesses, with a franchise arrangement. The local gang paid a fee or tribute to a ruling city-wide group, and kept 'books' recording its transactions. There were large differences in income between those at different levels. While the rank-and-file earnings were close to the level of wages that could have been obtained in an ordinary job, those at the top enjoyed very large incomes. There were frequent inter-gang wars and a 7 per cent annual death rate; for the foot soldiers the risk of being killed was 80 times higher than for the African-American population in general. After the arrest of its leader, this gang dissolved and its 'territory' was taken over by others.

By contrast, Decker and Chapman (2008) studied cocaine smuggling from Colombia to the USA, and found that the cartel arrangements that had dominated the trade in the 1990s had waned in importance. Decker and Chapman interviewed 34 individuals serving lengthy prison sentences (mostly greater than 15 years). While most were drug users themselves, the majority regarded themselves primarily as businessmen. Overwhelmingly, their motives were economic, and few gave much thought to the end-users of the trafficking trade. Recruitment into the process was mainly through personal contact, and the connections between participants were more akin to loose and flexible coalitions than centralised gangs. Individuals were only in contact with those either side of them in the transportation chain. This pattern appears to have evolved in response to the efforts of law-enforcement agencies, and a capacity to adapt and evolve to avoid detection or to minimise losses appears to have been a feature of the illegal drugs trade for a long time (Dorn, Murji and South, 1992).

Similar arrangements appear to be a hallmark of vehicle trafficking. For the year 2012, Interpol's database recorded 7.2 million vehicle thefts in 127 countries (Interpol, 2014).

In the opening years of the 21st century, half a million vehicles per annum (mainly sports and luxury cars) were stolen in wealthy countries and sold in less affluent ones (Clarke and Brown, 2003). Accomplishing this involved a series of separate tasks: after the initial theft, mechanics changed vehicle identities or appearance, others forged documents, and couriers moved vehicles between countries. But there would be only minimal contact between these 'specialists', and the people behind the whole operation might never meet any of them, thereby keeping risk as low as possible.

From a psychological standpoint, however, relatively little is known about those who commit these kinds of offences. There is some evidence that the pathways of those involved in organised crime differ to some extent from those of individuals involved in 'high volume' crime. This has been a neglected area of research as compared with most other types of offence, but van Koppen, de Poot, Kleemans and Nieuwbeerta (2010) have reported findings from the Dutch Organized Crime Monitor. This is a large-scale study of 120 criminal groups who were committing offences during a 12-year period (1994–2006), and comprises a total of 1,623 individuals. Organised crime in the Netherlands took particular forms, centred around trafficking of drugs, stolen vehicles, smuggling illegal immigrants, and human (including sexual) trafficking. Studying a subset of 854 offenders, van Koppen and colleagues (2010) found that a quite large fraction (40 per cent) of those involved could be described as adult-onset offenders. While there was a smaller group who had been involved in offending since adolescence, the adult-onset group committed their first offences at a mean age of 29. It has been suggested that participation in organised crime requires a particular skill set that differs from that involved in ordinary property or violent crime. While many offenders act alone, organised crime self-evidently involves communication and cooperation with a range of other people, often including contacts from different walks of life or of different nationalities. Some of the necessary skills are ones that could be used in running legitimate businesses, and indeed some who are found guilty of these offences have previously done so – perhaps an especially tempting opportunity arose, however, or presented itself at a time when the individual had need of additional funds. Alongside this, the type of social influences identified by Sutherland (1983) would also probably be operating.

Corporate violence

We saw in Chapter 2 that within criminology the familiar definition of crime as 'violation of criminal law' is more or less unanimously regarded as unsatisfactory, mainly because of its narrowness. It excludes numerous ways in which harm is caused in society, which for a variety of reasons are not categorised as crime. As we have just seen, however, there is evidence that a large swathe of illegal and harmful behaviour is carried on by individuals and by corporations, the total costs of this behaviour far exceeding those arising from 'ordinary crime'. The most sharply contested segment of this field of investigation concerns the concept of *corporate violence*. Let us look at what this term means and why it is a focus of dispute.

Hartley (2008, p. 27) argues that although business executives are not usually thought of as engaging in violence, 'corporations do engage in acts with violent outcomes. The belief that corporate crime is less harmful than street crime is a myth.' While corporate violence can take many forms, Hartley divides it into three major categories: poor working conditions and violations of safety regulations; the sale of harmful or defective products; and environmental pollution.

Safety violations and poor working conditions

There have been numerous industrial accidents in which the cause has been traced to safety practices that had been ignored or compromised in order to reduce running costs. They include the 1984 explosion at the Union Carbide Corporation's pesticide plant in Bhopal, India, in which toxic gases were released over a wide area. The official death toll was 3,787; but the disaster caused many thousands more deaths in its aftermath, and over half a million injuries due to the effects of the toxins. Another was the collapse in

2012 of a building used as a clothing factory in Dhaka, Bangladesh, which claimed 1,129 lives. But breaches of safety standards have also occurred in countries where we assume that such standards are more carefully monitored. Explosions at the Piper Alpha North Sea gas platform in 1988, which claimed 167 lives, and at the British Petroleum/ Deepwater Horizon platform in the Gulf of Mexico in 2010, which killed 11 workers and caused massive environmental damage, are only two of many possible examples. In these and many other cases, safety was given lower priority than cutting costs.

Yet these tragic events form only part of a much bigger picture. The International Labour Organization, an arm of the United Nations, estimates that on an annual basis worldwide there are 2.3 million work-related deaths, 340 million occupational accidents, and 160 million victims of work-related illnesses (International Labour Organization, 2011). While some of these incidents may not have been foreseeable or preventable, the majority were due to failures in applying appropriate safety standards, to the taking of shortcuts to save money, or to unhealthy working conditions such as dealing with toxic substances (e.g. asbestos) without sufficient protection. Brookman and Robinson (2012, p. 566) comment that 'deaths due to corporate negligence and neglect (much of it is wilful) dwarf all other kinds of homicides that are routinely counted'.

Sale of harmful or defective products

There have been many examples of companies holding back information about the harm their products might cause, or continuing to sell goods that were known to be defective. The deadliest of all in sheer numbers stems from the action of tobacco companies, which concealed evidence of the harmful effects of cigarette smoking for a 30-year period, and which have continued to target new markets (as already noted in Chapter 2). Many deaths and other problems have been caused by medicines, as in the case of the drug thalidomide, which during the 1950s was advertised to women as a cure for morning sickness during pregnancy, but led to deformities at birth in many thousands of children.

Other notorious cases include the production during the 1970s of the Ford Pinto car (Baura, 2006). This model was designed with the fuel line close to the back of the vehicle, where it could rupture and explode on impact during a collision. It was reported that accidents in which this happened led to an estimated 500–900 burn deaths. Investigative journalist Mark Dowie (1977) obtained internal memos that showed that the manufacturer had been well aware of this possibility. Improving the safety would have cost \$11 per car, however, totalling \$137 million across all units. Instead, Ford conducted a cost–benefit analysis, factoring in amounts of compensation to be paid in the event of an estimated 180 fatal accidents and 180 injuries a year, and since that cost totalled only \$49.5 million, the company decided not to alter the design for several years, expecting thereby to save \$87.5 million.

Environmental pollution

In discussions of the human impact on the environment, comparisons are often made between the amounts of pollution caused by different countries. Within countries, however, industrial corporations produce a large share of the pollution. Hartley (2008) considers this the most prevalent category of corporate harm as it has the most far-reaching effects. In a worldwide study by Pimentel *et al.* (2007), based on data from WHO and other sources, the authors estimated that chemical emissions and environmental degradation were responsible for 40 per cent of deaths globally per year. These deaths were the results of direct and indirect exposure to toxic chemicals used in manufacturing, to pesticides in agriculture, and to the longer-term impact of these and other compounds in contaminating the water supply and in fostering conditions that allow the growth of disease pathogens (such as the micro-organism that causes malaria).

There have been disputes over how problems such as the ones discussed in this section should be regarded, and the question has often been posed: are these really crimes? As regards some types of economic crime, the corporate world has tried to resist the 'crime' label, and the line between business practice that is clever and innovative ('sharp') and that which is criminal can be difficult to draw. Taking a moral perspective, Robinson and Murphy (2009) have analysed the differences between ordinary, conventional, traditional (or 'street' crime) and corporate economic crime or 'elite deviance'. The effects of violent crime, as conventionally defined, are mainly direct and immediate. There is usually an individual offender, and the action is one of commission and is considered wilful and voluntary. Corporate violence, on the other hand, is indirect, indeed usually distant, and in most cases its effects are delayed. There are often many people playing some part, and company employees probably do not set out deliberately to do harm; they may just never think about the consequences of their actions. Yet those individual employees (or the corporate body) are still culpable, as in many particular instances it has been shown that they acted not just negligently, or recklessly, but knowingly. The number of occasions on which this has led to prosecution, however, is extremely small in comparison with what occurs in ordinary criminal cases. The attitude of authorities and law-enforcement agencies to corporate misdemeanour appears at best to be 'ambivalent' (Nelken, 2012). For this reason, few if any forensic psychologists are likely to work with individuals who had been involved in these forms of harm-doing.

The junction of economic and violent crime

We can now travel full circle, as it were, and find our way back to the areas covered in some earlier chapters. To conclude this chapter, let us look briefly at a type of crime that partly reflects the theme of the present section, economic crime, but also links it to the subject matter of Chapters 7 and 8. *Contract killing* has features of an economic crime, since perpetrators carry it out for money; yet obviously this crime also involves homicidal violence. Despite its seriousness, there is very little research on this kind of offence. That might be because it is comparatively rare as a form of murder, but that is difficult to tell as it is not identified separately in legal statutes, so the absolute amount of this crime is unknown. In addition, the secrecy that surrounds this crime makes it difficult to identify when it has occurred.

Self-evidently, a contract murder involves at least three people. The first is the person who commissions and pays for it, the instigator or hirer, who wants someone dead. The second is the person who carries out the act, the hiree or assassin. The third is the intended target or victim, of which there is usually just one, though there could be more. It is worth noting that a 'contract' to kill is not written down and is not legally binding. If the hiree fails to carry out the job as agreed, there is little likelihood that he or she will be pursued through the courts. For this reason, fees are often paid in two instalments, one before and one after the work has been carried out.

Criminal justice statistics for Scotland (Scottish Government, 2003, 2013), covering the ten-year period between 1993 and 2002, show that for the most part only a small percentage of homicides were classified as contract killings, though this showed some variation and rose as high as 11 per cent in one year. Possibly as a result of fuller information becoming available and some crimes being reclassified, in the following ten-year period up to 2012–2013 very few murders were recorded under this heading. What did remain constant, however, was that almost all perpetrators were male – very few offences of this type are committed by women.

Mouzos and Venditto (2003) analysed a series of 163 contract murders committed or attempted in Australia between 1989 and 2002. These constituted about 2 per cent of the total number of homicides during that period. Amongst them, 69 were successfully completed, while 94 were failed attempts. Most victims were in the age range 25–49 and the majority were male. The age of instigators was on average slightly older, whereas the perpetrators were slightly younger. In 74 per cent of cases the murder weapon was a firearm, the remainder involving various weapons including knives, blunt instruments, drugs and explosives. In a small number of cases, instigators specified that victims were to be beaten to death. The fee that was paid showed a remarkably wide range: from a mere $500 (Australian) to $100,000, with an average of $16,500. There were numerous motives for taking out contracts to have someone killed, which the authors divided into nine categories; though in the second largest category (17 per cent of the offences), the motives were unknown. The other commonest motives, in descending order of frequency, were: the dissolution of a relationship (e.g. to prevent an ex-partner from forming a liaison with someone else, or to eliminate a current partner who was a barrier to a new relationship; 19 per cent); financial (usually to benefit from an insurance policy; 16 per cent); to silence witnesses (13 per cent); for revenge (10 per cent); and drug-related (6 per cent); with remaining categories (e.g. 'personal advancement') accounting for only a few killings each. There were similar kinds of motives for both completed and attempted homicides, though the frequencies differed.

In the UK, Cameron (2013) reported a study of 52 known paid murders carried out between 1972 and 2011, although it should be noted that his sources of information were newspaper reports and their accuracy is not guaranteed (though journalists often find information that is not found by anyone else). The objectives of the study were primarily economic and focused on how instigators made decisions to take out a murder contract. Again, given the risks involved, the median cost was perhaps surprisingly modest at £10,000, but there was a very wide range from a mere £200 to £1.5 million. Ages of hirers, perpetrators and victims were broadly similar. The largest group of victims comprised relationship partners (56 per cent) and in just under one-third of cases the primary motive was inheritance (the very high fee just cited was such a case).

Levi (1981) reported an interview with a professional 'hit man' (who used the pseudonym 'Pete'), who was serving a prison sentence for one of his crimes that had gone wrong. Pete had committed a number of contract killings – although the exact number is not disclosed, there are references to at least four – and saw himself as an independent freelance agent who took satisfaction in doing his job well. He was ashamed when one commission went badly awry, and it was this that led to his arrest. Levi describes the process whereby Pete had assumed a professional identity, and how he controlled his internal reactions to taking a life, especially after his first 'hit', in which the victim looked at him as he died, with an expression of incomprehension on his face. Following this, Pete was ill for two months; but he succeeded in forcing himself to 'reframe' the event, to extinguish his negative reaction. After that, the job became 'routine'. This man's motive was purely economic, and Levi illustrates his use of several neutralisation techniques, including a form of appeal to higher loyalties (pride in his skill and expertise), and denial of wrongfulness or injury (as he was an instrument of someone else).

As news reports often remind us, there are other types of planned assassinations that are politically motivated. It is usually assumed that they have a different origin from the kind discussed here, for example to stop an individual or group from gaining power, or to eliminate the leader of a competing party. This does not exclude the possibility, however, that those commissioning such crimes might not also have personal motives intermixed with factional or ideological ones.

Conclusion

Comparing the different topics covered in this chapter, there are evidently large differences between them in the amount of psychological research relevant to them. Substance-related offending is very extensively researched, and a psychological perspective is widely, if perhaps not universally, viewed as having something to contribute to theory, research and practice in this field. That is important also because substance use may be a risk factor for almost any kind of offending. In the other areas covered in this chapter, psychology has less of a presence, though the volume of work on arson or firesetting is substantial and in many ways leads developments in this area. On robbery, kidnapping or abduction, and economic crimes, psychological studies are considerably thinner, and it may not be unfair to say that psychology has yet to make its mark in relation to the study of these crimes and in guiding practice when working with these offenders.

Chapter summary

The chapter has covered a variety of types of offences, which in some respects are quite a disparate mixture. Apart from substance misuse itself, another thread that runs through the other offences discussed in the chapter, at least in some of the forms they take, is that of acquisitiveness or monetary gain. That is central to robbery, and to the economic offences discussed at the end of the chapter. But it also drives some forms of firesetting, and some forms of kidnapping and hostage-taking.

The issue of substance misuse can be of relevance in relation to almost any kind of offending, and while the focus here was principally on its possible links to violence, it is also an established risk factor for offending behaviour in the widest sense. An important reason for considering it here has been to present the argument for avoiding an exclusively biologically oriented approach to substance dependence and addiction. Despite strongly held views to the contrary, the ground beneath the Brain Disease Model of Addiction is not as firm as many of its proponents claim.

There is a close association between substance abuse and some forms of robbery, mainly street robbery. The chapter examined those associations, but also considered other patterns of robbery that are more likely to be planned, organised and committed by groups.

Further reading

» Statistics on drug use quoted in this chapter are from Home Office sources. For anyone interested in the health aspects of these data, such as hospitalisation rates, information can be obtained from the Health and Social Care Information centre website: www.hscic.gov.uk.

» On substance misuse, a highly recommended book combining accounts of personal experience with information on neuroscience is by Marc Lewis (2015): *The Biology of Desire: Why Addiction is Not a Disease*. New York: PublicAffairs.

» The European Monitoring Centre for Drugs and Drug Addiction, based in Lisbon, produces a wide range of documentation on all aspects of drug use, intervention and policy.

» The Arson Prevention Forum (APF) was established in the UK in 2012 as a result of merging the Arson Control Forum, established by the government in 2001, and the Arson Prevention Bureau, which provided advice to businesses and the public on behalf of the insurance industry.

» On kidnapping, Diana M. Concannon (2013), in *Kidnapping: An Investigator's Guide*, 2nd edition (London and Waltham, MA: Elsevier), gives an overview of the different patterns. Richard P. Wright (2009), in *Kidnap for Ransom: Resolving the Unthinkable* (Boca Raton, FL: Taylor & Francis), provides an account of the sequence of events in kidnap and the processes of negotiation.

» On arson, the best source is: Rebekah M. Doley, Geoffrey L. Dickens and Theresa A. Gannon (eds) (2016), *The Psychology of Arson: A Practical Guide to Understanding and Managing Deliberate Firesetters*. London and New York: Routledge.

» On economic, white collar, and corporate crime, see the book edited by Gregg Barak (2015), *The Routledge International Handbook of the Crimes of the Powerful* (London and New York: Routledge). On organised crime, see Klaus von Lampe (2016), *Organized Crime: Analyzing Illegal Activities, Criminal Structures, and Extra-Legal Governance* (Thousand Oaks, CA: Sage).

Mental Disorder and Crime

This chapter is concerned with the complex question of the relationship between criminal behaviour and mental health problems, focusing particularly on offences of violence. There is extensive evidence that the rate of mental health problems amongst prisoners is higher than that in the community in general, but the *nature* of any such links has been the subject of much debate. In many countries there is a proportion of offenders who are detained under mental health law rather than criminal law. Forensic psychologists work in both of the key settings where such problems come to the fore – prisons and secure mental health services.

Chapter objectives

- To outline some principal concepts relating to mental health problems and disorders.
- To present a critical analysis of currently dominant concepts and models in this field.
- To summarise findings from surveys of the mental health needs of prisoners.
- To review evidence concerning the relationship between mental disorder and crime, with particular reference to violence.
- To provide an overview of treatment and service arrangements for offenders with major mental health problems.

Many jurisdictions make provision for addressing the particular problems that arise when someone who has committed a criminal offence is also found to be suffering from a **mental disorder**. While many prisons have mental health units, the general environment of prisons is not designed with the needs of this group in mind. Many countries have therefore built specialised secure hospital units for persons whom it is thought necessary to contain, but who are seen as being in urgent need of treatment for mental health problems in addition to restraint of their criminal conduct.

Broadly speaking, there are two major aspects to these arrangements. First, some individuals who have committed offences are judged as not having been fully responsible for their actions when they carried them out. There can be several possible explanations for this, and in this chapter we will consider the explanations that are attributed to the presence of a disordered state of mind. Second, recognition by courts that those offenders are not fully responsible often leads them onto a separate route or track of services, which usually requires that the individual be detained in a secure mental health facility where the necessary treatment can be provided, rather than in a penal institution. All the services associated with mental health and offending are often governed by a separate strand of law pertaining to what is now widely called 'forensic mental health' (Bartlett and McGauley, 2009).

In some countries, such as the United States, forensic psychologists are extensively involved in the legal proceedings leading up to the court decision as to whether someone will be declared legally insane or made subject to mental health law (Rogers and Shuman, 2000; Skeem, Douglas and Lilienfeld, 2009). In other countries, including all parts of the United Kingdom, forensic psychologists are employed mainly in prisons, secure mental health units or probation services. Thus with a few exceptions (mainly independent experts working in private practice), they generally become involved only *after* court decisions have been made.

For the most part, individuals detained under mental health legislation are likely to have committed fairly serious offences, usually involving personal violence of some kind. Psychologists are involved in their assessment and treatment, in monitoring and evaluating their progress, and in advising on their suitability for transfer to different levels of security or eventual return to the community. A key aspect of this work in both prison and hospital locations is the assessment of risk of further violent or sexual offending. (These areas will be covered more fully in Chapter 18.)

This chapter is divided into several main sections. First, we examine in general terms the nature of **mental health problems** and disorders, but adopt a questioning stance towards the orthodox view of what such problems consist of using psychiatric diagnosis. Next, we survey evidence concerning the mental health problems of adult prisoners and young offenders. Following this, we address the key question of the extent to which there is a relationship between mental disorder and crime, and to what extent any such link is a causal one, with particular reference to violence. Within this, we consider the two major categories of mental disorder that have been studied most intensively: psychoses and personality disorders. We also examine what have been variously called disorders of sexual interest or preference. Finally, but more briefly, we survey the system of treatment services that has developed to address the needs that arise in this area, and the routes along which individuals travel on their journey through that system.

Mental health problems and disorders: some key distinctions

A useful place to begin is with some of the definitional problems and related issues that arise in this area. It is important to be aware of the problems that *many* people experience in response to adverse events, and to distinguish these from reactions or mental states that are more severe or more lasting. Some difficulties may continue for protracted periods, or spread outwards to cause other disruptions or personal suffering.

The two main features of such disruption are some level of *impairment*, and a sense of losing *control* – an inability to overcome one's problems (Haynes, O'Brien and Kaholokula, 2011). These do not, however, amount to a diagnosable mental disorder. In the study of the latter, some other terms are commonly used:

- *Syndrome* This term denotes a *cluster* of reported problems or symptoms that regularly co-occur, to such an extent that they appear to belong together.
- *Mental disorder* This term is used more strictly to denote difficulties that are frequent, severe or enduring. That is, they become highly salient, even dominant, in someone's life.
- *Disease* The concept of mental *disorder* is not the same as that of *disease*, or at least not in the way that that word is used in physical medicine. In some parts of psychiatry the two words are sometimes used interchangeably. Hyman (2010), however, suggests that the word 'disease' should be reserved for a medical problem where the cause is known, while 'disorder' should be used to refer to problems where the cause is unknown.

Estimating prevalence

Survey evidence suggests that a substantial number of people describe problems on one or other of these levels during the course of their lives. A report by the World Health Organization (2001) estimated that almost one in four people around the globe had been affected by a mental health problem at some stage of their lives, and that globally at that time there were 450 million people suffering from a mental or behavioural disorder. The WHO researchers found that approximately 1 million people commit suicide each year, and between 10 and 20 million attempt it. In the United Kingdom, surveys of mental health have been conducted at several time-points by the National Health Service Information Centre for Health and Social Care (McManus *et al.*, 2009). These surveys showed, for example, that in 2007 various forms of depression and anxiety, which together are classified as 'common mental health problems' (CMHPs), were reported by one in six (17.6 per cent) of the population in the age-group 16–64. When other problems such as *post-traumatic stress disorder*, eating disorders, alcohol and drug misuse and schizophrenia were added, the proportion screening positive for at least one condition rose to 23 per cent – almost one in four.

Some studies have yielded figures even higher than those. In the National Comorbidity Survey Replication (NCS-R) in the United States, with a nationally representative sample of 9,282 participants, Kessler *et al.* (2005) found a *lifetime prevalence* (up to age 75) of any disorder of 46.6 per cent. However, there have been concerns that using a retrospective method – asking people to recall health problems over a selected past period – can lead to an underestimate of true prevalence, especially after a long gap. To overcome this, as part of the Dunedin Longitudinal Study, which included health as well as behavioural outcomes, Moffitt *et al.* (2010) conducted a clinical interview with just under 1,000 participants at ages 18, 21, 26 and 32. This study generated lifetime estimates for every disorder category that were *double* those reported in the NCS-R study. There are also suggestions that mental health problems such as depression and anxiety are affecting more and more people over time. Indeed, there have been worries, particularly in the USA, that there was virtually an 'epidemic' of mental ill-health (Whitaker, 2005).

In the face of the growing alarm, however, are these reported problems really mental disorders? Researchers have protested that in fact what are natural and integral parts of the experience of being human have been classified as 'mental disorders' (e.g. Horwitz and Wakefield, 2007). Some psychologists have voiced concern that the net effect of that trend is such that normal human reactions have been transmuted into a kind of pathology. This has been described as the 'medicalization of misery' – the 'psychiatrization and psychologization of almost every aspect of human experience' (Rapley, Moncrieff and Dillon, 2011, p. 5).

The underlying problem that gives rise to these confusions and disagreements is that there is no objective means of categorising the varieties of distress which people experience that is based on an impartial or scientific standard. Many attempts have been made to define the difference between 'normality' and 'abnormality'. That can be done in statistical terms, as large departures from the mean; with reference to what is adaptive or maladaptive, functional or dysfunctional, for someone; by reference to individual distress, which is necessarily subjective; or by comparison with prevailing social norms. But such efforts invariably return to the basic discovery that normality can only be defined through the meanings assigned to it in a given community. The definitions of these terms are not independently verifiable according to any neutral standard: they are *socially constructed* (Maddux, Gosselin and Winstead, 2015).

Further evidence of this is that widely held beliefs concerning what constitutes insanity, and assumptions regarding what causes it, have changed quite dramatically over successive historical epochs. For example, *hysteria* was at one time thought to be a mental disorder of emotional excess, considered unique to women. The word is derived from the same lexical roots as the Greek word for 'womb', as the female anatomy was thought to be the source of the problem. In 1866 a British obstetrician, Dr Isaac Baker Brown, published a book advocating the use of clitoridectomy to cure epilepsy, catalepsy and hysteria in women, and a scandal erupted when it was discovered that he had been practising this at his London surgery (Fennell, 2010). Likewise, the notion of homosexuality as a form of illness was part of conventional thinking until not very long ago; in the USA it was diagnosable as a psychiatric disorder until 1973. It is still seen as unnatural or illicit (or both) by some sectors of the community, by some religions, and in some societies. For example, in Uganda, where homosexuality was already punishable by imprisonment, a 2009 parliamentary bill included clauses to introduce the death penalty for 'aggravated' cases. After a series of legal disputes, the proposal was dropped in 2014.

Similarly, ideas concerning schizophrenia – which corresponds to many people's stereotypical notions of 'madness' – have undergone some remarkable changes over the last few centuries (Read, 2004). For example, hearing voices is listed as one of the classic 'first rank' signs of psychotic illness. But community surveys found that 'hearing voices' was reported by 11–13 per cent of the US population, and by 6.2 per cent in a similar study in the Netherlands. Those affected were not troubled by what they heard. Van

Os, Hanssen, Bijl and Ravelli (2000) suggested that experiences associated with psychosis may have a continuous distribution in the general population, rather than a dichotomous pattern that divides psychotic from normal. The operative variable appears not to be the *experience* of hearing voices, but the individual's attitude to those voices and relationship with them (Bentall, 2009).

Psychiatric diagnosis

Nosology, the science of classification of disease entities, has proved to be invaluable in many fields of medicine. The concept of *diagnosis*, the detection of which disease is afflicting an individual, is central to medical practice. The concept was imported into the field of psychiatry in an effort to afford psychiatry the same status as other medical specialisms (Moncrieff, 2009). Thus diagnostic systems in psychiatry are a method for classifying mental health problems in a manner analogous to that which might be applied to physical ill-health. According to Widiger (2015, p. 97), 'the impetus for the development of an official diagnostic nomenclature was the crippling confusion generated by its absence'. Sets of criteria were developed in psychiatry from the 1950s onward in an effort to increase the reliability of the process of diagnosis (Hyman, 2010).

The primary objective of a psychiatric assessment is to gather enough information to enable a diagnosis to be made. Doing so is thought to offer four important advantages (Eastman, 2000):

- *Classification* The systematic description of patterns amongst mental health problems makes it possible to place them in groups that share common features. This initial step is seen as vital on the route to eventual identification and classification of 'disease entities' (Kendell and Jablensky, 2003; Wing, Sartorius and Üstün, 1998).
- *Aetiology* Having found identifiable syndromes, it should then be possible to develop an understanding of their pathological origins. For example, we might expect those who share common patterns to have a similar underlying cause (in medical terminology, the *pathogen*) and we would investigate accordingly.
- *Prognosis* If syndromes do share common roots, they may also be likely to continue along similar paths in the future. This opens up the possibility of predicting the average course and pattern of a disorder – for example, short term, episodic, chronic, or lifelong.
- *Therapy* Knowledge of causes, development and prognosis can also enable clinicians to determine the most suitable and effective treatment that could ameliorate, and maybe even eliminate, the problems diagnosed.

Considerable energy has been expended in attempts to devise a systematic and sound approach to the diagnosis of mental disorders. The results of this have altered over time, and systems of psychiatric classification are in a state of evolution. Two approaches are in current use, respectively known as the *International Classification of Diseases* (ICD) and the *Diagnostic and Statistical Manual* (DSM), as outlined in the 'Focus on ...' box on page 249.

For certain types of psychiatric disorder a specific organic origin has been established, and where that has occurred a diagnostic approach has been shown to work extremely well. One of the foremost examples is *Huntington's disease*, which is a genetically transmitted *neurodegenerative disorder* resulting in cognitive decline and other marked impairments, with a typical age of onset between 35 and 44 years of age. The cause of this disease has been traced to a specific genetic mutation, and while the mechanism of its action is not yet wholly understood, understanding of the disease is sufficiently well developed that diagnosis can be undertaken with a high level of accuracy (Walker, 2007).

For many other mental and behavioural problems, however, there is no known single origin or cause. In relation to schizophrenia, for example, there has been a long running and at times vociferous dispute over whether or not the disease has a genetic origin. Researchers have found a large number of gene risk factors for schizophrenia,

FOCUS ON …

Diagnostic systems in psychiatry

It is mandatory for anyone working in the field of mental health to be familiar with the concept of psychiatric diagnosis, with the basis on which it rests, and with the processes involved in undertaking it. Some initial confusion is almost inevitable, however, as there are two distinct, although intersecting, systems of psychiatric diagnosis in contemporary use.

One, developed in the USA by the American Psychiatric Association (2013), is called the *Diagnostic and Statistical Manual of Mental and Behavioral Disorders*, usually simply abbreviated to DSM. First published in 1953, it has gone through several revisions and is currently in its 5th edition (hence it is presently called DSM-5).

The other, developed by the World Health Organization (1992), an agency of the United Nations based in Geneva, is one part of a major project called the *International Classification of Diseases* or ICD. It is now in its 10th edition (hence ICD-10; the 11th is due in 2018).

The development and launch of the DSM-5 in May 2013 was accompanied by a high level of controversy and by widespread protests. There was a barrage of criticism concerning numerous aspects of it, portions of this criticism coming from authors of earlier DSM editions (Frances, 2013), and other vociferous objections coming from numerous professional groups, including the British Psychological Society, as well as from many service user groups.

Previously, comparisons between the two major diagnostic systems have shown that the extent to which the diagnostic criteria matched each other – meaning that individuals would be placed in the same disorder categories using either approach – varied from one category to another. In one study of this kind, Andrews, Slade and Peters (1999) used the Composite International Diagnostic Interview (CIDI), a highly structured clinical assessment, to examine 1300–1500 people from a 'disorder-enriched' population sample. Across all disorders, there was 68 per cent agreement (concordance) on diagnoses. However, this ranged from 87 per cent for dysthymia and 83 per cent for depressive episodes, to only 35 per cent for PTSD and 33 per cent for substance abuse.

Widiger (2015) provided a history of how the two diagnostic systems had evolved. Many commentators have expressed grave reservations about the expanding scope of psychiatric diagnosis. Following the appearance of the fourth DSM in 1994, there were repeated criticisms of its over-inclusiveness (e.g. Kutchins and Kirk, 1997). Satirical though earnest predictions were made concerning the likely content of the DSM-5, long before it began to be shaped (Blashfield and Fuller, 1996). As the DSM-5 Task Force proceeded with its work, numerous critiques were published in efforts to influence the final result. There have continued to be two fundamental issues at stake: (a) whether it is appropriate to extend the concept of 'psychiatric disorder' to apply to almost any form of human distress (such as shyness, or prolonged grief reactions), and (b) the doubtful status of the evidence adduced to support some of the proposed diagnostic categories.

Question

In your own experience, how useful is a psychiatric diagnosis in helping to make sense of an individual's behaviour?

but many of these are also risk markers for several other psychiatric disorders, including bipolar disorder, attention deficit hyperactivity disorder, autism, severe learning disabilities, and some forms of epilepsy (Doherty, O'Donovan and Owen, 2011; International Schizophrenia Consortium, 2009). A major study of genetic 'risk loci', in a very large sample of 33,332 cases and 27,888 controls, reported that four specific gene sites were significantly associated with five different psychiatric diagnosis categories

(Cross-Disorder Group of the Psychiatric Genomics Consortium, 2013). These major mental health problems have no distinctly identifiable causes at genetic level, and each seems likely to be a result of numerous factors acting in combination.

Alongside the problems of unknown or extremely uncertain aetiology, there are also three other significant difficulties with current diagnostic systems:

» *Comorbidity* In many instances, individuals who meet the criteria for diagnosis of one type of mental disorder also meet the criteria for another, and sometimes for several others (Clark, Watson and Reynolds, 1995). This confounds the idea that we might expect to find discontinuities of symptom profiles ('zones of rarity') between disorder categories (Hyman, 2010). On average, between 50 per cent and 60 per cent of those diagnosed with a mental disorder also met criteria for another disorder. For *generalised anxiety disorder* (GAD), for example, the figure is as high as 83 per cent. The resultant uncertainty in diagnosis detracts from the potential advantages of diagnosis listed earlier. It also calls into question the validity of the categories that have been created. 'At present there is little evidence that most contemporary psychiatric diagnoses are valid, because they are still defined by syndromes that have not been demonstrated to have natural boundaries' (Kendell and Jablensky, 2003, p. 11). Despite that drawback, those authors nevertheless thought diagnoses were useful concepts.

» *Heterogeneity* The criteria for diagnosing any given disorder usually consist of a list of symptoms or problem behaviours. Individuals may be diagnosed with the disorder if they satisfy *some* of the criteria. Taking *borderline personality disorder* (BPD) as an example, there are nine criteria specified; for the diagnosis to be applied, an individual needs to manifest any five of the nine. Two individuals diagnosed with BPD might thus have only one of these features in common; and there are 256 theoretically possible ways of meeting the criteria for diagnosis. In a study of 930 psychotherapeutic day-hospital patients in Norway, Johansen *et al.* (2004) found 252 who met criteria for a diagnosis of BPD. Within this group, researchers identified 136 different permutations of the criteria, and: 'The maximum number of patients with exactly the same combination of criteria was six' (Johansen *et al.*, 2004, p. 292). Individuals can therefore be really quite unlike each other in terms of their symptom presentations, so it seems reasonable to ask how much sense it makes to say that they have the same disorder. The members of the group diagnosed with BPD by Johansen *et al.* met an average of 6.1 criteria of BPD – but they also on average met 14.7 criteria for other kinds of personality disorder.

» *Prognosis* Some mental disorders, such as schizophrenia, are considered to be chronic conditions. However, follow-up of patients diagnosed in different countries shows marked discrepancies in the proportions having the 'best course' over a ten-year period (Desjarlais, Eisenberg, Good and Kleinman, 1996). While the figures for high-income countries such as the Czech Republic, Denmark, the USA and the UK ranged from 3.4 per cent to 32.2 per cent, the corresponding range for medium- and low-income countries such as Colombia, India and Nigeria was notably higher, from 27.2 per cent to 52.1 per cent. Schizophrenia is also thought to require lifelong treatment usually with 'antipsychotic' medication, in order to control what are called the *positive symptoms* of hallucinations, delusions and thought disorder. However, Harrow and Jobe (2007) contacted a group of 64 patients diagnosed with schizophrenia on five successive occasions over a total period of 15 years. Contrary to expectations, they found that in terms of global functioning those patients who remained off psychiatric drugs fared significantly better than those who took them. In the medicated group, the proportions showing psychotic activity were 79 per cent at the 10-year follow-up and 64 per cent at the 15-year follow-up. For the unmedicated group, the equivalent figures were 23 per cent and 28 per cent. Whitaker (2010) suggests that the standard medical response to some ailments, including the dispensing of neuroleptic drugs for schizophrenia, can often make matters worse.

Turning to *negative symptoms*, Evensen *et al.* (2012) charted the presence of a 'flat affect' (social withdrawal and emotional unresponsiveness) in a group of 184 people diagnosed with schizophrenia, who were assessed at several points over ten years. Only 5 per cent of the group showed the symptoms enduringly throughout that period; 29 per cent had never shown them to begin with; 16 per cent showed a deteriorating pattern and 10 per cent an improving pattern; and 40 per cent a pattern that fluctuated over time.

These kinds of evidence raise questions concerning both the scientific credibility and practical implications of the process of syndrome classification as it currently stands. One trenchant criticism of the medical-diagnostic model highlighted some of its difficulties by examining the extent to which *happiness* meets the criteria for a psychiatric disorder (Bentall, 1992) – which it was found to do, as well as some other syndromes: it is statistically abnormal, and involves cognitive and emotional aberrations. Despite these and many other objections, however, diagnosis remains the core organising principle in most mental healthcare.

None of this is intended to suggest that there are no circumstances in which diagnosis is valid and helpful. In one respect, the use of diagnostic systems that involve placing problems in categories works well at the interface between mental health and legal concepts (Eastman, 2000). The law typically deals with categories, often of a dichotomous nature (guilty or not guilty; fit or unfit to plead; having full or diminished responsibility), so diagnostic systems are well tailored to addressing medico-legal or psycho-legal questions.

By contrast, many variables in psychology are conceptualised as continuous in form, and evidence strongly supports the expectation that this is the most appropriate approach to understanding them. Cognitive, personality and behavioural measurement relies on conceiving of variables as lying on dimensions or continua, and the same applies to mental states such as anxiety, depression or paranoia. We can divide a spread of scores in some way by applying cut-off scores (sometimes simply called 'cut scores': Dwyer, 1996), but doing so is often arbitrary and there are not always satisfactory reasons for setting them at one point rather than another. Yet in diagnostic systems, variables are used to place individuals in clinical groups – principally 'normal' versus 'pathological'.

Biopsychosocial model

The variability of individuals' reported experiences of mental health problems reflects the level of complexity of the factors that contribute to them. The problem of causation has no simple solution, and can only be properly understood by resorting to a *multifactorial* perspective.

The leading contender in generating explanations within such a perspective, as outlined in Chapter 5, is the **biopsychosocial model** (Bennett, 2011). Within this, the numerous factors that may play a causal role are located under three broad categories:

11

- *Biological factors* These include the influence of genes; the impact of physical and learning disability; psychological effects of physical disease, the ingestion of toxins, or substance misuse; and organic factors such as brain injury or deterioration in later life.
- *Psychological factors* These include early socialisation, learning processes, and personality development; the formation of attitudes and beliefs; patterns of information and cognitive processing; self-awareness and self-management; and the effects of close relationships.
- *Social factors* These include demographic, social-structural and family factors; levels of income, wealth and power; neighbourhood, housing, employment and other life opportunities; the effects of mass media, language and culture; and the extent of shared meanings and values.

The biopsychosocial model has been a prominent influence in the field of mental health for a number of years. The pathways that connect possible causes to particular outcomes can often be very hard to track down, reflecting the dual problems of *mul-*

tifinality and *equifinality* (which we encountered in Chapter 5).

The limitations of diagnosis

Given the difficulties just outlined, we might wonder how the use of diagnosis has achieved its position of such dominance in forensic mental health services. Describing the history of psychiatry as a profession, Moncrieff (2009), as noted earlier, suggests that the use of diagnosis was introduced into a situation where it was not really applicable in order to remedy the uncertainties and insecurities felt by its practitioners relative to their colleagues in other branches of medicine.

According to Hyman (2010), the advent of the DSM-III in 1980 was particularly influential in the effort to improve the reliability of diagnosis. This was also a major turning point in the sense of confidence felt within psychiatry, which not long before had been reeling from the impact of the 'antipsychiatry movement' following critiques by Thomas Szasz in the USA, Ronald Laing in the UK, and Michel Foucault in France. While it achieved that purpose, however, the new diagnostic armature had the effect of creating an 'unintended epistemic prison' (Hyman, 2010, p. 157) for its users.

Psychologists have forwarded possible alternatives to diagnostic systems. One suggestion is to focus separately on specific symptoms of mental health problems, while another has been the development of *case formulation* which is designed to produce an understanding of the patterning of difficulties at the individual level. Neither of these has achieved the status of diagnosis, but case formulation is often used alongside it and we will examine it in Chapter 18.

Surveys of mental health problems in prisons

The previous discussion is designed to encourage a sceptical attitude towards diagnostic systems in mental health. Nevertheless, whatever reservations we might have about their scientific status, we cannot avoid their use as they continue to provide the prevailing terminology in both mental healthcare services and mental health law, and also in research on the possible links between mental health problems and crime.

One approach to investigating possible links between mental disorder and crime is to examine the extent to which people who are convicted of criminal offences show symptoms of mental disorder. This has been the focus of a number of epidemiological surveys in several countries. Such research has focused mainly on prison populations. Overall, these studies show that there are significantly higher levels of mental disorder in prison settings than in the outside community.

The largest study of this kind in the United Kingdom was conducted by Singleton, Meltzer and Gatward (1998), who interviewed 3,142 prisoners, drawing their sample from 131 different prisons. They found that 7 per cent of male sentenced prisoners, 14 per cent of female prisoners (remanded or sentenced), and 10 per cent of males on remand met criteria for diagnosis of psychotic illness. The corresponding figures for *antisocial personality disorder* (ASPD) in the same three groups were 49 per cent, 31 per cent and 63 per cent, and for the general class of neurotic disorders (severe anxiety, depression or other emotional problems) 40 per cent, 76 per cent and 59 per cent. Levels of harmful or hazardous alcohol and drug use were also very high. Overall, fewer than one in ten prisoners showed *no* evidence of the major diagnostic categories examined in the survey. Reviewing a series of studies conducted in the United States and Canada, Lamb and Weinberger (1998) concluded that the proportion of prisoners suffering from acute mental disorders in local city and county jails in the USA ranged from 6 per cent to 15 per cent, and in state prisons from 10 per cent to 15 per cent.

Adults

Epidemiological studies of mental health problems in adult prisoners have been conducted in a number of countries. In an initial review, Fazel and Danesh (2002) reported a meta-analysis of 62 interview-based surveys from 12 countries, drawing on an aggregate sample of 23,000 prisoners. Respective rates of diagnosis of psychosis, major depression or any personality disorder were: amongst men, 3.7 per cent, 10 per cent and 65 per cent; and amongst women 4 per cent, 12 per cent and 42 per cent. Fazel and Seewald (2012) later reported an expanded systematic review focused on psychotic illness and major depression, combining data from 109 samples in 24 countries, with a total sample of 33,790 prisoners. This found a pooled prevalence rate of psychosis of 3.6 per cent for men and 3.9 per cent for women, and of depression 10.2 per cent for men and 14.1 per cent for women.

Similar findings have been reported in other literature searches (Sirdifield, Gojkovic, Brooker and Ferriter, 2009; Steadman *et al.*, 2009). Cumulatively, these reviews provide strong evidence that levels of mental disorder are significantly higher in prisons than in the community outside. Extrapolating from the UK survey data, Peay (2012) estimated that at that time there were probably 5,934 prisoners with psychosis in England and Wales alone.

In a related systematic review, Fazel, Xenitidis and Powell (2008) integrated findings from ten surveys of the prevalence of intellectual disabilities amongst prisoners. Studies originated from five countries (England and Wales, the USA, United Arab Emirates, Australia and New Zealand), and had a combined sample size of 11,969 (92 per cent male). Most assessments involved use of a screening procedure, followed by administration of an intelligence test (predominantly the WAIS-R) and other clinical measures. Prevalence rates ranged between 0.0 and 2.9 per cent, though most estimates were in the range 0.5–1.5 per cent. While these are lower rates than those found for mental disorders, as Fazel, Xenitidis and Powell (2008) pointed out this is a highly vulnerable group that has been found to be significantly over-represented in prison suicide statistics.

Youth

Studies also show that adolescents in penal institutions report a higher rate of CMHPs and of diagnosable mental disorders than are found in the community (Fazel, Doll and Långström, 2008; Lader, Singleton and Meltzer, 2003; Penner, Roesch and Viljoen, 2011). In a large-scale overview, Casswell, French and Rogers (2012) integrated findings from nine surveys of young offenders' mental health. The proportions meeting criteria for at least one mental health problem were consistently higher in custodial settings. This may be because those sent to custody are a subgroup who have more serious underlying multiple problems to begin with. Alternatively, the stresses of incarceration may lead to deterioration in the mental health of individuals made subject to it. A third possibility is that young people in the community may 'self-medicate' as a way of coping with their problems, making regular use of alcohol or other drugs (Chitsabesan and Bailey, 2006).

However, young people under community supervision also exhibit higher levels of mental health problems than the population as a whole. In a study in New South Wales, Kenny, Lennings and Nelson (2007) administered a number of self-report measures to 800 young offenders (mean age: 17 years) under the supervision of the Department of Juvenile Justice. Some 40 per cent of the males and 38 per cent of the females reported symptoms within the 'severe' range on the measure used; in addition, 23 per cent of males and 38 per cent of females reported some form of severe trauma (marked forms of neglect or of abuse) in their lives. Similar findings have been obtained in England (Chitsabesan and Bailey, 2006; Chitsabesan *et al.*, 2006), where between one-third and one-half of young people supervised by Youth Offending Teams (YOTs) had significant needs in mental health (Carswell *et al.*, 2004; Stallard, Thomason and Churchyard, 2003; Walsh *et al.*, 2011). All studies suggest that there are large gaps in providing services to meet those needs.

Other data provide a possible link between survey findings on young and adult offenders and the prevalence of *attention deficit hyperactivity disorder* (ADHD) in imprisoned groups. Recall from Chapter 5 that in longitudinal studies of development a constellation of problems that included restlessness, impulsivity and hyperactivity was noted as being one of the strongest predictors of involvement in delinquency (Ellis, Beaver and Wright, 2009; Farrington, 2007; Sabates and Dex, 2012). Gudjonsson *et al.* (2009) reviewed nine studies in this area, which found that between 24 per cent and 67 per cent of adult prisoners had been diagnosed with ADHD in childhood and 23–45 per cent still met the diagnostic criteria in adulthood. This cluster of problems presents an elevated risk of criminality, and Retz and Rösler (2009) have mapped out possible interactions between genetic susceptibilities and both 'pervasive' and 'situational' environmental contributors to such risk. There are parallels here with the gene–environment (G×E) interaction models described in Chapter 5.

Schilling, Walsh and Yun (2011) reviewed 102 studies of the possible connections between ADHD and crime, attempting to draw it to the attention of criminologists on the grounds that people who meet the criteria for ADHD 'are present in correctional populations at rates exceeding their prevalence in the general population by at least a factor of three or four' (p. 9). They suggest that the syndrome may be a manifestation of the continuum of 'low self-control' postulated in some prominent criminological theories. When ADHD is accompanied by 'co-morbid' *conduct disorder* and *oppositional defiant disorder* during childhood, this may represent an extreme end of that continuum.

The available figures suggest that the rate of mental health problems in prison settings may be higher with respect to personality disorders (PDs). In one sense that is scarcely surprising, given that in most cases this consists of *antisocial* (DSM) or *dissocial* (ICD) personality disorder, definitions of which rely partly on evidence that an individual has violated the rights of others, for example by repeatedly committing acts that can lead to arrest. Accepting the 'partly tautological nature' of the link between *antisocial PD* and criminal offending, Roberts and Coid (2009) found that it was negatively correlated with age at first offence, and showed a strong positive correlation with numbers of previous prison sentences, and with a wider range of offence types – including violence, though this was the lowest correlation observed. There were also significant associations between a diagnosis of *paranoid PD* and robbery and blackmail; between *schizoid PD* and offences of kidnap, burglary and theft; and between *schizotypal PD* and arson. We will examine some aspects of the link between PD and crime more fully below.

Mental disorder and the risk of violence

Findings of this kind do not in themselves signify the presence of a cause–effect relationship between mental disorder and crime (including violence). Some prisoners may develop mental health problems as a reaction to incarceration, and there may not be any prior connection between those difficulties and their offending. A further interpretative difficulty arises from the often reported finding that many factors thought to play a causal role are also correlated with each other. Social deprivation, family dysfunction, parental neglect, childhood victimisation, low educational attainment, erratic lifestyle, a history of substance abuse and neighbourhood disorganisation have each been separately associated with both mental disorder and crime. These complications need to be taken into account; and, as recognised and analysed in some detail by Anckärsater *et al.* (2009), the criteria for properly demonstrating a causal connection between mental disorder and crime have rarely been unambiguously fulfilled.

While the pattern that has emerged from this is not yet entirely clear, there is a broad consensus on a number of general conclusions. The first is that there is powerful evidence that people suffering from severe and enduring mental health problems are much more likely to harm themselves than anyone else. According to reports by the World Health Organization (WHO) which draw on international surveys, a very high proportion of those who committed suicide – over 90 per cent – had a psychiatric diagnosis at the time of death (Bertolote and Fleischmann, 2002). The diagnoses associated with the highest risk in the general population were mood disorders (which includes major depression), followed by substance-related disorders, personality disorders and schizophrenia. The cohorts on which these results are based came predominantly from countries in Europe and North America. However, a similar pattern has been found in China, based on data from the National Psychological Autopsy study. The odds ratio for the association between mood disorders and suicide was 44.2, with a corresponding figure of 7.4 for psychosis (Tong and Phillips, 2010). The former figure far exceeds any available estimate of the risk that someone with a mental disorder will commit a serious crime, and the latter is above the highest found to date for a link between psychosis and crime. McLean *et al.* (2008) amalgamated findings from 23 systematic reviews of risk factors for suicide, together with other studies of protective factors. Many aspects of individuals' lives were found to have a differential impact on suicide, including gender, urban or rural residence, unemployment, and the extent to which there are firm cultural prohibitions against it. It is also influenced by the availability of the means to carry it out. Overall, however, there is a general agreement that mental disorder is the largest single risk factor for suicide, in addition to the heightened risk of self-harm already noted.

A second point of agreement is that there is relatively little evidence that mental health problems *in general* are associated with a heightened risk of committing crimes of violence. On the contrary, they typically appear to be less reliable predictors than other variables. Bonta, Law and Hanson (1998) undertook a meta-analysis of studies on this question. They identified 64 independent samples subsuming a total of 15,245 participants, and computed the predictive validity of categories of variables in four broad sets: *demographic*; *criminal history*; *deviant lifestyle*; and *clinical*. The most accurate were demographic and criminal history variables. Here the correlations with general and violent recidivism for demographic variables were both +0.12, and for criminal history +0.08 and +0.15 respectively. The overall pattern that was found showed close parallels to that typically obtained with 'mainstream' offender populations in the penal system. The weakest predictors of recidivism were *clinical* variables, where the corresponding correlations were –0.02 and –0.03. Only a DSM diagnosis of *antisocial personality disorder* was associated with a greater risk of future criminality, and psychosis was negatively correlated with future general and violent recidivism. Other studies since then have obtained analogous findings (e.g. Gray *et al.*, 2004; Phillips *et al.*, 2005).

Psychosis

However, more recent large-scale reviews have suggested that some symptoms of mental disorders are associated with an increased risk of violence. One principal area of interest has been symptoms of schizophrenia and other psychoses as possible risk factors, where several meta-analyses have been reported. In these reviews, an odds ratio of 1 indicates that violence is equally likely whether or not psychosis is present. Below 1, an association with violence is less likely; above 1, it is more likely.

Findings of these studies display a wide range. Some found no association at all, while others reported quite high odds ratios (i.e. a significantly heightened risk of violence). Tiihonen *et al.* (1997) conducted a 26-year follow-up study of a birth cohort (n=12,058) in Finland, and found the following odds ratios for the risk of violence: for schizophrenia, 7.0; and for mood disorders with psychotic features, 8.8. Fazel *et al.* (2009a) reviewed 20 studies with an aggregate sample of 18,423 individuals, and after discounting the influence of concurrent substance abuse, found a mean odds ratio of 2.1 for the relationship between schizophrenia and violence. Douglas, Guy and Hart (2009) reviewed a total of 204 studies, subsuming 166 independent samples, and concluded that 'psychosis was reliably and significantly asssociated with an approximately 49 per cent to 68 per cent increase in the odds of violence relative to the odds of violence in the absence of psychosis' (p. 687). If this sounds large, note also that 'the average effect size for psychosis ... is comparable to numerous individual risk factors' found in other research (p. 693). But as just noted, there was considerable heterogeneity in the findings surveyed, with one-quarter of the effect sizes obtained being below zero (with a mean odds ratio of 0.73), while another quarter were far larger (above an odds ratio of 3.30).

The discrepancies between findings might be partly explained by several moderator variables, some of them operating in combination. For example, high rates of mental disorder, abuse of alcohol or other substances, and violence may be a function of neighbourhood factors such as deprivation and social disorganisation (Elbogen and Johnson, 2009; Fazel *et al.*, 2009b; Silver, Mulvey and Monahan, 1999; Steadman *et al.*, 1998). Thus it is possible that even if people with psychoses do commit acts of violence, that might not be a result of any predisposition intrinsic to their mental state, but a reaction to events in their lives such as family conflict or repeated victimisation by others (Silver, 2006). Yet some high odds ratios have remained, even where other factors such as those have been controlled for in the analysis.

If individuals suffering from psychotic illness sometimes do have an elevated risk of acting violently, even when other factors have been taken into account, why might that be? Keep in mind first that the torment associated with such illness, in instances where it results in extreme forms of behaviour, is more likely to lead to suicide than to causing harm to others. The heterogeneity noted above may conceal some more specific routes whereby psychosis is a risk factor for personal violence. Bentall and Taylor (2006) suggested three possible connective pathways. First, there is tentative evidence that some delusional states such as paranoia could be a result of perceptual abnormalities, which result in affected individuals paying excessive attention to perceived threats. Second, some individuals may be prone to a kind of faulty reasoning in which, faced with an uncertain situation, they are prone to jumping to conclusions before having weighed up all the evidence. Third, there is evidence that paranoia is associated with low self-esteem, and there may be a mechanism whereby individuals protect the self by habitually attributing negative events to the actions of others.

Based on an integrative review of studies in this area, Bo *et al.* (2011) proposed that there are two main pathways linking features of schizophrenia to violent behaviour. One pattern was more pronounced amongst individuals who had little or no history of violence prior to the onset of the illness. First episodes of psychosis were most often associated with its positive symptoms (delusions, hallucinations and thought disorder), and the period of onset may also be one of higher risk for the perception of threat and the resultant occurrence of aggression. However, any such pattern may be present in only a proportion of cases. In an in-depth interview study in Sweden, Radovic and Högland (2014) asked 47 detained patients, all of whom accepted their diagnosis and admitted their offences, to what extent the two were connected. Only 4 thought that their severe mental disorder was the sole cause of the crime; 13 considered that it was a contributing factor; and the largest single group, of 15, thought that the disorder had nothing to do with the crime.

Another aspect of this which has been researched is the possible role of *command hallucinations* in prompting individuals to act violently. Hallucinations are not unique to any single type of diagnosis and are also experienced by people with no mental disorder. They can occur in any sensory modality but those of an auditory nature are the most common. A study of 103 psychiatric inpatients by McNiel, Eisner and Binder (2000) found that 30.1 per cent reported having heard voices telling them to hurt someone, and 22.3 per cent said they had complied with such commands, though only five said they had done this often. Following the commands issued by voices is by no means automatic and some people resist them. Research has suggested that compliance with commands is very variable and is an outcome of a complex combination of characteristics. In an Australian study of 75 forensic patients, Shawyer *et al.* (2008) found that these included more severe psychosis, having comorbid delusions, and low levels of maternal control in childhood. In a UK study Bucci *et al.* (2013) found that compliance with voices was associated with belief in the omnipotence of the voices, and with impulsivity.

In addition to these possibilities, it has also been found that, as in anxiety, paranoia induces individuals to engage in what are called *safety behaviours* – that is, actions in which they take steps to avoid or in some cases to neutralise feared events. In a study of 100 patients diagnosed with psychotic disorders, Freeman *et al.* (2007) found that a large majority of them (96 per cent) exhibited safety behaviours of some kind. Thus when faced with a perceived threat, or with a belief that one is being controlled by others, many individuals resort to preventive or defensive action, and there are instances where this can consist of aggression towards others to counteract the threat they are thought to pose. Such symptoms have been called 'threat/control override' (or TCO) symptoms (Link, Stueve and Phelan, 1998), but research on their relation to violence has yielded somewhat inconsistent results. Haddock *et al.* (2013) reported a study of 325 people with schizophrenia and substance misuse problems, of whom 32.3 per cent had committed at least one violent incident in the preceding two years. Amongst the study group, 48.0 per cent reported TCO symptoms and 11.9 per cent reported command hallucinations. However, neither of these was associated with violence to others, but both were associated with self-harm.

Personality disorder

The second type of connection identified by Bo *et al.* (2011; see above) is mediated by a separate factor, that of **personality disorder**. Where this occurs, a pattern of antisocial behaviour is likely to have been present before the emergence of psychotic illness. As we noted earlier, in one sense the connection between personality disorder and crime in general, and with aggressive or violent behaviour in particular, is almost axiomatic, because criteria such as 'violation of social norms' or 'a low threshold for the discharge of aggression' form part of the diagnostic definitions of some of these syndromes.

The DSM-5 system contains ten types of personality disorder (PD), which are divided into three clusters:

» *Cluster A: Odd or eccentric disorders* These include *paranoid*, *schizoid* and *schizotypal* PDs.

» *Cluster B: Dramatic, emotional or erratic disorders* These comprise *antisocial*, *borderline*, *histrionic* and *narcissistic* PDs.

» *Cluster C: Anxious or fearful disorders* These consist of *avoidant*, *dependent* and *obsessive-compulsive* PDs.

The ICD-10 system by contrast lists nine types of personality disorder. Some are fairly close equivalents of the DSM categories, while others correspond less well. McMurran (2009) provides a helpful side-by-side comparison of the two schemes. Both systems allow for an additional, but looser and less clearly specified category. In the DSM-5, for example, this is called 'Other Specified Personality Disorder'. For the equivalent concept in the DSM-IV, there was no consensus on the number of features that had to be present for the diagnosis to be applied. Different studies suggested five, eight, ten or fifteen criteria as being needed (Verheul, Bartak and Widiger, 2007; Verheul and Widiger, 2004).

An international network of researchers has provided estimates of the prevalence of PDs worldwide. Huang *et al.* (2009) collated WHO data from 13 countries, including some classed as economically less developed, with a total sample of 21,162. Data were based on the screening questionnaire that forms part of the International Personality Disorder Examination (IPDE; see the 'Focus on ...' box on page 258). The overall prevalence rate was estimated to be 6.1 per cent, with corresponding rates for DSM-IV clusters A, B and C of 3.6 per cent, 1.5 per cent and 2.7 per cent respectively. Note the slightly lower estimate for the second cluster, which contains most of the PDs commonly associated with offending behaviour. As the authors themselves suggest, these findings should be interpreted cautiously. Neither the IPDE nor the three-cluster model have been empirically validated in all the countries where the data were gathered.

When the prevalence of PD categories has been examined within offender populations, the most frequently found is the 'Antisocial' or 'Dissocial' type (in DSM-5 and ICD-10 respectively). The DSM-5 diagnosis requires evidence that an individual had some features of *conduct disorder* with onset before the age of 15. PDs are often assessed using a combination of interviews and structured clinical inventories. Widely used and well validated psychometric instruments for this purpose include the *Minnesota Multiphasic Personality Inventory* (MMPI-2), the *Millon Clinical Multiaxial Inventory* (MCMI-IV), and the *Personality Assessment*

FOCUS ON ...

The International Personality Disorder Examination (IPDE)

The International Personality Disorder Examination (IPDE) is a well-established clinical interview for the assessment of the presence of one or more types of personality disorder. It was originally developed by the World Health Organization (Loranger, Janca and Sartorius, 1997). There are two components to this assessment.

1 There is a Screening Questionnaire, presented in booklet form, and containing a series of items to which individuals respond on a *True/False* basis.
2 Depending on the results of this screening – which is not in itself designed for diagnostic purposes – an interview may then be conducted. There are two 'parallel' formats of the Examination, which correspond to the DSM-IV and the ICD-10 diagnostic systems.

The Screening Questionnaire comprises 77 items for the DSM-IV version and 59 items for the ICD-10 version. The full interview contains 99 questions for DSM-IV and 68 questions for ICD-10; of these, 52 questions overlap both versions. The interview can also be used in an abbreviated form, and the manual specifically allows employment of only the questions associated with whichever personality disorder categories have emerged from the screening as potentially present.

There is a detailed manual for scoring individuals' responses in the interview, and training is required prior to its use (Loranger, 1999).

Question

When trying to assess personality, under what circumstances would you accept what someone says about himself or herself, rather than what is recorded in file information?

Inventory, amongst others. Alongside interview, file-based and other kinds of information, these can allow comparison between individual score profiles and those of key reference groups.

In the initial meta-analysis of prison mental health surveys from 12 countries cited earlier, Fazel and Danesh (2002) found high rates of personality disorders in prison populations. While only a few surveys reported on personality disorder in general, we saw that no fewer than 65 per cent of men and 42 per cent of women were found to meet the criteria for some PD diagnosis. In 28 surveys focusing more specifically on antisocial PD, 47 per cent of men met diagnostic criteria. In seven studies reporting on the mental health of women prisoners, 21 per cent met criteria for antisocial PD and 25 per cent met criteria for borderline PD. There was, however, significant heterogeneity in the findings of these surveys, according to the size of the study sample; whether it was done in the United States or elsewhere; and whether or not the interviewers were psychiatrists, who were more than twice as likely to diagnose PD as other assessors (42 per cent as compared to 19 per cent).

Psychopathy

The position that was described earlier (in the 'Focus on ... Diagnostic systems in psychiatry' box) is more perplexing in this area, however, as a third approach has been developed for classifying severe personality pathology. *Psychopathy*, although not a psychiatric diagnosis as such, is regarded as a more severe version of the type of personality disorder labelled as 'Antisocial' in the DSM or 'Dissocial' in the ICD (Coid and Ullrich, 2009). It represents the classification of personality disorder most closely associated with serious criminal conduct or repeated involvement in violence. Ogloff (2006) sets out a useful conceptual analysis of the overlaps and distinctions between these three categories.

Several meanings have been attached to the word 'psychopathy' over the past 200 years or so, and Arrigo and Shipley (2001) provide a useful historical background to the use of the term. However, the one that current usage most firmly draws upon originated in the work of the psychiatrist Hervey Cleckley (1976), who, in a seminal book first published in 1941, which contained numerous case vignettes, described individuals who may present an outward appearance of being congenial and even engaging, but who are inwardly detached. This concept has had a substantial impact on present-day conceptualisations of a subgroup of people who are motivated by pursuit of their own interests to the extent that they have little or no regard for the interests of others, or indeed that they will use others to achieve their own ends. They are described as being emotionally callous and deficient in the capacity for empathy; likely to be impulsive, and to exercise little or no self-restraint; and to be prone to the use of deception on an almost casual basis. Some members of this group are prepared to use violence, or to instigate others to use it, *instrumentally*, with little concern about the impact of those actions other than their usefulness in achieving a goal. Recalling the distinction noted in Chapter 6, this type of aggression is premeditated and emotionless, and designed to serve some other purpose than simply the discharge of negative feeling associated with expressive or reactive aggression. Such a pattern is thought to be more typical of psychopathic individuals (Glenn and Raine, 2009), and many of the people who committed the kinds of extremely violent crimes described in Chapters 7 and 8, including crimes of a serial nature, were assessed as meeting criteria for inclusion in this group. Such an image has, amongst other things, given rise to some of the iconic film portrayals of the last 50 years, perhaps most chillingly that of Hannibal Lecter in *Silence of the Lambs*. However, many other individuals who are classed as 'psychopathic' have not committed offences approaching that level of seriousness.

While most of the research pertaining to psychopathy has been conducted in North America (mainly with Euro-Americans), with a smaller amount in Europe, similar syndromes are reportedly recognised in cultures outside 'the West', and in societies as far apart as the Yoruba of Nigeria and the Inuit of north-western Alaska (Murphy, 1976). Members of these societies give descriptions of individuals who are habitually self-seeking, exploitative and deceptive, and who, despite knowing that an action is wrong or that it hurts other people, repeatedly carry on doing it. Murphy (1976) relates the view of one informant to the effect that, after it became clear that someone manifested these characteristics, the traditional solution to the problem sometimes involved the summary despatch of such a person into the freezing Arctic waters when nobody else was looking. These problems were also regarded as something that a shaman or healer would not be able to change – that is, the afflicted persons were thought to be incurable. This perhaps parallels debates about the 'untreatability' of psychopaths.

The most influential psychological analysis of this, which extrapolates the ideas of Cleckley and which has generated a considerable quantity of research, is that of Hare (1993, 2003; Hare and Neumann, 2008). A key part of his work is the operationalisation of the definition of psychopathy with reference to a specially developed measure, the *Psychopathy Checklist*, of which there are three separate versions in use (see 'Focus on ... the Psychopathy Checklist' on page 260). The term 'checklist' is somewhat misleading here, as it may imply a simple box-ticking exercise: in reality, each item requires a considerable amount of thought and involves making some quite complex judgments.

The original model of what these checklists measure contained two main factors, scored separately as 'Factor 1' (Interpersonal/affective items) and 'Factor 2' (Deviant/antisocial-lifestyle items). On the basis of later research, each was further subdivided into two *facets*, yielding a set of four constructs, which together compose the definition of 'Hare psychopathy' (Hare and Neumann, 2008). The technical manual (Hare, 2003) includes tables for converting raw scores into standard or centile scores on both the factors and the facets.

Surveys of the prevalence of this personality configuration in the community, using the Hare measures, suggest that it is

FOCUS ON ...

The Psychopathy Checklist

Personality inventories such as those widely used in psychology are self-report instruments, and for forensic assessment purposes such methods have been criticised for their exclusive reliance on respondents who may have a vested interest in conveying to others a specific impression of themselves. Although they contain validity scales for the detection of inconsistent reporting or of malingering, these are not always sufficiently discriminating to detect some kinds of invalid responding.

The *Psychopathy Checklist* is a widely used format for the purpose of assessing what is thought to be the most severe form of antisocial personality. Usage of this assessment entails collection and review of information from case files, and it is recommended that this be accompanied by an interview. Comparison of the different sources of information enables assessors to arrive at more soundly based judgments and to check for misleading responses. It is also considered good practice for the scoring to be completed jointly by a team of assessors working together.

There are three versions of the measure:

- *Psychopathy Checklist – Revised* (PCL:R), used in assessing adults: 20 items.
- *Psychopathy Checklist – Screening Version* (PCL:SV): 12 items.
- *Psychopathy Checklist – Youth Version* (PCL:YV), for age range 12–18: 20 items.

Items in all three versions are scored 0, 1 or 2, according to detailed specifications contained in the manual (Hare, 2003). Thus the maximum score possible on the PCL:R, for example, is 40, with the conventional cut-off indicating the presence of psychopathy for North American males set at 30, and for European males at 25.

Hare and Neumann (2008) describe the Checklist as measuring two factors of psychopathy each subsuming two contributory facets, and organised as follows.

Factor 1: Interpersonal/affective items

- *Interpersonal items* Presentation of glibness and superficial charm; grandiose sense of self-worth; prone to pathological deception, and to con or manipulate others.
- *Affective items* A lack of remorse or guilt; shallow emotional experience; callousness and lack of empathy; failure to accept responsibility for actions.

Factor 2: Deviant/antisocial lifestyle

- *Lifestyle items* A pronounced need for stimulation or proneness to boredom; a tendency to be parasitic on others; a lack of realistic long-term goals; impulsivity; irresponsibility.
- *Antisocial items* Poor behavioural controls; early behaviour problems; a history of juvenile delinquency; revocation of conditional release; and criminal versatility.

Question

Based on assessments you have conducted or on your reading of files, which interpretation of the factor structure of the PCL:R appears to be most applicable in making sense of individuals you have assessed?

relatively low. In the United Kingdom, Coid *et al.* (2009a) used the screening format of the *Psychopathy Checklist* (PCL:SV) and assessed a sample of 638 participants in the age range 16–74 from a larger study of psychiatric morbidity. Using a cut-off score of 13 (out of a maximum of 24) as an indicator of 'possible' psychopathy, they found a prevalence rate of 0.6 per cent, with a male-to-female ratio of 4:1. There were significant correlations between PCL:SV total scores and separate clinical interview ratings for three types of personality disorder: antisocial, borderline and histrionic (all from DSM Cluster B, as noted earlier). As might be expected, given how psychopathy is defined, in prisoner and psychiatric inpatient samples the rates are much higher. Sullivan and Kosson (2006) summarised findings from 19 studies using the full version of the *Psychopathy Checklist* (PCL:R), conducted in prisons or secure hospitals in Scotland, England and Wales, Belgium, Netherlands, Germany, Norway, Sweden, Spain, Portugal and Argentina. The overall mean score for 2,046 prisoner participants was 17.5, though this was significantly lower than the mean score found amongst samples in forensic (19.5) and psychiatric (22.5) settings; again not unexpected, as the latter are often more highly selected groups. The proportions of prisoners above the cut-off score of 30 (used for defining 'Hare psychopathy' in North America) ranged from 3 per cent to 47 per cent; and even allowing for different cut-off scores, there was 'a great deal of variability in apparent base rates' (Sullivan and Kosson, 2006, p. 443).

In another study, in England and Wales, Coid *et al.* (2009b) found a lower prevalence rate: 7.7 per cent amongst men and 1.9 per cent amongst women prisoners. Studies of psychopathy have also been conducted outside the West. In a survey of 351 prisoners in Iran, 23 per cent were found to exceed the cut-off score for psychopathy on the PCL:SV (Assadi *et al.*, 2006).

The overall picture, then, is that although the exact proportions vary considerably, all published studies have found prevalence rates that were markedly higher in prisons and secure units than amongst general population samples. Other data confirming this were assembled by Sirdifield, Gojkovic, Brooker and Ferriter (2009). The assessment of personality disorder, and particularly of possible psychopathy, has understandably become a regular feature of the work of forensic and clinical psychologists and psychiatrists working in these settings.

Explaining psychopathic features

The patterns found in these studies might of course just reflect the presence of higher proportions of 'life-course persistent' offenders in adult samples, as identified in the work of Moffitt (1993, 2003) which we encountered in Chapter 3. Moffitt considered that members of this group may have some underlying disposition towards offending and that this might be partly attributable to neuropsychological vulnerabilities of some kind. There is some evidence of stability, for example, from the age of 13 to the age of 24 in the 'impulsivity' and 'antisocial' behaviour components of psychopathy, though less continuity in the 'arrogant' or 'deceitful' interpersonal style and deficient affective experience (Lynam *et al.*, 2007). Looking farther down the age-range, there are indications that some features, in the form of 'callous-unemotional' traits, can be identified at a fairly early stage, in children as young as seven (Viding, Blair, Moffitt and Plomin, 2005).

Other researchers, however, have cautioned against viewing psychopathic propensity as amounting to a general theory of crime (Walters, 2004), and it is more likely that it is only a subgroup even of that segment of the recidivist population who meet the necessary criteria. Several theories have been offered regarding the origins or 'aetiological mechanisms' of this category of mental disorder, and cover the usual range of factors: genetic, neurological, socialisation, personality trait, social-cognitive.

Various theories have been proposed concerning what might be called the 'core' of what constitutes psychopathy. One is that it results from low fearfulness, a suggestion forwarded by Lykken (1957) which has been refined into more specific hypotheses by many other authors. Related possibilities include that it has its roots in an inability to learn from experience, in pathological sensation-seeking, or in a deficit in the behavioural inhibition system. Each of these approaches involves the suggestion that all of the phenomena observed in the presentation known as 'psychopathy' can be traced to a single cause. Each of them has stimulated sizeable volumes of research. Two major groups of investigations that have been pursued in this area focus on the neurobiological and cognitive-affective aspects.

Neurobiological factors

There are suggestions that the psychological features of psychopathy may result from differences in brain structures or in the level of activation of different neural centres. Raine (2008) has reviewed neurobiological evidence linking genes, patterns of brain activity and antisocial behaviour. Several studies employing brain-imaging techniques have found what appear to be neurological differences between the brains of individuals with high PCL:R scores and non-clinical comparison samples. Studies generally concentrate on a small number of 'regions of interest' (ROIs) within the brain, including for example some loci within the pre-frontal cortex (the region just behind the forehead), which is well established within neuropsychological research as a centre of planning and decision-making or 'executive' control processes.

Yang and Raine (2009) conducted a meta-analysis of 43 studies in which comparisons were made between the pre-frontal lobes of individuals with histories of violence (including some diagnosed with antisocial PD, and some classed as psychopathic), and either non-offending psychiatric patients or healthy controls. The variables examined were either gross *structural* (anatomical) features or *functional* differences such as levels of activation (as measured by localised cerebral blood flow). Moderate-to-large effect sizes (Cohen's *d*) showing reduced structure and function were obtained for certain areas, including the *right orbitofrontal cortex* (nine studies, ES = −0.48) and the *right anterior cingulate cortex* (six studies, ES = −1.12). These regions are considered to have a principal role in decision-making, impulse control, and emotional regulation, though they also serve a number of other functions. The evidence is consistent with an explanation of the poorer self-control (of individuals who are repeatedly aggressive and violent) in terms of the reduction in structure and function observed. Clearly, however, this requires considerable further investigation and testing.

Another ROI is the *amygdala*, a structure located centrally in the brain which is one of several implicated in the formation of long-term memories and in the mediation of emotional responses. It is also believed to be important in social behaviour, and its volume is correlated with the size and complexity of individuals' social networks (Bickart *et al.*, 2010). Blair (2005, 2007; Blair, Mitchell and Blair, 2005) reviewed results suggesting that this nucleus plays a part in what might be called 'moral learning', alongside other evidence that it is less active in people classed as psychopathic. Compatible with this is the finding that adolescents assessed as high on 'callous-unemotional' traits have lowered amygdala responsiveness when presented with signals of emotional distress in others (Marsh *et al.*, 2008). Yet it is important to note that psychopathy 'is not associated with a lesion to a particular region' (Blair, 2007, p. 388), but is more likely to be reflected across a number of neural sites. A particularly striking result was reported by Craig *et al.* (2009), who used diffusion tensor magnetic resonance imaging (DT-MRI) to scan neural activity in a group of nine adult males, all convicted of serious violent and sexual crimes, who had a mean PCL:R score of 28.4. They were compared with a group of healthy male controls matched in age and IQ. Results showed a significant difference in white-matter integrity in the *right uncinate fasciculus*, a tract of neural fibres connecting the orbitofrontal cortex to the amygdala. This was also significantly negatively correlated with scores on Factor 2 of the PCL:R. For experimental control purposes, studies were also conducted of connective tracts with other brain regions, but no other differences were found.

All of this sounds very promising in terms of contributing to an understanding of the relationships between brain function, emotion and behaviour. But evidence emerging from neuroscience investigations is not wholly consistent, to an extent that makes it difficult to draw any clear conclusions. Patrick, Venables and Skeem (2012) reviewed a set of 18 studies using functional magnetic resonance imaging (fMRI) or other brain-scanning techniques with individuals obtaining high scores on measures of psychopathy or antisocial personality. In relation to the amygdala, for example, some studies found reduced levels of activation, whereas others found the opposite. Patrick *et al.* (2012, p. 68) comment that it is not so much that the findings are 'inconsistent' but rather that they are 'all over the map'. While this may be partly a result of the small samples typically used in such studies, a more fundamental problem might be that high scorers on psychopathy assessments have less in common than we think, and that what is measured by scanning instruments may bear only a distant relation to the features gauged in those assessments. There is also a major scientific and philosophical leap to be made in trying to connect the results of such experiments to an event (such as a serious crime, usually part of a complex sequence of behaviour) that occurred in very different circumstances perhaps a number of years earlier.

Some authors have raised broader questions over the validity of conclusions that can be drawn regarding links between brain function, cognition, emotion and behaviour from studies that use scanning methods. Vul, Harris, Winkielman and Pashler (2009) locate some of the problems in what, in an earlier unpublished version of their paper, they called 'voodoo correlations'. Vul *et al.* (2009) carried out a literature review and surveyed authors of 55 papers so found, asking them for details of their data-collection and analysis methods. Brain-imaging technology generates a vast amount of correlational data, to an extent that in many studies only results that exceeded specified thresholds were included in published reports. Ioannidis (2011) identified similarly worrying problems in an even larger set of studies, in which variations in the volumes of different brain structures had been associated with different mental disorders. Using specially developed software to test for 'excess significance' in statistically under-powered samples, Ioannidis (2011) examined 461 datasets concerning seven different psychiatric conditions. There was strong evidence of bias in published studies, suggesting that 'the number of positive results is way too large to be true' (2011, p. 777). Both of these trenchant reviews suggest that there is a need to be cautious when evaluating claims about direct associations between brain structures, psychological processes and antisocial conduct.

Cognitive-affective processing

Another related set of proposals focuses more closely on the possibility that the kernel of a psychopathic personality resides in disrupted patterns of cognitive-affective processing. Baskin-Sommers and Newman (2012) compared the evidential support for three hypotheses, each postulating a different mechanism as central. One is that psychopathic persons show a deficient *violence inhibition mechanism*: (VIM: see e.g. Blair, Monson and Frederickson, 2001). Another is that they have a farther-reaching *paralimbic dysfunction* affecting many brain structures (Kiehl, 2006). Both of these imply that psychopaths fail in some respect to experience emotion as others do. A third idea, the *response modulation hypothesis* (RMH: Newman, Curtin, Bertsch and Baskin-Sommers, 2010; Vitale and Newman 2007) suggests that the problem resides elsewhere, in the focus of attention, and that when psychopaths' attention is directly centred on fear-related stimuli, they react like anyone else. There are some research findings in support of each of these mechanisms, but no 'critical experiment' that would allow us to choose between them. It is equally possible, however, that the models are complementary, and that each has a role to play in explaining cognitive-affective deficits in different individuals assessed as psychopathic.

Although some of the proposals in these areas have been in circulation for a number of years, relative to the formidable challenge that they present – of understanding the problem designated as psychopathy – research is still at a comparatively early stage. Perhaps as a result of the sheer scale and complexity of that challenge, to date evidence gathered in relation to them has not been wholly consistent. This may not be surprising, given that individuals are usually selected for research studies on the basis of their PCL:R or PCL:SV scores, and these measures themselves assess several different kinds of variables – that is, there are different ways to obtain a score above the prearranged cut-off.

Other difficulties arise from the discovery that the scoring of the PCL:R may be influenced by the position of the assessor in the forensic or legal system. Murrie, Boccaccini, Johnson and Janke (2008) found fairly large discrepancies between the scores of two psychologists on opposite sides of 'Sexually Violent Predator' civil commitment trials in Texas, in which an individual may be compulsorily detained if considered dangerous on the basis of personality and other assessments. One psychologist worked for the state as 'petitioner' (prosecution) and the other was retained by the respondent (defence). The observed disagreements in scores lay outside the range that would be comprehensible as standard error, suggesting that 'partisan allegiance' may have influenced the assessments. Instances such as these call into question the reliability of the PCL:R: it may be that the foundations of the elaborate edifice that has been built by means of it are not as firm as they at first appear.

Disputes on the assessment and structure of psychopathy

More fundamentally, there are also debates over what PCL-R measures and what is the underlying composition of psychopathic personality. Disagreements persist over precisely what the checklists developed by Hare actually assess. The underlying factor structure of the PCL:R continues to be a matter of uncertainty, and in contrast to the four-factor model described by Hare and Neumann (2008; see the 'Focus on ...' box on page 260), other analyses have yielded three- and five-factor solutions. Combining and analysing datasets from eight Canadian and two American samples, Cooke and Michie (2001; Cooke, Michie, Hart and Clark, 2004) contended that a two-factor model could not be sustained, and that a three-factor solution proved superior. The factors thus identified were: (a) an arrogant and deceitful interpersonal style; (b) deficient affective experience; and (c) an impulsive and irresponsible behavioural style. Skeem and Cooke (2010) expressed a concern that the PCL:R as an assessment tool has become too closely identified with violent crime. The measure and the concept are thereby conflated, resulting in confusion regarding the meaning of psychopathy as a personality variable. Skeem and Cooke argued that personality and criminal lifestyle need to be kept separate rather than somehow being combined into a single score, the meaning of which then becomes difficult to interpret.

Other instruments have been devised for the assessment of those features of psychopathy thought to underpin the Hare checklists. They include the *Antisocial Process Screening Device* (Frick and Hare, 2001), used for assessment of callous-unemotional traits and impulsive conduct problems in younger age-groups, and the *Psychopathic Personality Inventory* (Lilienfeld and Widows, 2005), a self-report questionnaire for adults. However, it is unclear to what extent the latter measures the same dimensions as the PCL:R (Copestake, Gray and Snowden, 2011).

When academics have disagreements, the disputes are generally conducted in relatively sober tones in the pages of scholarly journals, or occasionally in verbal sparring at conferences. For the most part such exchanges are civil and polite (though we have no way of knowing how academics describe each other in private – after all, they are only human). Now and then, however, things may become publicly acrimonious, and one or other may even threaten legal action. The dispute over the status of the PCL:R provides an illustration of this. The article just cited by Skeem and Cooke (2010) was accepted by the journal *Psychological Assessment* more than two years before it finally appeared. Professor Robert Hare, author of the PCL, claimed that their article misrepresented his work and was defamatory. Publication of the paper was delayed while this litigation was in progress. Hare (2010) provided his views on this controversy; Poythress and Petrila (2010) offered an overview and reflections on the dispute.

Another possibility that has been mooted for some time, and which might explain several of the discrepancies in research results, is that there may be subtypes of psychopathy. Extending an earlier 'classic' twofold distinction between primary and secondary psychopathy, which essentially differed in levels of anxiety, Blackburn (2009) describes four possible subtypes, called 'primary', 'secondary', 'controlled' and 'inhibited' psychopaths. Some psychometric data supports these distinctions, and the groups may also differ in the kinds of violence in which they engage and their likelihood of being aggressive while in institutions.

Approaching the concept from a different direction, other authors contend that, given the complexity of the construct, it is possible that some of the features traditionally considered integral to psychopathy may not in fact be essential. Poythress and Hall (2011) reviewed evidence calling into question whether impulsivity is indeed the prominent feature of psychopathy it has long been believed to be. Overall, surveying the diverse results, it seems unlikely that there is any single variable that is central to psychopathy or that there can be a unitary explanation of the various facets the definition of it is thought to encapsulate, at least using PCL measures as the yardstick.

Psychopathy and the category–dimension debate

There is another fundamental issue which echoes those we encountered earlier when discussing the conceptualisation of mental disorder in general. This is whether personality disorders, including psychopathy, are best represented in terms of *categories* or of *dimensions*.

On the one hand some researchers claim that psychopathy is a *category*, 'a real phenomenon (essentially a restriction of that described as antisocial personality), and psychopaths comprise a discrete natural class of individuals (even though the boundaries of this class may be indistinct)' and that psychopathy is 'not merely the end of a continuum of natural variation' (Harris, Skilling and Rice, 2001, pp. 197, 226). Use of phraseology that describes psychopaths as being 'among us' implies that they are a distinct group, perhaps not quite full members of the human species; and authors of some studies in this area, such as Hare (1999), do refer to them in such terms, and appear almost to subscribe to that view. A separate approach is that we are dealing with differences along a *dimension*, and the research of Coid and Ullrich (2009) suggests that the differences between psychopaths and others are a matter of degree. To try to resolve this question, some researchers have employed *taxometric analysis*, as described in the 'Focus on ...' box below.

FOCUS ON ...

Mental disorders: categories or dimensions?

Taxonomy is the process of classifying natural phenomena into groups. A *taxon* is a general term for any identifiable group discovered by this process. Examples include the classification of rock types in geology, and of plant and animal species in biology. The Swedish botanist Carl Linnaeus (1707–1778) devised the system of species classification in current use, though it has been considerably modified by the findings of research informed by the theory of evolution.

Applied to psychology, the question arises as to whether people belong in naturally occurring groups. Are there different types of people? Or do they vary along different dimensions such as traits? Diagnostic systems in psychiatry rest on a basic premise that mental disorders are discrete categories. That is, they are each presumed to have an identifiable form and capable of being distinguished from one another, with gaps between them. Many practitioners and researchers, however, find that this view does not correspond well to the observed patterning of mental health problems, in which symptoms appear to run along a continuum of severity. Thus there has been disagreement over whether such problems are best understood by means of a *categorical* model or a *dimensional* one. Should we think in terms of 'kinds' or of 'continua'?

Paul Meehl and his colleagues (Meehl, 1992; Ruscio, 2007) developed a set of statistical techniques to enable researchers to test which of those models provides a better 'fit' for the data on any selected type of problem. *Taxometric analysis* applies a model of measurement based on the investigation of *latent variables*. These are variables hypothesised to underlie a psychological measure, and they can be detected using a series of specially devised computer programs. Several different types of analysis are available for this, and in order to decide whether a dataset best fits a categorical or a dimensional shape, there should be a consistent pattern emerging from at least three of them.

A large number of studies have now been conducted to test whether the distribution of features of a disorder better fits a continuous or a categorical pattern. Recent reviews of this area indicate strongly that most of what are often regarded as *categorical* variables actually have an underlying *dimensional* structure. Haslam, Holland and Kuppens (2012; Haslam, 2011) carried out a wide-ranging review of 177 research studies, together involving over half a million participants and producing 311 separate sets of findings for analysis. The studies were on a wide range of mental health problems: mood, anxiety, or eating disorders; substance abuse; externalising problems; schizotypy; and personality disorders. Some studies focused on variations within the normal range of personality functioning.

Based on careful analysis of the studies, and taking methodological differences into account, Haslam *et al.* (2012) concluded that only 14 per cent of the studies produced evidence supporting a taxonic interpretation of the data available. Most of these emerged in studies of schizotypy and substance abuse. As statistical methods in this area have developed and have been applied to more datasets, the proportion of findings that emerge as indicating the presence of underlying categories has gradually declined. For the majority of the problems that have been studied in this way, the allocation of people into diagnostic categories is not soundly evidence-based.

Question

Applying this to your own experience, do the people you have worked with appear to belong to identifiable types, or does a dimensional model fit better with what you have observed?

The initial conclusions regarding the categorical nature of psychopathy were based on a study by Harris, Rice and Quinsey (1994), in which they analysed PCL:R scores for a sample of 653 male offenders with mental disorders who were detained in secure psychiatric hospitals in Canada. However, other studies in this area have reached opposite conclusions (Edens, Marcus, Lilienfeld and Poythress, 2006; Guay, Ruscio, Knight and Hare, 2007; Marcus, John and Edens, 2004). Edens *et al.* (2006) questioned several aspects of the Harris *et al.* (1994) study. For example, the PCL:R scores they reported were based on file review data only; and the PCL:R was scored dichotomously rather than using the standard three-point scoring (0, 1, 2: see the 'Focus on ... The Psychopathy Checklist' box on page 260). A large portion of the sample were men who had been found 'not guilty by reason of insanity' (NGRI), and while Harris *et al.* conducted some analyses with those men removed, doubts have been expressed regarding whether this was satisfactorily achieved. An implication of the resultant composition of the sample is that where Harris *et al.* believed they had found a taxon, it was the inadvertent discovery of one based on *schizotypy* rather than on psychopathy as such. In any case, a taxonic result was obtained only in relation to Factor 2 of the PCL:R (antisocial lifestyle), and not for Factor 1 (interpersonal and affective items). There was also an anomaly in that the cut-off between the two groups identified – psychopaths versus the rest – was at a score of 19 or 20, whereas in the PCL:R manual (Hare, 2003) this is given as 30 for North American and 25 for European samples.

In an effort to remedy these problems, Edens *et al.* (2006) administered the PCL:R, incorporating an interview, to a group of 876 prisoners and patients with substance-abuse problems. They were also able to analyse the resultant data using several taxometric methods developed since publication of the Harris *et al.* (1994) study. In one method, the four facets of the PCL:R were systematically compared. Each one in turn was used as an *input variable*, and its score distribution was divided (cut) into 50 regular segments. Taking the other facets in turn, the mean score of the cases *below* the cut was subtracted from the mean score of the cases *above* the cut. This procedure is known as *MAMBAC* ('mean above minus below a cut'). The resultant *output variable* is then plotted on a graph against the input variable. If the latent distribution is *categorical* (or *taxonic*), the graph will have a single peak (an inverted V-shape). If the construct is *dimensional* (or *continuous*), the graph will instead have a concave shape. It is possible to average and combine these plots across several variables. Figure 11.1 shows the results of doing so, as obtained by Edens *et al.* Here the actual scores are compared with sets of simulated data – how they would look if the underlying variable were either categorical (taxonic), on the left, or dimensional (continuous), on the right. The distribution is fairly clearly one of the latter kind. This is just one of several analyses that were undertaken, all yielding results that were more consistent with a *dimensional* than with a *categorical* latent variable.

Similar findings have been obtained in other studies of different aspects of assessed psychopathy. Walters (2014) analysed PCL:YV scores, and scores on a separate measure, the Youth Psychopathic Traits Inventory, of 1,162 young male serious offenders (mean age 16) from the multisite Pathways to Desistance study. Walters, Knight, Looman and Abracen (2016) reported a taxometric study of psychopathic traits in a sample of 1,404 sex offenders against children, adults, or both in Canada. Walters, Ermer, Knight and Kiehl (2015) undertook an analysis of the distribution of one of the hypothesised biomarkers of psychopathy, grey-matter concentration in specific brain areas, obtained from MRI scans of a sample of 254 maximum security prisoners. In all three studies the results supported the picture of psychopathy as a dimensional rather than as a categorical variable, with individuals showing gradations of difference rather than evidence of separate categories.

These findings have several implications. Extrapolating from them, most researchers doubt whether there is an identifiable 'core' of psychopathy to be discovered, regardless of whether it is proposed to have a genetic, neurobiological, or social-cognitive mechanism. There are almost certainly several factors operating, and the kind of personality functioning that qualifies as 'psychopathic' involves several of those factors in combination. Psychopathy is therefore highly complex and unlikely to be under the control of a small number of genes or of any single defectively wired brain area.

The resolution of this debate also has ramifications for the wider concept of what it means to say that someone has a personality disorder. Issues arising from this played a pivotal part in efforts to place the DSM-5 on a firmer empirical footing than was the case with its predecessor, the DSM-IV (Frances and Widiger, 2012; Livesley, 2012; Widiger and Trull, 2007). Proposals to revise the con-

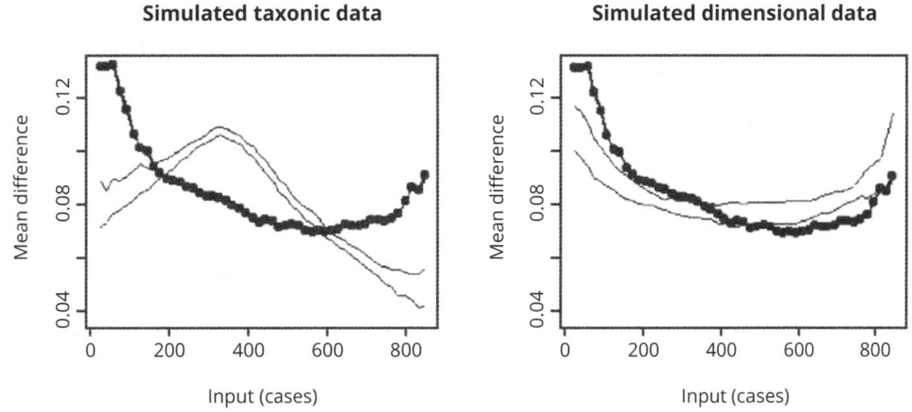
Simulated taxonic data
Simulated dimensional data
Mean difference
0.04
0.08
0.12
0
200
400
600
800
Input (cases)

Figure 11.1
Taxometric analysis of Psychopathy Checklist scores. The lighter lines represent sets of simulated data; the darker lines show an underlying variable. As can be seen, the line for the underlying variable clearly matches the dimensional (continuous) distribution, not the categorical (taxonic) one.

Source: Figure 2. From Edens, J. F., Marcus, D. K., Lilienfeld, S. O. and Poythress Jr., N. G. (2006). Psychopathic, Not Psychopath: Taxometric Evidence for the Dimensional Structure of Psychopathy. Journal of Abnormal Psychology, 115 (1), 131–144. Copyright © APA 2006. Reprinted with permission. DOI: 10.1037/0021-843X.115.1.131

ceptualisation of personality disorder and to replace the categorical system with a dimensional system were not fully implemented in the DSM-5, however. Instead, an 'alternative model' was outlined, centred on the use of personality traits and impairments in personality functioning, to produce a diagnosis of *personality disorder – trait specified* (PD-TS). Proposals were also made for a 'hybrid' model that combined categories and dimensions, based on distinguishing different levels of personality functioning, with the hope that this would generate research findings and allow its validity and usefulness to be tested.

Do some clusters of personality features predispose individuals to violence?

If linear connections between specific personality traits and violence are hard to establish, could it be that some *combinations* of these give more reliable predictions? An early version of such a concept was the *MacDonald Triad*, named after the psychiatrist who proposed the idea in 1963. He suggested that three kinds of child behaviour – persistent enuresis (bedwetting) beyond the age of five, cruelty to animals, and an urge to set fires – were predictive of a later tendency to commit acts of violence. This has become part of the historical folklore of forensic psychiatry and psychology, but evidence supporting it has been fairly weak (Patterson-Kane and Piper, 2009). Some studies have found evidence linking animal cruelty in adulthood to an increased risk of violence, including partner assault (DeGue and DiLillo, 2009; Febres *et al.*, 2014). A study in Switzerland found a strong association between animal cruelty and increased risk of serious violence and of vandalism (Lucia and Killias, 2011). However, on the basis of two related meta-analyses, Walters (2013) questioned whether animal cruelty was any more closely associated with violent than with non-violent offending.

More recently, another combination of traits has been suggested: what has been called the *Dark Triad*. This is the proposal that narcissism, Machiavellianism and psychopathy in combination are associated with a marked propensity towards violence (Paulhus and Williams, 2002). This has stimulated a substantial amount of research, including development of a specially designed measure, perhaps fittingly called the 'Dirty Dozen' (Jonason and Webster, 2010). Furnham, Richards and Paulhus (2013) have reviewed evidence concerning the Dark Triad and concluded that there is a moderate degree of support for the existence of a relationship between this configuration of personality variables and violent criminality.

Disorders of a sexual nature

Another major category of problems that are classed as psychiatric disorders and that are directly linked to criminality are those associated with sexual offences of various kinds. While committing such offences is not in itself indicative of a mental disorder, a proportion of individuals who act in this way may do so as a result of motives and interests that deviate significantly from the norms of society and that may therefore have been classified as mental disorders. They may also cause significant distress to the persons so affected.

In psychiatric terminology, these disorders are grouped under the heading of **paraphilias**, which have as an essential feature 'any intense and persistent sexual interest other than sexual interest in genital stimulation or preparatory fondling with phenotypically normal, physically mature, consenting human partners' (American Psychiatric Association, 2013, p. 685). A *paraphilic disorder* results when this interest causes distress or impairment to the individual experiencing it, or when it entails personal harm or risk of harm to others. This general category subsumes eight types of problems, which are: *voyeurism*, *exhibitionism*, *frotteurism*, *sexual masochism*, *sexual sadism*, *paedophilia*, *fetishism* and *transvestism*. In ICD-10 there are six 'disorders of sexual preference', some of which, if expressed, are likely to lead a person into conflict with the law: fetishism, fetishism-transvestism, exhibitionism, voyeurism, paedophilia and sadomasochism, which may also exist in various combinations. In DSM-5 there are also 'other' and 'unspecified' categories, and these include a range of rarer problems, such as necrophilia, telephone scatalogia, zoophilia and coprophilia (Kafka, 2010).

The foregoing list contains a very wide range of behaviours, so we should also note that people with convictions for superficially similar types of sexual offences are likely to be a heterogeneous group. For example, even amongst those who have committed sexual offences against children, there is a spectrum of motives and only a proportion can be accurately described as 'paedophilic'. In a study of sexual offending in England and Wales, Grubin (1998) estimated that proportion to be somewhere between 25 per cent and 40 per cent. It is further worth recalling (from Chapter 9) that not all of those diagnosed with paedophilia necessarily commit sexual offences: *having* such a preference is not illegal, but *acting* on it is. Where sexual offenders who are detained in secure hospitals or who are serving prison sentences have been diagnosed, that diagnosis is more likely to be of a personality disorder rather than a disorder of sexual interest, and a proportion are diagnosed with multiple comorbid disorders.

Paedophilia – persistent sexual interest in prepubescent children – is probably the most frequently encountered problem of this type in penal and secure mental health settings. It is described as emerging early in life, and may take heterosexual or homosexual forms (Seto, 2008). It affects a far larger proportion of males than females, but little is known about its overall prevalence rate, or of its pattern across the life-course, though it is believed to decline with advancing age. There is evidence that sexual arousal decreases with increasing age, and that recidivism rates gradually reduce with increasing age at release (Barbaree, Blanchard and Langton, 2003). For extra-familial child molesters, however – a group that may contain a higher proportion of paedophiles – there may be a plateau effect until the fifties (Craig, 2008), though data directly pertaining to this are sparse. Seto (2008) reviews three principal theoretical accounts of the aetiology of paedophilia: one based on learning theory; another in terms of a cycle of sexual abusiveness; and a third suggesting that it has a neurodevelopmental origin.

Comorbidity is described as being frequently found amongst members of this group, with anxiety, depression and personality problems often diagnosed (Seto, 2008). As just suggested, studies generally have found a range of other diagnosable mental disorders in those convicted of sexual offences. In a Swedish study of men convicted of sexual offences (n=1,215), the rates were relatively low (Långström, Sjöstedt and Grann, 2004): the most frequent diagnosis was alcohol dependence (7.8 per cent), followed by drug dependence (2.8 per cent), personality disorder (1.8 per cent), and psychosis (1.4 per cent). Other studies have found higher rates of personality disorders: in a US study of those detained under 'sexually violent predator' laws, 23.6 per cent obtained scores of greater than 30 on the PCL:R (Vess, Murphy and Arkowitz, 2004). Although the data are not provided, the proportion meeting diagnostic criteria for antisocial personality disorder would almost certainly have been somewhat higher. Indeed, amongst those found guilty of sexual homicide, fairly high rates have been found (Carter and Hollin, 2010), and it has even been suggested that the overwhelming majority would meet the criteria for antisocial PD. Studies reviewed by Chan and Heide (2009) did find extremely high rates.

A small proportion of sexual offenders may meet criteria for a diagnosis of sexual sadism, with rates thought to range between 5 per cent and 10 per cent, though some studies have produced higher estimates, highest of all where assaults are fatal (Marshall and Kennedy, 2003). Although perpetrators of sadistic sexual crimes understandably give rise to considerable alarm, and there is a sizeable volume of writing on this topic, reviewers of this area have called for more methodical and soundly based research (Yates, Hucker and Kingston, 2008). Once again clear definitions are elusive, but a key issue to attend to in assessments is that the individual obtains pleasure and excitement from engaging in acts of sexual cruelty and from the suffering of the victim – and in a way that is distinct from a sexual assault that also contains elements of physical brutality, but which may have other explanations. There are several subtypes of sexual sadism, and several competing theories as to its aetiology, but again its origins are not clearly understood (Yates *et al.* 2008). The continuity of most deviant sexual interests over time is thought to be maintained through engagement in fantasy, and while this need not necessarily be accompanied by masturbation, it often is (Ward and Beech, 2006, 2008).

Treatment of mental disorders

The pattern of delivery of services to address mental health problems is very uneven around the world. In the richest countries, the numbers of people treated in psychiatric hospitals have dramatically declined in the period since 1960–1970, with a growing emphasis on outpatient community treatment (the 'community care movement'). A similar trend is occurring in other countries, though much more slowly. In many places, even allowing for the overestimation of prevalence alluded to above, there are large shortfalls in service provision. According to the most recent edition of the WHO *Mental Health Atlas* (World Health Organization, 2011b), based on a survey of 184 member states, 'Globally, spending on mental health is less than two US dollars per person, per year and less than 25 cents in low income countries' (p. 10). Even in England and Wales, although almost half of all ill-health amongst those under the age of 65 is *mental* ill-health, only a quarter of sufferers are receiving any treatment (Centre for Economic Performance, 2012). It seems likely, therefore, that there remains a sizeable level, indeed potentially an enormous level of unmet need in many communities (Kazdin and Blase, 2011).

In Chapter 19 we will examine the evidence relevant to the impact of treatment or other types of intervention on offending behaviour and criminal recidivism. The evaluation of therapy for mental health problems is a parallel but virtually separate field. There is a very extensive literature within it, and only a brief overview can be given here. Most of the therapies for mental health problems in widespread use today fall into two major categories: they are either *pharmacological* or *psychological*.

Pharmacological therapy

Pharmacological therapy, involving psychotropic medication or drug therapy, is by far the dominant approach. According to the National Institute of Health and Care Excellence (NICE) in the UK: 'The most common method of treatment for common mental health disorders in primary care is psychotropic medication. This is due to the limited availability of psychological interventions, despite the fact that these treatments are generally preferred by patients' (2011a, p. 5). It is not an exaggeration to say that across the world tens of millions of people are receiving drugs for the kinds of CMHPs discussed at the outset of this chapter. In England, for example, the numbers of psychiatric drugs prescribed increased on average by 6.8 per cent per year between 1998 and 2010, by which point the total number of such prescription items reached 79.8 million (Ilyas and Moncrieff, 2012). Globally, the pharmaceutical industry, even just that part of it dealing with psychiatric medicines, is a business with a total annual turnover running into hundreds of billions of US dollars. Its leading companies (Johnson & Johnson, Pfizer, Roche, GlaxoSmithKline, Novartis, AstraZeneca and Eli Lilly, sometimes collectively referred to as 'Big Pharma'), are highly profitable enterprises. It has been suggested that the competition between these companies and their sponsorship of comparative 'head to head' outcome studies of different drugs may explain some of the anomalous findings of medication trials (Heres *et al.* 2006; Lexchin, Bero, Djulbegovic and Clark, 2003).

At various points in the past, other somatic procedures have been used within psychiatry, including *insulin coma therapy* (based on the theory that this would rid the nervous system of schizophrenia); the use of *malaria* to treat the 'general paralysis of the insane' caused by syphilis (in the belief that the resultant fever would kill the pathogen); and various forms of *psychosurgery* (such as *leucotomy* or *lobotomy*, removal of parts of the frontal lobes). However, these and many other procedures have now been abandoned. Those still used today include the administration of *electroconvulsive therapy* (ECT) for depression; and some forms of *neurosurgery* are still employed, but only very rarely, in the treatment of mood disorders (Sachdev and Chen, 2008).

The conventional and received view of the action of psychotropic medication is that specific drugs have been developed that have selective impact on neural events or sites associated with particular psychiatric disorders. For that reason, these drugs are described as belonging to groups such as *antidepressants*, *antipsychotics* and *anxiolytics*. These terms in themselves imply that the cause of the associated disorder is known, and that the drug counteracts it.

However, this explanation is at odds with the bulk of the evidence. It has simply not been established that the mental disorders treated by most psychiatric prescription drugs have their origins in a neurochemical imbalance; nor is it the case that any drug has an action so precise as to be able to remedy a specified problem of this kind (even assuming that that had indeed been the cause to start with) without also having other, unwanted effects. An alternative view of the mechanism by which drugs operate has been developed by Moncrieff (2009; Moncrieff and Cohen, 2005), who has called the sequence of supposed causes and effects just outlined the *disease-centred model*. Within that model, the process of treating a mental disorder is likened to that of treating a physical health problem, as when administering insulin to control diabetes, or antihypertensive drugs to relieve high blood pressure. However, the medical knowledge that has been acquired of the pathophysiology of those ailments has no equivalent in relation to mental disorders. The labelling of a category of substances as 'antipsychotic' (or 'antidepressant') has been done to convey an impression that the substances have those effects, when closer examination reveals that this is not really what they do. This amounts, in Moncrieff's words, to a 'huge collective myth' (2009, p. 237).

Moncrieff (2009) therefore typifies the disease-centred model of drug action as highly misleading, and proposes that it be replaced with a *drug-centred model* which more accurately reflects the available data on the effects of psychotropic medications. The drug-centred model suggests that most psychiatric drugs have a general effect of dulling an individual's reactions to the surrounding world or to his or her inner disturbance or anguish. Such therapeutic effects as are seen in controlled research and in clinical practice are a result of what is in fact, overall, an intoxicating action. In relation to some aspects of mental illness experience, this action may have partial benefits, for example in dampening down some features of some symptoms. Nevertheless, the drug does not directly or differentially 'treat' the causes of a disease. Some further details, relevant in comparing the two models, are given in the next 'Where do you stand?' box.

11

WHERE DO YOU STAND?

What are the effects of psychotropic medication?

Whether we are professionals or laypeople, many of us tend to take for granted that different psychotropic medications have specific kinds of effects. Their very names – antidepressants, anxiolytics, antipsychotics – directly suggest that they do, and it comes as no surprise, therefore, to find a correspondence between the syndrome from which a person is diagnosed to be suffering and the corresponding type of drug prescribed.

However, the psychiatrist Joanna Moncrieff (2009) has raised some searching questions regarding these matters, and has examined both the history of psychiatric drugs and how they were introduced, alongside clinical data about their pharmacological effects. Moncrieff distinguishes two distinct models of psychotropic drug action, which she calls the 'disease-centred' and the 'drug-centred' models of drug action. Some comparisons

Disease-centred model	Drug-centred model
Drugs help to correct an abnormal brain state	Drugs create an abnormal brain state
Therapeutic effects of drugs derive from their effects on disease pathology	Therapeutic effects derive from the impact of a drug-induced state on emotions and behaviour
Drug effects may differ between patients and volunteers	Effects do not differ between patients and volunteers
The outcomes of drug research consist of effects of drugs on measures of the disease and its symptoms	Outcomes are a non-specific effect caused by drug ingestion and how this interacts with behaviour and experience

Source: adapted from Joanna Moncrieff, The Myth of the Chemical Cure: A Critique of Psychiatric Drug Treatment published 2008 by Palgrave Macmillan, reproduced with permission of SCSC.

between them are shown in the accompanying table.

A paradigmatic illustration of the disease-centred model is the use of insulin for treatment of diabetes, where there is a known metabolic effect directly linked to the cause of the problem. Psychiatric medication is offered on the basis that it is an essentially equivalent process. Moncrieff, however, argues that there is no actual parallel between the two. All that psychotropic drugs have in common is that they induce a generally intoxicating effect. They may reduce levels of some distressing symptoms, but at the same time they often cause very adverse reactions. Crucially, most psychotropic drug actions are not specific to the symptoms of one illness any more than to those of any other. A closer analogy to their effect, in fact, would be to say that their use resembles drinking alcohol to overcome social anxiety.

Where do you stand on this issue?

1 How much evidence is there that psychotropic medicines have specific effects?

2 Which of the two models in the table gives a better account of psychotropic drug effects?

Several psychiatric drugs, mainly in the neuroleptic group, are often prescribed both to reduce the symptoms of severe mental illness and also to control anger, impulsivity and aggressiveness. A review of randomised controlled trials of medication for the reduction of violence found some positive effects (Hockenhull *et al.*, 2012). Other substances are used specifically in sex-offender treatment, and a separate group of hormonal anti-libidinal agents are used for the reduction of sexual urges. These treatments have been found to be effective in reducing sexual reoffending (Lösel and Schmucker, 2005), though other summaries are more equivocal (Association for the Treatment of Sexual Abusers, 2012). Running counter to this, there are also documented cases of some types of medication being associated with increased violence, as documented in a review by Moore, Glenmullen and Furberg (2010).

Psychological therapies

The other major type of therapy, though accessed by far smaller numbers of people, is *psychological*, and essentially involves the service user working with a practitioner such as a counsellor or a psychologist. The bulk of such work is done individually, though it can also be delivered in group format; and most of it entails direct face-to-face contact, though a small proportion has been devised for computer-assisted use. Psychological therapy can take various forms, depending on the theoretical allegiance of practitioners, and might consist of *behavioural*, *cognitive*, *psychodynamic*, *systemic*, or other types of approach. There are many variants, to an extent that even more than two decades ago Kazdin (1986) suggested that it was possible to identify over 400 named types of psychological therapy, including some major approaches and numerous blends or permutations of those. While some were substantially grounded in scientific theory and research, regrettably others had very little evidence either to support the model that allegedly informed them or to demonstrate that they had any useful effects. However, there is now extensive evidence that soundly based psychological therapy for mental health problems is both effective (Roth and Fonagy, 2006) and cost-effective (Layard, Clark, Knapp and Mayraz, 2007). Despite such findings, in a context of steadily rising total expenditure on mental health services, surveys have suggested that the percentage of mental health service users in receipt of these therapies has been declining relative to the numbers receiving medication (Mark *et al.*, 2007; Olfson and Marcus, 2010).

Forensic mental health services

Individuals who have committed offences and who also suffer from diagnosed mental disorders are likely to be detained under mental health legislation. If their offences are of a serious violent or sexual nature, or if they have marked substance-abuse patterns, they are likely to spend a number of years in secure hospitals. The level of security (in the UK, 'high', 'medium' or 'low') will usually be determined by assessing the level of long-term risk, but it could also be chosen to address ongoing serious management problems. There is likely to be an extensive period of assessment, and individuals will usually be offered some combination of both of the main types of therapy just described, pharmacological and psychological. In some cases, medical treatment may be made compulsory and medication may be administered by injection. Individuals' progress is likely to be managed by a multidisciplinary care team that includes a psychiatrist, a clinical or forensic psychologist (or both), nursing staff, and a social worker. There may be a wider team, including occupational therapists (or other specialists such as art, drama or music therapists), teachers, advocacy services, and possibly a chaplain or an imam. Clinical (including psychological) services will be delivered through a care plan based on the assessment of risk and need, and the plan should be formulated within the framework known as the *Care Programme Approach* (Department of Health, 2008), which entails regular review.

For those detained for any length of time as a result of having committed offences, return to the community will generally be carried out in a phased, stepwise process, and will involve several components. It might entail increasing amounts of time in the community during short periods of community leave, initially escorted by a staff member; and then, depending on progress and the assessment of risk, unescorted. It is generally regarded as vital that individuals refamiliarise themselves with the outside world before release, as even in a few years it may have changed in crucial ways. Therapeutic work to address mental health problems and to reduce risk is usually joined to a range of other social care and rehabilitation services, such as sheltered housing, hostels, day centres, financial support or family support, according to individual need.

Post-discharge follow-up

With respect to those who have been detained in secure (forensic) mental health units in the UK, there is an expanding amount of research reporting outcomes in the years after discharge from such institutions. Prior to 1980, most individuals in this category (who had committed serious offences, and were diagnosed with major mental disorders) were detained in high security hospitals. Medium secure units were introduced following the publication of the *Butler Report* in 1975, but the first of them did not open until the early 1980s (Snowden, 1983; Stocking, 1992). Coid *et al.* (2001) provide descriptive information on those detained in medium security in the period 1988–1994, but it is likely that the profile of patients detained in such units has gradually changed since then. Table 11.1 summarises some key findings of post-discharge follow-up studies published since 1990. Some studies report data on patients from a single unit, while others analysed data from several units. Several earlier follow-up studies were reviewed by Bailey and MacCulloch (1992b);

Authors (date)	Discharges from	Sample size	Maximum follow-up period (years)	Percentage reconvicted in categories as reported
Bailey & MacCulloch (1992a)	High secure hospital	112	14.0	Whole sample: 36.6 Mental illness: 21.0 Personality disorder: 54.9 Serious offence: 17.0
Buchanan (1998)	High secure hospitals	425	10.5	Any offence: 34.0 Serious offence: 15.0
Friendship, McClintock, Rutter & Maden (1999)	Medium secure unit	234	14.0	Any reoffence: 23.9 Violent reoffence: 10.0 Sexual reoffence: 2.0
Jamieson & Taylor (2004)	Medium secure unit	197	12.0	Any reoffence: 38.0 Serious reoffence: 26.4
Maden *et al.* (2004)	Medium secure units	959	2.0	Any reconviction: 14.6 Violent reoffence: 6.0
Coid, Hickey, Kahtan & Zhang (2007)	Medium secure units	1,344	9.9	Any reoffence: *Men:* 46.8 *Women:* 16.3 Violent reoffence: *Men:* 7.4 *Women:* 2.5
Davies, Clarke, Hollin & Duggan (2007)	Medium secure unit	550	20.0	Any reconviction: 49.0 Readmitted: 38.0 Serious reoffence: *Mental illness:* 13.7 *Personality disorder:* 15.0
Gray, Taylor & Snowden (2008)	Medium secure units	996	5.0	Any reconviction: 34.2 Violent reconviction: 10.6
Ho, Thomson & Darjee (2009)	Medium secure unit	96	2.0	Minor reoffence: 40.6 Serious violent reoffence: 4.2
Clarke *et al.* (2013)	Medium secure unit	550	20.0	Readmitted to hospital: 61.6 Readmitted to secure unit: 37.6

Table 11.1 Follow-up studies of people discharged from secure mental health services in the United Kingdom. These studies have all been published since 1990.

and McGuire, Mason and O'Kane (2000) tabulated some of their findings.

In several respects, there are some broadly consistent trends emerging from these studies. Discharged patients who are younger, male, and unmarried, and who have a diagnosis of personality disorder and larger numbers of previous convictions, are more likely to be recalled to hospital or convicted of a further offence. Conditional discharge – which involves adherence to supervision and other requirements, and is also more supportive – has better results. The rate of serious reoffending and of general reconviction for those discharged from high security hospitals is on average lower than that for those released from prison; and for discharges from medium security, it is lower still.

These findings could be interpreted as showing that the forensic mental health system is reasonably effective. However, members of the samples studied here have generally spent longer in hospital than most prisoners spend in prison, and without relevant comparative outcome data, such a conclusion is somewhat speculative: we are not really comparing 'like with like'. Furthermore, given that discharge is less likely the higher the predicted risk, it is not easy to see how meaningful comparisons can be made.

Chapter summary

Many people experience mental health problems at some stage of their lives; and for a proportion of people who break the law, such problems are a factor associated with their offending behaviour.

- This chapter has outlined the systems of diagnosis used in psychiatry, and also indicated some difficulties with them when considered from a psychological perspective.
- There is evidence that prisoners report higher rates of such problems than are found amongst the community as a whole, and many prisons have additional services to address these needs. In other cases, where problems are more severe, individuals are detained under mental health law rather than being sentenced under criminal law. Both groups are highly vulnerable, and their problems are often worsened by an association with substance misuse.
- The relationship between criminal or antisocial behaviour and mental health is a complex one, and many aspects of this have not yet been fully resolved. However, some symptoms of severe mental illness, and some personality patterns, are associated with a heightened risk of violence, and a task often performed by forensic psychologists is the assessment of the levels of such risk. The chapter also examined some of the complexities of assessment in this area.
- There is also evidence that mental health problems can be reduced through psychological therapies, and that these can have the associated benefit of reducing the risk of reoffending.

Further reading

- There are many texts that provide an overall introduction to abnormal psychology, analyse key concepts, and provide information on the range of mental health problems. Good examples include the books by Ann M. Kring, Sheri L. Johnson, Gerald C. Davison and John M. Neale (2017) *Abnormal Psychology: The Science and Treatment of Psychological Disorders* (13th edition, Hoboken, NJ: Wiley) and by Paul W. Bennett (2011), *Abnormal and Clinical Psychology: An Introductory Textbook* (3rd edition, Maidenhead: Open University Press).
- In medical terms, organic psychiatry is the most highly developed area of the discipline. The authoritative volume on it is this one: Anthony S. David, Simon Fleminger, Michael D. Kopelman, Simon Lovestone and John D. C. Mellers (2012), *Lishman's Organic Psychiatry: A Textbook of Neuropsychiatry* (4th edition, Chichester: Wiley-Blackwell).
- For a highly readable overview of some of the controversies in psychiatry, see Richard P. Bentall (2009), *Doctoring the Mind: Why Psychiatric Treatments Fail* (London: Penguin); while further analysis of those issues and arguments can be found in the volume edited by James E. Maddux and Barbara A. Winstead (2015), *Psychopathology: Foundations for a Contemporary Understanding* (4th edition, New York, NY: Routledge).
- For information on global issues in mental health and services, visit the World Health Organization (WHO) website on mental health, at: http://www.who.int/topics/mental_health/en/index.html
- A broad-ranging overview of the field of forensic mental health is provided in an edited volume by Annie Bartlett and Gill McGauley (2009), *Forensic Mental Health:*

Concepts, Systems and Practice (Oxford: Oxford University Press).

» There are several handbooks providing in-depth coverage of the study of personality disorders, including W. John Livesley and Roseann Larstone (eds) (2018). *Handbook of Personality Disorders: Theory, Research and Treatment* (New York, NY: Guilford Press) and on psychopathy Christopher J. Patrick (ed.) (2018), *Handbook of Psychopathy* (2nd edition, New York, NY: Guilford Press).

Offences: Investigation, Evidence and Sentencing

Once an offence has been committed, the perpetrator must be identified and then escorted along a route through the criminal justice system. Part 3 considers the work of the police and the courts, the need for reliable evidence, and the nature and purposes of sentencing.

Investigating Offences: Gathering Information and Interviewing

Interviewing is a complex process. At the very least, it is a relationship between two individuals who are unlikely to know one another, and in which, typically, one is trying to gather information from the other. There are many situations when someone might carry out an interview: for example, with a client who wants to have some kind of support, a witness who wishes to help with an inquiry, or someone who has been arrested for an offence and does not want to be prosecuted. In each situation the dynamics between the interviewer and the interviewee, the context, and the attributes that each person brings can all make a difference. So although on the surface interviewing might appear to be a relatively simple process, when we begin to examine it more closely we can see that there are a range of other issues to consider: for example, the possible power difference between interviewer and interviewee; the potential consequences of what is revealed during an interview; and whether or not the interviewee is willing. We also need to consider whether the interviewee is a victim, a potential perpetrator, or a witness to a highly stressful event; and whether the interviewee is very young, might easily be persuaded, or has some kind of learning disability. Finally, we need to consider how elements of memory function could impact on how accurately events are remembered.

Chapter objectives

- To have a broad perspective of the range of different circumstances relevant to a forensic psychologist in which interviews might take place.
- To gain an understanding of some different approaches to interviewing.
- To understand some of the important issues that surround the interviewing process.
- To identify some of the important skills that can assist in good interviewing.

The investigative process

Once there has been a complaint that an offence has or may have been committed, the process of gathering information, referred to as an *investigation*, will typically begin. At its simplest, this will be a matter of speaking with the alleged offender or the person pleading guilty to the offence. Such a case may occur if an individual is caught shoplifting and that person's details are passed on to the police. Where there is a lack of certainty about the nature of the offence (or indeed whether an offence took place at all), about the identity of the offender (especially if, when located, a suspect denies the offence), and where there may be a need to gather information from other sources (typically suspects, victims, or witnesses), a variety of considerations and issues may arise.

These are partly issues of how to elicit information accurately, and partly issues of evidence and how the legal system allows evidence to be gathered. Shepherd (2007) writes: 'Investigation in the criminal context involves the *lawful* search for detail enabling reconstruction of an actual or intended illegal act, and of the mental state accompanying it' (p. 3). As an example, there have been discussions in recent years about how evidence in relation to terrorist activity might have been obtained (notably, whether or not *torture* has been used), and these discussions reflect both moral and ethical concerns (Thienel, 2006) and the reliability of that evidence (Ratner, 2003). Both areas of literature suggest that torture leads to evidence that is inadmissible and is likely to be flawed. The section below will deal with the latter issue; for further ideas about ethical issues, see Thienel (2006) and Costanzo, Gerrity and Lykes (2007) as a starting point. It might also be useful to try to access the United Nations *Convention against Torture and Other Cruel, Inhuman or Degrading Treatment or Punishment* (the 'Torture Convention') for further arguments against the use of torture in obtaining information.

Torture

Torture (or what some of its proponents refer to as *enhanced interrogation*) is likely to be the most extreme method used to extract information from an individual. Typically we would expect that torture would be considered only in the case of an individual who is thought to be lying, so most likely an offender or, conceivably, a reluctant witness (for example, a witness withholding evidence, who was being required to testify against a colleague or **co-conspirator**). However, is torture likely to provide the interrogator with reliable information?

By the very nature of torture, there is no empirical investigation (in the public domain) that can shed light on its effectiveness, but subsequent interviews with victims of torture have suggested that they would have been prepared to say anything just to bring the torture to an end (McCoy, 2006). Perhaps more worrying is that although it is not possible to demonstrate that torture works, research does suggest that trained interviewers believe they are more accurate at recognising deception than they actually are (Kassin and Fong, 1999). Given that there is also a tendency to believe that people are lying more frequently than is actually the case (Masip, Alonso, Garrido and Anton, 2005), it is likely that under conditions where torture is an option, it might be applied. Thankfully, as far as we are aware torture is not an issue for the typical investigative situation in most countries, and we now turn our attention to those practices that are more commonly used.

Researching the investigative process

There is little empirical literature that is concerned with the investigative process (Stelfox, 2009), and much of the process has developed through professional practice rather than being driven by scientific evidence. To some extent this is because it is difficult to think of a situation where one could compare practices for investigating comparable crimes, because crimes are different in many subtle ways. Certainly, science has played a role in the development of new techniques, such as the use of fingerprints and DNA, and psychology has played a role both in the evolution of interview techniques (Bull and Milne, 2004) and in the refinement of ideas concerned with criminal profiling (Canter, 2004b).

Prior to there being a police force, *individuals* were responsible for the investigation of crimes against them, and it is likely that a vast range of approaches were used, dependent on the crime, the individuals' characteristics, and the resources available to them. With the advent of professional policing – which was an evolution of the Bow Street Runners, a group of professional crimefighters set up in 1750 by a Justice of the Peace, Henry Fielding (Reiner, 2000) – there was a gradual refinement and standardisation of approaches. The greatest impact upon standardisation was the number of changes brought about by concerns over miscarriages of justice (Walker and Starmer, 1999) during the latter part of the 20th century, which resulted in clear definitions of police powers, the roles of investigators, and the processes of investigation. The most well known of these is probably the **Police and Criminal Evidence Act 1984** or **PACE** (Stelfox, 2009). One consequence of these new definitions was the recognition of a need to professionalise the process of investigating, which resulted in the 'Professionalising Investigation Programme'. Amongst other skills of investigation, this directly trains officers in aspects of interviewing, through two modules: 'Investigative Interviewing for Volume and Priority Investigations' and 'Investigative Interviewing for Serious and Complex Investigations'.

Given that a major concern of the investigative process is possible **miscarriage of justice**, a variety of methods have been developed to create a record of the interview process so that factors such as coercion could be examined. Recently these have included the use of video-recordings, which in some cases might be used both as evidence of a confession and as proof that the confession had not been forced. Interestingly, research has

WHERE DO YOU STAND?

Torture

The Torture Convention states:

> For the purposes of this Convention, torture means any act by which severe pain or suffering, whether physical or mental, is intentionally inflicted on a person for such purposes as obtaining from him or a third person information or a confession, punishing him for an act he or a third person has committed or is suspected of having committed, or intimidating or coercing him or a third person, or for any reason based on discrimination of any kind, when such pain or suffering is inflicted by or at the instigation of or with the consent or acquiescence of a public official or other person acting in an official capacity. It does not include pain or suffering arising only from, inherent in or incidental to lawful sanctions.

Given that this is the basis for identifying torture, it is worth considering some issues that it raises.

First, how do we define 'severe pain or suffering'? This definition suggests that there is continuum of pain and suffering; and we need to keep in mind that individuals may not experience and perceive pain and suffering in the same way. Second, *physical* pain and suffering are easy to understand, but what is meant by *mental* pain and suffering? Some authors (e.g. Bufacchi and Arrigo, 2006) equate this to *psychological* pain and suffering, but are 'mental' and 'psychological' necessarily the same thing? What counts as mental pain? (Presumably this would not include headaches, as they are physical pain.) What about suffering that might occur later, such as flashbacks? Therefore, we could try to develop a clearer idea of the concept of torture, both so that we know when torture is and is not being committed, and to tighten the definition to make it less likely that torture will be condoned.

The Torture Convention also makes it clear that there are no circumstances under which torture can be justified. Do you agree? A variety of authors have suggested that if the torture of one person leads to information that prevents the harming or death of others, then this might be considered a defence (see for example Parry, 2004). How many others would need to be saved for torture to be acceptable? Does that number depend on who it is who is saved? Would we consider that torture is reasonable in order to save 1 president, or 15 children, or 100 women? Does it matter what we are saving them from, such as a bomb, a fire, or infection with a life-threatening disease?

Even if we can determine some metric whereby torture can be judged acceptable, we are still left with another issue: that we may not know whether or not the person being tortured has the information we need.

Where do you stand on this issue?

1 Are there any conditions under which you think that torture could be condoned, even if there is some doubt as to the quality of the information that might be gathered?

2 What issues would you consider in the decision-making process so that you might feel justified in your position? For example, would you consider legal, ethical, or psychological issues, and if so what might they be?

12

demonstrated that what the video depicts in these interviews plays an important role in mock-jury decisions and their assessments of the extent to which a suspect has been coerced. Lassiter and Irvine (1986) conducted a study where groups of participants were each shown a videotaped confession showing one of three possible scenes: the interviewer only appearing on-screen, the suspect only appearing on-screen, or the suspect and the interviewer together on-screen. These were compared to one another and to a group who read a **transcript** of the interview. Lassiter and Irvine found that interviews were considered by participants most likely to have been coerced when what they viewed was the interviewer-alone recording, and secondly when they viewed the suspect and the interviewer together, and with the lowest assessment of coercion in the suspect-alone condition. The transcript condition led to assessments of coercion similar to the interviewer-only condition.

A later study showed that these manipulations impacted upon mock-jury decision-making: convictions were found to drop by 35 per cent in a group watching an interviewer-alone video compared to an interviewer and suspect together video (Lassiter *et al.*, 2002). Research such as this demonstrates that the use of technology needs to be carefully considered in legal settings, rather than assuming that it will always be of benefit. One might also consider how the use of video could impact upon forensic psychologists' understanding both of clients and of assessment processes if the forensic psychologists are unable either to be at the original interviews or to interview the clients later for themselves. Equally, video is often used in assessing the skills of various psychologists who are being trained – or who are demonstrating existing skills – in, for example, the use of a particular psychometric test. As with the attributions of coercion above, it is possible that similar biases may impact upon these assessments too.

Investigative interviewing

When carrying out interviews, the police in England, Wales and Northern Ireland use what is referred to as the *PEACE model* of investigative interviewing. The aim of this model is to ensure both that the maximum amount of information is elicited from an interviewee and also that this information is obtained legally and ethically (which reduces the likelihood that its provenance can be contested at trial). Research has shown that the behaviour of the interviewer during an interview has an impact on the information elicited, which could include eliciting false confessions or confessions that are ruled as inadmissible in court (e.g. Baldwin, 1993). The idea of maximising the quantity and quality of the information obtained is quite different from the earlier aim of interviews as an exercise in seeking confessions (Shawyer, Milne and Bull, 2009).

PEACE consists of the following five stages: *Preparation and planning*, *Engage (and explain)*, *Account*, *Closure* and *Evaluation*:

» ***Preparation and planning*** This occurs before the interview takes place. It requires that all the relevant and available evidence is collected, allowing the questions to be used in the interview to be planned in advance, and the purpose of the interview to be defined.

» ***Engage and explain*** Here the essence of the model is to develop rapport with the interviewee and to build an understanding of the interviewee's motivatation. Additionally, the process of the interview should be explained, including its importance, issues of timing, when breaks have been scheduled, and so on.

» ***Account*** This stage is concerned with managing the interview so that the interviewee will provide information. There are two specific techniques that may be used at this stage: the *Cognitive Interview* and *Conversation Management*. It may be necessary to challenge the interviewee, to examine the interviewee's account in more detail, and to remain observant as to whether there is a shift in the interviewee's cooperativeness.

» ***Closure*** At this stage the interviewer provides a summary of the interview, allowing any further information to be given if the interviewee has anything to add. This stage is important, to ensure that the interviewee will be willing to be interviewed again if necessary.

» ***Evaluation*** This refers to an evaluation of the interview itself and of the quality of the information elicited. It allows the interviewer to determine whether the interview goals have been achieved, and what further steps might be required.

As the above description makes clear, PEACE really provides a structure for the interview process rather than detailing technical aspects of interview technique, but it does assist in ensuring that each interview is comprehensive and fair. The PEACE protocol also advocates the use of the Cognitive Interview.

In using PEACE, officers in England and Wales work within a tier system: Tier 1 is the most basic form of interviewing, incorporating the Cognitive Interview; and Tier 5 is the level of the most experienced and most highly trained officers. Tier 1 officers typically make use of three of the components of the Cognitive Interview (described below), omitting the 'recall from a variety of different perspectives' component.

The Cognitive Interview

The *Cognitive Interview* (Fisher and Geiselman, 1992) is based on psychological principles drawn from an understanding of human memory and how best to support accurate recall of events during interviews. Typically, it is intended for use with witnesses and victims (Memon, Wark, Bull and Koehnken, 1997), although a cooperative offender may also be able to provide more accurate information through these processes. A variety of modifications have been developed, resulting in approaches that are considered as effective as the original format, but also in some respects better – for example, newer approaches are shorter in duration (Dando, Wilcock, Milne and Henry, 2009).

The Cognitive Interview consists of four stages:

» *Context reinstatement* This is concerned with attempting to have the witness re-experience the external, emotional and cognitive factors that were present at the time of the event, as research has suggested that this enhances recall (e.g. Tulving and Thomson, 1973). External factors include the weather, smells, and other sensations; the emotional factors include feelings such as surprise and fear; and cognitive factors include thoughts at the time of the event.

» *Recall in other than forward temporal order* Interviewees are encouraged to recall information in a variety of orders. This has two primary aims: one is that some information may be more accessible when memory is interrogated in this way; and the second is that the memories may be more accurate as when reporting in reverse order, for example, interviewees are less likely to fill in details according to their expectations and biases. This follows on from the work of Schank and Abelson (1977), which was concerned with schema theory.

» *Recall from a variety of different perspectives* This may be from the perspective of another witness (recalling what you think another bystander might have seen), if the matter under investigation is a crime, but other perspectives are possible. Milne and Bull (2002) give the example of asking the interviewee to consider a robber's hairstyle from the perspective of a hairdresser. This idea developed from the work of Anderson and Pichert (1978).

» *Recall as much information as possible* Also known as the 'report everything' instruction, this stage allows interviewees to report incomplete information and matters that they may believe are irrelevant. In part this simply allows more information to be collected; but another idea is that the recall of incomplete information may lead to other information being recalled also.

Research has suggested that the Cognitive Interview results in the elicitation of more information than would be obtained through other forms of structured interviewing, and that this information is still of high quality (Köhnken, Milne, Memon and Bull, 1999). Similar effects have been found when using this technique with children (Milne and Bull, 2003); with older adults (Wright and Holliday, 2007); with victims of crime (Fisher, Geiselman and Amador, 1989); and, to a lesser extent, with people who have mild learning disabilities (Milne, Clare and Bull, 1999). Overall, the Cognitive Interview appears to be useful in a number of contexts and with a variety of groups of individuals in helping interviewers to gather useful information.

One concern raised about the Cognitive Interview is the amount of time it takes for interviewers to carry it out. Research with British police officers has indicated that time pressure is one of the reasons why a

WHERE DO YOU STAND?

Cognitive Interview

The four different phases of the Cognitive Interview are based on research demonstrating how memory may be enhanced via a range of techniques. Some may not be particularly useful in specific cases – for example, young children are not particularly good at perspective-taking, and individuals with poor 'theory of mind' skills may not be able to imagine how another person may have been thinking and feeling, and how that might influence what that person would see, hear, feel, and thus remember.

Research (see Brown and Geiselman, 1990; Milne and Bull, 2001) has looked at another group of individuals who may benefit from the use of the Cognitive Interview: people with learning disabilities (known in the USA as 'people with an intellectual disability'). Given that it is estimated that there are nearly 1.5 million people in the UK who could be described as 'learning disabled', this is not an inconsequential population.

People with learning disabilities can find recalling information more difficult: learning disabilities are often associated with issues of encoding and recall, which results in the process of accessing information being less complete and taking longer. However, the Cognitive Interview appears to improve the recall of correct information in people with a learning disability (though still less than in a non-learning-disabled population interviewed using the Cognitive Interview), without increasing the number of errors (getting facts wrong), but with an increase in the amount of extra information reported that was not present in the event.

There are other important factors to consider in addition to simply using an appropriate interview strategy – for example, one might consider the complexity of the questions used – but it is clear that it is possible to improve recall by using a supportive strategy based on an understanding of how memory works.

Where do you stand on this issue?

1 With your knowledge of memory, are there are any other techniques that you could imagine might be useful for enhancing investigative interviewing for a learning-disabled or otherwise vulnerable population? For example, what factors might be useful when interviewing children?
2 Are there ways to reduce the reporting of events or facts that were not present in a situation without further unintended consequences? Is it enough that people try to imagine what they were feeling at the time of an event, or should they be placed in a situation that evokes those same feelings?
3 If the latter did work, what are the ethical issues concerned with possibly asking that witnesses re-experience strongly negative feelings, such as fear?

Cognitive Interview will not be undertaken with a witness (Kebbell, Milne and Wagstaff, 1999). In order to provide an interview strategy that incorporated the positive aspects of the Cognitive Interview but was also practical in terms of time, Davis, McMahon and Greenwood (2005) carried out a study examining what they refer to as the *Modified Cognitive Interview* (MCI). The MCI omits two elements of the original Cognitive Interview, the 'Recall in other than forward temporal order' stage and the 'Recall from a variety of different perspectives' stage. In their study, Davis and colleagues compared this version with the Cognitive Interview and with a structured interview. Their results suggested that the MCI was statistically as good as the Cognitive Interview in eliciting correct information, and they suggest that the MCI takes less time to complete. Dando *et al.* (2009) produced another modified version in which participants were asked to provide a sketch of the event being recalled, and they found that this led to similarly high levels of recall and to reduction in time compared to the standard police Tier 1 version of the Cognitive Interview (as described above).

Clearly, there are elements of the Cognitive Interview that are beneficial to eyewitness recall, which is important for the investigative process, and researchers are developing newer approaches so that this strategy can be applied practically in real police interviews. Another method that has been described as a useful interview strategy, though it has been less empirically scrutinised, is Conversation Management.

Conversation Management

Conversation Management is a technique that has been developed in order to elicit information from uncooperative people (see Shepherd, 1986). It involves using three core strategies, which Shepherd has termed 'reciprocity', 'RESPONSE', and 'management of conversation sequence'.

» *Reciprocity* Similar to rapport, the idea here is that if interviewers disclose something about themselves, this may develop trust with the interviewee, and in addition the social pressure of sharing may encourage an interviewee to share too (Cialdini, 2001).

» *RESPONSE* This strategy consists of *Respect*, *Empathy*, *Supportiveness*, *Positiveness*, *Openness*, *Non-judgmental attitude*, *Straightforward talk*, and *Equals* talking to one another. According to Shepherd (2007), using these approaches will help to maintain the dialogue between the interviewer and the interviewee by expressing an appreciation of the relationship between the two. Shepherd also provides guidelines for aspects of the interview such as the greeting the interviewee at the beginnning, monitoring the interviewee's emotional state during the interview, and closing the interview. Research has demonstrated that when murderers and sex offenders interpret the interviewer's behaviour during the interview as expressing more 'humanity' – as opposed to 'dominance' – they are more likely to admit their crimes than to deny them (Holmberg and Christianson, 2002).

» *Management of conversation sequence* This consists of four areas of management: managing the contact with the interviewee; managing the course of the interview; managing the conduct of those present; and managing the content of the interview. In each of these four areas the interviewer plans the interview in order to ensure that, for example, aims are achieved and each stage of the interview is followed (and is explained to the interviewee).

The general purpose of this approach is that it keeps the interviewer in control of the process, without allowing it to become an interrogation instead of an interview. However, what makes this approach particularly useful is the extent to which interviewers using these strategies are able to notice areas of inconsistency, contradiction or missing detail, and any gaps in the interviewee's account. These can then be focused on to aid the investigative process.

FOCUS ON ...

Good cop, bad cop

There are a number of interview techniques that one could use when working with an individual, and potentially the ones we have described are new for the reader. One that might be more familiar, and may be an approach that some psychologists might consider employing, is a favourite of crime drama. Given that it is generally known and is a recognised interviewing technique, if now somewhat outdated and probably illegal in its most extreme forms, we will consider it here.

Detective films frequently depict the 'good cop, bad cop' dynamic within interviews. Also known as 'friend-or-foe', this is a technique whereby one police officer intends to intimidate the suspect by, for example, acting aggressively or showing disbelief, and a second police officer is friendly, kind (e.g. providing tea and cigarettes) and understanding. The intention is presumably that having been made to feel frightened, disregarded and not believed by the first officer, the suspect will more likely respond to the kindness and rapport of the second officer, and will confess or provide important information. It is not a new technique – a passage in Homer's *The Iliad* describes Odysseus and Diomedes acting in this way – but as it is so frequently portrayed (for examples, see episodes of *Waking the Dead*, *NCIS* and *Law and Order: Criminal Intent*), it would be useful to consider the psychology and the evidence for its efficacy.

On the face of it, such a technique might work in the same way that torture is thought to work: an individual is so frightened at the possibility of the 'bad' cop returning that she or he will say anything to the 'good' cop in order to prevent that happening. Alternatively, the future that the 'bad' cop is offering (life in prison, being convicted of other crimes, loss of family, loss of status, etc.) may be in contrast to the 'good' cop's offer (which may actually reflect reality) of how cooperation might lead to a lesser sentence, that the media do not need to be informed, that maybe the prison would be an open prison, and so forth, and this may make cooperation seem to offer benefits.

In both of these hypothetical models we can understand the interview as a form of negotiation or bargaining, in which the suspect wants the best outcome (possibly release, perhaps the lowest sentence) and the officers want information that will lead to a conviction. Indeed, Kamisar (1980) refers to 'good cop, bad cop' as a distributive bargaining tactic. Research concerned with organisational processes and negotiation has considered this approach and suggests that it can be effective. For example, Brodt and Tuchinsky (2000) have demonstrated that the use of this technique can influence an individual's acceptance of taking on a task that she or he was previously not inclined to accept. They also showed that two people both enacting the same role, whether both 'good' cops or both 'bad' cops, did not increase the likelihood of acceptance, thus suggesting that the important element of this technique is the *contrast* between the two roles.

A more recent study (Sinaceur, Adam, Van Kleef and Galinsky, 2013) has shown that emotional inconsistency in a single negotiator can lead to concessions in negotiation, in part because the other person in the negotiation feels less in control. Again it seems that the contrast in the negotiator's emotions is important. So, within the legal and ethical requirements of your jurisdiction, perhaps such a technique might be useful. However, we need to examine the details of what may actually be going on if 'good cop, bad cop' tactics alter an individual's behaviour: does it do so in a way that, in the investigative process, is of benefit? That is, does becoming more compliant necessarily mean that an individual is becoming more open and honest, and as such there are not increased concerns regarding miscarriages of justice?

A recent study suggests possibly not (Mann *et al.*, 2013). Mann *et al.* examined how the demeanour of a second, non-interacting person involved in an interview (displaying supportive, neutral, or suspicious expressions) might impact on the ways in which individuals, whether telling the truth or lying, respond to a neutral interviewer's questions. They found that a second interviewer showing a supportive demeanour produced greater detail in truth-tellers than in liars, despite the fact that the interviewees appeared to pay very little attention to the second interviewer. In essence, this means that it is easier to detect deceit when a second interviewer is supportive than when that interviewer is acting as if suspicious. In this study the contrast, although more subtle, seems to play a role when the contrast involves a negative element.

Of course, the main differences here are that in the Mann *et al.* study the second interviewer is silent rather than being actively negative (a 'bad' cop), and that the study was not directly concerned with issues of compliance as lying participants were not expected to change their stories. However, it does raise a question concerning how the details of the contrast between interviewers might be influencing behaviour in ways that are less productive than desired. It would be interesting to examine the potential impact of a second interviewer on the outcome from other interview techniques, such as the Cognitive Interview. For the forensic psychologist, these are the kinds of issues that might be considered when assessing interviews, providing advice on interview techniques, or thinking about one's own interview style.

Questions

1 Do you think there are any ethical issues with the 'good cop, bad cop' approach? If it leads to a confession or yields important new information, would you be able to set your ethical concerns aside?

2 How easy do you think it would be to take on either of these roles? Would this depend on the attributes of the person being interviewed (e.g. their age, their gender, their alleged offence, their vulnerability) or your age, gender, your personal history?

Issues with eliciting information in investigative interviews

Although both of the techniques described above – the Cognitive Interview and Conversation Management – rely on the ability of the interviewee to recall information, the difference is that in one situation it is assumed that the interviewee *wants* to recall information and to share it, whereas in the other it is assumed that the interviewee may wish to keep some information secret, or possibly to confound it in some way, or generally doesn't wish to provide it.

In both cases, however, the issue of eliciting information is impacted by general issues of memory. How good are we at remembering the kind of information that would be of most use to an investigation? Primarily, this question is concerned with aspects of **eyewitness memory** (although there is research concerned with **earwitness memory** too: see Olsson, Juslin and Winman, 1998). There may, for example, be specific issues concerned with identifying an individual, such as issues of face recall or recognition, gender, or race, and these may all impact on the reliability of identity parades and recognising people from **mug shots**. Another issue is the impact on memory of factors such as the presence of a weapon or of violence during an event.

In addition, there are also specific offence-related issues in interviewing, such as those that arise when working with particularly vulnerable groups, for example abused children, individuals with mental illness or learning disabilities, or victims of particular kinds of crime (such as rape). We will deal with each of these issues below.

Memory

Numerous psychological textbooks can provide a sound background in the current state of knowledge regarding human *memory*, including how it impacts upon daily life, and how vulnerable it is to subtle shifts in context (see, for example, Frenda, Nichols and Loftus, 2010; Loftus, 2011). As this chapter relates to the investigation of crime, however, we will focus on a number of the most relevant areas, rather than attempting to provide an exhaustive and detailed coverage of all of the literature on memory.

Memory and face recognition

It is well established that human beings are remarkably good at recognising faces, to the point where it is claimed that *face recognition* is the *most* well developed of human perceptual skills (Avidan *et al.*, 2013), and that this is true even under less than optimal conditions (as, for instance, in looking at low-resolution photographs: Harmon and Julesz, 1973). Nevertheless, face recognition is not without its limits and, according to Wells (1993), it can be highly inaccurate in eyewitness identification situations.

This is both interesting and frustrating for the forensic psychologist, especially given that some researchers suggest that the brain may have evolved specifically in order to recognise faces. This is demonstrated by the neuropsychological deficit **prosopagnosia**. Research has shown that even people whom one has known well *prior* to a head injury, may become unrecognisable *after* it; and yet the ability to recognise *other* objects may remain intact, suggesting that face recognition involves a separate mechanism within the brain (see Avidan *et al.*, 2013;

Behrmann, Avidan, Thomas and Humphreys, 2009). However, it is important to remember that some of the elements of natural face recognition and those required during the process of formal identification may be quite different. For example, natural face recognition typically happens with a moving face and with a context of some sort, whereas recognition during an investigation may depend on a drawing, a motionless picture, or a computer graphic. Further, research has demonstrated that the ways in which information about a face is gathered may impact on how useful that information is in later identification. One study (Wogalter, 1996) demonstrated that the free descriptions of a face that people give are more useful than the results of asking them to use either a rating scale for the presence of particular features or a feature checklist. This is true despite the fact that many of the free descriptions given when remembering the face of an individual who is absent seem to be of poor quality (e.g. 'The man had thin lips'). Moreover, research has shown that even when the person being identified is actually present and compared to an identification photograph of that person's face that only *resembles* that individual, supermarket cashiers – who presumably are trained in comparing identity (ID) photographs with the people presenting them, as for example when checking the photographic ID of someone wishing to buy alcohol – only questioned the photograph in 40 per cent of cases (Kemp, Towell and Pike, 1997). Bruce and colleagues, in a number of studies, have shown that despite the presence of high-quality CCTV images, people are relatively poor at identifying faces, even when the video image and the target photograph are similar in angle and lighting (Bruce *et al.*, 1999; Henderson, Bruce and Burton, 2001), and particularly when the person to be identified is unfamiliar to the witness. Further, there is evidence to suggest that when a witness is using photographs to identify a person, the more pictures the witness has seen before reaching the one to be identified, the lower the likelihood that the target face will be identified – and the likelihood is even lower if the faces seen before were similar (Lindsay, Nosworthy, Martin and Martynuck, 1994). There is also evidence to suggest that there is a positive bias in recognising faces within one's own age-group (Anastasi and Rhodes, 2006) or within one's own race (Tanaka and Pierce, 2009), and that there is also an own-gender recognition bias in women (Lovén, Herlitz and Rehnman, 2011).

Along with these biases, there are situational factors that will impact on the accuracy of face recognition, such as the ambient light, the exposure time, and the use of masks or disguises by the person one is trying to identify. This combination of factors, along with the possibility that the face was only seen for a short time and during a period of stress, and that some time may have elapsed before the process of re-identification takes place, all have an impact on the witness's accuracy in identifying an individual's face. This raises important questions for the use of technology such as CCTV in comparing an image with a defendant, and indeed for the value of eyewitness identification in general.

Witness recall and event memory

Identities are not the only elements that witnesses may be asked to recall: they may also be required to provide descriptions of *events*. In the discussion of the Cognitive Interview, mention was made of the benefit of using different temporal orders in order to reduce biases. The biases of concern are our tendency to fill gaps in our memories with events that did not actually happen but that our schemata of such events suggest would *typically* happen. Research has demonstrated that the errors made in such circumstances are particularly prevalent in remembering actions (Garcia-Bajos and Migueles, 2003), and seem to be based on prior knowledge of crimes. This work is linked historically to the work of Bartlett (1932), whose research, which was concerned with remembering and retelling stories, demonstrated that there is a tendency to *remove* information that does not fit our own perspective (e.g. our culture) and to replace it with information that does. The research of Anderson and Pichert (1978) demonstrated that what we recall is also strongly determined by the perspective we take. In their research, participants were asked to read a story, half of them being required to take the perspective of a burglar, and half the perspective of a house buyer. The results demonstrated that perspective impacted on the kinds of details remembered by the two groups. More surprisingly, when asked during a second recall phase to *change* their perspective, participants remembered new material that they had not previously reported. This provides support for the technique used in the Cognitive Interview when asking witnesses to try to recall events from a different perspective. Importantly, this does not suggest that memory *storage* is necessarily impacted by perspective, but it certainly does show that *recall* can be. The Cognitive Interview makes use of Anderson and Pichert's work to develop the idea of changing perspective to enhance recall, and it is useful to be aware that critics of the Cognitive Interview point out that Anderson and Pichert's study requires what is referred to as a change in *conceptual* perspective (that is, a change in the way one understands the situation), whereas the Cognitive Interview asks that interviewees change their *perceptual* perspective (how the situation is perceived by another person), which is a quite different cognitive task (see Davis, McMahon and Greenwood, 2005).

Research has also suggested that the very process of interviewing may be responsible for aspects of events being forgotten. Bäuml and Kuhbandner (2007) have shown that if a subset of a word list is repeatedly retrieved – which is similar in some ways to what may occur during an investigative interview – this can lead to the *non-retrieved* words being forgotten. MacLeod (2002) has shown the same effect for events. Crucially, Bäuml and Kuhbandner (2007) demonstrated that the effect is mood-dependent, and that a temporary negative mood appears to prevent forgetting from taking place. The reason for this effect may be linked to a change in the way that the items are processed when a person is in a negative mood – specifically, that items are processed individually – and this may help to reduce inter-item interference (see Storbeck and Clore, 2005).

Change blindness

The foregoing discussion is based on the idea that the witness has perceived the event and that that event is therefore available for recall. A range of studies have demonstrated, however, that we do not always perceive *changes* in events, even when to another observer those changes may be strikingly obvious. This effect is known as **change blindness** (Simons and Levin, 1998), or what Douglas Adams (1982), in *Life, the Universe and Everything*, described as an 'SEP', or 'Somebody Else's Problem'. It is hard to believe that we are so unaware of change around us. (You might like to search for 'change blindness' on your favourite internet video channel to find some examples.) One of the most curious examples is that provided by Simons and Chabris (1999), where a film of people playing with basketballs is interrupted by an actor, dressed in a gorilla suit, who walks on, stands centre screen, and thumps her chest. In their study, only 50 per cent of participants (who are asked to count the number of passes of the ball) noticed this. Although there does not appear to be research investigating whether specific interview techniques might be able to induce recall in these situations, this does seem to be a case in which attention to one task (counting the number of passes of a basketball) supersedes attention to unexpected and unusual events. Further work has indicated that there may be a cultural element to this effect. Masuda and Nisbett (2006) have shown that there are differences between Americans and East Asians in sensitivities to focal and contextual information. In one of their studies concerned with static images, American participants were far less sensitive than East Asians to changes in the context (e.g. buildings in the background of a scene), but both groups were equally able to detect changes in focal information (e.g. the colour of a truck in front of a building). Where animations were used, American participants detected more focal changes than the Japanese participants, but the Japanese participants detected more contextual changes than the Americans. Masuda and Nisbett hypothesise that this may be an effect of East Asians taking a more holistic approach in perceiving the world.

Weapon focus

As the above description of change blindness indicates, attention can play a major role in what a witness might be able to report. A further example of this is known as the *weapon-focus effect* (Loftus, Loftus and Messo, 1987). This refers to the fact that when a weapon is present in a crime scene, this appears to draw people's attention, to the detriment of other features of the event, such as the weapon-holder's features (Pickel, French and Betts, 2003). In 2009 the National Crime Victimization Survey in the US (NCVS, 2009) estimated that a weapon was used in 22 per cent of all incidents of violent crime (approximately 946,000 incidents) and that the most frequent type of offence in which a weapon was used was robbery. It follows that the presence of weapons may be having a serious impact on the prosecution of nearly 1 million offences in the US. From 1993 to 2001, however, NCVS (2003) data suggest that there was a gradual reduction in weapon use in the US. According to the Office for National Statistics in the UK, in the period 2011–2012 firearms were used in 9,555 recorded incidents in England and Wales, and the police recorded 30,999 incidents where knives and sharp instruments were used (ONS, 2013). We need to keep in mind that in both countries these figures record *official* rates of weapon use in crime, and the figures may also underestimate the frequency of weapons being present but not used in the commission of an offence.

Interestingly, despite the common-sense view that a weapon might draw attention to itself and away from other aspects of the event, research has indicated that it might not be the effect of a weapon *per se* but rather that in some circumstances the weapon may be considered to be unusual or threatening. In an ingenious study, Pickel (1999) was able to examine these issues by presenting participants with a weapon in either a consistent situational context or an inconsistent situational context (a gun in a firing range or at a sports match) and where the person holding the weapon did or did not provide a context (e.g. an American police officer or a vicar). Pickel's findings suggested that it was the consistent, out-of-context weapon that resulted in the most interference, so it was the *unusualness* of the weapon, rather than its threat, that was important. However, later work (Hope and Wright, 2007) has suggested that the weapon too may play a significant role in the memory decrements observed in such studies, possibly because the presence of a weapon signifies something about 'importance' (and thus grabs attentional resources) or because it may induce negative emotions due to assumptions regarding threat. To complicate matters, Shaw and Skolnick (1994) have generated data suggesting that in responding to objects there might also be an effect associated with gender, which might mean that issues of unusualness and threat cannot be generalised. In their study they found that females were more likely to identify a target person when there was a weapon (a gun) present. They also showed that there is an own-gender bias in identification (similar to the own-race bias described by Brigham and Malpass, 1985, and Wright, Boyd and Tredoux, 2003), which they suggest may be due to differential levels of processing. When viewing a target of our own sex our processing may be deeper as we consider such questions as 'What kind of person is this?', whereas with other-sex targets we may focus on a more superficial judgment, such as 'How attractive is this person?' This is quite likely an oversimplification, however, reflecting a purely heterosexual conceptualisation of the world.

Although the exact psychology of the weapon-focus effect may not have been mapped, it is clear that elements of the offence (e.g. weapons, context, unusualness and gender) play a role in determining what people pay attention to and how well they remember, and this in turn influences how reliable someone will be as a witness. However, it is not just what a witness might see and how well they remember it that will influence the reliability of their evidence: this also depends on how the identification process is carried out.

Reliability of line-ups (identity parades)

ID parades and their photographic equivalent are an important part of the investigative process as they allow witnesses to identify a person whom they think they saw, and to do so in a context where the investigators know who the innocent 'foils' are. Beyond the impact of an identification on the investigative process, where it may help in restricting the focus of an investigation (thereby saving time and money), there is the acknowledged fact that evidence of an individual's identity is considered to be very persuasive in court (Wright, 2007). Of course this can work both ways – if the actual offender is not *recognised*, or if an innocent person is wrongly identified, then this will have serious consequences for an investigation and, possibly, for justice.

For the purposes of this section, a *line-up* – where there are people standing together in a room, – and a series of *photographs* of people, will be considered as one and the same, because to date there does not appear to be strong evidence that either method of presentation is better than the other (for a review, see Cutler, Berman, Penrod and Fisher, 1994). Obviously, all the issues that are true for facial recognition will also be relevant in identification, and the same biases of age, gender and race need to be considered in determining the reliability of the process.

The process of constructing a line-up can influence the likelihood of a correct identification or a misidentification. A line-up could consist of different numbers of people, and among them, different proportions of suspects and innocent people. If a line-up includes only one person who fits the witnesses' description, the line-up should be considered as biased – for example, if the witness has identified a white male and all but one of the members of the line-up are *Asian* males, that line-up is clearly biased against the white male. Brewer and Palmer (2010) provide another example: of having one individual in a line-up with blue eyes and the rest with brown, when the witness's report has indicated that she or he believes that the offender has blue eyes. Given that there are a number of people who share similar features, however, then the absolute number of people in a line-up does not appear to make a difference to identification accuracy (Nosworthy and Lindsay, 1990). See Malpass, Tredoux and McQuiston-Surrett (2009) for guidelines regarding the constitution of line-ups.

The person responsible for supervising the witness may inadvertently play a role in the accuracy of an identification – and, to view this more cynically, a person in this position could influence the witness on purpose. The expectation or hope that a witness will identify a particular individual may lead that person consciously or unconsciously to give off subtle non-verbal cues, as was found to be the case in the famous 'counting horse', **Clever Hans** (Pfungst, Rahn, Stumpf and Angell, 1911). Just as Hans's counting ability was shown to be completely dependent on almost undetectable cues unconsciously provided by his owner, research has demonstrated that individuals can be influenced by, for example, the wording of an identification task. If in their description of the identification task the police hint that they have already successfully identified the offender, then witnesses may be biased to select from a line-up even if they don't believe that the person they are looking for is actually present (Brewer and Palmer, 2010).

Issues with interviewing vulnerable people

The issues that have been considered thus far are based on research concerned with the 'average' man or woman, although there is evidence that the Cognitive Interview has also proved successful with members of some vulnerable groups (Milne, Clare and Bull, 1999). Something one comes to appreciate as a psychologist is that there are all manner of reasons why a given individual may be more or less vulnerable, either in relation to specific events (such as being interviewed) or more generally (such as having general communication difficulties, as for example may people with Asperger's syndrome; see Schall and McDonough, 2010). Vulnerabilities may impact on how well witnesses are able to represent themselves, how they respond to being interviewed, and how reliable is their evidence.

Research has been carried out that deals specifically with some of the more obvious vulnerabilities that have been identified, and in the following section we consider some of these issues and how they have been approached.

Victims of child sexual abuse

Victims of crime are likely to feel vulnerable, and perhaps those who are victims of sexual crimes even more so. Where that victim is a child those vulnerabilities are likely to be compounded still further, not only by the child's response to an offence that may not be within their frame of reference – not having a concept of 'sex' – but also by the particular cognition that is evident in different stages of childhood (Feiring, Taska and Lewis, 1999). For example, adolescents report experiencing more negative life events than children (Larson and Ham, 1993). Child victims of abuse report feeling socially isolated, depressed, and experience low self-esteem (Tyler, 2002). These overriding cognitions may impact upon both the information that can be elicited from a child and, on account of that information, the consequences for the alleged offender (Bruck and Ceci, 1995).

While there is evidence to suggest that the Cognitive Interview may be useful in interviewing children (Milne and Bull, 2003), such studies are not typically carried out with children who have been sexually abused, so the results may not be generalisable. Even in studies where this has been done, there is an inherent problem: how can we determine whether a particular approach produces more reliable information when we cannot compare it to 'the truth'? For example, Cyr and Lamb (2009) looked at the use of a particular interview technique in Quebec (the National Institute of Child Health and Human Development (NICHD) investigative interview protocol: see Cyr and Lamb, 2009). They compared the format of the interviews before and after interview training, and the detail elicited in the interviews. Neither of these measures could prove that the protocol was helpful other than in changing the interview practice and in eliciting 'more' information – this did not necessarily imply that the information elicited was accurate or honest. Pipe and colleagues (2008) demonstrated that using the NICHD protocol does have an impact on the number of cases that go to trial and result in conviction, but these decisions are influenced by so many factors other than factual accuracy that this is also not a reasonable test of an interview technique's abilities.

Other approaches have been used to supplement interview techniques. Using the same method described by Cyr and Lamb (2009), Teoh, Yang, Lamb and Larsson (2010) looked at the use of gender-neutral diagrams of the body to examine whether these might help children in their accounts of sexual abuse. They found that the use of the interview protocol and the diagram resulted both in reports of new aspects of abuse (e.g. touches on the body not previously reported) and in reports giving more detail regarding the touches described. However, the use of anatomical props has been criticised in the past. Research has suggested that it may lead to no improvements, and that under certain circumstances it may lead to fabrication and exaggeration (Steward *et al.*, 1996; Thierry, Lamb, Orbach and Pipe, 2005). For a compelling overview of research concerned with children as witnesses, and discussion of some of the techniques used in some infamous child-abuse cases, see Ceci and Bruck (1993). As with all human interaction, the picture is complicated by other issues. For example, the gender of the interviewer has been shown to impact on how vulnerable a child is to suggestive questions and on how much detail is provided (Lamb and Garretson, 2003); and the age of the child also impacts on how much detail she or he can provide (Lamb and Garretson, 2003). This last finding is important as 'level of detail' is one of the criteria on which the veracity of an account is based (Haskett, Wayland, Hutcheson and Tavana, 1995).

In response to the complications that have been identified with interviewing vulnerable children, a number of techniques have been developed. Specific details can be found elsewhere; but some of these techniques may be less commonly known but worthy of consideration when working with children, and those will be considered here:

» *The allegation blind interview* With this technique, the interviewer is ignorant of offence-specific information prior to the interview. Some evidence suggests that this can lead to greater disclosure and that it may help to reduce interviewer bias and the possibility of increasing **suggestibility** (Cantlon, Payne and Erbaugh, 1996). One potential issue with this approach, however, is that without knowing in advance what issues might be involved, the interviewer cannot be certain that the necessary material has been covered, cannot know what areas might need to be challenged, cannot be aware of particular sensitivities, and so on.

- *Truth–lie discussions* This technique, which has been shown to have some impact, involves having a discussion with the child about the difference between the truth and a lie. Various authors have recommended this as part of the interview process (e.g. Wyatt, 1999). Huffman, Warren and Larson (1999) demonstrated that in a sample of 67 children who were asked about a staged non-sexual event, truth–lie discussions on their own did not lead to more accurate reports; but with the addition of discussions regarding the possible consequences of lying, the accuracy of the children's reports was found to have increased. A potential *caveat* here is that it is not clear whether such discussions would be similarly effective in cases of sexual abuse or other offending behaviour.
- *Touch Survey* This technique is based on discussions with the child about the nature and forms of touching, how it feels to be touched, where they have been touched, and who has touched them (Hewitt, 1998). The author suggests that it is useful for examining physical, sexual and emotional abuse in children over the age of four. It does not seem that this approach has been heavily researched, however, and some of the concerns raised regarding the use of anatomical dolls may also be relevant here, although Hewitt states that the ways in which the questions are asked are neither leading nor suggestive. The survey allows children to identify the location of touch on a drawing and to provide a drawing of a facial expression of how it made them feel. Additionally, a drawing can be used to examine whether another person has asked a child to touch him or her.

People with an intellectual disability

As we have seen, there are many challenges for the professional when interviewing children, and the same is true of other vulnerable groups. One such group is people with an intellectual or learning disability (also known in the US as people with mental retardation). The British Institute of Learning Disabilities (BILD) provides a definition of learning disability (LD), suggesting that this involves having difficulties with 'understanding, learning and remembering new things, and generalising any learning to new situations' (Northfield, 2004), and it is clear that someone with such difficulties should be considered as vulnerable when being interviewed. Finlay and Lyons (2001) provide a good overview of the issues that need to be considered when interviewing an individual with an LD; three that are particularly relevant to the forensic domain are highlighted below.

Research has suggested that many people with LD find dealing with abstract concepts quite complex. Smith (1993) found that from a sample of 45 defendants with LD, 16 per cent could not understand the term 'guilty' and 20 per cent could not understand the term 'not guilty'. Other work has demonstrated that people with LD may struggle with issues regarding emotions (e.g. McVilly, 1995), and where concepts may be more or less boundaried (e.g. the concept of 'friends'; see Barlow and Kirby, 1991). Each of these issues means that interviewers – and those who interpret interviews – need to exercise caution when making assumptions about the answers given to queries related to these and other abstract concepts, and interviewers should attempt to express their questions in a style that reflects sensitivity to the person's range of skills and needs. A second issue, linked to this, is that people with LD may provide answers to questions that appear irrelevant or contradictory. These answers may be taken as an indication that the person is struggling to understand the questions. However, they may also be an indication that the person is preoccupied with something and may not be willing, or able, to move on to the new topic (Biklen and Moseley, 1988; Dempster and Corkill, 1999). Note that care should be taken to try to separate out these two possibilities without making the assumption that perseveration is necessarily linked to some kind of traumatic experience – there may be other reasons why a person becomes preoccupied (for example, the topic's novelty or personal embarrassment). Finally, and again linked to the above, is the finding that people with LD may be particularly sensitive to questions that focus on sensitive material (which is likely to be the case with the commission of offences or being the victim of offences). Research has demonstrated that anonymous questionnaires result in greater admission of risky behaviours by adolescents with LD than confidential interviews (Pack, Wallander and Browne, 1998). It has also revealed that the responses given to questions tend to be biased by the *content* of the question – for example, questions concerning negative behaviours lead to a 'no' response, regardless of how the question is phrased (e.g. 'Are you allowed to *X*?' or 'Is it against the rules to do *X*?' – where X is a negative behaviour: Shaw and Budd, 1982).

Each of these examples demonstrates again the complexity of interviewing a vulnerable population. Milne and Bull (2001) provide an overview of approaches developed to assist in working with this population while minimising the impact of suggestibility on their accounts. They consider the impact of aspects of questioning, interview context (e.g. duration, setting and time spent building rapport) and specific memory issues, ultimately suggesting that the Cognitive Interview may be a sound overall approach in dealing with the complexity of LD. A variety of studies have likewise given support to the idea that the Cognitive Interview is useful in working with people with LD, and not just for the process of investigative interviewing (Milne, Clare and Bull, 1999).

Interrogative suggestibility and false confessions

Much of the earlier material in this chapter has indicated that the process of interviewing has potential pitfalls. Of greatest concern, perhaps, is the fact that under certain conditions some people may report that they have been involved in offending behaviour when in reality they have not. Not only can this have severe consequences for them, but it may also lead to a waste of resources by the legal system either because the reported event did not happen or because it did happen but someone else was responsible.

As discussed at the beginning of the chapter, the use of torture is one situation where we might expect that people might make false confessions, but there are other circumstances too where this may happen, due to aspects of the person or aspects of the interview. Kassin (2008) provides some examples where people confessed to crimes, which he suggested was an indication of a need for attention or self-punishment, or that the person in question would gain something (for example, by protecting someone else). One cited example is that of the murder in 1947 of Elizabeth Short (also known as 'the Black Dhalia'), which allegedly resulted in confessions by 50 men and women. However, often in these situations it appears that people are confessing without having been interviewed, and often where there is evidence to suggest that they *cannot* have been involved (e.g. because they were not within the area at the time of the offence, or because they were unaware of important details of the offence). Kassin suggests that there are three types of false confession: *voluntary confessions*, as described above in relation to Elizabeth Short; *compliant confessions*, which are a result of individuals believing that if they confess they will escape punishment or unremitting questioning; and *internalised confessions*, whereby an individual is vulnerable to particular interrogation techniques and comes to believe that he or she *did* commit the offence. Kassin provides a number of examples of real cases in which false confessions were made and the outcomes were negative for the confessor, such as the case of Jeffrey Deskovic, who was imprisoned for 15 years for a murder he did not commit.

False confessions through suggestibility

A number of factors have been identified as potential reasons why an individual under interview might falsely confess to an offence. The most obvious, perhaps, is individuals' vulnerability, defined in terms of their limited ability to understand either the interview or the possible consequences of their responses. Children and people with a learning disability would fall into this group. Bain and Baxter (2000) define a number of other factors that might play a role in suggestibility. For example, interviewees come to the interview with a set of biases and expectations about the interview, the interviewer, and their own innocence, and these may make them more resilient or more suggestible. How an individual perceives negative feedback (e.g. as criticism) and how they respond to such a perception (by either rejecting it and thus being unaffected by it, or by accepting it and thus increasing their feelings of anxiety, loss of self-esteem, and so on) may make an individual more or less likely to display suggestibility. Finally, the concept of *compliance* – the idea that some individuals, in an effort to avoid confrontation with the interviewer, may admit to things when they know that their admission is false – should also be considered. An example of a reason for this would be a belief that if the interviewer is happy with one's responses, this will result in release. This may make some individuals more likely to agree to an interviewer's assertions, even though they know that their responses are inaccurate.

Gudjonsson has developed scales in order to measure suggestibility, with the aim of identifying individuals who may be particularly suggestible and who may therefore require particular support if interviewed, and also with the aim of being able to examine the reliability of confessions that are subsequently retracted (Gudjonsson Suggestibility Scale-Gudjonnson, 1984). A variety of studies have looked at these scales to examine the way in which interview styles, for example, impact upon suggestibility. Bain and Baxter (2000) reported a study comparing the friendliness with which an interviewer conducts an interview and the impact this has, which demonstrated that style did not affect recall of an event but that a more 'abrupt' style led to greater levels of suggestibility (as measured by the Gudjonnson Suggestibility Scale). Drake and Bull (2011) demonstrated a relationship between negative life events – such as work difficulties, problems at school, or problems within relationships – and suggestibility.

It is quite likely that suggestibility is not confined to making false confessions, but may also influence false accusations of others, and this has subsequent consequences for police investigations, further interviewing, and the possibility of innocent people being taken before the court.

Credibility of children's testimony

Research has suggested that for the most part adults do not consider children to be reliable witnesses. For example, children's memories have been found to be less reliable than those of adults (Cole and Loftus, 1987); they are considered to be more suggestible than adults and remember less than adults (Goodman and Reed, 1986); and they are less able than adults to separate fact from fiction (Goodman, Golding and Haith, 1984). Duggan and colleagues (1989) found that these pervasive attitudes are likely to become exaggerated during jury deliberations. Golding, Dunlap and Hodell (2009) reviewed the accumulated research concerning this.

The value of children's evidence in court has therefore been negatively stereotyped, and this has serious implications for legal processes – particularly in cases of child abuse, where the child may be the only witness. One possible explanation for their difficulties with providing evidence is that children, along with other vulnerable people, might find the process of appearing in court confusing and stressful, and this might lead to a reduced ability to represent themselves. A number of approaches have been developed in response to this, including the use of **video-links** and videotaped interviews. Although the use of a video-link may be helpful in minimising the anxiety that court proceedings can produce in vulnerable witnesses and defendants, and although it may encourage children to give evidence where they otherwise might not have given that evidence (Plotnikoff and Woolfson, 2004), the approach is not without its problems. Eaton, Ball and O'Callaghan (2001) demonstrated that, in simulated trials, the evidence from video-links was considered less credible than that provided either in court or via a pre-recorded video. This is in contrast to research that indicates that children are actually more resistant to **leading questions** when interviewed over a video-link than face to face, and that face-to-face interviews of children result in more incorrect information than video-link interviews (Doherty-Sneddon and McAuley, 2000). Similarly, Swim, Borgida and McCoy (1993) showed that for some elements of an offence, the style of witness presentation does make a difference (in this case, video resulted in a lower conviction rate), even though the mock jurors in the video condition reported more pro-prosecution thoughts throughout the trial. Ross and colleagues (1994) also showed that under certain circumstances the use of video evidence resulted in lower conviction rates, and this may partly combine with the issues presented concerning child credibility (as the Goodman *et al.* (1984) study suggests).

Nevertheless, it appears that this negative stereotype about the reliability of evidence given by children is unfounded. Studies have suggested that in *real* cases of child abuse, children are able to identify perpetrators accurately and to describe the details of the offence (Johnson and Foley, 1984; Jones and Krugman, 1986). It therefore seems that in court a child's *actual* credibility may be at odds with the impact of video evidence on a jury's *belief* in the child's credibility, which has clear potential implications for the outcome of a trial.

In the UK, the recognition that appearing as a witness may be difficult for a child has been identified by the Youth Justice and Criminal Evidence Act 1999, which provides a number of measures intended to assist young people (defined as being under 17 years of age) including, in Section 28, the use of pre-recorded, pre-trial cross-examinations. The Act specifically sets out to support individuals who may be considered vulnerable to the court process because of their age or incapacity, known as *vulnerable witnesses*, and those who are likely to be distressed due to giving evidence, known as *intimidated witnesses*. Video-links are just one of the special measures that can be allowed, along with the use of screens to hide witnesses from other court attendees, the removal of wigs and gowns by judges and barristers and the use of intermediaries who can help the vulnerable person in understanding and communicating. Further consultation has been carried out by the UK government, based on work examining the needs that young people identify (Plotnikoff and Woolfson, 2004), with the aim of further supporting people during the court process. However, as research has demonstrated, some care needs to be taken in considering the possible impact such measures may have on juries' thinking and decision-making.

Basic principles of interviewing

As should be apparent, the process of interviewing is not simple and depends on a variety of factors. However, there are four basic principles that are considered to be at the heart of any investigative interview, as described by Powell, Fisher and Wright (2005):

1. Good rapport between the interviewer and the interviewee.
2. A clear description of the investigative aims of the interviewer. (This is considered crucial, because an investigative interview is not a context that most people have experienced, and thus they are unlikely to know what is required and wanted from them.)
3. The use of open-ended questions.
4. A willingness to explore alternative hypotheses – that is, a willingness not simply to seek confirmation for what the interviewer already believes, as this is likely to introduce bias.

These four principles are a good basic set of skills to develop, and on which to build effective interview technique.

Chapter summary

Interviewing is a complex process and a variety of factors may impact on the usefulness of information obtained from the interview.

- The fact that human memory and perception are fallible will come as little surprise to the student of psychology, and nor should it be a surprise that research is endeavouring to discover ways in which to enhance interview techniques and the presentation of information to witnesses. Note, however, that any such developments are likely to bring further areas for consideration, as demonstrated by juries' hesitation in trusting information given by a child using a video-link.
- Less obvious, perhaps, is the complexity of the various factors that might interact and together determine how effective and informative an interview may be. For example, the effectiveness of torture in gathering accurate information is not clear; whereas other techniques, such as Conversation Management, are asserted to be helpful in interviewing reluctant witnesses, and the Cognitive Interview appears to result in eliciting more useful information, even in situations where a witness is vulnerable.
- Interviewers too are challenged by the need to construct and to communicate coherent accounts of events, which affect how they design their interviews and present their findings. It is important for the forensic psychologist to be aware of these various issues in order that she or he can take an appropriately informed view when working with individuals, be they victims, perpetrators, or witnesses. For example, some biases may impact on the accuracy of identification of potential suspects, such as gender and age biases; we seem to be particularly poor at remembering actions; what we remember can be biased by the perspective we are taking at the time of looking at the information (e.g. a house buyer or a burglar); and culture may impact upon the kinds of change that we notice (we may experience change blindness).
- It is likely that many of these biases cannot be managed within an interview – is it reasonable, for example, to ask a female witness to try to report what she would have noticed had she had a male perspective, perhaps thereby reducing the same-gender bias in women? Even though these biases cannot be managed within the interview, they are still important issues to be aware of.

12

Further reading

The following texts would be good initial sources of information to learn more about interviewing:

- Bartlett, F. C. (1932). *Remembering: A Study in Experimental and Social Psychology*. London: Cambridge University Press. One of the classic studies in memory.
- Gudjonsson, G. (2003a). *The Psychology of Interrogations and Confessions*. Chichester: Wiley. An important book for understanding the psychology of the interview process.
- Stelfox, P. (2009). *Criminal Investigation: An Introduction to Principles and Practice*. Cullompton: Willan Publishing. A useful book in understanding the practicalities of investigation, including investigative interviewing.

Profiling Offenders: Methods and Results

Profiling has been defined as 'the combination of analysis of available information and the application of relevant psychological theories to provide investigators with clues about the likely characteristics (such as where they might live or their occupation) and the type of person who would have committed the offence' (Tong, Bryant and Horvath, 2009, p. 70). Despite this definition, profiling is not clearly understood within psychology, and this chapter considers some of the ways in which profiling in conceptualised.

Chapter objectives

- To consider the issue of criminal profiling.
- To understand the historical development of profiling.
- To compare deductive and inductive profiling.
- To consider the issue of geographic profiling.

From the definition given above, it is clear that the fundamental role of *profiling* is to help investigators by reducing the possible pool of individuals they need to consider when seeking to identify an offender (in the case of *forensic* profiling). This is a point that Canter has made repeatedly (e.g. see Canter and Allison, 2000): that the *value* of profiling is in the practical implications it can have for police investigations, and therefore that its use in that context should influence decisions about what information to include in a profile. Hypothesising the internal state of an individual who might have committed a particular crime is not of enormous investigative value unless we can be sure that this state is *permanent* – or at least long-lasting – and that it predicts other more identifying factors, such as someone's profession or location, or other crimes that they may have committed (Duff and Kinderman, 2008).

The process of profiling can be considered to consist of two methods, which can broadly be understood as one that is *inductive* or *scientific* and one that is *deductive* or *intuitive* (although see Hicks and Sales' (2006) critique of both methods, which highlights some commonalities). For each there are authors who provide support for their favoured method and critiques of the other. Here our aim is provide an overview of both without favouring either. First we will consider some of the important basic issues for profiling.

How is profiling possible?

The basic principle that underlies profiling is that behaviour is determined by a *range* of factors, some of which are correlated to a high enough degree that we can begin to make predictions about other aspects of an individual's existence. For example, if an offence involves a break-in through a window that demonstrates a degree of skill (i.e. the glass has been cut, not smashed), then this skilled behaviour is very likely to have been determined by that individual having spent time practising that skill. The chances that an unskilled person could carry out this skilled action are low. With such evidence, the first step might be to consider investigating people with those skills. Some of these people might not be readily identifiable, however – there might be undetected criminals who are skilled in this way, or individuals other than **glaziers** who have developed the same abilities – but it does provide a direction for the investigation. Similarly, if there is evidence of a car being used, this is likely to rule out children; and if the type of car can be identified, the pool is restricted further to people who have, or have access to, that make and model. (The access might have been gained by stealing the car.) So it is possible that evidence at a crime scene may indicate certain behaviours, and those behaviours may be able to provide guidelines that allow an investigation to proceed.

The same idea applies when profiles are used to guide interviews or to determine the legitimacy of a document such as a suicide note. If we can identify regularities in behaviour, then we can use those regularities to predict how people will respond to questions in an interview and how they will express themselves in their writing. Reduced to its simplest description, profiling really consists in getting to the point where you believe that you know enough about an individual's behaviour, from their past, to make predictions about ongoing or future behaviours. In some respects, this is exactly what a goalkeeper will do when facing a penalty or what a batter will do when facing a bowler, which is why sportspeople spend so much time reviewing previous games and the behaviour of their opponents.

In non-forensic contexts, there is a great deal of evidence supporting the idea that our behaviour is strongly influenced by external factors. For example, evidence from consumer behaviour suggests that if one makes a decision to buy financial services, the order in which those services are bought follows a predictable pattern (Paas and Kuijlen, 2001). Similarly, there is the concept of **permeable barriers** (Rengert, 2004), which suggests that features in the environment such as rivers and motorways impact upon the decisions people make when planning shopping, entertainment (see Hillier, Burdett, Peponis and Penn, 1987), and the commission of crime (Greenberg, Rohe and Williams, 1982; Newman and Franck, 1982). It is also the case that our preconceptions of our environment have an impact on how we perceive it (and thus how we might behave in it). Mattson and Rengert (1995) have demonstrated that research participants travelling through an area perceive distances differently depending on how dangerous they believe that area to be – the more dangerous they perceive it to be, the greater the distance they infer. Thus our movement within our environment is neither random nor entirely self-determined. It is not unreasonable to suggest, therefore, that the location of offences is determined by, for example, where individuals work, live and know, and also where they feel that they might easily be recognised, expect to find potential victims, or from which they believe they can easily escape. (For some examples, see Brantingham and Brantingham, 1999.) That is, there are explanations for *offences* being committed in particular places, because there are explanations for why *people* are in particular places.

What this also makes clear is that one can profile both victims and offenders, so that an understanding of someone who has already been a victim may provide some useful information for an investigation, particularly when the victim is still alive. For example, if one determines that the victim had no apparent reason to have been at the crime scene, that would suggest that she or he was transported there in some way. Equally, it suggests that the offender must have had some reason to be in locations where the victim *did* have reason to be. Such information may be useful in developing an accurate picture of the timeline of an offence, and aspects of that offence that might inform the investigation.

A brief history of profiling

The **FBI** (the Federal Bureau of Investigation) in the US is widely accredited with being the first organisation to develop a systematic approach to criminal profiling, though there are earlier individual examples (Brussel, 1968). Initially, the approach was deductive, based on the experience of FBI investigators and a sense that this experience allowed the investigators to 'get inside the heads' of the offenders (Douglas, Ressler, Burgess and Hatman, 1986). However, perhaps the first examples of profiling are to be found in the work of Galton, Lombroso, and Snow. What is interesting about these three examples of what we can think of as profiling is that they each demonstrated a scientific, *inductive* approach to the problem of profiling, yet when profiling became more widely used in the investigative process, it tended to be *deductive*.

Francis Galton and Cesare Lombroso

Francis Galton was of the view that mental abilities would be inherited along with physical characteristics, both for offenders and non-offenders (Galton, 1877). He suggested that he was able to identify physical characteristics that could be associated with the kinds of crimes that men in English prisons had committed. He referred to 'special villainous irregularities' of offenders' faces, suggesting that this is a commonality amongst individuals who commit crimes and that these irregularities might therefore be useful for investigators to seek out when searching for perpetrators (Galton, 1883, p. 224). Similarly, one element of Cesare Lombroso's work was concerned with identifying the physical features that he suggested were associated with offending (Lombroso, 1876). Over the course of his five volumes of *Criminal Man* the story does become more complex, but the initial idea was that offenders are 'atavistic' (i.e. primitive) and possess physical characteristics that parallel their immorality. For example, Lombroso suggests that in comparison to non-offenders, offenders tend to have foreheads that slope more, bigger ears and jaws that protrude more. Lombroso's original work, published in 1876, may be considered one of the earliest attempts at criminal profiling, whereby investigators would be guided to look for individuals with particular physical traits and also styles of tattoo, which thus restricted the pool of individuals who could have committed the offence. In neither case – Galton or Lombroso – is there evidence that the ideas these authors espoused were tested for their ability to predict that an individual would offend or that they were successful in the apprehension of offenders. However, it is clear that there was some belief that offending is linked to other characteristics of an individual, and that these characteristics could thus be used to identify that person.

Some modern writers have continued in this vein. For example, Benis (2004) described the characteristics of certain personality types. He suggested that the 'aggressive type' is typically short and promiscuous, and the leader of a militant, genocidal movement. Similarly, Carré and McCormick (2008) suggested that facial structure may reliably predict aggressive behaviour; and Cantor and colleagues (Cantor *et al.*, 2007) found that differences in physical height are linked to types of sexual offending. This is explored in the next 'Where do you stand?' box.

WHERE DO YOU STAND?

Are behaviour and physical features related?

A number of studies have suggested that there are reliable relationships between physical features and behaviour. As mentioned, Carré and McCormick (2008) have suggested that a specific element of facial structure, the width-to-height ratio, reliably predicts aggressive behaviour in men, when studied either on the hockey field or in the psychological laboratory. In their 2009 paper, Carré, McCormick and Mondloch provide examples in which faces allow participants to accurately predict other aspects of individuals' behaviour – for example, cheating at games – and they demonstrate in their studies that people can use facial structure to accurately predict the likely aggressive tendencies of others. Cantor and colleagues (2007) have demonstrated, in a sample of Canadian men, that paedophilic sexual offenders are statistically significantly shorter than non-offenders. Finally, Hanoch, Gummerum and Rolison (2012) demonstrated, after comparing a sample of 44 male offenders and 46 male non-offenders, that the right-hand second finger to fourth finger length ratio predicts criminality.

These are interesting findings and fit well with the ideas of Galton and Lombroso, although perhaps the physical features that do seem to be predictive of behaviour are more subtle than those earlier authors suggested. The explanations given for these relationships are that the genetic information for the physical and the behavioural characteristics is linked; or that whatever circumstances influence one characteristic (typically in the developing foetus) also, independently, influence the other.

From an evolutionary perspective, one could argue that being able to identify people who might cheat or who are likely to be aggressive is useful: it allows us to avoid losing resources or being harmed, and thus we are more likely to survive. From a forensic perspective, such characteristics could be useful in profiling if police are aware of the various anatomical and behavioural correlations and as long as these can be shown to be usefully predictive. Even if not completely accurate, such correlations could potentially speed the identification of an offender and thus reduce criminality.

Taking this idea further, if physical features are predictive enough – and how much is 'enough' will be open to debate, given the potential consequences of getting it wrong – could you imagine a situation, akin to that portrayed in the film *Minority Report*, in which criminals could be apprehended *before* their crimes, in this situation on the basis of their physical features? Could we even make such assessments before birth? How different would this kind of decision be in comparison with, for example, decisions based on detecting genetic differences via amniocentesis, such as Down's syndrome?

Where do you stand on this issue?

1 In your view, how accurately would a physical feature need to predict criminal behaviour for you to consider including it in a profile to help a police investigation? What are the potential ethical issues?
2 Similarly, how accurately would a physical feature need to predict criminal behaviour for you to consider using it as a means of preventing crime? What are the potential ethical issues?
3 Are there any circumstances whereby you would consider this as an approach in making decisions about abortion policy? What are the potential ethical issues?

John Snow

Johnson (2006) recounts the first example of profiling, although it was concerned with an outbreak of **cholera** in 1854 and is therefore more concerned with *geographic* profiling (where best to look for something) than with *individual* profiling (who best to look for). A London general practitioner (a medical doctor), John Snow, mapped the reported deaths from the cholera outbreak and determined that there was a large concentration of deaths in one particular area of London. From this he determined that the *source* of the outbreak was likely to exist in this area. Coupling this hypothesis with his theory that cholera was a water-borne disease, he located and turned off the water pump that supplied the identified area, and the outbreak of cholera rapidly ceased. Clearly, Snow had been able to identify a pattern in what was happening and he had inferred from that something about cause and effect. It is important to note that without the underlying theory that cholera was water-borne – the favoured theory at the time was that it was transmitted through the air – it is likely that the pattern of deaths would not have been as meaningful as it turned out to be, particularly as it allowed Snow to account for why some pockets of the community were *not* affected (e.g. for various reasons they preferred water from another source).

The idea of profiling had thus been clearly demonstrated by Snow and proposed by authors such as Galton and Lombroso, and yet it was some time before the practice came into use during investigations. It is not entirely clear when the first investigative profile was developed, or when profiling first assisted in the successful identification of an offender. The most commonly identified first appearance of a profile is that of Langer (1972), who was asked to provide a psychological profile of Adolf Hitler in order to help the Americans to predict his behaviour. Working from a psychodynamic perspective, Langer suggested a number of different outcomes, one of which was that Hitler might commit suicide. His work was clearly deductive in nature, relying as it did on descriptions of Hitler and interviews with people who knew him. Perhaps the best-known profile is that ascribed to a psychiatrist, James Brussel, who, it is claimed, even accurately predicted that the perpetrator of a number of bombings in New York City would be wearing a buttoned, double-breasted suit when he was apprehended (see Schlesinger, 2009).

Once profiling was being used in the identification of offenders, its value was perceived differently by different proponents. Some authors recognised it as offering insight into behaviour (Douglas, Ressler, Burgess and Hatman, 1986), whereas other authors considered that it provided information for the identification of personality traits (Rossmo, 2000). As suggested earlier, behaviour that is suggestive of skills and knowledge may be of practical use if that skill reduces the pool of people who could have been involved in a crime; using a rock to break a window reduces that pool rather less than the use of a glass-cutter, and the use of a glass-cutter suggests experience rather than luck. The identification of a personality type may not be as direct nor as helpful. For example, evidence of unnecessary aggression at a crime scene might indicate an aggressive personality or it might indicate that the perpetrator was angered (either by something that occurred before or during the offence). Either way, it may be less useful for the police to be searching for angry people.

West (2000) presents an interesting overview of what he sees as the role of clinical psychologists in providing support to the police from their analysis of a crime scene. His view supports both behavioural and personality aspects. For instance, he suggests that it may be possible to make judgments about the relationship between the victim and the perpetrator, about the expectations that the perpetrator brought to the crime scene, and about the extent to which harm to the victim was incorporated into the offence in order to reduce an unpleasant emotional state in the perpetrator.

Kinds of profiling

Deductive profiling

According to Turvey (1999), **deductive profiling** 'bases its inferences on the behavioural evidence in a particular case, or a series of related cases' (p. 183). The idea is that experience in solving crimes allows an individual, and thus an institution (such as the FBI), to develop a real-world understanding of what crime-scene behaviours mean, and what these can tell us about the perpetrator. This information, or profile, can lead to the identification of the responsible individual. As Napier (2010) writes: 'behavior is left at a crime scene and can be read for the traits of the criminal, which in turn will be used by the investigator for each aspect of his investigation' (p. 24). So there is a sense in which we can develop an important understanding of a person from their behaviour – which requires both that a person's behaviour does indeed allow that and, in particular, that behaviour at a crime scene can fulfil that function.

As crime has taken place throughout human history and as there have been police forces for many decades, there have been many opportunities for investigators to learn from crime scenes and perpetrators. One might assume that over time a series of inferences would have developed that linked useful behaviour to evidence, but this does not appear to be the case. In Turvey's examples (1999, p. 185), the deductions that can be made appear simplistic (e.g. if an offender wears gloves, this suggests that the offender is aware of the value of fingerprints) and not of great investigative value, or the process of identifying the evidence and then forming a part of the profile from it is not clear. For example, Turvey seems to imply that if there is evidence of a victim having suffered, this suggests that the offender was seeking or achieved sexual gratification. This assumes that there must be a link between one individual's suffering and another's sexual gratification, which is not necessarily true – the evidence base for this assertion is not clear, and again the investigative value is not immediately apparent. Also, presumably it is only possible to accurately identify the presence of suffering for the victim if the victim is still living and can provide that information – care needs to be taken in assuming that someone suffered if we will be drawing important conclusions based on that assumption. Similarly, from an example report (p. 386) concerned with the deaths of three male children, Turvey variously describes characteristics of the offender as someone who 'projects a macho, heterosexual, in-control image', 'must be dominant in all relationships with women', and has 'a potentially violent temper'. Unfortunately the report does not indicate how these conclusions have been reached.

Deductive profilers claim that the strength of their approach comes from the fact that their conclusions are drawn from their premises, and that these relationships have developed through experience of crime and through the insights offered by offenders as to why they did what they did, what it might mean, how it reflects their personalities. However, many of these premises are untested in that it is not known how frequently they are true – for example, that aspects of the multiple killing of boys are linked to a need for dominance in relationships with women. This means that there is a statistical element to deductive profiling – something that is frequently seen as a criticism of inductive methods – but it does not appear to have been tested. Of course, this does not prove that there are *no* examples of behaviour that link to personality or any other features of an individual (such as their goals and plans, and intentions), but two questions remain: if there are such links, what are they, and how useful are they in the profiling process?

Holmes and Holmes (2009) write that 'the profiler is aided by an intuitive sense in the profiling process. That is, he develops a feel for the crime' (p. 13), and this is in line with film and literature portrayals of profiling. Linked to this intuition is a view that crime-scene behaviour provides a 'truth' about the offender: that is, that the behaviour provides an accurate description of the individual. Napier (2010) exemplifies this view: 'Offenders are often skilled at concealing aspects of who they truly are and what their value systems are. However, in the commission of a crime for which he does not anticipate being caught, the offender releases his hidden nature via his criminal behaviour and his interaction with the victim' (p. 24). The first identified example of deductive profiling in literature, according to Holmes and Holmes (2009), is in a story by Edgar Allan Poe in 1814 (*The Murders in the Rue Morgue; an Interesting Account of Profiling*), which describes the approach to solving crime as having, 'in truth, the whole air of intuition' (p. 75). Crucially, although Holmes and Holmes do not suggest that deductive profiling should not rely on psychological theory, they do explicitly state that what separates the deductive profiler from the inductive profiler is that the latter has no need of knowledge of the works of Freud, James, Watson and Skinner, thereby hinting that psychodynamic and behavioural approaches provide a suitable conceptual basis for developing a profile.

Despite such concerns about deductive methods of profiling, it is true to say that this intuitive approach was the starting point for criminal profiling, and various descriptions of these profilers, their processes, and often their remarkable successes can be found in the literature (Brussel, 1968; Kessler, 1993). However, one must keep in mind that there may well be less well-known examples in which the profiles were not in fact particularly helpful. Indeed, it has been suggested that in some early profiles the detail was reflective of the time and culture, rather than being specific in identifying an individual based on their behaviour (Snook *et al.*, 2008).

More recently, the FBI, who are often portrayed as intuitive profilers, began to accumulate data to support their typologies of crime and criminals (see Kessler, 1993). Based on their work, authors such as Turco (1990) have suggested that the crime scene can be thought of as 'a symptom of a behavioural act and in a broader perspective as a projection of the underlying personality, life style and developmental experiences ... of the perpetrator' (p. 150). However, analysis of data from crime scenes that had been described as either 'organised' or 'disorganised' (which is part of the FBI's originally deductive typology: see Ressler, *et al.* 1986) indicated that crime-scene behaviour did *not* fall within these two distinct categories, which suggests that there is not a strong link between the breadth of behaviours found at a crime scene and the categorical description of the criminal as determined by deductive profiling (Canter, Alison, Alison and Wentink, 2004; and for a further example see Melnyk, Bloomfield and Benell, 2007). See the 'Focus on ...' box on page 304 for more information on the FBI's work.

Interestingly, Holmes and Holmes (2009) suggest from their examples of profiling that both deductive and inductive methods are used, but it is clear that their use of the term 'inductive' is based on the individual experiences of officers rather than on inferences

FOCUS ON ...

Organised and disorganised offenders

Early FBI profilers considered that, on the whole, violent sexual offenders and sexual murderers left crime scenes that were either organised or disorganised. An organised crime scene might best be described as 'neat and tidy': there is little evidence of unplanned behaviour. In contrast, the disorganised crime scene is described as chaotic and suggestive of spontaneity and impulsivity.

Various authors have identified characteristics that they believe are linked to the different kinds of crime scene and that therefore contribute to profiles (see Ressler and Burgess, 1985; Schlesinger, 2009). For example:

Disorganised	**Organised**
Below average IQ	Average to above-average IQ
Unskilled work	Skilled work
Lives alone	Lives with partner
Known victim or location	Victim a stranger
Demands submission from victim	Sudden violence to victim
Strange-looking	Physically attractive
Leave the body where killed	Transport the body
History of psychiatric treatment	History of behaviour problems

Questions

1 If we take the view that a useful profile will assist the police by helping to focus an investigation and to reduce the pool of potential people to investigate and interview, which of the above characteristics do you think might fulfil this criterion?

2 Is it possible that with additional information some characteristics might be more useful? (For example, if there is evidence of a skilled break-in, the 'skilled work' element of the organised crime scene might suggest someone with a locksmith's or glazier's skills.) Taking that approach, which factors above, with further investigation of the crime scene, might prove helpful?

drawn from scientific investigation, and they do not explicitly include research as contributing to the inductive process. Turvey, a proponent of the deductive approach, is so adamant about the value of behavioural evidence, and so against what he refers to as the 'scientification' (1999, p. 257) of profiling, that he suggests profilers should be concerned only with what an offender *did* and should place no value on interviews and psychometric tests. For a useful discussion of concerns with non-scientific profiling approaches, see Chapter 3 of Hicks and Sales (2006).

Inductive profiling

Inductive profiling stems from efforts to identify regularities between criminal behaviour and the source of that behaviour. Indeed, Canter and Youngs (2003) have suggested that the term 'profiling' should be replaced by the title **investigative psychology**, to make clear that the aim of the work is to provide empirically supported models and inferences that contribute to police work, and that it is just one of a number of investigative tools (see also Vandiver, 1982). The basic principle is that through the investigation of offences and offenders it may be possible to develop a database of the characteristics of individuals that are linked to offending behaviour. Comparing the behaviour present in a new crime scene with such a database is intended to provide an outline of the characteristics of the kind of individual who might have committed the offence, thereby guiding the investigation. This will only be useful, however, if those characteristics can be identified. For example, a prediction regarding where the individual might live, what profession that person might have (through skills shown at the crime scene) and what other crimes he or she might have committed would be useful, whereas predicting the offender's mental state at the time, or the motive that led to the offence, might be less so. Canter (2007) provides an example of how the regularities in our behaviour are used to identify possible instances of crime. Credit-card companies build up profiles of individual customers, based on what they spend, where they spend and so on, and a particular transaction that stands out from this pattern alerts the company to the possibility that a fraudulent transaction may have taken place. This example also demonstrates that profiling is not without error, as anyone who has had their credit cancelled whilst they have been on holiday will attest.

Previous research has suggested that it is possible to develop categories of offenders, as, for example, Fritzon (2001) has done with regard to arsonists. These kinds of profiles have found regularities in the behaviours of offenders which, when subjected to statistical analysis, can be interpreted as indicating that different categories of offenders – in Fritzon's case, 'Despair', 'Display', 'Damage' and 'Destroy' – tend to behave in different ways. Similar work has been carried out with regard to rapists (e.g. Canter and Heritage, 1990) and murderers (Santilla, Häkkänen, Canter and Elfgren, 2003). However, such models rely on the 'homology assumption' (Mokros and Alison, 2002): that 'the degree of similarity in the offence behaviour of any two perpetrators from a given category of crime will match the degree of similarity in their characteristics' (p. 26). Tests on characteristics of 100 stranger rapists by Mokros and Alison (2002) and robbers and arsonists (Doan and Snook, 2008) suggest that there is only weak evidence for this assumption.

Another concern with the models that are developed concerns their statistical reliability. Many of the models (Canter and Heritage, 1990; Fritzon, 2001) have made use of a technique known as *multi-dimensional scaling* (MDS), which provides a plot showing, for instance, how closely certain behaviours co-occur. For example, in some rapes the offender will talk to the victim and steal an item of clothing. MDS shows how likely these and other acts are to co-occur, and the clusters of behaviours that emerge are used to categorise different kinds of offenders. The difficulties with this approach are firstly that it assumes accurate recall on the part of victims (or of investigative teams) and secondly that the decision concerning where the categorical boundaries lie is not statistically determined but is instead the responsibility of the person interpreting the output. Some examples that support the inductive view are provided by the work of Davies (1997) and House (1997). In the former case, rapists who broke into properties were more likely to have convictions for property offences; and in the latter, rapists who showed high levels of aggression were more likely to have convictions for aggressive offences. More recently, Tonkin, Bond and Woodhams (2009) showed that the more expensive the footwear evidenced at a crime (by, for example, the shoe imprint), the more likely an offender was to be unemployed and living in relative deprivation.

In some situations this kind of profile has great potential value, for example in helping to compare crimes in order to determine whether they are connected. It is not so clear that profiles of this kind are particularly useful in identifying the perpetrators if the information that is offered is concerned only with offence-related acts (e.g. in the case of rape, information about kissing, conversation, or stealing something from the victim). However, as these models rely on the accumulation of research in order to refine them, it is plausible that other characteristics, identified in future research, may also be related, such as how far the offender is likely to have travelled from home to commit the offence.

A variety of criticisms can be levelled at inductive profiling. For example, the information on which the databases are built all comes from convicted offenders (Wilson, Lincoln and Kocsis, 1997), and those who are caught and convicted may be a unrepresentative subset of all offenders. Turvey (1999) has pointed out that the databases on which the analyses are carried out include only a very small number of cases in relation to the number of actual offences (which is also true of the FBI's database of serial murderers). As was suggested for deductive profiles, care must be taken when reading descriptions of cases in which inductive profiling is described as having successfully contributed to an investigation, as there may also have been many cases where this profiling was not helpful. Also, we must consider what counts as success. For example, (Godwin, 2008; Godwin and Rosen, 2005) provides a case history in which his geographic profile predicted that a killer lived within a circle with a diameter of approximately one mile. Although he was arrested within that area, the killer's home was *not* within the predicted area, yet Godwin's description implies that the profile was successful.

Geographical profiling

Work has been carried out to look at the importance of location in an offender's decision-making (Canter and Larkin, 1993; Godwin and Canter, 1997). It is suggested that some behavioural characteristics indicate whether an individual might be a 'marauder' or a 'traveller', and this in turn provides information about the offender's tendency to be at a distance from home before committing offences. Of course, issues of travel also link back to the material concerned with how geography impacts upon behaviour (Brantingham and Brantingham, 1999), and how our experience and knowledge of our environment biases our decision-making. Clearly, geographical information has the potential to influence investigative decision-making if it can reduce the possible area of searching for a possible offender. The use of information to provide clues as to a location that might be important to an individual offender led to the development of *geographical profiling*, whereby the profile seeks to reduce the area on which an investigation will concentrate, rather than identifying a type of individual. This has the benefit of combining psychological information with information on police databases recording where known offenders live and work. Geographical profiling is another example of an inductive process – research is required to demonstrate the possible relationships between, for example, offence type and distance to crime, crime sites and disposal sites, multiple offenders and crime sites, and locations of an offender's workplace or home.

A practical example of geographic profiling is the work of Canter on the cases eventually linked to John Duffy, known as the Railway Rapist (Canter, 2007; also see Godwin and Rosen, 2005, for US examples). Based on the spread of rapes and murders around an area of London (see Figure 13.1) and on how that map changed over time, Canter suggested that the offender was likely to live in a particular area of the city. This led the police to pay particular attention to an individual who was already on their list of suspects. Eventually they gathered enough evidence to prove that Duffy was indeed the man they were after.

Canter (1995) has produced similar maps for other offenders, such as Peter Sutcliffe, to demonstrate the potential value of geographical approaches, but it is important to keep in mind that in some cases, including Sutcliffe's, it was not geographical profiling that led to his identification but lucky policing. A source for information on Peter Sutcliffe is Burns' (1984) book: *Somebody's Husband, Somebody's Son: The Story of Peter Sutcliffe.*

The process by which geographical profiling is now carried out is via a variety of mathematical techniques that consider the distances between linked crimes (Canter, Coffey, Huntley and Missen, 2000), and a number of software packages have been developed to support these calculations (e.g. *DRAGNET* and *Predator*).

The descriptions of profiling above have assumed that there are relationships between certain characteristics of a person (or personality) and how that person might behave. The concept of personality is based on the idea that categories of characteristics – whether 'normal' as in extrovert, or 'disordered' as in histrionic – are predictive of biases in thinking and behaving. Indeed, Child (1968) defined personality as 'more or less stable, internal factors that make one person's behaviour consistent from one time to another, and different from the behaviour that other people would manifest in comparable situations' (p. 83). Personality covers a broad range of material and is described by a wealth of theories. However, personality

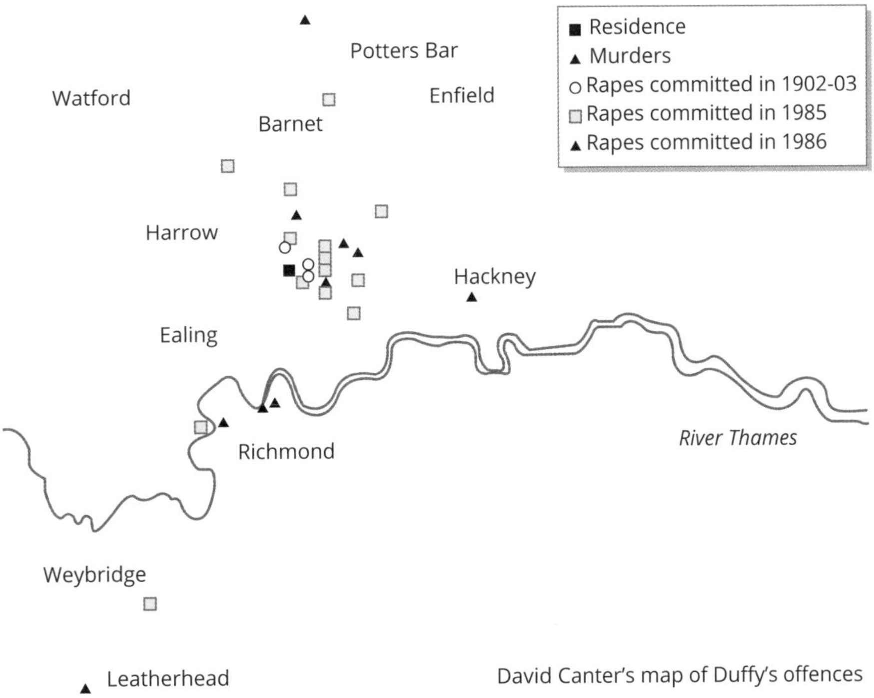
Residence
Murders
Rapes committed in 1902-03
Rapes committed in 1985
Rapes committed in 1986
Potters Bar
Watford
Enfield
Barnet
Harrow
Hackney
Ealing
Richmond
River Thames
Weybridge
Leatherhead
David Canter's map of Duffy's offences

Figure 13.1
Geographic profiling: a depiction of the pattern of rapes and murders showing time and location.

Source: Canter, D. V. (1994). Criminal Shadows: Inside the Mind of the Serial Killer. London: HarperCollins. Copyright © 1994 Professor David Canter.

theorists broadly agree that personality is determined by both internal factors and by external, situational factors (for example, the behaviour of another person within a relationship: see Zayas, Shoda and Ayduk, 2002). The combination of internal and external factors increases the complexity of determining how personality impacts upon the utility of profiling. A profile of an individual describing their personality that had been generated from purely internal factors would probably not link an individual's crimes – their behaviour might differ according to their circumstances; and a geographical profile might not be useful as the particular circumstances that trigger a crime may occur independently of location. If personality was based entirely on the person, then we might expect that profiles would be incredibly accurate.

If we accept that personality is in effect a form of bias, then this suggests that it will certainly be important in profiles. The difficulty is that many aspects of personality have not been examined to determine the extent to which personality does bias behaviour, and whether it does this in ways that would be useful to investigators. For example, we have an intuitive sense of what an 'introvert' is like, but we do not know how introversion might be expressed during the commission of a rape. If we assume that an introverted rapist would not be talkative, we might deflect attention from the fact that the rapist may be forensically aware and have a distinctive accent or speech pattern. Similarly, one might assume that profiling could be used to investigate any form of crime, but profiling requires that the offence is sufficiently demanding that it restricts the pool of suspects. For example, low-level shoplifting doesn't require a great deal of skill, so a profile is unlikely to be more helpful than suggesting that the offender is probably someone local. (For more information regarding profiling and shoplifting, see Dabney, Dugan, Topalli and Hoolinger 2006.) Some authors (e.g. Wilson, Lincoln and Kocsis, 1997) have suggested that profiling is useful only 'where there is some evidence of psychopathology in the offenders, such as lust killings or those where extensive mutilation is present' (p. 8). This suggests that non-psychopathological people behave in less predictable and understandable ways and that those with psychopathology are more predictable and understandable.

With regards to psychopathological individuals, Duff and Kinderman (2008) have argued that it is not necessarily possible to diagnose psychopathology from an individual's behaviour *in absentia*; and that in the case of personality disorders, at least, the presence of psychopathology does not imply behaviours that are remarkably different from the norm, but rather that the content of thoughts that *led* to those behaviours may be quite different. This contradicts the views of some authors (e.g. Holmes and Holmes, 2009) who suggest that chaos at a murder scene indicates a disorganised personality, which allows for certain assumptions about that individual's 'social core variables' (p. 47). Indeed, they state that: 'As certainly as a psychometric test reflects psychopathology, the crime scene reflects a personality with pathology' (p. 48). There is evidence to suggest that psychopathology is linked to regularities in behaviour. For example, research has demonstrated that individuals diagnosed with schizophrenia show a preference for turning left, and that this tendency correlates with the severity of the symptoms (Bracha *et al.*, 1993). However, would there be evidence at a crime scene of such a preference?

The overwhelming *caveat* is that the condition of the crime scene may be as it is as a result of the offender, or of the interaction between the offender and victim (e.g. the victim may have fought hard), or its condition may have predated the offence, or events may have occurred post-offence that have impacted the crime scene, such as the presence of animals, the effects of weather, the actions of the individuals who found the crime scene, and suchlike. This last possibility, that evidence might change between the commission of a crime and its detection, is referred to as **Evidence Dynamics** (Chisum and Turvey, 2000). As Alison, Bennell, Mokros and Ormerod (2002) write: 'The notion that particular configurations of demographic features can be predicted from an assessment of particular configurations of specific behaviors occurring in short-term, highly traumatic situations seems an overly ambitious and unlikely possibility' (p. 132).

This links in with another concern of investigative psychology: that the intent or reason for the behaviour is not particularly useful in directing police inquiries. In part this is because the intent is unknowable during the investigation, but it is also because studies have suggested that intent is not particularly predictive. For example, one might assume that the motivation for fraud is to achieve greater wealth, and one might therefore suppose that likely fraudsters would have money troubles. However, as Stotland (1977) suggests, 'sometimes individuals' motivation for crime may have originally been relative deprivation, greed, threat to continued goal attainment and so forth. However, as they found themselves successful at this crime, they began to gain some secondary delight in the knowledge that they are fooling the world, that they are showing their superiority to others' (pp. 186–7).

The value of profiles

The aims of a profile

Canter and Alison (2000) identify four fundamental questions on which the foundations of profiling are based:

1. What are the important behavioural features which may help identify (and prosecute) an individual?
2. What inferences may be made about the characteristics of that individual which may help in identification?
3. Are there other offences which are likely to have been committed by the same person?
4. Can we discriminate between different offending individuals?

Usefully for psychology, these are generally important questions for understanding any form of behaviour and as such the psychology that underpins profiling need not be considered as a special, separate type of psychology. Further, what these questions begin to suggest is that large groups of the population can be discounted as potential suspects quite early on, without needing to involve a great deal of psychology but based rather on simple practicalities. So what can a psychological profile add?

What is the value of a profile and can this be determined?

From the perspective of the media, one might assume that a profile is intended to identify a perpetrator, but despite some of the remarkable cases where this *does* appear to have been the result, what we know about psychology suggests that this is usually not a realistic expectation. Even if it were possible to define the personality of an offender precisely through a profile, investigators would still need to be able to identify that personality in a specific individual. If it were possible to predict the behaviour of an individual through a profile, that individual would have to have been known already so that his or her behaviour could be monitored to observe and record the predicted behaviour.

In some ways this is oversimplifying the situation, as in reality it is very rare that an individual variable is used to form the basis of a profile. In practice, profiles commonly consider ten variable groups, as shown in the list below. They were extracted by the CTN ('Coals to Newcastle') project from the analysis of 111 profiles that had been written for the police (Copson, 1995), and these groups were the ones considered to best categorise the kinds of information routinely presented in profiles:

1. Features of the offence.
2. Character of the offender.
3. Origins of the offender.
4. Present circumstances of the offender.
5. Criminality of the offender.
6. Geographical location of the offender.
7. Predicted future behaviour of the offender.
8. Interview strategy to be adopted.
9. Threat assessment.
10. Specific recommendations to the police.

Clearly, information about these groups of variables (some more than others) could help to focus an investigation, but the information available would have to be incredibly specific to identify a particular person. Indeed, even if all ten elements were available, it is still unlikely that they would identify a particular individual.

Table 13.1 shows an example of a profile offered by Strentz (1988), who suggested that a profile of a leading member of a radical right-wing group in the US would include the following information. By way of illustration, we have noted in the second column the profile categories from Copson, identified by their respective numbers, to demonstrate how those categories might be used. Apart from those characteristics that we might be able to infer from our stereotype of a radical right-wing group member, it is not clear that the remaining characteristics would be particularly useful in identifying an individual – for example, how would we recognise a 'Strong controlled paranoid type personality'? – nor how they could provide some form of direction rather than just a potential description.

13

Profile (Strentz)	Groups of variables (Copson)
Male	2, 8
White Protestant	2
College educated or attendance	2
35–50+	2, 4
Middle class	3, 4, 6, 8
Urban sophisticated	3, 4, 6, 8
Literate in English	2, 4, 8
High verbal skills	2, 4, 8
Well-trained perfectionist	1, 2, 4, 8
Strong controlled paranoid type personality	1, 2, 4, 8
Politically active and articulate	1, 2, 4, 8, 10

Table 13.1 Elements of a profile. This table compares a profile provided by Strentz with the variable groups identified by Copson.

Similar concerns could be raised about the use of **crime-scene analysis**. The idea here is that examining how the victim was treated, how the victim is displayed, and the way in which the location of the crime is presented will together provide insight into the nature of the offender. Turco (1990) has suggested that the crime scene can be thought of as 'a symptom of a behavioural act and in a broader perspective as a projection of the underlying personality, life style and developmental experiences ... of the perpetrator' (p. 150). However, there is little empirical evidence to support the view that offending behaviour is a projection of, for example, lifestyle – and, equally, it is not clear what would constitute a 'projection'. This principle appears to be a psychological equivalent of **Locard's Exchange Principle**, which can be described in this way: 'Any action of an individual, and obviously, the violent action constituting a crime, cannot occur without leaving a mark' (Locard, 1934). Locard was referring specifically to contact, for example when someone touches another person or an object, and noting that whenever such a contact occurs there is a transfer from one to the other, which can later be identified. With crime-scene analysis, it seems that there is a parallel assumption that what is identified as part of the crime scene can also be thought of as the offender leaving his or her mark, and that that mark provides important psychological and investigative information. As mentioned earlier, the principle of Evidence Dynamics alone, whereby the crime scene may be altered between commission of the offence and the scene being investigated, suggests that the idea of a one-to-one mapping between the scene and characteristics of the offender will be difficult to resolve.

The more realistic value of a profile is, as suggested earlier, simply in reducing the possible sample of individuals on whom investigators need to focus. This is demonstrated by the work of Snow (Johnson, 2006) already mentioned: Snow was able to estimate the probable location of the source of cholera outbreaks, but he was not able to precisely identify what in that location was responsible for the outbreak. To reach his conclusion, Snow relied on his own theory of the transport of disease.

An issue for profiles, and indeed any form of forensic report that deals with issues of probability, is how those probabilities will be interpreted. If an individual is described as 'likely to reoffend', or in the case of a profile if it is said that 'it is very likely that the offender will have a manual, unskilled occupation', what is the impact of those probabilities on the way in which that information might be used? A study by Villejoubert, Almond and Alison (2008) has demonstrated that certain expressions of probability lead to variation in how they are interpreted and that the way in which the probabilities were framed also has an impact. Thus, care should be taken not only in how a profile is developed, but also in how it is communicated.

Interviewing suspects

Psychology has turned its attention to determining methods for successful interviewing of a range of individuals. These methods consider the needs of those who might be classed as vulnerable (children, individuals with learning disabilities, and so on), and to take into account what we know about the reconstructive nature of memory, making use of such techniques as the Cognitive Interview (see Chapter 12; and Milne and Bull, 1999). In addition to these psychological approaches, which are empirically based, investigative psychology has broadened its scope to cover all aspects of the investigative process, including interviewing suspects.

For example, work by Arnold, Gozna and Brown (2007) examined the compliance of suspected offenders during police interviews and how this related to those individuals' behavioural characteristics. Additionally, individuals who define themselves as profilers have also suggested strategies to work with particular categories of offender. Holmes and Holmes (2009), for example, suggested that there are *typologies* of offenders. In the case of lust murders these are asocial and non-social. Not only do Holmes and Holmes suggest that these two types differ in their personal characteristics and post-offence behaviour, but they also propose different interview techniques. For example, they suggest that asocial offenders respond best to having empathy shown to them, with the interviewer using a counselling approach and the interview being held at night. For the non-social offender, they advise that one should use a direct strategy based on details about which one is certain, and that the offender 'will only admit to what he must' (p. 84). Turvey (1999) also suggests that profiling is useful in developing interview strategies. Napier (2010) provides an interesting description of one approach to using profiling in the interview process, referred to as *Targeted Subject Interviewing* (TSI): it is an 'interview plan tailored to the vulnerabilities and psychological weaknesses of the suspect as revealed by the subject's criminal behaviour and interaction with the victim' (p. 2). However, Napier's book is predominantly aimed at the interviewing and interrogation of individuals accused of serious crimes, and who are assumed to be without learning disabilities or mental health difficulties: this might explain the strong tone used in the explanation.

In the UK, perhaps the best-known case of a profiler being involved in interview strategies (and in information-gathering) is that of Paul Britton in the Rachel Nickell murder, although debate continues as to the success and appropriateness of that case: see the 'Focus on ...' box below. However, strategic thinking based on personality types is not limited to profiling. For example, Walters (2003) suggested that for what he referred to as the 'introvert-oriented personality', a subtype of 'primary dominant personality types', an interviewer should 'avoid all forms of overt hostility' as these individuals do 'not handle intimidation well and will shut down' (p. 264). These latter approaches appear to be deductive in nature, with the personality being deduced from background and behaviour, for example, rather than from psychometric testing.

FOCUS ON ...

Profiling in the Rachel Nickell case

Rachel Nickell was a 23-year-old woman who was murdered in July 1992 on Wimbledon Common in London. At the time of the murder, it stood out as taking place in daylight, in a public space, and whilst Rachel was with her two-year-old son. The coroner, Dr Paul Knapman, described it as a 'frenzied attack', and by February 1993 the police had taken over 1,000 statements but had not charged anyone.

This case is both interesting and frustrating: interesting because it has been written about by various authors, and frustrating because there does not appear to be a consistent account of the case. The various accounts can be read in books by the man initially accused of the murder, Colin Stagg (*Who Really Killed Rachel*); the profiler, Paul Britton (*The Jigsaw Man*); and one of the senior police officers, Keith Pedder (*The Rachel Files*). Ultimately, Robert Napper was convicted of this crime. Rather than be concerned with the details of the crime, however, we will consider accounts of the profile and how that impacted upon the case.

There is some debate as to whether Stagg had already been identified by the police as a likely suspect before the profile was constructed, or whether the profile was constructed first. Either way, at least part of the profile focused on the idea that the perpetrator would experience sexually sadistic fantasies. (Much of the rest of the profile would not have potentially distinguished Stagg from many other men, 20–30 years old, and living alone not far from the crime scene.) As this chapter has tried to make clear, information about preferences is not useful for an investigation because that aspect of the offender is not necessarily observable; but in this case the profiler and the police worked together on Operation Edzell, a specific plan whereby this aspect of their suspect, Stagg, would become apparent. In order to achieve this, they had an undercover police officer pose as a woman who was sexually interested in Stagg, who had an interest in deviant sexual fantasy and behaviour, and who discussed this with Stagg both in letters and in person. Although Stagg was interested in developing a sexual relationship with this undercover officer, and to some extent did go along with the fantasies, he did not acknowledge having been involved in the Nickell murder and he apologised if she felt his fantasies had gone too far.

Although it might have been useful to develop a profile of the murderer, there are a number of issues worth examining here. Firstly, it appears that the profile did little to help reduce the potential pool of suspects beyond what common sense might have achieved – that is, in identifying that the offender was a young male living nearby. Secondly, the profile suggested in addition some kind of deviance from the norm, but this was something that would not necessarily be apparent to investigators, so it would need to be examined at interview, rather than it being a characteristic that could help with making the investigation more targeted (unless only individuals identified by police records as having a specific deviance were to be considered).

Perhaps the most important issue is that in order to do this, the decision was made to employ a young woman, described as attractive, to pose as someone with an interest in a young male who was living alone, and to indicate that she found deviance sexually arousing. Even if the profile of the killer was accurate, an equally accurate profile could be constructed to suggest that if an attractive young woman tells a young man that she finds murder sexually alluring, there is a high chance that he will fake that too in order to achieve his sexual goals, whether or not he finds the idea and act of killing a thrill.

The idea that an individual's characteristics might interact with an interviewer's style, location, gender, age and so forth is based on the psychology of personality. As it has been demonstrated that there are indeed consistencies within personality types, there is evidence supportive of the approach. As with criminal profiling, so too with interviewing: it appears that there are *deductive* and *inductive* camps, and the same pros and cons need to be carefully considered with each approach to reach a conclusion as to how it works and how well it works.

Conclusion

Snook *et al.* (2008) suggest not. In their discussion of profiling, in which they openly do not include geographic profiling, they suggest that to date there is no evidence to support the idea that profiling is reliable, valid, or useful. In studies that have compared the accuracy of trained profilers with university students, researchers have found no differences in the quality of the profiles produced or in the accuracy of the profiles. As discussed above, one important consideration is how we might *measure* value. Despite descriptions to the contrary, the idea that a profile can identify one particular individual is perhaps optimistic, so holding profiling to that level of performance may be unreasonable. Instead, it might be more reasonable to consider cases where profiles have made a helpful contribution to operational decisions, either in novel ways or as part of the evidence supporting a particular focus or direction. Taking this approach might more fairly test both deductive and inductive approaches and might also help to dispel the myth of profiling: that it is somehow more powerful than anything else that psychology offers. Indeed, profiling is very much like formulation in clinical and forensic practice, in which evidence is acquired and hypotheses are developed in seeking to understand the person, the behaviour, and how to manage it. We do not expect our formulations to be wholly accurate, but simply to point us in the right direction.

Chapter summary

- Profiling in forensic psychology has a particular goal: to reduce the potential number of individuals whom investigative authorities might need to examine in the course of identifying the perpetrator of a crime. To be of practical use, the information within a profile must be both accurate and predictive, and it must include features that can be identified, such as a gender, a profession and particular behaviours.

- There is evidence that human behaviour is, within limits, predictable, and this is the basis for profiling. Behaviour in the ways that we move around where we live and shop, the order in which we purchase particular items, and the impact of architecture on our behaviour, amongst other examples, all demonstrate that behaviour is shaped by our experiences, our knowledge and our surroundings, and that there is a degree of *consistency* in that behaviour. If we can identify what factors influence *criminal* behaviour, and if those factors are identifiable, then we can build up a profile of the kind of person most likely to exhibit that behaviour.
- In suggesting that the process faultlessly identifies an individual, media portrayals of profiling are likely to be inaccurate. Nor is profiling a recent concept: the earliest examples we can examine are from the 19th century, and include the work of Lombroso, Galton, and Snow. Galton and Lombroso both suggested that physical features may be indicative of behaviour and that criminals in general could therefore be identified by their villainous irregularities, but such features would not necessarily pinpoint a specific criminal. Snow provides perhaps the first example of geographical profiling, but with the difference that he identified an object (a water pump) rather than a person as the source of the spread of cholera. He also went further in identifying a *specific* water pump, but at that time there were few sources of publically available water, which may have made his task easier.
- Profiling can be broadly split into two approaches. The *deductive* one, which might be considered as the more 'clinical' approach that one sees in films and on television (consider examples such as *Cracker*, *Wire in the Blood*, *Criminal Minds* and *Profiler*), relies primarily on crime-scene evidence to lead to deductions about the perpetrator. The *inductive* approach relies on the scientific identification of behavioural regularities. There are few media portrayals of inductive profilers, although David Canter has appeared in his own television series, *Mapping Murder*. Both approaches have their advocates and their critics, and it is important to engage critically with the various literatures to understand fully the potential value of each approach, both in developing profiles and in developing the psychology of offenders and of offending behaviour.
- Beyond the identification of an offender, profiling has also been used in the development of interview techniques with particular individuals. The choice of technique is based on the idea that different personality types respond differently to different interviewing styles. For example, some interviewees will feel reassured by expressions of empathy from an interviewer. The basic principles are the same; and although they may be less explicit, there do appear to be both deductive and inductive approaches to interviewing suspects, too. In a parallel development, there is work looking at the characteristics of witnesses and how these might influence interview style, and this has led to developments such as the use of the Cognitive Interview with vulnerable witnesses.
- The value of profiling, whether deductive or inductive, is hard to ascertain as data from real cases are not easily obtained. The popular literature tends to present the successes, whereas in the academic literature one finds criticism and concern. From a practical perspective, it is important that the ideas and their value are tried and tested; and an academic approach requires that we consider the underlying psychology and ensure that there is evidence to support our conclusions.

Further reading

It would be useful to read a range of views of profiling. To start that process, we suggest:

» Douglas, J. E., Ressler, R. K., Burgess, A. W., and Hatman, C. R. (1986). Criminal profiling from crime scene analysis. *Behavioral Sciences and the Law*, 4, 401–421. Despite being rather old, this article gives a helpful overview of what was the traditional FBI approach to profiling.

» In contrast: Canter, D. V., Alison, L. J., Alison, E., and Wentink, N. (2004). The organized/disorganized typology of serial murder: myth or model? *Psychology, Public Policy, and Law*, 10, 293–320. This article presents the case *against* this kind of approach.

» Canter, D. and Fritzon, K. (1998). Differentiating arsonists: a model of firesetting actions and characteristics. *Legal and Criminological Psychology*, 3, 73–96. This paper presents an example of multi-dimensional scaling, which has been a frequently used tool in the profiling literature.

» Another form of analysis, Principal Components Analysis, is presented in the work of Santilla concerning the investigation of burglary: Santilla, P., Ritvannen, A., and Mokros, A. (2004). Predicting burglar characteristics from crime scene behaviour. *International Journal of Police Science and Management*, 6, 136–154.

» Finally, an article by Muller is a useful point of consideration as to the value of profiling: Muller, D. A. (2000). Criminal profiling: real science or just wishful thinking? *Homicide Studies*, 4, 234–264.

Going to Court: Processes and Decision-Making

Across the world there are a variety of legal systems and the bodies that are responsible for the administration of justice according to those legal systems are the courts. In the United Kingdom there are different legal systems for England and Wales, Scotland, and Northern Ireland (although some laws apply throughout the UK), and for different aspects of the legal system there are different courts. For example, the military has its own courts, and there are also specialist youth courts. In the United States there are similar divisions, for example the Supreme Court and the Alien Terrorist Removal Court, and individual states have their own courts. It is within the courts that decisions are made as to how the relevant law will be applied in particular cases, and thus how it will impact on the various parties involved – typically, in forensic situations, on offenders.

Chapter objectives

- To gain an understanding of the basic structure of the court system in England and Wales, as an example of a court system.
- To develop an understanding of the various courts in which a forensic psychologist would typically expect to appear, or with which a forensic psychologist would need to work.
- To understand some areas of complexity within the legal system that might impact upon a forensic psychologist's clients.
- To be aware of some factors that may impact upon sentencing.
- To appreciate the issues that an expert witness may have to consider when involved in a court case.

This chapter provides an overview of the *court* system, focusing primarily on the English and Welsh systems. Although there are many similarities with other systems, such as those of Scotland, Northern Ireland and Australia, an attempt to cover the whole range of similarities and differences would require a book in itself. Two differences in the Scottish system are worth mentioning, however. First, Scottish courts attach importance to the concept of *corroboration*: the requirement that at least *two* sources of evidence support the facts that might lead to the conviction of an individual. (Corroboration in this form is not required under English and Welsh law.) Second, whereas in England and Wales there are two possible verdicts – 'guilty' or 'not guilty' – in Scotland there are *three* possible outcomes from a trial: 'guilty', 'not guilty' and 'not proven'. While the latter two have the same effect – that the person is acquitted – a 'not proven' verdict can be interpreted as suggesting that the person may actually be guilty, but there was insufficient evidence to prove this. Indeed, some other countries have wanted to adopt this third verdict for just that reason, including the US (see Bray, 2005).

Across the world court systems differ markedly and can be enormously complex, so we have chosen to concentrate on those areas in which forensic psychologists are most likely to be involved during their careers. We have therefore not included some elements of the UK court system, such as the Supreme Court, Coroners' Courts, Courts of Chivalry, Courts-Martial, Courts-Martial Appeal Courts, Ecclesiastical Courts and Election Courts. Texts dealing specifically with the court system can be consulted for information about these.

The structure of the English and Welsh court system

Passage through the court system is not, as one might imagine, easily defined by the type or seriousness of the crime, for example, and there are numerous further complications in setting out the structure simply and accurately if one were also to consider **appeals**. Numerous legal texts provide a thorough overview of the complete and complex system (e.g. Slapper and Kelly, 2009) and these should be consulted for a thorough grounding in this area. McMurran, Khalifa and Gibbon (2009, p. 3) provide a useful flowchart overview of the court system, which is reproduced in Figure 14.1.

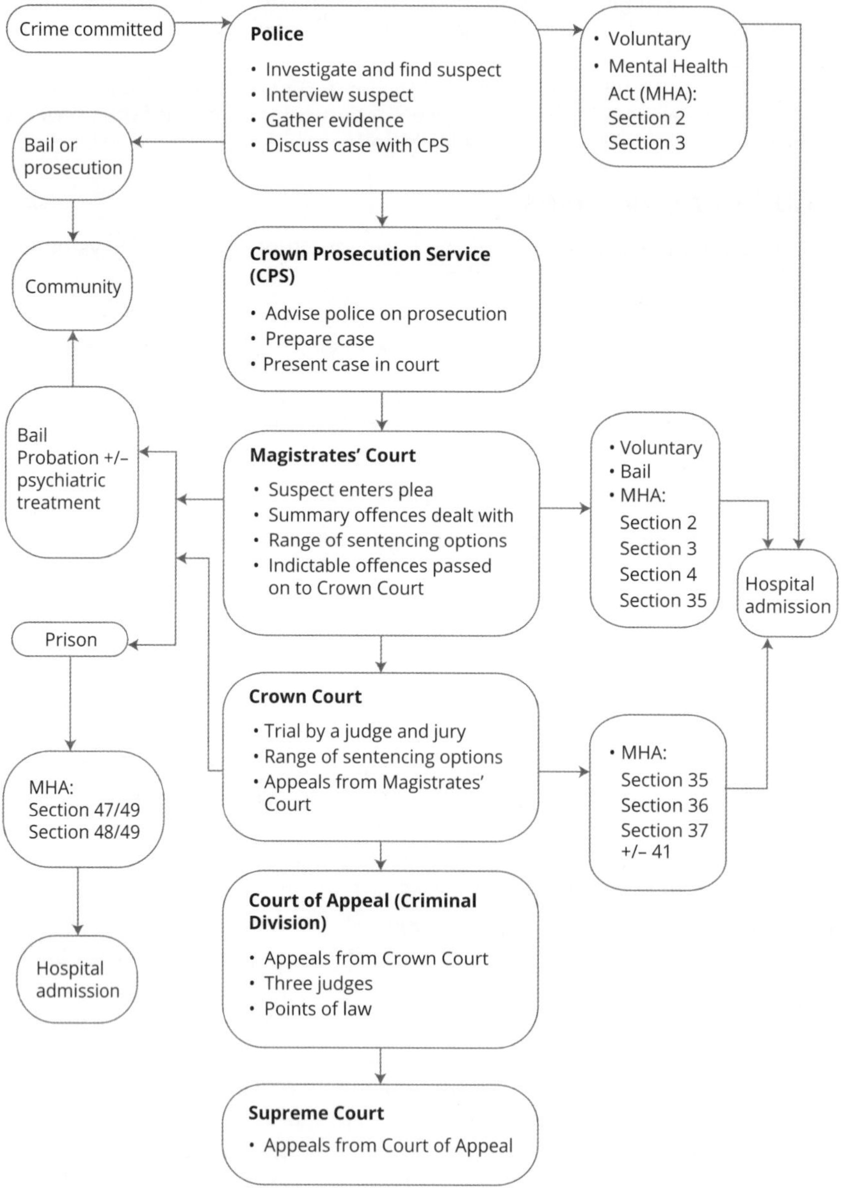
Crime committed
Police
• Investigate and find suspect
• Interview suspect
• Gather evidence
• Discuss case with CPS
• Voluntary
• Mental Health Act (MHA): Section 2 Section 3
Bail or prosecution
Community
Crown Prosecution Service (CPS)
• Advise police on prosecution
• Prepare case
• Present case in court
Bail Probation +/– psychiatric treatment
Magistrates' Court
• Suspect enters plea
• Summary offences dealt with
• Range of sentencing options
• Indictable offences passed on to Crown Court
• Voluntary
• Bail
• MHA: Section 2 Section 3 Section 4 Section 35
Hospital admission
Prison
Crown Court
• Trial by a judge and jury
• Range of sentencing options
• Appeals from Magistrates' Court
MHA: Section 47/49 Section 48/49
• MHA: Section 35 Section 36 Section 37 +/– 41
Court of Appeal (Criminal Division)
• Appeals from Crown Court
• Three judges
• Points of law
Hospital admission
Supreme Court
• Appeals from Court of Appeal

Figure 14.1
Flowchart of the English and Welsh court system.

Source: adapted from Figure 1.1 The criminal justice process and diversion mechanisms. From McMurran, M., Khalifa, N., and Gibbon, S. (2009). Forensic Mental Health. Cullompton, Devon: Willan Publishing. p. 3. Copyright © 2009 Willan Publishing, reproduced by permission of Taylor & Francis Books UK.

The following material seeks to provide an overview of the system as it applies to criminal cases, to help you develop a sense of how the court structure may impact upon outcomes for offenders. What happens in court impacts upon, for example, individuals' freedom, their perceptions of their risk, and their opportunities to receive intervention. The forensic psychologist may play a part in the decision-making process and may come into contact with some of the people processed by the court, depending on what that outcome is. In this way the legal system can be seen as a filter which determines the different paths, or journeys through the system, that individuals may take.

Courts

Introduction to the courts

The court system exists to settle disputes with authority, but in many areas of the law the courts are not the only setting, nor indeed the major setting, in which disputes are resolved (see Cownie, Bradney and Burton, 2007).

The basic structure of the courts in England and Wales can broadly be thought of as determined primarily by two factors. One factor is the type or seriousness of the case. **Summary cases** can only be heard at the Magistrates' Court, and these include most motoring offences and less serious cases of public order and assault. There are a range of cases that may be heard either at a Magistrates' Court or at the Crown Court, such as drugs offences, and more serious criminal offences are heard at the Crown Court. The second factor is whether the case is being brought by a **plaintiff** (an individual, a company, or a public authority) or by the State. In the former situation, the case would be dealt with by the Civil Court; in the latter, the case would be dealt with by the Criminal Court. This section will deal only with criminal cases, so it will not touch on family or civil cases.

However, one interesting issue worthy of mention relates to a difference between the Civil and Criminal Courts: the level of proof required is different. In *civil cases,* the level of proof required is that the individual is guilty on the 'balance of probabilities'. One way to understand this concept is to consider that the court is trying to determine whether or not an event happened. If the evidence provided suggests that the event is more likely to have happened than not, then this satisfies the test of 'the balance of probabilities'. A consequence of this level of proof is that as different events are more or less likely to occur – for example, accidental injuries are more common than intentional harming – this means that the balance of probability is not constant for every case. This point was presented by Lord Nicholls (*In re H (Minors) [1996] AC 563 at 586*) as follows:

> The balance of probability standard means that a court is satisfied an event occurred if the court considers that, on the evidence, the occurrence of the event was more likely than not. When assessing the probabilities the court will have in mind as a factor, to whatever extent is appropriate in the particular case, that the more serious the allegation the less likely it is that the event occurred and, hence, the stronger should be the evidence before the court concludes that the allegation is established on the balance of probability. Fraud is usually less likely than negligence. Deliberate physical injury is usually less likely than accidental physical injury ... Although the result is much the same, this does not mean that where a serious allegation is in issue the standard of proof required is higher. It means only that the inherent probability or improbability of an event is itself a matter to be taken into account when weighing the probabilities and deciding whether, on balance, the event occurred. The more improbable the event, the stronger must be the evidence that it did occur before, on the balance of probability, its occurrence will be established.

In *criminal cases*, on the other hand, the level of proof required is described as 'beyond **reasonable doubt**'. Here it is up to the prosecution to show that there is no reasonable explanation, given the facts of the case, other than that the defendant committed the crime. This does not mean that there will be *no* doubts, just that these doubts must not be stronger than the reasonable belief that the defendant is guilty.

Types of court

Magistrates' Court

The *Magistrates' Court* can be understood as the first part of the court process for criminal proceedings (although it also deals with some civil cases, such as failures to pay fines, along with granting licences for businesses, and Youth Courts). It deals with an estimated 97 per cent of criminal cases in England and Wales. Thus, although Magistrates' Courts might be considered as the least important of the courts, from the perspective of the seriousness of the matters that they can consider and the severity of the consequences that they can impose, they carry the heaviest burden.

Magistrates – also known as Justices of the Peace – decide whether a case should be heard at the Magistrates' Court or the Crown Court, making this decision on the basis of whether the offence is considered to be 'summary' (as discussed above), 'either way', or 'indictable'. 'Either way' cases are considered to be more serious and can be dealt with either in the Magistrates' Court or the Crown Court and include burglary and drugs offences. If the magistrates decide that the case should go to the Crown Court, meaning that they themselves do not have the necessary legal power to deal with the case, the defendant cannot appeal this. As an example of the limitations of magistrates' legal power, a Magistrates' Court can only sentence an individual for up to 6 months for burglary (although if there are two offences, then two consecutive sentences of 6 months may be imposed, resulting in a sentence of 12 months), whereas the Crown Court has available to it a limit of 14 years. On the other hand, if the magistrates decide that the case is to stay in the Magistrates' Court, then the defendant can *ask* for the case to be heard in a Crown Court, provided that he or she is pleading 'not guilty' to the offence. This course of action may be chosen if a defendant and his or her legal advisers consider it more likely that a jury will find the defendant 'not guilty' of the offence. 'Indictable' offences include the offences of murder, robbery and rape. Prior to 2013 an additional hearing was held to make a decision regarding whether a case should be transferred to the Crown Court (*Committal proceedings*). However to speed up the process, in 2016 this was replaced with a Plea and Trial Preparation Hearing at the Crown Court.

It is the less serious criminal cases that are dealt with by summary trial in a Magistrates' Court, which means that there is no jury. The trial is held in front of two or three magistrates, who are not professionally employed by the legal system and do not need any formal legal qualifications. The *magistrates* are members of the public who have been appointed to their position by advisory committees, who judge individuals on the basis of six characteristics: good character; understanding and communication; social awareness; maturity and sound temperament; sound judgment; and commitment and reliability. Magistrates are unpaid and work part time. There is a second group of magistrates, known as *district judges*, who are qualified lawyers and who are paid for their work. They tend to be found in larger cities and can hear cases on their own.

There are guidelines for Magistrates' Courts (Sentencing Council, 2017) that outline the decision-making process for magistrates. The process consists of five stages, including the consideration of harm, of any mitigating factors, and of sentence reduction on the grounds of a 'guilty' plea. If the defendant pleads *guilty*, the magistrates may decide to impose a sentence immediately, or they may decide to gather further information, such as a pre-sentencing report from the National Probation Service, in order to help them determine an appropriate sentence. If the defendant pleads *not guilty*, then typically the court will set a date for a hearing, after which the defendant may be placed on **bail**, may be kept in custody, or may be released until summoned to appear again before the court.

Neither the legal system nor the law are simple systems. One consequence of this complexity, and a factor that also adds to it, is the fact that *appeals* can be made in relation to court decisions. Where magistrates have made a ruling, this can be appealed in a number of ways. The original magistrates may decide to review the case again, if they believe there are issues of justice to consider; or appeals may be made, for a variety of reasons, to the Crown Court, the

High Court, or for a judicial review. A judicial review may be undertaken if there are concerns that the magistrates may have exceeded their powers or made some form of legal error (see Keogh, 2010). The High Court considers appeals that are based on a challenge to the outcome, or the verdict, of the case.

Crown Court

The *Crown Court*, a part of the Supreme Court of England and Wales, is a relatively new addition to the court system, having been established in 1971 to replace a number of previous courts (**Assizes** and **Quarter Sessions**). It is legally construed as being a single entity, despite being represented in different offices across the two countries. It is here that more serious criminal cases are tried, along with appeals from Magistrates' Courts concerning criminal and civil proceedings. Trials are held on the basis of a document called a *bill of indictment* (or just *indictment*), which describes the criminal charges brought against the defendant. These are categorised as shown in Table 14.1.

Class of indictment	Offence examples
Class 1	Murder, treason
Class 2	Manslaughter, rape
Class 3	All others
Class 4	Those offences that could be tried in a Magistrates' Court but have been passed to the Crown Court

Table 14.1 Examples of Crown Court indictments.

The indictment is constructed by the prosecutor who, in most cases, acts on behalf of the Crown (the State) and is employed by the **Crown Prosecution Service** (CPS). The CPS takes the case over from the police, who have already carried out their investigation. It is the prosecution that is required to prove its case – the guilt of a defendant must be proven by the prosecution (not the defendant's innocence by the defence), and the proof of guilt must be 'beyond reasonable doubt' (as discussed above). Rock (1993) provides a useful, in-depth, ethnographic account of the workings of a Crown Court – see the 'Focus on …' box.

14

FOCUS ON …

Crown Courts

Rock's (1993) work aimed to explore the experiences of witnesses in a Crown Court in England with a view to informing decisions regarding the necessary support for victims of crime. In doing so he was able to provide fascinating insights concerning an important part of the legal system, which has mostly remained unexamined.

Rock's analysis provides an interesting view of the formality and ceremony of the Crown Court process, which he describes as 'conflict' – due to the adversarial nature of the trial system – and as deliberately simplifying the complexity of human experience to focus on the nature of the alleged offence under consideration. Another area of conflict Rock acknowledges is that, in the nature of the trial process, alleged wrongdoers and their victims (or families) are brought together in one place and their situation is examined in public, whether related to fraud, rape, assault, theft, or murder. On this basis one can understand why a court could be perceived as a place of conflict.

In his book there are numerous transcripts of court cases where it is plain to see the various tactics used by barristers, defendants and witnesses in the process of giving evidence, and how this process can veer away from the simplistic idea of uncovering the truth of a situation. Thus, although the trial process attempts to simplify an event so that it can be understood by a jury, it may actually *add* complexity through the interactions of the various parties involved. Additionally, the possibility that a victim may find the process retraumatising when subject to examination in court is clear from the transcripts and Rock's analyses.

Media representations of trials suggest a formal and quite definite progression in a trial (for examples, one could see the films *Anatomy of a Murder*, *To Kill a Mockingbird* and *A Few Good Men*). As Rock's analysis makes clear, however, and despite there being a strong structure in place to manage the process, within that structure there is much variation and – although Rock does not reach this conclusion – quite possibly a degree of chaos for witnesses and defendants.

Crown Courts have public galleries, and it would be of great value to attend a trial in a Crown Court to observe the process, and then to contrast your experiences with the ethnographic work of Rock and with the formal descriptions of legal process provided in academic texts.

In the Crown Court, the case will be heard by a jury consisting of twelve people and will be overseen by the trial judge. It is the *jury* who come to a decision concerning the guilt or innocence of a defendant, whereas the role of the *judge* is to ensure that the legal processes are upheld in the court – for example, that the case is fair – and to act as a legal mentor to the jury. If a defendant pleads guilty, then there will be no trial and the Court will impose a sentence.

The Crown Court has guidelines similar to those described for magistrates, although the range of sentences is greater and the kinds of offences considered are different. For example, the Sentencing Council has outlined the issues to be considered in respect of the *Sexual Offences Act*, indicating that in a case of an adult raped by a single offender, where there are no aggravating factors, then the starting point for a sentence should be five years (Sentencing Council, 2014).

Before court

Before an individual is brought to the court charged with a criminal offence, there must have been a complaint made about the offence, followed by an investigative process which begins to identify the individual or people responsible. Although it is not our intention to focus on these aspects of the process here, it is important to note that there is a wealth of psychology involved in these initial stages, which may play a crucial role in who comes into contact with the legal system and how they are dealt with – and, ultimately, in deciding the role of the forensic psychologist with that individual. Each of the facets of that process – the willingness of one or more individuals to make the initial complaint, the gathering of witness statements and the interviews undertaken by the police (see Chapter 12), and how evidence is used in order to make operational decisions – has its own research literature detailing the ways in which psychology impacts upon it. The research also considers questions that arise, such as, 'Why would an individual who has been raped *not* go to the police?' or 'How might we best interview a potential suspect who appears to be uncooperative?' The next 'Where do you stand?' box will consider the issue of victims in court.

In criminal cases, once a crime has been reported and a suspect has been apprehended, the police must make decide whether or not to charge that person with a crime. It is possible for the police to decide to issue a *caution* – only adults can receive a caution: young offenders receive a *warnings* or a *reprimand* – or not to respond at all to that person's behaviour. This means that the police have a powerful impact upon who

WHERE DO YOU STAND?

Victims in court

When an individual makes a complaint to the police, it is not just the suspects who come under scrutiny but also the *victim*, as the police seek to understand the circumstances of the crime. During this process it is quite possible that a victim will feel revictimised. They will have their account checked and be asked personal questions, and they may decide that taking their complaint further will be too difficult, particularly if they have concerns about the likelihood of a conviction. Yet if a victim decides not to proceed with a prosecution, then an offender may be free to continue committing further crimes and generating more victims.

If the complaint reaches a Crown Court, the victim may be cross-examined by the defence barrister, whose task is potentially to discredit the victim's ability to describe the offence and the offender accurately, and even to question the fact that a crime was committed at all. One frequently considered area of crime where this is contentious is rape. Data show that in the UK there are a small number of false allegations of rape when compared to the number of prosecutions of rape (0.6 per cent; CPS, 2013), and the number of prosecutions itself is small in relation to the number of rapes committed (as we saw in Chapter 9).

Clearly it is important to ensure that innocent defendants are not convicted, but English law also allows, with the court's permission, the introduction of evidence of 'bad character' regarding *victims*. 'Bad character' is indicated by evidence of, or a disposition towards, misconduct; and misconduct includes issues of culpability or blameworthiness. It is therefore possible that victims of rape may be questioned in order to suggest that they themselves may be culpable or blameworthy of the rape they have experienced, or that their allegations of rape are false. For example, they may be asked, amongst other things, about their sexual history, whether they had been drinking, and whether they had actually *consented* to sex.

So there is a dilemma, arising from the importance of ensuring both that victims of serious crimes are treated fairly and not retraumatised, and that defendants are suitably represented, so that as far as possible the reality of the situation becomes apparent to the jury. However, it is also important that offences are identified and offenders suitably managed to try to reduce future offending.

Where do you stand on this issue?

1 Do you think that the legal process might determine whether a victim of a serious crime will report it to the police?
2 Are there any changes that might impact on the reporting of crime, so that real victims *would* report crimes and so that there would be fewer cases of *false* reporting?
3 Should victims of crime be legally compelled to support prosecutions and to give evidence in order to increase conviction rates?
4 Is it reasonable to question victims in a way that might imply blame? If not, how should defendants be protected from false allegations?

comes before the courts and what offences the courts consider, thereby influencing an individual's journey through the legal system. The basis for the decision-making process will be police procedure. The decision-making policies of police forces are not routinely available, presumably because this might impact on their ability to conduct police work. However, redacted copies of the Metropolitan Police's *Standard Operating Procedures* for the primary investigation of crime can be found on the internet. Of note here is that the guidelines clearly state that, 'When considering the necessity to arrest, officers should make a clear note of their reasons. It is insufficient to only state, for example, "to allow the prompt and effective investigation of the offence".' This implies that the officer must make an informed decision about the need to arrest an individual and, as with all decisions, this will be influenced by many factors.

A highly controversial fly-on-the-wall documentary shown on the BBC, *Police*, concerned with the Thames Valley Police in England in the 1980s, provides various examples of their influence. In one instance, in the episode 'A Complaint of Rape', three officers were trying to persuade a woman who was making accusations of rape that she hadn't actually been raped. Although the officers may genuinely have believed that no offence had been committed, the documentary demonstrated the way in which, even at the very early stage of the legal process, the police were able – as they still are, to some extent – to impact on which offences and offenders were taken further along the legal pathway. The behaviour of the officers in that documentary led to a series of complaints and ultimately to the development of female-only rape teams in the Thames Valley force. It is probably unlikely that the police would *not* charge a person for a serious offence, but it is important to be aware that even at this early stage in the process decisions are being made that influence the ways in which society is made aware of and protected from offending, and how those who offend are dealt with.

Once an offender has been charged, a decision is made as to whether or not to prosecute. This decision is made by the Crown Prosecution Service, and is based on two factors:

1. Is there a realistic prospect of conviction?
2. Is the prosecution in the public interest?

Again, therefore, a degree of filtering is possible as to which people and which cases come before the courts. The CPS maintains a comprehensive website, where outlines of their decision-making processes can be found (see http://www.cps.gov.uk/). The information available there also describes the kinds of evidence that the police are recommended to collect for certain offences. For instance, in the event of a complaint of harassment, the CPS legal guidance suggests (in Section 9.29) that 'In cases of stalking and harassment, the police should encourage the use of Victim Personal Statements (VPS) when dealing with these cases.' While it is not unreasonable to *assume* that these guidelines are based on principles that have been tested – that is, that the CPS knows that such evidence clarifies issues in the case and is useful in building a case against an alleged offender – there is no real research data to support this. Also, the very existence of these guidelines could influence, and thus bias, the ways in which the police work, the material that they gather, and the assumptions that they make. Again, there is the possibility of a degree of filtering within the legal system.

FOCUS ON ...

The Crown Prosecution Service

The Crown Prosecution Service (CPS) is a government department that has responsibility for prosecuting criminal cases in England and Wales. It came into existence in 1985 in response to a number of criticisms regarding the criminal justice system. The three main criticisms were that the police were bringing too many weak cases to court (leading to acquittals), that the standards operated by different police forces in deciding whether or not to prosecute were inconsistent, and that the police should not both be investigating crimes and then deciding whether to prosecute.

The CPS can be thought of as a law firm dealing exclusively with criminal cases. It has five roles:

1. Advising the police on cases for possible prosecution.
2. Reviewing cases submitted by the police.
3. Determining any charges in more serious or complex cases.
4. Preparing cases for court.
5. Presenting cases at court.

In order to fulfil these roles, the CPS follows the Code for the Crown Prosecution

Service (see below), which is made up of two stages: the evidential stage and the public interest stage. At the evidential stage the decision is concerned with whether there is enough usable, reliable and credible evidence that there is a realistic prospect of conviction. The CPS defines a realistic prospect of conviction thus: 'a jury or a bench of magistrates, properly directed in accordance with the law, will be more likely than not to convict the defendant of the charge alleged'. If the CPS is not convinced at this stage then the case will not progress to the second stage, regardless of how serious the case may be.

During the second stage, concerning 'public interest', the CPS decides whether a prosecution is warranted, based on the following seven factors:

1 How serious is the offence committed?
2 What is the level of culpability of the suspect?
3 What are the circumstances of, and the harm caused to, the victim?
4 Was the suspect under the age of 18 at the time of the offence?
5 What has been the impact on the community?
6 Is prosecution a proportionate response?
7 Do sources of information need to be protected?

Each of these factors consists of elements that may argue for or against the public interest in prosecuting a case.

It is also worth noting that the CPS does not necessarily prosecute an individual based on the most serious of the charges against that person. Instead, they may select charges:

- that reflect the seriousness and extent of the offending that is supported by the evidence
- for which the court has adequate powers to sentence and to impose appropriate post-conviction orders
- that enable the case to be presented in a clear and simple way.

Questions

1 In what specific ways can the CPS be seen to be acting as a filter in the criminal justice system? To what extent do you think this is reasonable?
2 Are there circumstances in which serious crimes might not be prosecuted by the CPS? Should this be understood as a failing of the CPS or a reasonable consequence of having a fair criminal justice system?

Reference

- Based on *The Code for Crown Prosecutors*, 7th edition, www.cps.gov.uk/sites/default/files/documents/publications/code_2013_accessible_english.pdf. © Crown copyright 2013. Contains public sector information licensed under the Open Government Licence v3.0: http://www.nationalarchives.gov.uk/doc/open-government-licence/version/3

In court

The legal process can determine the eventual outcome for someone charged with an offence. Just as a police force may have an effect on an alleged rape case (as described above), the behaviour of barristers may impact upon whether a case is successfully heard in court. One of the makers of the *Police* documentary, Charles Stewart, made a related documentary, *The Doncaster Rape*, which followed the case of a 14-year-old rape victim. The film and the subsequent reports in the media indicated how intimidating a defence barrister's questioning of a witness could be. We might understand such questioning as being a consequence of the adversarial legal system that exists in many countries, a system that has been portrayed in numerous films, such as *A Few Good Men* and *Anatomy of a Murder*, and that has been experienced by forensic psychologists in their role as expert witnesses. Less consciously on the part of a barrister, perhaps, is the psychological phenomenon of the **misinformation effect**, whereby inaccurate or biased questioning after an event can impact the accurate *recall* of that event (see Itsukushima, Nishi, Maruyama and Takahashi, 2006). It is possible that a particular line or style of questioning may lead to witnesses misrecalling events that they have seen or heard or experienced, and this may also play a role in determining the outcome of a court case (e.g. Klemfuss, Quas and Lyon, 2014). Similarly, in a situation of being questioned it is possible that people may become scared, upset or angry, and this too may impact on their ability to recall events accurately. We might expect that many issues of bias, misinformation and misunderstanding could be pervasive also in relation to members of the jury. A recent study showed that US jurors who experience increases in anger during the sentencing phase of a murder trial are more likely to support a sentence of death (Nuňez, Schweitzer, Chai and Myers, 2015). Clearly the psychologist can do little about these issues, but it is useful to be aware of them. The next 'Where do you stand?' box considers trial by jury.

WHERE DO YOU STAND?

Trial by jury

Trial by jury in serious cases is considered to be one of the most important features of the English legal system and jury service is a legal responsibility that most of us have (if we are 18 years or older, are on the electoral register, and have lived in the UK, Channel Islands, or Isle of Man for a period of at least five years since the age of 13). If you receive a summons and do not attend you can receive a fine of £1,000, unless you are excused for some reason.

Although the legal system attempts to exclude individuals it considers unable or unlikely to be able to discharge their duty to the court appropriately, there are also guidelines through which individuals may be removed from the jury if good cause is demonstrated, and jurors may also be vetted. However, the vast majority of people who are summoned do become jurors. They are then involved in making decisions in matters about which they may not be considered to have any expertise, and are expected to base their decisions purely on the evidence presented in court.

Where do you stand on this issue?

1 Do you think that a jury system like that in the UK is inherently fair or unfair?
2 Jurors may lack relevant expertise, both in the legal and criminal justice system and perhaps also in the specifics of a particular case (such as fraud, or wounding with intent). Is this a disadvantage or advantage for them?
3 Is it possible that defendants will receive unjust sentences because of this system? Or do you believe that because it is the legal system it is necessarily just?

As was the case for the Magistrates' Court, a defendant who has been sentenced by the Crown Court may appeal to the Criminal Division of the Court of Appeal. Further appeals are possible, for example, to the Supreme Court. For countries that are members of the European Union, the highest court is the European Court of Justice.

Legal systems

In the UK, many European countries and the USA, the legal system is referred to as being *adversarial*. This is in contrast to the *inquisitorial* system, as employed in France. There are a number of differences between these two systems that influence sentences and treatment received by an offender. The primary difference is that in an adversarial system the defence and the prosecution can be thought of as being in competition to provide the most convincing case, which is then decided upon by the jury, the judge, or the magistrates. That is, the court may be thought of as impartial, basing its decision on the facts presented. In the inquisitorial system, in contrast, it is a judge who is responsible for asking the questions and weighing up the evidence, and then she or he determines whether a trial is required. If it is decided that a trial *is* required, then that trial is adversarial, with a different judge presiding. In essence, therefore, both systems maintain an adversarial element, but with different methods of determining whether or not a trial will take place. There are two other differences that are important. Firstly, the rules of evidence in adversarial proceedings are stricter because the decisions are not being made by legal professionals. Secondly, in adversarial systems a 'guilty' plea prevents the case from continuing, and may come about as a result of 'plea bargaining' (see below); whereas in the inquisitorial system a 'guilty' plea is simply considered as a part of the overall evidence.

Sentencing

As has been mentioned earlier, the different courts have different sentencing powers, with those of the Magistrates' Court being more restricted. Magistrates' Courts can only impose a maximum custodial sentence of six months and a maximum fine of £5,000 (2017 figures). Just as the *structure* of the courts is not simply described, so the *decision-making* process for sentencing is also complex. This section will briefly outline some of the legal aspects that are taken into consideration when sentences are determined by judges.

It is important to keep in mind the implications of sentences. Clearly, prison sentences remove an individual from society, which should reduce the risk to society. However, a prison sentence also removes that individual from some potentially negative and positive influences in society and may expose them to negative and positive influences in prison, which might contribute either to further offending or to desistance. Sentence length may impact upon whether an individual will be able to access any form of intervention whilst in prison (for example, for anger issues or sexual offending; shorter sentences make it harder to access support due to waiting lists and the time it takes to complete a programme), and decisions about detention under the *Mental Health Act* may result in indeterminate incarceration and the imposition of treatment involving medication. Finally, the debate about the value of imprisonment against the value of community service and other forms of reparation needs to be considered. If the person is considered low risk should society bear the financial burden of putting someone in prison? Can society benefit from having low-risk offenders provide useful services?

Potentially, forensic psychologists may become involved in two places. They are frequently involved in the *assessment* of offenders, either before a trial or before sentencing, and these assessments may play a role in the trial itself (with the forensic psychologists serving as an expert witness) or in the sentencing decision by the judge. Secondly, and depending on the sentence imposed, an offender may become a forensic psychologist's client. For example, when offenders are only fined they are unlikely to see a psychologist; but if they receive a custodial sentence or a community sentence, a forensic psychologist may become involved in further assessments or interventions, such as with a sex-offender treatment programme within prison or in working alongside probation officers or other agencies within the community.

Life sentences

The mandatory life sentence for murder in the UK can be understood as a reaction to the removal of the death penalty in 1965. Such a sentence does not necessarily mean, in fact, that individuals will stay in prison until they die; it means rather that the sentence is indeterminate, with a specified period to be served in prison before an individual can be considered for release. This is to allow for what can be thought of as different levels of 'seriousness' of murder – a strange concept, perhaps, given that in each case the person is responsible for having taken another's life. However, consider the difference between one individual who plans and carries out the killing of a partner for reasons of jealousy, and another who kills a partner with a terminal illness (a so-called 'mercy killing'). In each situation one person causes another's death, yet the motivations are quite different. Depending on our assumptions about behaviour, the former is also likely to be considered as posing a greater risk to society than the latter, in the sense that that individual might offend again. In both these situations, the minimum period that must be served before an application can be made for parole serves the purpose of *punishment*. The period of time served beyond this minimum and until release has been sanctioned serves a *preventative* purpose. Offenders who have been convicted of murder but later released (referred to as 'on licence') can be recalled if a reassessment suggests that they still pose a risk.

Section 269 of the Criminal Justice Act 2003 provides a three-tier system setting out sentencing principles for different classes of murder, but there are also other situations where individuals may receive a life sentence, for example if they are considered to be 'dangerous'. In part this is determined by the nature of the offence (e.g. rape or manslaughter), and in part by a consideration of the risk to the public if that person were to offend again.

Other sentences

Judges usually have a degree of flexibility in determining the sentence they pass. There are a number of factors to be taken into account which may lead a judge to consider that a crime should be viewed as more serious (such as evidence that a rape was planned in advance) or that provide an explanation for why an individual may deserve leniency (such as evidence of provocation). This mirrors the situation described for individuals sentenced for murder: the judge can consider the nature of the offence and take that into account.

Despite this flexibility, some other offences do have what could be thought of as a starting point for the consideration of the eventual sentence. For example, the trafficking of a Class A drug attracts a minimum sentence of seven years and domestic burglary a minimum of three years. Not all sentences are prison sentences: individuals can instead receive Probation Orders or Community Orders, whereby responsibilities and restrictions are placed on the offender, requiring them to undergo some kind of intervention or to take part in work aimed at reparation.

Another possibility is for an individual to receive a **Hospital Order** under the Mental Health Act 2007: in this case, although the individual has been convicted of an offence, the court believes that she or he is suffering from a mental disorder that could be treated appropriately through medical intervention. There are four criteria which must be met for an individual to be detained under this Act:

1. An individual must have, or be suspected of having, a mental disorder.
2. The mental disorder must be of a degree or a nature that requires detention in order that the individual may receive treatment in hospital.
3. The reason for detention must be to protect the public and for the good of the individual.
4. Suitable treatment must be available.

The Act contains a number of sections that deal with the transfer of individuals from prisons, and restriction of leave, for example, and there are provisions that determine who can challenge an order or apply to have one placed on an individual. An individual may, if considered well again, be transferred back to prison. If the person remains unwell, he or she may not go back to prison, and ultimately may spend more time in hospital than might have been the case if he or she had gone to prison.

Plea bargaining

Plea bargaining is a method by which people charged with crimes may try to reduce the seriousness of the charge or the seriousness of the penalty they are facing. There are two circumstances in which this process could be used.

Firstly, a guilty plea, particularly if made early on in the legal process, is taken into account when determining a sentence: this leads to what is referred to as a **sentence discount**. This is now part of law (Criminal Justice Act 2003) and courts are required to consider a guilty plea when determining an individual's sentence. There is some flexibility in how this is calculated, although there are also guidelines. For example, it is recommended that a guilty plea entered as early as possible should lead to a maximum of a one-third discount. Once the trial has begun, however, it is recommended that a guilty plea should result only in a one-tenth reduction.

The second situation occurs when an individual agrees to plead guilty to a lesser charge, which is known as *charge bargaining.* An example would be where an individual originally charged with murder agrees to plead guilty to manslaughter, on the understanding that the change in charge and the guilty plea will both be taken into account in sentencing. In both cases the plea is made without knowing what the difference between the two outcomes might be. The individual's legal team might certainly make informed guesses, but the judge does not provide this information in advance because this could be seen as exerting pressure on a defendant, and pleas must be seen as having been made freely.

Plea bargaining is a controversial issue, as it can be seen as rewarding the guilty who plead guilty and adding further punishment for the innocent who plead not guilty. On the other hand, an early guilty plea can reduce costs and court time.

Issues of appearing in court

Research has demonstrated that both children and adults, whether appearing as witnesses or the accused, find the experience of attending court difficult (for transcriptions of court proceedings where this is apparent, see Rock, 1993). Freshwater and Aldridge (1994) interviewed children and adults, and most of the words they used to describe their appearances in court were negative, such as 'scared', 'intimidated and 'nervous'. There are also reasonable concerns that such experiences may impact on the accuracy of witnesses' recall.

Shuman *et al.* (1994) provide an overview of popular reports of the impact on jurors of traumatic cases, such as the case against Jeffrey Dahmer (an infamous necrophiliac and cannibal in the US who committed offences until 1991). They also provide an account of others' and their own research concerned with the impact on the public of jury service. The anecdotal evidence they report suggests that where cases involve graphic information jurors may experience nightmares, mood swings, and even vomiting. Empirical studies have demonstrated a range of effects, from psychological to physiological illness, including post-traumatic stress disorder (PTSD). Shuman *et al.*'s own work was concerned with the effects of sitting on a jury and compared groups exposed to traumatic evidence (e.g. concerning murder or child abuse) and non-traumatic evidence (e.g. concerning drug possession or burglary). They considered a number of other factors, but in essence they demonstrated that jurors exposed to distressing cases were more likely to experience self-reported symptoms of trauma than those exposed to non-traumatic cases.

Another issue is recall by witnesses. Saywitz and Nathanson (1993) demonstrated that simply questioning children in a mock court about an experience in which they had taken part two weeks previously produced greater memory impairments for recall than with children of the same age who were questioned in their school. A later study (Nathanson and Saywitz, 2003) showed the same memory decrement in the mock courtroom and also an elevated heart rate, suggestive of an experience of greater stress. Given that psychology has already demonstrated the fallibility of eyewitnesses (see Wells and Olson, 2003, for an overview), as well as the inability of juries to detect inaccurate eyewitness accounts (McConkey and Roche, 1989), it is not unreasonable to presume that eyewitness accuracy may become even more impaired under courtroom conditions.

Miller and Flores (2007; see also Chamberlain and Miller, 2008) provide an overview of the stress experienced by juries and judges. The most obvious source of stress is the potential impact of evidence and witness testimony that may be graphic and disturbing, and there is also the additional stress that may be produced by complicated cases which may last for long periods of time and require those involved to process large amounts of information. Additionally, some jurors experience stress simply because of being summoned to be a jury member, because of the disruption to their work and home lives, and through the process of reaching a verdict.

For the alleged offender, too, appearing in court is likely to be stressful, almost regardless of whether or not they plead guilty. An offender who pleads not guilty will face cross-examination, and also the possibility that being convicted after a not-guilty plea may result in a longer sentence. The court environment, concern over the outcome, and the eventual tariff are all likely to impact on offenders' ability to function, particularly for first-time offenders, and that may lead to the same kinds of memory issues found by Saywitz and Nathanson (1993) in children. Further evidence of the impact of court, and indeed of the impact of the entire process of the investigation and court examination, is the existence of *voluntary false confessions* (as opposed to false confessions brought about by coercion), in which innocent individuals plead guilty to offences they did not commit.

Gudjonsson (2003b) provides a good overview of how this may occur during police investigations where, for example, 'reality monitoring' (Johnson and Rye, 1981) may break down under stress. *Reality monitoring* is our capacity to know the difference between memories for events that have actually occurred to us and events that we may remember because we have been told about them or imagined them. If this capacity becomes compromised, people may admit to actions that they did not make, and possibly even to crimes that they did not commit, believing that their memories are accurate. Similarly, witnesses may believe that they have seen, heard or experienced events that did not happen to them. It is plausible that similar effects may occur under the stress of a court appearance. It has been estimated that the number of false guilty pleas is greater than the number of false confessions (Gross *et al.*, 2005), in which case there may be a significant number of individuals who plead guilty to a crime that they have not committed and are in consequence exposed to the subsequent impact of the legal and penal system. Research by Redlich, Summers and Hoover (2010) shows that from a sample of over 1,000 offenders with mental illness, the rates of self-reported false guilty pleas ranged from 27 to 41 per cent across the six sites where participants were recruited. On this basis, they suggest that over 400 members of their sample had made guilty pleas when they were in fact innocent; and approximately 2 per cent of these cases were for serious crimes such as murder and rape. In an earlier paper, Redlich (2006) discussed the potential impact of other factors, such as age, on the likelihood of a false guilty plea, although she suggests that to date there is not enough evidence to know the extent of this impact.

Clearly, the court system has an impact on the individuals who work within it. As this may influence the available evidence, how it is understood, and how it is used in the decision-making process, there are good reasons for psychology to investigate these effects and to attempt to develop a system that is more stable. Unfortunately, aspects of the court system are not routinely open to investigation (although see Rock, 1993), so we are currently unclear about the exact influence of factors such as stress.

Expert witnesses

Psychologists may be called to provide evidence to the court. Primarily, this will be through the provision of reports regarding a particular person, and the psychologist may be directed from either side of the adversarial process. The report is not intended to favour either side, however, but rather to present an impartial opinion and facts. The role of the expert witness is to help in the decision-making processes, both that of the jury and that of the judge, and as such may play an important role in determining the outcome of a trial. The expert witness therefore has both legal and personal responsibility in carrying out that role, and must be scientifically rigorous and also just. Importantly, in England and Wales, it is the judge who decides whether someone is suitable to act as an expert witness – simply having qualifications and experience does not entitle you to act in that role. In 2011 the Law Commission produced a report, *Expert Evidence in Criminal Proceedings in England and Wales*, which provided a comprehensive description of the issue of expertise used in court and a range of recommendations for the use of experts. Some of these recommendations were accepted into the Criminal Procedure Rules in 2014, including the necessity for an expert's report to include information that will allow the court to decide whether the expressed opinion is sufficiently reliable to be admitted as evidence.

As described in Chapter 1, both Münsterberg and Marbe had written about the use of psychology in the legal process in the early 1900s, and the legal profession has gradually recognised the value of psychological expertise, in much the same way that medical expertise was already recognised. It is important to be aware that this shift was not due entirely to the increasing science-base of psychology. As Goodman-Delahunty (1997) suggested, changes in the law allowed for claims of psychological injury, and this necessitated the use of psychological evidence. The history of expertise in the legal process is rife with poor practice (see Ireland, 2010) and in order to overcome this, the Daubert developed guidelines (Daubert, 1993). Although they are not legally binding, these outline a set of principles through which best practice may be preserved in the testimony and reports of expert witnesses. The criteria, known as the **Daubert Trilogy**, are:

1. The testimony is based upon sufficient facts or data.
2. The testimony is the product of reliable principles and methods.
3. The expert has applied the principles and methods reliably to the facts of the case.

Point 2 concerns the scientific basis of data. The work on which tests are based should have been peer-reviewed, have standing in the psychological community, and the level of error should be known. Being guided by such principles has become even more important since a ruling that expert witnesses are no longer immune from claims that there has been negligence or dishonesty in the expert's work (Dyer, 2011; *Jones v. Kaney, 2011*). Forensic psychologists should pay particular attention to this so as not to stray beyond their skills or areas of expertise. Examples of poor practice include using psychometric tests with which one is unfamiliar or that one does not fully understand, or assessing or commenting on an area of psychology (or any other profession) when that would be better done by another expert.

The Criminal Procedure Rules were developed with the aim that criminal cases would be carried out justly. Part 33 of these rules deals specifically with expert witnesses and what is required of them. Freckelton and Selby (2002) have provided five rules that they suggest have become commonly accepted in guiding expert evidence, which cover expertise, common knowledge, the area of expertise, the 'ultimate issue', and the basis for giving an opinion, as set out in Table 14.2.

Rule	Explanation
Expertise	The individual should be an expert on the basis of their knowledge and experience so that they will be able to assist the court
Common knowledge	The knowledge and expertise of the individual must surpass that which might be considered common knowledge or common sense and thus it is required by the court
Area of expertise	The knowledge and expertise of the individual should be recognised as credible by their peers
Ultimate issue	Expert evidence should express an opinion that is the role of the court to decide. It is important to note that this has been abolished as an issue within the courts in England and Wales since 1972
Basis	The expert opinion must be based on that individual's own observations

Table 14.2 Five rules for the admission of expert evidence proposed by Freckelton and Selby.

Source: adapted from Freckelton, I. & Selby, H. (2002). Expert Evidence: Law, Practice, Procedure and Advocacy. Sydney: Lawbook Co. Reproduced with permission of Thomson Reuters (Professional) Australia Limited, legal.thomsonreuters.com.au

Ultimately, the expert is providing information to help the court make its decision, and that should be kept in mind during both the assessment and the report-writing stages. During the preparation for an assessment this is a non-trivial matter. Although the expert will be asked to address certain issues concerning an individual and the legal case to come, until the assessment has started it is not always apparent what may be necessary to fulfil one's duty to the court. It is also important to see the direct link between the assessment and the report, ensuring that the issues to be addressed in the report are included in the assessment, and that the assessment is coherent.

Once the assessment has been performed, the report must be written. A report is important in a number of ways (see Melton *et al.*, 2018). Not only does it provide a detailed account of the findings and opinions of the psychologist, with the intention of assisting the court, it also provides a record of, for example, an individual's qualifications for being a suitable expert, the sources used in compiling the report, meetings with the client, the scientific bases of the tests used and so on. As such it should be considered an important source of information providing the context for the report, what was involved, and what was concluded. According to Melton *et al.* (2018), a well-written report may negate the need for a court appearance (and the consequential stress involved). The Criminal Procedure Rules of 2007 describe the components of a report from an expert witness in England and Wales, as set out in Table 14.3.

• Give details of the expert's qualifications, relevant experience and accreditation
• Give details of any literature or other information which the expert has relied on in making the report
• Provide a statement setting out the substance of all facts given to the expert which are material to the opinions expressed in the report, or upon which those opinions are based
• Make clear which of the facts stated in the report are within the expert's own knowledge
• Description of who carried out any examination, measurement, test or experiment which the expert has used for the report and (i) give the qualifications, relevant experience and accreditation of that person, (ii) state whether or not the examination, measurement, test or experiment was carried out under the expert's supervision, and (iii) summarise the findings on which the expert relies
• Where there is a range of opinion on the matters dealt with in the report (i) summarise the range of opinion, and (ii) give reasons for their own opinion
• If the expert is not able to give an opinion without qualification, state the qualification
• A summary of the conclusions reached.
• A statement that the expert understands their duty to the court, and has complied and will continue to comply with that duty
• A declaration of truth as a witness statement

Table 14.3 The content of an expert report, as described by the Criminal Procedure Rules, 2007.

Source: adapted from The Criminal Procedure Rules; The Criminal Practice Directions (October 2015 edition as amended April, October & November 2016 and February, April, August & October 2017), Ministry of Justice. © Crown copyright 2017, licensed under the Open Government Licence v3.0: http://www.nationalarchives.gov.uk/doc/open-government-licence/version/3

The use of these guidelines as a template for a court report should help to prevent many of the possible shortcomings of such reports. A report may not be used, particularly if it does not add to the position that the solicitors are taking. If it *is* used, however, there is a possibility that the expert may be called to court and may be required to defend the report against cross-examination.

Of course, being involved at any of the different stages of the court system has the potential of exposing professionals to stressors, such as appearing in court, working to the often tight deadlines that legal work can require, and assessing individuals with distressing backgrounds who have committed distressing offences. It is important to remain mindful of factors and to reflect on how they might impact on our work and on how we perceive the world and interact with it, both in the short term and in the longer term.

Conclusion

The preceding material provides an overview of a part of the English and Welsh court system, the part with which forensic psychologists are most likely to deal in carrying out their work. It is fairly clear that the system is not straightforward, and there will be many occasions when the nuances of the law and the legal system may contradict our assumptions concerning law and justice. It is useful to understand the basics of the legal process in order to have some understanding of how one's clients may have come to be in their current situation (the journey that they have taken through the system), to have a sense of what possible impact that situation might have had on their lives (e.g. their education or their relationships), and the impact of any ongoing legal issues they may face. For the forensic psychologist involved in private assessments and expert witness work, it is essential to have some knowledge of the ways in which the courts work, and also of the demands placed on those who do this kind of work.

This chapter has examined a number of structural features of the English and Welsh legal system, providing an overview of some of its important structures and how psychology is interwoven, sometimes unknowingly, into these structures. Our aim has been to give the forensic psychologist a sense of how the legal system may influence outcomes for an individual, with the idea that this leads to consideration of the implications for that individual as to their circumstances and their contact with psychology. In Chapter 15 we will consider some further aspects of the legal system.

14

Chapter summary

» Movement through the court system of England and Wales (and indeed through any national court system) is complex and depends on a vast array of factors.

» At its most basic, we can think of courts as differing in the seriousness of the cases they can consider, and thus the seriousness of the sentences they can impose.

» The imposition of sentences is a complex decision-making process. It is one of the factors that will determine the kinds of people whom a forensic psychologist may assess and for whom the forensic psychologist may provide interventions.

» If involved in the legal proceedings, the forensic psychologist may be called to act as an expert witness, a role that has important responsibilities and consequences.

Further reading

The following texts would be good initial sources of information in learning more about the English and Welsh legal system.

» Cownie, F., Bradney, A. and Burton, M. (2007), *English Legal System in Context*, 4th edition (Oxford: Oxford University Press). This, along with the Slapper and Kelly reference below, provides a good overview of the English legal system using language and examples that should be suitable for those without a specific legal education.

» Ireland, J. L. (2010). Legal consulting: providing expertise in written and oral testimony. In Ireland, C. A. and Fisher, M. J. (eds), *Consultancy and Advising in Forensic Practice: Empirical and Practical Guidelines*, pp. 108–122 (Chichester: BPS-Blackwell). This chapter provides a forensic psychologist's perspective, from an experienced forensic practitioner and academic, of the issues of appearing in court.

» Slapper, G. and Kelly, D. (2009), *The English Legal System*, 10th edition (London: Routledge-Cavendish). As noted above, this is a useful text in gaining a deeper understanding of the English legal system.

Considering Evidence: Witnesses, Experts and Juries

We have already considered a number of issues concerned with the structure of the legal process (see Chapter 14), which relies on legal professionals, witnesses, defendants and juries, and the specific orientation that each brings to the setting. Whereas the previous chapter dealt primarily with issues of the structure of the court system, this chapter deals with other aspects of the process, including cross-examination, juries and standards of evidence. At the conclusion of this chapter the reader should have a good overview of many of the factors that can impact on the outcome of a trial. Forensic psychologists need to be aware of these issues for two reasons: firstly that they may become expert witnesses, and secondly that they are relevant when working with other professionals involved in this part of the forensic journey – for example, in preparing court reports and in understanding the experiences of their clients.

Chapter objectives

- To understand some of the more detailed aspects of working within the court system.
- To recognise the importance of language in the court process.
- To appreciate the different standards of evidence that may be applicable in different situations.
- To learn about jury decision-making.
- To be aware of the areas where the forensic psychologist may be able to work, and the knowledge that is necessary in order to do that work in an informed way.

Cross-examination in criminal trials

As was mentioned in Chapter 14, in both the UK and the USA the legal system is referred to as being an 'adversarial' system, in which the defence and the prosecution can be thought of as in competition with one another. The role of each side is to present the most compelling case it can, with a view to persuading the jury or the judge that its own portrayal of the case is the best representation of what is most likely to have actually happened. In such a situation, the legal professionals from both sides are able to ask questions of any witnesses and of the defendant (or defendants). Where that questioning is being carried out by what could be construed as 'the other side', it is referred to as **cross-examination**. Doak (2005) wrote: 'The entire criminal process is designed to culminate in a confrontational showdown between the prosecution and the accused' (p. 297).

The same adversarial relationship may be assumed to occur between the defence attorney and the witnesses for the prosecution or the victims, and we might expect that such a confrontational approach could have negative consequences for them. Indeed, Walker and Louw (2005) demonstrated that *some* victims of sexual offences did report having felt intimidated by the defence attorney during cross-examination (20 per cent from a group of adult and child victims in South Africa), whereas the majority felt that sufficient steps were taken to protect them during this process (85 per cent). Thus, although victims felt that they were suitably cared for and supported during the trial process, some of these, even with that level of support, still felt intimidated.

As some individuals do feel intimidated by the legal process, it is important to consider the impact that this might have on how people interact with the legal system, and the extent to which this might be responsible for *changes* in the reporting of crime, the prosecution of crime, and the conviction for crime. Early research has suggested that positive attitudes regarding how victims believe that the police will treat them increase the likelihood of reporting sexual offences (Dukes and Mattley, 1977). In a more recent study, Fisher, Daigle, Cullen and Turner (2003) found that in a sample of American college women who had been raped, 17.4 per cent chose not to report this to the police because they were concerned that the police would be hostile in their treatment of them. Some studies have shown that where cases have gone to trial, the rape victims report an increase in fear, depression and anxiety (Sales, Baum and Shore, 1984); and where the victims feel that their experience within the legal system has been difficult, they report higher levels of symptoms of post-traumatic stress (Campbell *et al.*, 1999). Although it is not clear from this research that it is the adversarial approach itself that results in individuals feeling fearful about becoming involved in the legal system – there might be other concerns, such as a fear of being targeted by the accused at a later date, or not wanting the details of one's experience being publically reported – it is likely that this approach plays a part. Indeed, the passing in the US of **rape shield laws** in the early 1970s (which limited the extent to which the sexual history of someone making an accusation of rape can be presented in court) are an acknowledgement of this possibility, and similar laws have been adopted in a variety of other countries too. (In the UK, this is covered in the Youth Justice and Criminal Evidence Act 1999.)

From a US perspective, Lininger (2005) provides an accessible overview of some of the issues that cross-examination in an adversarial setting may raise. He identifies that cross-examination may be characterised as '**revictimization**', particularly in cases of sexual assault and domestic violence, and stems from what Estrich (1987), a professor of law and a victim of rape, has described thus: 'the law's abhorrence of the rapist in stranger cases like mine has been matched only by its mistrust of the victim who claims to have been raped by a friend or a neighbour or an acquaintance' (p. 4).

The role of language

Smith (2006) suggests that cross-examination is the most difficult part of a barrister's job, and provides a number of reasons why this is the case. Mostly he suggests that this is because successful cross-examination requires a high degree of preparation, during which the barrister seeks to identify potential weaknesses in a witness's evidence. Smith also writes that one question is the key to building a successful cross-examination: 'What do I want this witness to say?' By the end of the cross-examination, says Smith, 'Hopefully you will have weakened, damaged or even destroyed, by skilful questioning, the effect of the evidence' (p. 17). Further, Haydock and Sonsteng (1994), in their manual on advocacy – the act of arguing a particular position or point – suggest that the barrister should be attempting to control the responses of the witness so that she or he portrays events in the way the *barrister* prefers, rather than according to the understanding of the witness. Often this will include phrasing questions so that they are closed questions that demand simple or *Yes/No* answers (Smith, 2006), which research has shown is the form of questioning that most easily results in manipulation (Lamb *et al.*, 2002). For example, Tourangeau and Smith (1996) showed that in response to a closed question asking about the number of sexual partners, a closed format with an emphasis on lower numbers led to significantly lower reporting than a closed format with an emphasis on higher numbers, suggesting that respondents may be biased by the boundaries that closed questions may imply. Thus responses can be biased by barristers in favour of their client's position. Schaeffer and Presser's (2003) review of the science of asking questions provides a useful overview of some of the issues about how questions may impact upon responses.

Eades (1995) has also suggested that lawyers use language to manipulate individuals in the court, and research has demonstrated that this may be more powerful when the person under questioning is vulnerable in some way (Brennan and Brennan, 1988). As an example of the use of biased language, Schmid and Fiedler (1998) carried out a study demonstrating that in a simulated courtroom setting, defence and prosecution representatives differed in the linguistic strategies adopted in their **closing speeches**. Those acting for the defence emphasised the more positive aspects of defendants and tended to ignore their negative aspects, but did the opposite when referring to the victim of the offence. Those acting for the prosecution showed the opposite pattern. This might seem fairly obvious, given what the two sides are trying to achieve. However, the authors analysed the *ways* in which the different representatives talked about the victim or the defendant. They found that prosecutors tended to be negative towards the defendant, implying that the defendant had intended to cause the crime and that this was *internally* driven; whereas the defence representatives tended to imply *external* causes for defendants' negative attributes. A second study by the same authors demonstrated that some of these strategies do indeed have an impact on verdicts and punishments, as determined by the individual decisions of people asked to act as jury members.

The use of language in courts is an interesting area to consider, given that the process of making a decision requires assessing the *evidence*, most of which is presented verbally, and – although it may be uncomfortable to accept this – assessing the *person* who gives that evidence. Taslitz (2006) presents an interesting review of how language in the courts plays an important role in outcomes, with jurors making decisions that are based at least partly on the perceived credibility and competence of witnesses, as portrayed by the witnesses' use of gendered language, identified as either 'women's language' or 'men's language'. Taslitz suggests that there are stereotypical language differences between males and females, and that assumptions about these differences lead to women mistakenly being assumed to be more caring than men, but less intelligent, competent and credible. The potential ramifications of this are quite alarming, particularly when considered in the light of convictions where the victims of the offences that are themselves gendered, such as rape (here considering the rape of a female by a male). If females are considered to be less credible on the basis of the language they use, how is that likely to influence a jury? There is a recognised problem of *case attrition* – few cases of rape are prosecuted; even fewer lead to convictions (see Campbell, 2006); and in some instances these conviction rates are falling (Larcombe, 2011). To what extent might this be a result of the effect of gendered language? Equally troubling is that even though we know that language *might* be influencing jurors' decision-making, it is not clear how that influence could be mitigated. It is also important to consider the effect language might have on the forensic psychologist who is assessing a victim, and the extent to which such language influences might play a role in impacting upon the assumed credibility of professionals when they are acting as expert witnesses.

Given the facts that the court process is adversarial, and that barristers clearly plan that by the end they will have 'weakened, damaged or even destroyed' some individuals' evidence (see above), it is not surprising that children, adults and even trained professionals find the process of cross-examination uncomfortable (see Reder, Lucey and Fellow-Smith, 1993). Westcott and Page (2002) have suggested that for children who have been sexually abused, cross-examination, if not conducted appropriately, may produce some of the same effects as the original abuse. Chapter 12 considered suggestibility and false confessions, and the same concerns arise here too, as with greater pressures and greater publicity, and fewer restrictions on interviewing techniques in the court, the possibility increases that people could become more suggestible. For example, Schooler and Loftus (1986) discussed barristers' use of negative feedback during questioning: a technique whereby the barrister implies that the witness's previous response may have been inaccurate, such as 'Is it possible that you might be mistaken, and that what you actually heard was ... ?' They demonstrated that such feedback may negatively influence witnesses' confidence in their own memory, and also make them more suggestible. As with many aspects of psychology, this idea is not new; Stern (1939) provided an interesting case example of a witness who appeared to be basing her testimony on the questions that were asked of her during her initial interviews. Research by Zajac and Hayne (2003, 2006) showed that cross-examination leads to children changing both previously incorrect and previously correct answers, which seems to support this concern. However, the Royal Commission on Criminal Justice (Home Office, 1993a) included the advice to judges that they should be wary of, and should intervene in, cases where bullying or intimidation was used during cross-examination. While that should be of some help, it is not clear how this advice is to be enacted. One approach to supporting vulnerable people in the UK came from the Youth Justice and Criminal Evidence Act 1999 (see Ellison, 2001), which allowed 'intermediaries' into the court to help explain questions and to provide support to the witness. A subsequent study demonstrated that prosecuting barristers were positive about their experiences of intermediaries being used during preparatory interviews of victims of sexual offences (see Walker and Louw, 2007).

Regardless of the science of examination and cross-examination, there may be an issue of greater concern: to what extent are witnesses being manipulated towards a particular description of events (or at least to imply such a version to the jury) rather than towards the truth? This issue is considered by Summers (1999), who provides two reasons why legal truth and actual truth may diverge: through issues of the legal process (e.g. some evidence being declared inadmissible, for example because it was found during an illegal search) or through court procedures (e.g. one side having a more highly skilled legal team). Additionally, one may consider that the very existence of an adversarial process could result in a desire to win, irrespective of the truth. The realisation that justice and truth may not always be the same has been expressed in the mass media, as exemplified by a line from the 2009 film, *Law Abiding Citizen*, spoken by Jamie Foxx: 'It's not what you know, Clyde, it's what you can prove in court.'

Expert witness evidence

As mentioned above, one of the areas on which cross-examination might focus is the evidence used in the case. For example, a barrister might challenge either a witness's competence – particularly in the case of expert witnesses: a variety of professionals such as psychiatrists, forensic psychologists, firearms experts and so on – or how evidence was obtained.

Whether an individual is deemed to be an 'expert' is determined by the trial judge, although this decision is guided by the law: experts are considered to be such on the basis of the expertise they have have gained through formal study and training or experience, or a combination of both, and that their expertise will add value to the evidence. The history of expert witnesses in the UK is both lengthy and complex. In the 1500s, 'experts' could be called to be jury members or to provide advice to the court, or they could be witnesses for the plaintiff or the defendant. For example, a jury of women might be called in cases of disputed pregnancy; language scholars to advise the court on contracts written in Latin; or a tradesman defendant might call another tradesman if he were being sued over poor workmanship, as for example in the tanning of hides (see Learned Hand, 1901). However, none of these individuals had any special status as an 'expert' – knowledge of the facts under discussion was sufficient for someone to be considered able to provide testimony and to effectively act as a jury.

Lord Mansfield (1782, in *Folkes v. Chadd*) suggested a change to this procedure, which can be seen as the first attempt at clarifying the legal status of expert witnesses and what was acceptable from them with regard to evidence. He said: 'On certain matters, such as those of science or art, upon which the court itself cannot form an opinion, special study, skill or experience being required for the purpose, "expert" witnesses may give evidence of their opinion' (Durston, 2011, p. 461). It is thus considered that the case to which Mansfield was referring, which was based on deciding whether some artificially constructed embankments had resulted in the eventual silting up of a harbour, provided particular status to individuals who had specific, scientific knowledge (see Golan, 2007) that allowed them to provide informed opinions. Of course the idea was not simply that experts could provide opinions, but rather that their opinions, based on their knowledge, experience and investigations (for example, testing materials or assessing clients), would be based on scientific facts. In practice, we might see the real difference as being that experts were permitted to give conclusions, based on their analysis of the evidence, which is not something that other witnesses were permitted to do.

Forensic psychologists, like their medical colleagues and many other professionals, are admitted to court to provide expert evidence. However, expert opinion in the courts has not been without its critics, as an example provided by Golan (2007, p. 256) from a 19th-century US judge, Judge Eindlich, highlights:

> Indeed, it is difficult to conceive of language within the bounds of decent and temperate criticism, which ought to be regarded as excessively severe in commenting upon the expert testimony nuisance as it has, of late years, been infesting our courts. In the way of wasting the public's time, in the way of burdening litigants with expense, and in the way of beclouding the real issues to be tried and effecting miscarriages of justice, it has grown to the proportions of an offensive scandal. Instead of being an aid in the administration of the law, it has become a positive hindrance to it. Instead of assisting in the approximation of the truth, it has become the means of obscuring it ... expert testimony is today discredited and rightly discredited by the courts, and ridiculed by the hard common sense of the people.

Although this extreme view has not resulted in the banning of expert witnesses, it does raise some important issues for the professional to consider. Having been asked to provide expert testimony, one might consider the extent to which the assessment and the subsequent report might 'obscure' or 'becloud' the real issues and the truth. Additionally, one would want to consider the possibility that the trial process might be difficult for the professionals themselves. In a study concerned with criminal barristers' views of psychology in the courtroom, the barristers identified a number of favoured techniques for discrediting expert witnesses, including highlighting factual errors and contradictions with other sources (including evidence from other expert witnesses), and suggesting the presence of bias in the report (Leslie, Young, Valentine and Gudjonsson, 2007).

In the UK, the status of expert witness testimony was reviewed by The Law Commission (2011), in response to the view that 'expert opinion evidence was being admitted in criminal proceedings too readily, with insufficient scrutiny' (p. 1). This parallels an earlier comment by Freckelton and Selby (2002), who described the English approach to allowing novel psychological evidence as 'benevolent acquiescence' (p. 79). The guidelines that were published are very similar to those currently in use in the US Federal court system and a number of individual states, which are known as the **Daubert Standard**. These guidelines replace the earlier standards for scientific evidence (though still used in some states) known as the *Frye Standard*, based on an American court case concerned with the admissibility of polygraph evidence: it was determined that expert opinion had to be based on scientific methods that were established and accepted within the particular field (see Greve and Bianchini, 2004). The Daubert Standard is somewhat more demanding in requiring that the theory has been or could be tested, that there has been peer review of studies (based on the idea that this should identify any substantive flaws), that error rates are known, and that the theory is generally accepted within the relevant scientific community. However, these four factors are not considered necessarily to be exhaustive; instead they may be seen as the *minimum* level that evidence must reach if it is to be considered acceptable to the Court.

The Daubert Standard grew from a case in 1993, in which a US chemical company (Merrell Dow Pharmaceuticals) was sued on the basis that one of its products was alleged to have resulted in birth defects. Since then, the Daubert Standard has been added to by the outcome of two further cases, *Joiner* and *Kumho Tire*, resulting in what is referred to as the Daubert Trilogy for codifying the rules of admissibility of expert testimony in US Courts. Where the trilogy has been accepted in its entirety by states – and it has not been accepted by all states (see Bernstein and Jackson, 2004) – the new rules state that expert testimony is acceptable if:

1. The testimony is based on sufficient facts or data.
2. The testimony is the product of reliable principles and methods.
3. The expert has applied the principles and methods reliably to the facts of the case.

Canada too has adopted the Daubert Standard and, as mentioned above, the UK is moving towards something similar. This is in response to a number of cases where scientific evidence has been called into question, for example the cases of Clark (EWCA, 2003) and Cannings (EWCA, 2004), both involving the deaths of children. In both cases the convictions of the mothers, Sally Clark and Angela Cannings, for killing their children were quashed, but for quite different reasons. In the case of Sally Clark the conviction was quashed because of evidence of misconduct and non-disclosure by an expert witness, and the suggestion that statistical evidence from another expert witness had been found to be flawed. The Cannings case linked more directly to issues of expert evidence: in that case the conviction was eventually quashed when the Court of Appeal found that the convictions were unsafe. This was because the original expert evidence had suggested that the deaths of *three* children from unexplained causes – Cannings had been convicted of two murders – was so rare that it could come about only if a parent were involved in the deaths (in this case, through asphyxiation). With the publication of new research suggesting that such a pattern of deaths from natural causes *was* possible within a single family, the Appeal judges decided that there was disagreement between experts as to how likely such a series of events might be. As there was a possibility that three children from the same family could all die unexpectedly and with no identifiable cause (such as harm from another person), Cannings could not be convicted of murder. Thus what is counted as expertise, as facts or as reliable methods may all change over time as we develop a greater understanding of matters such as sudden infant death, for example, or genetics, or disease, or a range of other areas about which experts may be called to give evidence in court. The status of expertise is considered in the following 'Where do you stand?' box.

WHERE DO YOU STAND?

The status of expertise

For the forensic practitioner, the status of expertise is not simply an academic issue. When the guidelines for expert evidence do change in the UK (or in individual states in the US), this could have important implications for the assessment and reporting practices of professionals presenting at court, and for the extent to which their expertise could be challenged. This in turn will require that thought is given to the criteria for acceptable expert testimony. Where the Daubert Trilogy has been accepted in the US, the issue of something being generally accepted within a scientific community appears to have been dropped, but it may be retained in the UK. This could be important, as shown by the case of Angela Cannings relating to the idea of what is generally accepted, as the original experts were of the opinion that it is generally accepted that multiple unexplained child deaths in a single family are indicative of a crime having taken place. Newer evidence influenced what is now generally accepted in these kinds of cases. However, the Trilogy standards raise a number of questions. For example, what would count as 'sufficient facts or data' and how do we characterise reliability when considering principles and methods and their application?

Within forensic psychological assessments, psychometrics are often used. If our reports are used in court, we may be expected to provide expert testimony and to support our choice of psychometrics, interpretation, and so on. Questions might relate to the reliability of psychometrics in general or of a particular test, the extent to which a particular interpretation fits with a specific individual, and how the test was administered.

Where do you stand on this issue?

How do you think that forensic psychologists might be able to ensure that their work will continue to be accepted by the courts?

The rationale offered by the Law Commission as to why there was a need for new guidelines in the UK is that expert witnesses are permitted to express opinions and that – in the nature of the fact that they are experts – their knowledge will be *outside* what might be expected of a juror. There is therefore a concern that jurors may be influenced by an expert's professional *status* rather than by the reliability of the *evidence* (an issue raised in the case of Sally Clark – see above). Some studies do indicate that factors such as the expert's gender may have an impact on the jury's decision (e.g., Schuller, Terry and McKimmie, 2001), and in mock-jury studies – see the 'Focus on …' box – if an expert has been paid impacts on the extent to which they are considered to have been 'bought' rather than being impartial (e.g. Cooper and Neuhaus, 2000). Boccaccini and Brodsky (2002) have demonstrated in a survey study that the public are more likely to believe experts who do practical work in the field of their expertise rather than those who are non-practising academics or experts for the court, and that they are more likely to believe experts who are not being *paid* for their expertise.

FOCUS ON …

Mock juries

Research on real juries is not permitted in England and Wales – any systematic observation of processes and substance of jury decision-making in real criminal cases is prohibited by the Contempt of Court Act 1981 (HMSO, 1981). Instead, **mock juries** have been used to simulate the processes that occur in real-life juries.

In typical mock-jury studies, part of a trial is presented either in written form or via videotape. Participants take on the role of jurors, deliberating and eventually reaching a decision on the case using the evidence presented (see Memon, Vrij and Bull, 2003). There are some advantages associated with this method. One is that it allows a high degree of control in the manipulation of variables; another is that it allows insight into the deliberation process and the information on which jurors base their decisions.

Research suggests that mock-jury research is effective in evaluating how individuals reach legal decisions (Freeman, 2006). A number of studies have found few differences between the verdicts of mock juries and those of real-life juries (Kerr, Nerenz and Herrick, 1979), so such studies do provide useful insight into what goes on in real-life juries (Ellison and Munro, 2010). However, one needs to be vigilant in assessing the research, as there are some studies that are described as mock-jury designs in which only individual decisions are analysed (e.g. Dunlap, Hodell, Golding and Wasarhaley, 2012), and these ignore the possible impact of the group decision-making process on individual decisions.

Questions

1 The mock-jury method has been criticised on methodological grounds (Breau and Brook, 2007). To what extent do you think mock-jury studies cannot replicate real juries because the mock-jury decision has no real impact on a defendant's life (or that of victims)?

2 To what extent do you think that the setting of a real jury and studies carried out in psychology laboratories might differ in important ways? Could the setting have an impact on the decisions of a jury?

Standards of evidence

Having considered some of the issues relating to expert evidence, we now consider some more general principles that cover what is considered as evidence within a case. Evidence consists of three categories:

- witness evidence
- documentary evidence
- 'real' evidence (or physical evidence).

The last term refers to items other than documents – for example, an alleged murder weapon. For each piece of evidence that falls into one of these categories, three areas are considered: its *relevance* (whether it proves or disproves a fact), its *admissibility* (whether it relates to the facts, and was obtained in an appropriate manner, for example during a legal search of a property or an appropriately conducted interview), and its *weight* (the extent to which the evidence can be relied on by the court).

In criminal cases, evidence is used in order to demonstrate 'beyond reasonable doubt' the elements of the offence, and it is for the prosecution to provide the information necessary to reach this standard. There is one situation where this is not true, and that is when the defendant is attempting to use a defence of 'diminished responsibility' – and in those situations the defence is required to provide proof 'beyond reasonable doubt' that there are grounds for accepting that defence: see the 'Focus on ...' box below.

FOCUS ON ...

Diminished responsibility

In England, **diminished responsibility** is known as a *partial defence*, and can be used in cases of murder. If successful, the offence of *murder* is reclassified as **manslaughter**, which has the effect of changing the likely sentence.

The principal argument in making this defence is that at the time of the murder, the individual's behaviour was influenced by an 'abnormality of mental functioning', and that this significantly contributed to the defendant's behaviour. The 'abnormality' must have arisen from a recognised medical condition. For example, an individual who was experiencing delusions as a result of a psychotic disorder such as schizophrenia may not be found guilty of murder if it can be shown, beyond reasonable doubt, that at the time of the murder the delusions significantly contributed to the murder.

The actual definition of 'diminished responsibility' leads to some interesting outcomes. A murder committed when a person is drunk would not result in a successful diminished responsibility plea, unless it could be shown that the drunkenness came about due to an abnormality of mental functioning that substantially impaired the offender's mental responsibility. Alcoholism, however, *is* a recognised medical condition that could impair one's mental functioning, and alcoholism may of course lead to drinking. As such it is not the *drunkenness* that is the issue, but the *mental functioning* that resulted in drunkenness.

Prins (1995) considered the issue of diminished responsibility in relation to three well-known cases, those of Peter Sutcliffe, Dennis Nilsen and Jeffrey Dahmer. Each was a multiple murderer, Sutcliffe and Nilsen from the UK and Dahmer from the US.

Nilsen was convicted in 1983 of the murder of six young men and the attempted murder of two more, although some sources claim that he murdered fifteen people and Nilsen himself, in a 1993 interview, claimed to be responsible for the deaths of twelve people. He is described as having strangled and drowned his victims, then cleaned their bodies and in some cases performed sexual acts on them, before eventually dismembering the bodies, discarding some parts and keeping others. He was eventually caught when blocked drains running from this house were found to contain human flesh and bones. As Prins (1995) notes, Nilsen's legal team suggested that, given the acts that he had committed, he must have had a mental abnormality; but the psychiatrists involved in the case were unable to agree on a diagnosis or on whether it resulted in the required abnormality of mind. At the same time part of Nilsen's diagnosis was that he had a personality disorder and that this was considered untreatable. As there seemed little value in Nilsen receiving hospital treatment, he was imprisoned on the basis of multiple counts of murder, rather than being sectioned to a secure hospital.

Question

Why do you think it might be important to maintain diminished responsibility as a partial defence?

This standard – 'beyond reasonable doubt' – is the standard used in most adversarial systems, for example in the UK and in the USA, but it is somewhat vague. It suggests that if a reasonable person has no reasonable doubts about the guilt of a defendant, then that defendant should be found guilty. As has been recognised in various jurisdictions, this can lead to certain problems. For example, in Canada the courts have recommended that jurors are given an explanation as to what 'reasonable doubt' means; whereas in England it is less usual that jurors are explicitly told to consider a person's guilt in relation to reasonable doubt; and in the US, according to Greene and Bornstein (2000), jurors receive 'precious little guidance' (p. 743) as to the standard expected by the court. So what is a 'reasonable person', and what counts as 'reasonable doubt'? Woody and Greene (2012) provide two descriptions of reasonable doubt: one quantitative, the other qualitative. Their quantitative example is that 'the defendant is presumed innocent unless the evidence against him has at least 91 per cent probability of truth'. Their qualitative description is: 'proof that leaves you firmly convinced of the defendant's guilt' (p. 859). This may not greatly help, if we require a precise decision about how we measure that the evidence meets at least 91 per cent probability, and given that we cannot know whether one person's firm conviction is of the same standard as someone else's.

As for the 'reasonable person', Miller and Perry (2012) debate this issue with regard to civil actions, highlighting that it is an issue that has 'bedeviled and divided courts and scholars for centuries' (p. 323). They compare two positions: whether reasonableness should be defined by *morality* (that is, reasonable people are people who act in a moral way), or whether it should be defined by *reality* or statistics (that is, how the majority of people would be expected to act in a particular situation). Although these authors state that they do not wish to endorse either position, they also argue that defining reasonableness through reality is impossible, and in effect they therefore endorse *morality* as the basis for judging reasonableness. Such a definition may be useful in allowing the law to recognise that someone has done wrong (that is, that she or he has harmed someone), but given the circumstances that the person's behaviour was not *immoral* (for example, that she or he harmed the other person in self-defence) – is society primarily moral? Niebuhr (1963) suggests not; individuals are *able* to be moral, says Niebuhr, but when groups form this capacity may be reduced. Another issue raised by the concept of the 'reasonable person', as discussed by Eastman (2000), is that of 'legal artefacts' (Eastman, p. 90). How the law defines this individual and what this would actually mean psychologically may differ greatly. Eastman considers the example of murder. Someone accused of murder could have that charge reduced to manslaughter on grounds of provocation. Such a reduction is based on the idea that if a *reasonable* person is *unreasonably* provoked, that person's reaction might be to kill the provocateur. This may make sense in law, but psychologically is this how we understand reasonable people to react? Statistically, murder as a response to unreasonable provocation, whatever that might be, is unlikely. As Eastman suggests, rather than there necessarily being any psychological truth behind the idea, this thinking is based on the law's need to identify different kinds of murder as having different levels of 'badness'. Similar arguments can be made for other artefacts on which the law relies, such as an individual being 'irrational' or 'acting automatically'.

Such a discussion might be intellectually interesting, but does an awareness of these issues have any important implications for psychology? Two examples suggest that there are elements that it *is* useful to be aware of. The first example is the existence of different *standards of proof*. In criminal law the standard is 'beyond reasonable doubt'; in civil cases (see below), the standard is 'the balance of probabilities'. This is not simply different wording: it is also a different standard of proof. The assumption is that juries in different kinds of cases, where the standard of proof differs, are able and willing to apply these different standards in their deliberations. A mock-jury study by Woody and Greene (2012) demonstrated that in their deliberations related to awarding damages jurors tend *not* to consider the standards of evidence, the authors' conclusion being that for most people these are novel concepts and that real understanding of them demands a high degree of thinking. As these different standards of proof may be too complex for most people to understand, they play only a small role in determining how evidence is considered. The second example is based on a study that considers 'noise' in information, which can be thought of as adding doubt about the accuracy of the information. In this study, 'noise' impacted on participants' decisions to punish one another. An interesting study by Grechenig, Nicklisch and Thöni (2010) used an online game of cooperation that allows individuals to use sanctions in order to manage cooperation and enforce prosocial behaviour. A degree of 'noise' was programmed into the game environment so that an individual's behaviour might be misrepresented to the other players, in such a way that they might mistakenly construe that person's behaviour as non-cooperative and might then choose to punish him or her for non-cooperation. If people have a tendency to make decisions based on doubt, or conversely how certain they can be that the information they have is accurate, then we would expect that the more inaccurate, or noisy, information is about a person's behaviour the less likely we should be to punish them as we are less sure of their guilt. In fact, however, the more the environment was likely to be providing inaccurate information, the more severely participants tended to punish one another. In other words, in this study, the less certain participants could be that the information they received was a true representation of another person's behaviour, the more likely they were to punish that person when the information indicated (possibly erroneously) that she or he had not cooperated. These two studies highlight the possibility that although the law identifies the central importance of issues such as levels of *proof* and *certainty*, it is entirely possible that within courts these are not the issues that accurately and consistently drive the deliberations of jurors.

In civil cases, the standard of proof is described as being 'on the balance of probabilities', which is considered to be a lower standard of proof than 'beyond reasonable doubt'. Here the idea is that if a judge is persuaded that one description of events is more likely than the other (and that neither is improbable), then the decision will be made in favour of the *more likely* description. Lord Nicholls explained it as follows (*re H (Minors) [1996] AC 563 at 586*):

> The balance of probability standard means that a court is satisfied an event occurred if the court considers that, on the evidence, the occurrence of the event was more likely than not. When assessing the probabilities the court will have in mind as a factor, to whatever extent is appropriate in the particular case, that the more serious the allegation the less likely it is that the event occurred and, hence, the stronger should be the evidence before the court concludes that the allegation is established on the balance of probability. Fraud is usually less likely than negligence. Deliberate physical injury is usually less likely than accidental physical injury.

The explanation of why the standards of proof are different is that in criminal cases a defendant who is found guilty may lose her or his liberty; whereas in civil cases, a defendant who is found guilty is likely to face only a fine. Additionally, the idea of harshly punishing an innocent person is considered far worse than allowing a guilty person to go free. (For an interesting discussion using decision theory to understand standards of proof, see Kaplan, 1967–1968.)

Admissibility of psychological evidence

Psychological evidence has been permitted in the civil courts for some time, for example in cases of trademark infringement (see Bartol and Bartol, 2006). In criminal cases, psychological evidence may play a role in a number of different areas, such as sentencing, risk assessment and **fitness to plead**, but it has not been so easily accepted as other forms of expertise, such as medical expertise. Golan (2007) provides some interesting examples of early cases where psychology played a part in the courtroom, including a case from 1906 that involved Münsterberg (see Chapter 1).

In part this difficulty for psychological evidence has been due to the Frye Standard in the USA and the Turner Rule in the UK (see above, and Colman and Mackay, 1995). The *Frye Standard* stated that expert opinion had to be based on scientific methods that were established and accepted within the particular field, and psychology has struggled to become identified with the use of scientific methods that are established and accepted. (In part this is historical, due to the relative youth of psychology as a discipline; and in part it is because psychology has not always been considered as meeting the rigorous standards set by the physical sciences regarding scientific method.) In contrast, the *Turner Rule* states that expert testimony is not required when it deals with matters considered to be 'of common knowledge and experience', a decision first made in a case where a man called Turner killed his girlfriend after she told him of her infidelities (*R. v. Turner*, 1975). The defence intended to prove provocation through the testimony of a psychiatrist, but that testimony was ruled as inadmissible because 'jurors do not need psychiatrists to tell them how ordinary folk who are not suffering from any mental illness are likely to react to the stresses and strains of life' (p. 841). The Turner Rule was overturned by a later case in which a mother, Sally Emery, appealed a conviction for failing to protect her child. In that case the judge allowed two expert witnesses, a psychologist and a psychiatrist, to provide evidence suggesting that Sally Emery was suffering from PTSD and battered woman syndrome, and would therefore not have been able to protect her child. The Emery decision led to a relaxation of the Turner Rule, as it was recognised that in some circumstances it was unlikely that jurors would have an in-depth understanding of psychology – that the necessary level of understanding might go beyond 'common knowledge'. Despite this decision, there have still been cases where expert psychological testimony has been deemed inadmissible; and if the UK does adopt a Daubert-style standard, it will be interesting to see how psychology fares under such scrutiny (see the earlier section concerned with cross-examination).

Mackay and Colman (1996) provide some examples of psychology not being permitted in original trial hearings (although on appeal this decision might have been changed). In one case a defendant tried to argue that as he was particularly vulnerable to threats – and he provided evidence of this psychological vulnerability – the fact that he had acted illegally but whilst under threat should be taken into consideration. This was not allowed in court, although the reasoning was not that the evidence itself was in any way improper, but rather that the basis of this defendant's vulnerability could not be proved to be due to some form of mental illness. It is not clear whether in part this ruling was based on the idea that a jury would not be able to comprehend how else a person might be vulnerable to threats if there were no diagnosable 'cause', and that it might be difficult to explain this without also implying that *everyone* might be more or less vulnerable to threats. However, research has demonstrated that if evidence is presented to jurors but found to be inadmissible, that evidence may still influence the jury if they believe the evidence to be reliable (e.g., Hodson, Hooper, Dovidio and Gaertner, 2005). Great care needs to be taken in relation to *when* a decision is made about the admissibility or otherwise of evidence.

The situation has changed over the last twenty years (see Gudjonsson, 2006; Gudjonsson and Haward, 1998) as psychological research has become more widely accepted in general, and as its impact on legal issues has become more broadly recognised. A study by Leslie *et al.* (2007) indicated that criminal barristers have developed a view of the roles of clinical psychologists in legal proceedings (e.g. in diagnosing personality disorders or in making an assessment of an individual's social skills), and where a clinical psychologist would be preferred to a psychiatrist (e.g. as in the case of confession reliability – see below). One of the reasons given for preferring one or the other profession related to how jurors and judges view individuals with medical qualifications; another was concerns about psychometric tests. However, the preference for psychology over psychiatry with regard to confession reliability is likely to be that if there is no diagnosable condition, psychiatrists are not as able as psychologists to comment on what *other* factors might impact upon the reliability of a confession – issues of personality, social skills, IQ and mental faculties are not their area of expertise. Although the study by Leslie *et al.* (2007) suggests that there is still a bias in favouring (or assuming that judges favour) medical qualifications over others, this research does give a sense that *clinical psychology* has carved out a recognised niche in legal settings. It is not unlikely that, given time, *forensic* psychology will be similarly regarded, which – given the definition of forensic psychology provided by Gudjonsson and Haward (1998), as 'that branch of applied psychology which is concerned with the collection, examination and presentation of evidence for judicial purposes' – should not be surprising. See Gudjonsson (2003b) for a description of the process that clinical and forensic psychology have gone through in order to be accepted in legal proceedings.

How is forensic psychologists' work used in court?

Depending on the settings in which forensic psychologists are employed, their work may be used in court in a number of different ways. For example, a forensic psychologist working in a community service for sexual offenders may be required to put together a report or expert evidence. This may be based on an assessment, or on the outcome of some form of intervention. This work may then be used by a referrer to help to prevent the individual concerned from having contact with his or her children, or to assist in *increasing* contact with the children, or to suggest that further psychological work would be advised. Within **secure services,** similar psychological reports could be used to help inform decisions regarding an individual moving to a lower level of security or regarding changes to an individual's leave restrictions, if they are permitted to be away from the hospital for periods of time. In the US, prior to sentencing a forensic psychologist might provide a report on an individual's drug abuse, with the possibility that this report might influence the sentencing decision (see Krauss and Goldstein, 2007).

Sometimes reports may be used in ways that conflict with the intended purpose of the report, because the referrer may have a particular goal and that may not be the same as that of the psychologist. For example, a forensic psychologist may identify a risk of harm to a child living at home and therefore recommend that work could be done to reduce the risk, with the long-term aim of the family being reunited. This report might then be used to identify that there is a current risk, and that a child should therefore be protected by being moved into care. In some ways, the role could be thought of as working either for the prosecution or for the defence, although the psychologist cannot decide how their work may be used. However, forensic psychologists may also be asked by legal professionals to carry out an assessment, specifically for a court case, and in those circumstances it is clear whether it is the defence or the prosecution that is requesting the work, and the psychologist can take that into account in choosing whether or not to take it on. This choice raises an interesting dilemma, as discussed in the next 'Where do you stand?' box.

WHERE DO YOU STAND?

Should you take the case?

Once the decision to carry out an assessment has been made, it is crucial to be aware of the exact requirements of the instruction. That will lay out the questions that are to be addressed and will very tightly define, or start to define, how the assessment might be approached.

It is also important to be aware of any dynamics that might already exist between you and the client. Greenberg and Shuman (2007) describe a case in which a Dr Bell was acting as expert witness for an individual, had been treating that individual, and was also that individual's sister.

Note that it is not the psychologist's role to comment on whether an individual is innocent or guilty, but rather to provide information that will assist the court in understanding important psychological factors that may be linked to issues such as witness accuracy, risk, or particular behaviours.

The expectation is that psychologists will at all times work within the ethical guidelines of their service and those of their professional bodies. In the UK, these would be both the British Psychological Society and the Health and Care Professions Council. In the US this would be the American Psychological Association (APA).

As an expert witness, the forensic psychologist's duty is to the court, regardless of who is paying. Even so, as forensic psychologists are able to choose which cases they take, is there a danger of showing (and making explicit) some kind of bias? For example, if one only accepts cases that are paid for by the defence, is there a reason for this? It is useful to think through the rationale for taking each particular case so that any potential conflicts of interest can be identified and managed before they impact on the work being undertaken.

Where do you stand on this issue?

If you were asked to provide a report for and possibly testimony to a court, how would each of the following issues impact on your decision? What are your reasons?

1 You are asked by the defence.
2 You are offered a substantial sum of money for your assessment and report.
3 The client's offence is particularly gruesome.
4 The client's offence reminds you of past events that happened to you.
5 The client has many convictions for sexual offences against children.
6 You have been working therapeutically with this client.
7 The client made a complaint about you in the past.
8 During your work with this client, you have shared details of your family.
9 You are struggling financially.

Ethical issues in court

Although the issue of ethics is, as will be seen in Chapter 20, applied very broadly throughout psychology, it is particularly important in the consideration of work in court. It is essential during assessments that the client is fairly treated and engages with the assessment having been fully informed of the purpose of the assessment. Indeed the APA, the NCME (National Council of Measurement in Education), and the AERA (American Educational Research Association) jointly produced guidelines for the ethical use of assessment (American Educational Research Association, American Psychological Association, & National Council of Measurement in Education, 1999).

Given that the psychologist is attempting to provide a true and accurate appraisal of someone, it may seem counter-intuitive that the individual should be fully informed about the nature of testing, allowing him or her the opportunity to try to **fake good**. However, a true and accurate appraisal by the psychologist cannot be achieved through coercion, subterfuge, or dishonesty. The APA provides an overview of the rights and responsibilities of test takers and of testers. For example, testers are expected to adhere to the test requirements as laid out in the manual, which may determine how the test is administered, the context in which should be administered, and the qualifications of the person administering it. If the tester does not follow these guidelines, the validity and reliability of the test may be compromised. Test takers have rights, such as the right to understand the purpose of the tests and the right to have test results kept confidential. Test takers' responsibilities are that they should follow the test instructions and represent themselves honestly during the testing. Although individuals may lie and 'fake good' on psychometrics and in interviews, forensic psychologists have recourse to the various 'lie scales' provided with some tests and can consult research and other sources of background information, and are thus in a position to comment on the likelihood that each test taker is – or is not – representing himself or herself honestly and openly. It is important to be aware of the rights of clients to have access to their scores, their responses, and any notes made by the psychologist during the testing process, and also the situations where this disclosure may be legally refused.

One would expect that similar ethical guidelines relating to the assessment of individuals would also apply to the treatment of offenders, and in principle this is the case. However, as Glaser (2003) points out, individuals working in the treatment of sex offenders may not be able to adhere to these ethical regulations. (Note that Glaser is referring specifically to treating sexual offenders where in some cases offenders are *obliged* to accept treatment.) Glaser offers six examples in which traditional ethical values may be broken, one of which is offenders having to accept treatment from non-clinicians or unqualified staff (i.e. not qualified psychologists, but psychologists in training), and another is when the main concern of treatment is the good of society rather than the good of the individual. Glaser's proposed solution to this problem is to consider professional behaviour in the light of a therapeutic jurisprudence model, which seeks to be fair and proportionate, and with the minimum infringement of an individual's rights, whilst using the legal process to support and assist individuals in managing their offending behaviour (for more details, see the section below on 'Therapeutic jurisprudence'). With this approach it is possible, according to Glaser, to deal with the otherwise hypocritical and ethical dilemma whereby 'clinicians abandon any pretence to have a primary or even a principal interest in their clients' personal needs' (Glaser, 2003, p. 152).

So far we have considered a variety of aspects that are essential to the court and the importance of psychology within court proceedings, looking at these from the perspective of barristers and witnesses. Now we will briefly consider another central component of criminal courts: the jury.

Jury decision-making

The jury is an important part of the justice system. The modern jury system has its historical roots in 12th-century England, having evolved from a group of individuals who *investigated* crimes to a group who are told about investigations and then make decisions regarding guilt and innocence. Originally, juries' decisions were based on what the jurors already knew, rather than on the presentation of evidence. It was not until the *Magna Carta* of 1297 that the idea of 'trial by one's peers' became standard practice in England (as remains so today), and that then became the purpose of the jury. In different countries juries have different responsibilities; and the size of the jury may differ too – whereas the standard in England is 12, as often portrayed in film and television, the number is 15 in Scotland. In the US, a Grand Jury can consist of 16–23 individuals – Grand Juries decide whether there is enough evidence that a person has committed a crime and should go to court – whereas a trial jury may have 6–12 people.

Despite the differences that may exist, the basic purpose of trial by jury is the same: to determine the guilt or innocence of a defendant. However, research has demonstrated that the size of juries does matter. Saks and Marti (1997) published a meta-analysis of US studies and found that larger juries are more likely to be accurate in recalling the information presented during the trial, they take longer to reach a decision, and they are more likely to be representative of the local community. (This may suggest that a Scottish jury is likely to have more reliable outcomes than others.) Unfortunately, however, the nature of group decision-making is not so clear-cut: in *non-jury* situations such as focus groups, smaller groups may be more effective (Kao and Couzin, 2014). It is not yet clear whether there is an optimal size. It may well prove that the determining factor is not the size of the jury but the individuals available to sit on the jury and the nature of the case that is on trial.

As a form of decision-making, the work of the jury is open to the same kinds of biases and influences as are other forms of decision-making. It is also open to the influences of group processes, as was well presented in the 1957 film, *12 Angry Men*, in which a jury are determining the guilt or innocence of an 18-year-old boy alleged to have stabbed his father. The film depicts the jurors battling with the process of decision-making, and highlights how preconceptions might influence their deliberations and conclusions. This fictional account is particularly powerful, but reality too provides us with some interesting examples to consider. Kassin and Wrightsman (1988) described a case from the USA in which the majority of a jury believed in demonic possession and because of this a defendant was not convicted; and McEwan (2000) mentions a UK case where jury members took part in séance to divine an individual's guilt. Clearly these are unusual cases, but they demonstrate that the jury is not immune to some of the vagaries that impact on life – and as the jury is not required to provide a rationale for its decision, the examples above were discovered only by chance.

As juries play such a crucial role, it is important to have some idea of the other factors that may play a part in a jury's decision, over and above consideration of the facts of the case. However, the process of the jury's work is not open to direct study. Even so, some studies conducted in the US have investigated aspects such as information load (e.g. Heuer and Penrod, 1994). Heuer and Penrod found that jurors self-reported that the greater the amount of information presented, the less they felt able to understand the issues considered at trial, and the less confidence they had in their verdict. More recently, Horowitz *et al.* (2001) found in mock-jury studies that the information load impacted upon verdicts, as did the level of technicality of the testimony. High information loads led to plaintiffs being disadvantaged, and high technicality was judged as more credible and therefore had a greater impact on the verdict than information that was less technical. In the UK, research has mostly been concerned with the behaviour of mock juries or investigating individuals after the fact, and this may not be a fair reflection of what really goes on during deliberation. Most obviously, perhaps, within a jury there is a combination of *individual* decision-making and *group* decision-making. At the level of the individual, we are concerned with basic psychological principles concerning attention, comprehension, recall, biases brought about by preconceptions and previous knowledge (see Carlson and Russo, 2001), and the impact of emotions (Feigenson, 2010). Further, there are additional forms of information (other than evidence) that may impact upon a juror's thinking, such as publicity regarding the trial, any instructions that a jury might be given by the judge, the inclusion of expert testimony, and potential exposure to evidence that is ultimately ruled as inadmissible. Daftary-Kapur, Dumas and Penrod (2010) provided a useful review of the ways in which these and other events may impact on juries, and suggested some ideas about how these impacts might be remedied. For instance, they detailed evidence indicating that pre-trial publicity can influence factors such as the credibility of defendants, their likeability, and the eventual trial verdict. Equally concerning is evidence from studies concerned with pre-trial publicity which suggests that participants mistakenly perceive this information as being part of the evidence in the trial. One possible solution suggested by the authors is for the trial to change location to a venue where there has been less publicity. In large countries and with cases that focus on local issues, this might have a beneficial effect; but where cases are of national importance or the country is small, such a move may not have much value, as the authors acknowledge.

With these factors at play there can be a wide range of opinions after a trial within a jury. Research has demonstrated that in almost 90 per cent of trials the initial majority verdict at the start of deliberations is the eventual verdict of the jury (Bornstein and Greene, 2011), thus it is plausible that the group dynamics are less important than the individual processes at work. Indeed, research suggests that jurors are more likely to be swayed by evidence than by pressure from the majority of the jury (Salerno and Diamond, 2010), although recent evidence suggests that the use of 'Victim Impact Statements' (where victims or their families can address the jury through a letter), which are not strictly evidence, increase the likelihood that a death penalty will be imposed in capital cases in the USA (Paternoster and Deise, 2011). One study of jurors' thinking is offered by Finch and Munro (2006) concerned with the interpretation of the Sexual Offences Act 2003 in relation to rape, providing some useful insights into the deliberation process. Their research indicates that some of the ideas on which the Sexual

Offences Act rests are not universally understood. For example, regarding the issue of consent in cases of rape, some participants believed that despite the complainant being so drunk that she was barely able to move and could only slur her words, if she did not consent to the defendant undressing her she would have been able to communicate this. Similarly, it seemed that consent was assumed based on events that occurred prior to the undressing, such as the woman had been at a party and had been drinking, rather than specifically linked to the events at the time of the alleged rape. We cannot assume that these prejudices are peculiar to individuals who participate in studies and as such they may impact on deliberations in courts. They also inform us about how some members of society construe issues such as women's behaviour and implied consent, the effect of alcohol on one's ability to interact effectively and meaningfully in the world, and what constitutes harmful, immoral, or illegal behaviour.

Another interesting issue in the case of juror decision-making is the extent to which a decision can be seen as an expression of a juror's judgment. There may be occasions when an individual's overt decision is in conflict with a decision that is in their own interest (see McLean and Urken, 1995). By this we mean that a juror may decide, based on the evidence, that an individual should be found not guilty of a sexual assault on some kind of legal technicality (rather than being innocent on the balance of probabilities), but may also have the view that people who commit sexual assaults should not be in the community. However, Shelton (2006) recommends that although not exactly the same as other examples of group decision-making, a thorough understanding of general group decision-making processes would be helpful in improving the jury process and that this is an important endeavour given the consequences of a jury's decision. The following 'Where do you stand?' box considers issues of jury service.

WHERE DO YOU STAND?

Jury service

In the UK, jury service is a requirement of citizens, other than in a few exceptional cases. For example, you must be between 18 and 69 years of age, be registered to vote in the UK, and have lived in the UK for more than 5 years after the age of 13. You may not serve if you are on bail, if you have been to prison or on a Community Order in the last 10 years, if you have received a prison sentence of 5 years or more, if you are regularly receiving treatment for a mental disorder, or if you do not have the capacity to manage your own affairs. Full-time serving military personnel, coroners and their staff can be excused. (For a video from the Ministry of Justice, see to the right.)

The process for becoming a jury member in the UK is as follows. You will receive a Jury Summons in the post, having been randomly selected to take part in jury service. You will need to fill in information on two pages and return those, keeping the remaining pages to have available when you appear for service. Failure to do so can result in a fine. You will wait in the jury area with the other members of the public selected for that jury period and names will be drawn at random for each trial. For any one trial approximately 15 people are randomly selected from the larger pool and from this smaller group the jury of 12 is again randomly selected.

Ministry of Justice Video

www.youtube.com/watch?v=yQGekF-72xQ&t=9s

Jury service in the US

In the US, potential jury members go through a process referred to as *voir dire* in which they are questioned in order to determine whether they have any biases or prejudices that might threaten their ability to remain impartial. The barristers – referred to as attorneys in the US – are responsible for this process and in theory they are seeking to ensure that the trial is fair for their side of the case. One might wonder if this process might not also be a strategy through which attorneys try to influence the likely outcome of a trial into the courtroom.

Some books and films do depict this process as one in which attorneys try to influence the outcome of the trial by choosing jurors likely to be sympathetic to their client.

Where do you stand on this issue?

As people called for service are identified randomly, a jury may consist of a broad range of people.

1. Do you think that such a system is likely to result in fair trials?
2. Do you think jurors need to be specifically trained? If so, what should they be trained in?
3. Are there any other criteria you would suggest should be included so as to prevent particular individuals from serving on juries?

Trauma in jury members

The jury is a crucial element of many legal systems and its decisions have important consequences for defendants. In order to reach these decisions jurors are exposed to descriptions of events, victims, photographs, and the consideration of complex material. Given this, to what extent are jurors affected by what they are exposed to in their role and might this impact upon their decision? A study by Thompson and Dennison (2004) looked at this issue in relation to effects of graphic evidence of violence on mock jurors. They demonstrated that the graphic evidence did not directly influence the verdicts, but that it did interact with the jurors pre-existing biases, and increased the level of stress they experienced. Previous studies have demonstrated an impact of graphic evidence on verdicts (e.g., Douglas, Lyon, and Ogloff, 1997) where the use of pictures both increases the likelihood of a guilty verdict and the extent to which mock jurors report distress. However, when compared to a group who did not receive pictures on how fair they thought they were being in their decision both groups report an equal level of fairness, suggesting that we may not be aware of material that biases us. An earlier study by Shuman and colleagues (1994) examined questionnaire responses from jurors who had been involved in either traumatic (e.g., murder, aggravated sexual assault) or non-traumatic (credit card abuse, unauthorised use of a motor vehicle) trials. Their data suggest that there are general health issues linked to more traumatic trials and a greater risk of depression, but no higher likelihood of PTSD. Jurors sitting through traumatic trials were six times more likely to meet DSM criteria for depression than the other jurors. Miller and Bornstein (2004) provide a useful overview of some of the causes and possible interventions for juror-related stress (typically provided by counsellors or clinical psychologists) and suggest that in some cases jurors may experience the same levels of stress as victims of crime.

The judge's summing-up and directions

At the end of a criminal trial the judge provides a summary for the jury and provides them with a degree of direction with the aim of helping them understand the nature of the task that they have before them. The summary includes the law concerning each of the charges against the defendant, what the prosecution must prove in order for the defendant to be found guilty, the key points of the case, and the strengths and weaknesses of each side's arguments, along with their duties to the court. Clearly this may have some impact upon the jurors and as such the idea is that this should be impartial. However, at the very least the summary contains what this particular judge considers the key points and the strengths and weaknesses. A recent study has demonstrated that, unsurprisingly, judges are prone to the same kinds of biases as the general population, and that these can impact upon their judgments. Rachlinski, Johnson, Wistrich and Guthrie (2008) have demonstrated the presence of racial bias in American trial judges in a sample of 133 judges, and found that the extent of the bias played a part in the harshness of their judgments. There are also trial examples where the judge has been perhaps less than impartial. Burgess (2009, p. 65) provides one example of a judge's summary in a case of murder: 'you have before you two different stories, one of which sounds highly probable, and fits in with all the known facts, and the other is so utterly ridiculous as to be an obvious fabrication'. Moreover, judges and juries do not seem to be similarly influenced by evidence, suggesting that there are at least two different approaches being adopted in this part of the process. Eisenberg and colleagues (2005) have demonstrated that judges tend to have a lower conviction threshold than jurors, thus they are more likely to convict an individual than jurors would be, based on the same evidence. Boniface (2005) gives some examples of judicial directions and points out that there are a number of potential problems with this system that has been developed in order to assist the jury. Firstly is the issue that the jury must understand and apply the directions of the judge, even if this is contrary to their own beliefs, and it is not possible for the judge to test this because juries do not have to provide a rationale for their verdict. A study by Kassin and Sukel (1997) sheds some light on this issue. They were interested in the impact on mock juries of the circumstances under which a confession was obtained, either freely or with the possibility that it was under pressure. In the latter case, some participants received information that the judge instructed them that the confession was either admissible or not (due to coercion). They found that the presence of a confession, regardless of the judge's instruction, was more likely to lead to a guilty verdict. A second concern is the potentially contradictory nature of a judge's summary. The example Boniface provides is where there has been a delay in a complaint being made against a defendant, as perhaps may happen in an allegation of rape. For a variety of reasons, such as injury and trauma, there may be a reasonable delay and the jury would have to be informed that such a delay is not necessarily an indication that the allegation is false. However, they may also be warned that they can take the evidence of delay into account when deciding if the alleged victim can be believed. In such situations the summary may be adding confusion to the jury's deliberations.

In countries and states where there is no longer a death penalty for crime the ultimate sanction is the life sentence (Hood and Hoyle, 2015). Many of the factors discussed earlier in this chapter and in previous chapters may impact on a decision as to the suitability of any given sentence but in the UK there is a mandatory life sentence for a conviction of murder. In the next section we will consider some of the issues related to life sentencing.

Sentencing

Life sentences

In the UK, once an individual has been convicted of murder, a *life sentence* is the only sanction available. However, few of the individuals who are given a life sentence receive what is known as a *whole life order*. The few who do represent exceptional circumstances in which the offence is considered particularly serious, such as the murder of a child, if the child was abducted or if there was a sexual or sadistic motivation, or a murder carried out for a political, a religious, or an ideological cause (Criminal Justice Act 2003). A life sentence in the UK usually comes with a *minimum term* which must be served before parole can be considered, and this takes into account the type of offence, factors such as an early guilty plea and any mitigating factors (e.g. a lack of premeditation). For different kinds of offences, there are different minimum term starting points. For example, the killing of an on-duty police officer by an individual over 21 years of age attracts a minimum term of 30 years; whereas if a murder is committed and a knife was involved, the minimum starting point is typically 25 years. As an example, the multiple murderer Dennis Nilsen, who was convicted of six murders and two attempted murders, received eight life sentences to be served concurrently, with a minimum of 25 years. Three years later the Home Secretary changed this to a whole life order. Whole life orders do not apply to offenders between 18 and 21: for offences that would attract a whole life order for an adult offender (someone over 21), the younger offender would attract a starting point of 30 years.

It may seem contradictory to refer to a sentence as 'life' when there is a possibility of release once the minimum time has been served. In practice, the minimum is a guideline, and the time actually served is also dependent on the inmate's behaviour, whether the offender has taken part in any mandated treatment, and (prior to release) the assessed level of risk of recidivism and danger to the public, for example. Even when they have been released, 'lifers' may be recalled to prison if they breach the conditions of their release, without the requirement of a further trial, and these conditions may be imposed for life.

Griffin and O'Donnell (2012) have suggested that the ways in which life sentences are managed within a country provides useful information about a nation's approach to criminal justice, and in a 2009 survey they presented, the UK had the highest percentage of 'lifers' (in relation to sentenced prisoners overall) in a wide range of countries, including the USA, Germany, New Zealand and Australia. Griffin and O'Donnell also highlighted the issue of the release of long-term prisoners. With an extended period of incarceration it is likely that a large range of factors come into play, including changes in relationships, society and technology. Ardley (2005) presented an overview of one particular open prison (a type of prison with minimum restrictions allowing inmates time to re-engage in society by working, spending time at home because they are believed to pose a low level of risk) which is responsible for preparing lifers for reintegration back into society. She identified a number of areas that the prison targets in order to achieve successful reintegration, including personal development (such as education, vocational training and unescorted leave), relationship counselling and stress management, along with what might be considered more offence-focused work which looks at, for example, victim empathy and anger management. Another issue of concern is to what extent these kinds of sentences are beneficial or therapeutic for the offender, and to what extent they are simply punishment or 'warehousing' in order to protect the public. (We consider this below in the section on 'Therapeutic jurisprudence'.)

Although previously in the UK the Home Secretary was responsible for determining whether a whole life order was appropriate, this responsibility has since been taken away. Initially, in 2000, this power was removed in relation to offences committed by anyone under 18; and in 2002 the same decision was made with respect to adult offenders. Now only judges can set tariffs, and only the Court of Appeal or the United Kingdom Supreme Court can make changes to a tariff. In the US, first-degree murder comes with a mandatory sentence of life without the possibility of parole, whether the state has the death penalty or not (and assuming that the death penalty is not imposed: Appleton and Grøver, 2007). Appleton and Grøver (2007, p. 599) provide an example of the outline of one state's description of its law. Washington State makes it absolutely clear that such a person will remain in prison, regardless:

> A person sentenced to life imprisonment under this section shall not have that sentence suspended, deferred or commuted by any judicial officer and the board of prison terms and paroles or its successor may not parole such prisoner nor reduce the period of confinement in any manner whatsoever including but not limited to any sort of good-time calculation. The Department of Social and Health Services or its successor or any executive official may not permit such prisoner to participate in any sort of release or furlough program.

The 'tariff'

When there is no mandatory sentence, the sentence imposed is intended in some way to reflect the severity of the offence. A problem is how such a scale of severity can be developed when there are many different types of crime, and in addition there are other issues to be considered such as the presence or absence of violence. Moreover, is

15

it reasonable for acts to be scaled by severity without considering the impact on the particular victim? This problem was made obvious by work that looked at how different groups of people understand the concept of justice, and how one might construct a scale of just consequences – something that Serba and Nathan (1984) referred to as a 'standardised justice model' (p. 221). In their study they asked different populations (e.g. prisoners and police officers) to rate the severity of a variety of different possible tariff outcomes, from the death penalty to small fines. Interestingly, although there was consistency in the *orders* of severity of the tariffs, the populations differed in how *serious* they perceived different outcomes to be. For example, police officers considered the death penalty to be more serious than life in prison, but to a much lesser extent than the prisoners. Serba and Nathan hypothesise that the prisoners might see a death sentence as a possibility for them, whereas the police might consider it as another form of justice.

In the UK the Sentencing Council provides a number of guidelines for sentencing (see 'Further reading'), which cover different kinds of offences, the Magistrates' Court, and circumstances that might reduce a sentence (e.g. an early guilty plea). The Council is a part of the Ministry of Justice, and along with developing guidelines it is also responsible for related research. For example, in 2011 the Council examined the public's attitude to sentence reductions for a guilty plea (Dawes *et al.*, 2011). In this work the authors noted that the public are of the view that reductions should come into force only if the guilty plea is entered early, and not once the trial has begun; and that the reduction should not be applied generally but should be dependent on other factors, such as whether the offender is a recidivist or a first-time offender. Additionally, they are concerned with the impact of sentencing decisions on victims and on the general public.

The former point addresses, to some extent, the question raised earlier about whether it is possible to develop a scale of severity without understanding the impact on the victim. It is certainly true that numerous cases have been highlighted by the media in which victims have suggested that the punishment given to an offender does not fit their own view of the punishment that would be appropriate, and this reflects the perceived view that prison is not punishment at all (e.g. Ardley, 2005). For example, in one case of assault the victim considered that his attacker should have received a sentence of 2 years, not just the 12 weeks he actually did receive ('12 weeks? Jack should have been locked up for two years', *The Sun*, 15 April 2009), and a family whose son was killed considered that the 10-year sentence his killer received was not sufficient ('10 years in jail isn't enough for Brandon's killer', *The Sun*, 9 February, 2009). Of course, one must consider the possibility that the view of justice and sentencing held by readers of UK tabloids may not be representative of the view held by people in the UK as a whole, but even if that were true they are nevertheless representative of a *part* of UK society. A 2013 report by the Ministry of Justice identifies that there is indeed variation in UK attitudes, but it states that most people believe that the courts are too lenient, whilst also underestimating the severity of sentencing practices (Ministry of Justice, 2013a). In a linked report, it identified ways in which public knowledge could be improved (Ministry of Justice, 2013b) by, for example, providing clear and consistent information about sentences, and ceasing to use the term 'life' as the public consider this to be an example of misbranding.

Legal systems have a number of goals: to reduce the danger to society by removing dangerous individuals from within it; to provide interventions for dangerous people so that they may be reintegrated into society; to inform perpetrators and society of the consequences of illegal behaviour, so that this awareness acts as a deterrent; and to redress harm that has been visited upon victims (or their families). Different nationalities and cultures see these goals as being met by the sentence received within their own legal system, be that community work, prison, or the death penalty. However, some writers have suggested that the legal process itself may also act in a therapeutic manner, and this is an aspect we will now consider. The following 'Where do you stand?' box will consider the death penalty.

WHERE DO YOU STAND?

The death penalty

According to Amnesty International, in June 2016 there were 58 countries who still used the death penalty. (An additional 31 countries had not abolished the practice, but had not used it for the previous 10 years. Although the last execution in Mongolia was 2008, Amnesty International included it on the list.) Amnesty estimated that in 2015 1,634 people were executed, nearly 600 more than recorded in 2014.

The argument that the death penalty works as a deterrent is not supported by research literature (e.g. Kovandzic, Vieraitis and Boots, 2009), despite some research suggesting that for every execution lives are saved (8 lives, according to Ehrlich, 1975; 18, according to Dezhbakhsh, Rubin and Shepherd, 2003). Early work by Marquart and Sorensen (1989) showed that of 558 individuals who had been on death row for murder but were released when the US Supreme Court cancelled all death sentences in 1972, 1 per cent committed another murder - a figure that suggests that the death penalty might not be required to keep society safe.

Although the death penalty may appear to be targeted at the offender, it is important to consider the potential impact on that person's family (see Sharp, 2005), on the family of the person who was offended against, and on those whose responsibility it is to carry out the sentence.

Finally, it is important to consider the possibility of a wrongful conviction. In the case of wrongful imprisonment people can be released and receive financial compensation, but there is no obvious manner to respond if someone has been executed. The UK abolished the death penalty in 1965, it is still available as a sentence in some US states and in various other countries.

Where do you stand on this issue?

1 Given what is said above, do you believe that the death penalty has a place in society?
2 Do you think that there are any circumstances in which the death penalty is an appropriate response to crime? If so, what are those circumstances, and why is it appropriate?
3 Regardless of your views above, what arguments could you present to support or refute the death penalty?

Therapeutic jurisprudence

As should be clear by now, there is a wealth of psychology involved in the court process, in relation to biases, decision-making, persuasion and so on. To some extent the impact that these processes may have on jurors (discussed in this chapter), witnesses and defendants (see Chapter 14) has been informally recognised by the courts and the wider legal system, and that awareness is demonstrated, for example, when judges allow breaks after distressing testimony has been given or if a cross-examination has been particularly gruelling (for an interesting comparison of judges' behaviour with witnesses who have or do not have a learning disability, see O'Kelly, Kebbell, Hatton and Johnson, 2003). In addition to these influences, another psychological element of the legal process has been identified and that is the possibility that the legal process might be able to act as a 'therapeutic agent' (Winick, 1997, p. 185). Such thinking may also be considered a response to the finding that imprisonment *per se* does not appear to impact upon recidivism, at least in the UK (see Lloyd, Mair and Hough, 1994).

Winick (1997) suggested that the various legal professions and the rule of law, acting as social forces, have an *impact* on individuals; and that as that is the case, they may have either negative or positive consequences for those individuals. In order to maximise the positive influence the legal system might have on prosocial thinking and behaviour, it is imperative that the consequences of this impact, and how they come about, be fully investigated. As examples,

Winick wondered whether aspects of the legal system might impact on factors such as an individual's acceptance of responsibility, compliance with an order, or victim empathy. Kavanagh (1995) used the American military's former 'Don't Ask, Don't Tell' rule to show how an apparently simple rule can have huge consequences for an individual's well-being; and thus how the legal system can, as in this case, act in an *anti*-therapeutic manner. This rule – repealed in 2010 – is concerned with the fact that as homosexuality was a cause for 'administrative separation' (in effect, being fired from military service), senior officers were not permitted to investigate a person's alleged homosexuality unless there was evidence of it, and gay individuals were barred from talking about homosexual relationships. Kavanagh points out that although this was intended to be a very specific rule, it contributed to issues such as social isolation and marginalisation because it inadvertently restricted discussion of other topics or at least the depth to which they could be discussed.

In contrast to the above example, Casey and Rottman (2000) described a number of innovative attempts to promote the therapeutic elements of the legal process. The development of specific 'drug courts', with the aim of supporting individuals through court-monitored detoxification programmes rather than sending them to prison, is a later example of such innovation (see Cooper, 2003). The purpose of this approach is to address the underlying *cause* of criminal behaviour in these individuals by providing them with opportunities to change. (However, the actual underlying cause may be deeper than at first appears – it is possible that substance misuse is just one part of a more generally antisocial approach to dealing with the world, and may thus be an indication of other difficulties too.) A similar approach is taken with some 'Mental Health' courts in the US, where decisions regarding sentencing may be made in order to ensure fast assessment and treatment of mental health issues – treatment which, as long as there are no immediate risk concerns, may take the place of a custodial sentence. Both versions of a court may allow individuals to access services, be exposed to more positive role models, and begin to escape from the cycle of crime and incarceration. Another example, which recognises the importance of maintaining close relationships, is the use of **therapeutic jurisprudence** concepts in 'family courts', where approaches such as dispute resolution and family support may be more advantageous than incarceration. Erez and Hartley (2003) outlined a range of ways in which the legal process could support immigrant women who have experienced domestic violence – from the initial process of reporting that violence (or being reluctant to report it) to the provision of testimony – by recognising the important cultural and gender issues that these women experience.

In the UK there is a structure through which the court is able to impact directly upon issues of well-being using the Powers of Criminal Courts Act 1973, as described by McGuire (2000). Under this Act, a judge can delay sentencing for up to six months, which would allow time for other assessments and work to be done that may directly impact upon recidivism. However, as McGuire reported, that power was being used very infrequently. A similar idea has been applied in the US at the end of a served sentence through a body referred to as a 're-entry court', which manages the gradual reintegration of an individual through the use of sanctions and reinforcement (Maruna and LeBel, 2003). Both approaches allow the court to play a more thorough and constructive role in what might otherwise be a purely punitive intervention.

It is in this area that forensic psychology could play an important role in the assessment of risk, identifying opportunities for intervention and then carrying out such interventions, based on accurate understanding of the individual and the range of services that might be available for that person. With that in mind, we will consider a number of areas where forensic assessment may play a role.

Areas of forensic psychology assessment

According to Grisso (1986), mental health professionals may be able to offer the legal system a number of different forms of assessment, including assessment of general competency to stand trial or be involved in the court process, assessment of the impact of any identified deficits that are relevant to legal proceedings, and assessment of issues regarding sentencing. As the legal system is concerned with human behaviour, it is possible that these assessments may contribute to the consideration of *any* offence, from fraud to physical harm, and everything in between. In this section we provide some general principles that you could extrapolate to your own particular areas of interest or concern.

Assessment for the legal process

Psychologists may be involved at several points in the legal process in assessing whether an individual can be considered **competent**. This may occur before individuals are charged, when they have been charged, or during the processes within court. It is important to consider these in the contexts of the court process and of therapeutic jurisprudence, because the outcome of these assessments might impact on decisions to divert an individual from court, from prison, towards particular services, or (if there are concerns related to diminished responsibility) to hospital. For example, Grisso (1998) developed a number of tests concerned with the ability of an individual in the US to understand their **Miranda rights** at arrest, which are concerned with the right to remain silent, the right to have legal representation, and the use of any material disclosed during interview. If an individual does not *understand* these rights, that person cannot be expected to comprehend the implications of *waiving* them. For the police this is important, as any evidence gathered might then be called into question during decisions to prosecute or during the trial. It is also important more generally in considering how such individuals should be managed when they have committed offences.

Once an individual has been charged, then assessments may be made as part of the defence case, including aspects of personality, intellectual ability, suggestibility, and any number of factors that might be considered to mitigate the offending behaviour or that might influence a judge's decision regarding sentencing. It is important to note that these are not tests of guilt or innocence, but they may address questions related to the reliability of the defendant's testimony, the defendant's understanding of the consequences of her or his behaviour, the defendant's ability to make rational decisions when under stress, and so forth.

Prior to the court case taking place, an assessment may be made as to the individual's competence to stand trial, based in the UK on the idea that no one should be brought to trial unless they are *capable* of standing trial. In a Crown Court in the UK, a judge alone determines (based on expert opinion) whether a defendant is unfit to face trial. A number of tools have been developed to look at this issue, one example being the *Fitness Interview Test – Revised* (FIT-R; Roesch, Zapf and Eaves, 2006). The FIT-R considers factors such as individuals' capacity to communicate with their lawyers, their understanding of the charges against them, and the possible consequences of the trial.

After a verdict and prior to sentencing, the court may require that an individual is assessed for a number of reasons, including their mental health, the presence of personality disorders, their likelihood of engaging in intervention, and their level of risk to themselves and others. This assessment would be used to assist the judge in determining an appropriate sentence (e.g. custodial or within the community); and, if it is to be custodial, whether prison or hospital is more appropriate. Magistrates are able to make a Hospital Order (but without recording a conviction), which would allow the individual to be admitted to some form of service that could address their mental health issues.

Injury compensation

There is a vast range of possible areas in which personal injury might occur, and which might subsequently require psychological input. Walfish (2006) provides a list of examples of personal injury cases, including a slip and fall in a grocery store, a cruise ship almost sinking, and the loss of an eye due to a malfunctioning toy. In situations such as these, the psychologist is attempting to determine the presence or absence of a psychological injury, the extent to which the event under scrutiny is the cause of that injury, and the extent to which the injury impacts upon the person. This means that the psychologist is also considering the possibility that an individual is **malingering**. Just as there are tests concerned with assessing specific consequences of personal injury, such as tests for post-traumatic stress disorder (PTSD), so there are tests that deal with specific areas of malingering. For example, there are tests specifically concerned with malingering of neuropsychological complaints (see Iverson, 2008), and there is a developing set of criteria for identifying this kind of malingering (Slick, Sherman and Iverson, 1999).

Walfish's (2006) chapter provides a useful overview of the areas that need to be considered when conducting a psychological examination of personal injury, along with a number of case studies which highlight some of the important issues. He identifies that the one element that sets psychological assessment apart in this area is the use of psychometric tests, and the benefits that these tests can offer over and above the observational accounts that might be offered by GPs, social workers, or other professionals. Crucial to such testing is the psychologist's ability to identify the appropriate tests and then to administer them correctly, and finally to be in a position to competently interpret and report the test results. These points are further amplified in a more recent review of the issues by Piechowski (2014).

Chapter summary

- This chapter has been concerned with factors that might impact on the outcome of a trial, considering these from the perspective of general psychological principles and specific issues for forensic psychologists. It has described one of a number of pathways through the system that an individual may travel having committed an offence.
- Many of these factors cannot be managed in any way during a particular court case; rather they should be seen primarily as areas for further research and potentially areas for training and legislation.
- We have considered some of the elements linked to cross-examination and expert witnesses, which are central elements of the adversarial legal system, and we have indicated the complex interplay between knowledge and bias. These elements are crucial to the ability of jurors to make informed decisions, based on the evidence. In relation to jurors, too, there are issues linked to bias, including how they may react to different kinds of evidence and to different kinds of witnesses, and the impact this may have on the outcome of the trial.
- We have considered issues related to the judge's decision-making, and how this part of the process may also support individuals by being therapeutic. We have identified some of the areas in which forensic psychology might influence the passage of the individual through the court process. This is a complex area at the interface between two specialised areas of human endeavour, the law and forensic psychology, each with its own vocabulary and its own premises from which the professionals work.
- It is important that professionals are aware of the factors that may have an impact on decisions taken in court. Awareness of these factors may help to focus assessments, to advise on how evidence should be presented in court, and to influence other areas of work that can, to some extent, be controlled.

Further reading

For more specific reading we recommend the following:

- Kapardis, A. (2014). *Psychology and Law*, 4th edition (Cambridge: Cambridge University Press). This provides a good overview of where psychology and the law meet, and presents an interesting perspective on the pros and cons of their union.
- Prins, H. (1995). *Offenders, Deviants or Patients?* (London: Routledge). Although now relatively old, this book presents a succinct overview of many important issues that psychology faces in working with individuals in the legal system.

And for an American view:

- Barsky, A. E. (2012). *Clinicians in Court: A Guide to Subpoenas, Depositions, Testifying, & Everything Else You May Need to Know* (New York: Guilford Press). Barsky's book is a useful overview of the practicalities for psychologists working within the legal process.

In relation to sentencing, the UK's Sentencing Council provides a number of guidelines. For more information, see their website:

- https://www.sentencingcouncil.org.uk

Sentencing: Principles and Procedures

We arrive at that point on the route through the system where some crucial and far-reaching decisions are made. Our working assumption is that the person we are tracking has committed at least one offence and will be found guilty as charged. Several options are then available as to how that person can be dealt with. Sentencing is ultimately an expression of society's view of what an individual has done, enacted through judges or magistrates in a court of law. This chapter examines the factors that influence sentencing decisions, and surveys what is known about their most important effects and outcomes.

Chapter objectives

- To outline the framework of sentencing decisions made by criminal courts, the objectives of sentencing, and the principles that inform sentencing decisions.
- To review the evidence on the outcomes of sentencing, with particular reference to the effectiveness of punishment.
- To examine factors taken into account in assessing criminal responsibility, and conditions under which individuals are not held fully culpable of offences they have committed.

A brief history of penal law

Archaeological research suggests that the world's earliest system of laws, which expressly forbade certain acts and prescribed penalties for them, was the *Code of Urukagina*, originating from ancient Mesopotamia and dating from around 2,360 BCE. King Urukagina is thought to have been a socially reforming ruler who set out to fight the corruption that had flourished under the ruler who preceded him. Unfortunately there are no extant remains of this code: its existence has been inferred from other materials. Considerably more is known of the *Code of Hammurabi*, which dates from *c.* 1,850 BCE in Babylon. (Babylon, like Mesopotamia, was located in what is present-day Iraq.) This code was engraved on an eight-foot-high *stele* (an upright stone slab) and was placed in public view so that citizens might acquaint themselves with it, though it is thought that few would have been able to read it. Figure 16.1 shows a side view of this almost 4,000-year-old object. (You can see the original in the Louvre Museum, Paris – Room 3 in the Department of Near East Studies, Richelieu Wing, if you are pushed for time.)

The Hammurabi Code is not quite like any present-day legal statute. It simply lists a series of 282 laws, which govern a wide variety of transactions, including marital and family relationships, and prices to be paid for certain services, like the hiring of a ferryboat. But it also specifies some rather grisly penalties for a range of crimes such as murder, robbery, abduction and burglary – yes, you guessed correctly: death in each case. For some lesser crimes, ears, tongues or breasts were to be cut off. There are also crimes for which the first penalty was a fine. That sounds lenient, until you realise that for those unable to pay, the outcome reverted to the standard penalty: death (Avalon Project, 2008).

For a lengthy period thereafter, across many other emergent civilisations, crime was viewed as a largely private matter. Issues were resolved not by arrest, prosecution and trial, but by families waging war on each other. In Europe, that is how things remained for several millennia until the early Middle Ages, when the state progressively took over

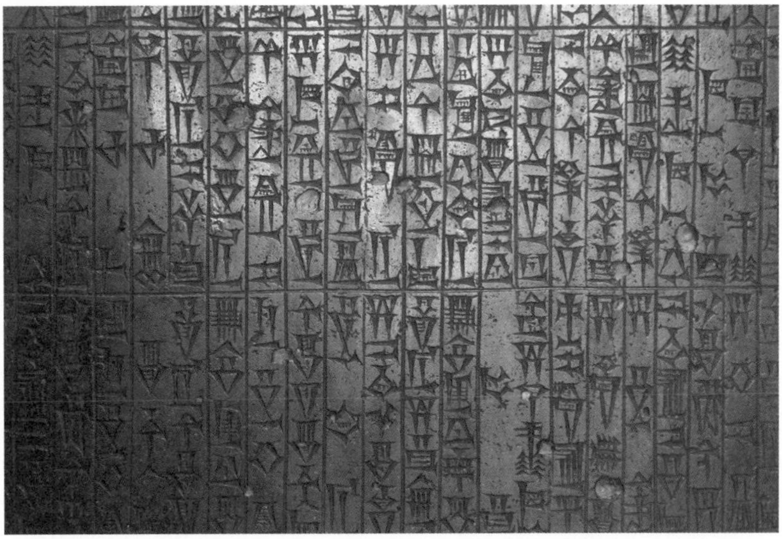

Figure 16.1
The Legal Code of Hammurabi, c. 1,850 BCE. One of the world's earliest systems of criminal law.

Source: iStock.com/jsp

responsibility for the judging and punishment of those who broke the law. From that point on, something distantly resembling the contemporary criminal court grew up. The response to many crimes remained harsh, however, and centred on the infliction of physical pain and public humiliation. The pillory, the stocks, the ducking stool, trial by ordeal, trial by combat, and burning at the stake were all in use at that time (Hanawalt and Wallace, 1998).

As we saw in Chapter 4, what is generally called the modern era of thinking on the subject of crime and justice only began to be ushered in over approximately the last 200 years. There were parallel changes in how crime was understood, in what was thought to cause it, and in the nature of society's response to it. Such forward steps were unsteady and lumbering, of course, with controversy erupting at numerous points along the way. Some scholars, such as the sociologist Norbert Elias, have viewed what has happened over the last few centuries as evidence of a 'civilizing' process (Elias, 2000), resulting from a growing revulsion at the practices of the past. Over the last three centuries, slowly and haltingly, we have also witnessed the advent and widespread acceptance of the concept of *human rights* (Grayling, 2007). Some fundamental change in sensibility seems to have occurred, although it is hard to reconcile that idea with the appalling record of the 20th century, and its record of genocide (as discussed in Chapter 8).

In England and Wales in the 18th century there was no centrally managed, state-controlled penal system as there is now. Prisons did not become fully the responsibility of the Home Secretary until 1878. The local prisons that existed were owned privately or by municipal or rural councils, and held debtors or persons who were awaiting trial. Individuals convicted of minor crimes were fined, placed in the stocks, or received corporal punishment, usually by being whipped with the branches of a birch tree ('birching') or sometimes a hazel tree. Birching was not abolished in Britain until 1948. Corporal punishment by caning, flogging or limb amputation is still used in some countries. Those who had committed more serious crimes were either executed or transported abroad, initially to the American colonies but then, after the unfortunate incident of the Declaration of Independence (1776), to Australia (Davies, Croall and Tyrer, 2010). During the 1770s the Sheriff of Bedfordshire, John Howard (1726–1790), inspected prisons throughout the country and also in several parts of Europe. His landmark work *The State of the Prisons*, published in 1777, drew attention to the disgraceful conditions

16

in which prisoners were kept. Those conditions were vigorously challenged by Howard, and later by other penal reformers such as Elizabeth Fry (1780–1845).

To most citizens of Europe over several hundred years, the very concept of what is now sometimes called 'rehabilitation' of a person who had offended against society would have made little sense. At the same time, the Judaeo-Christian tradition, which has been predominant in Western thought, has always promoted the view that the 'sinner', the person who had broken society's moral boundaries, could be redeemed and reformed. This was the origin of the late-18th-century idea of the penitentiary, an institution where by being kept separate from others and induced to concentrate on reading the word of God, errant individuals could realise the error of their ways, and repent.

Thus the founding of the modern prison, where individuals could be coerced into work routines and could learn to improve themselves, is 'a relatively recent social experiment which began 200 years ago' (Davies *et al.*, 2010, p. 430). It is generally traced to the early 19th century, when large penal institutions were established in Britain, France, the United States and other countries. Their arrival coincided with that of the factories and mills that were multiplying as the Industrial Revolution gathered pace.

In one sense, although the rhetoric was one of penitence, what was articulated then was the more concrete, optimistic, modernist idea that someone who had broken the law could change. There was a belief that his or her behaviour could be altered and become more socially acceptable, through means that were initially religious but became progressively more secular. This suggestion, although a recognisable aspiration of criminal justice systems today, is still a surprisingly fragile one. Even now it appears to have gained only partial acceptance in society. There remains a widespread populist view that certain patterns of behaviour are immutable, and that some types of people, such as those labelled 'habitual criminals' or classified as 'psychopaths', are incapable of change.

In relation to crime and punishment it has been suggested that the arrival of the modern prison was accompanied by a gradual shift of emphasis, from focusing on punishing/chastising the body to focusing on changing/reforming the behaviour and the mind of the person who has broken the law. According to this view, as argued by the French philosopher Michel Foucault (1979), from roughly 1800 onwards the ethos of societal control changed from one that entails imposing bodily hardship and discomfort to one that intrudes far more upon the daily activities and even the inner experience of the individual. 'At the beginning of the nineteenth century ... the great spectacle of physical punishment disappeared; the tortured body was avoided; the theatrical representation of pain was excluded from punishment ... during the 150 or 200 years that Europe has been setting up its new penal systems, the judges have gradually, by means of a process that goes back very far indeed, taken to judging something other than crimes, namely, the "soul" of the criminal' (pp. 14, 19). Furthermore, the high degree of surveillance undertaken in modern penal institutions is merely one end of a 'carceral continuum' whereby progressively greater control has been exercised over citizens through different phases of their lives. Schools, hospitals and workplaces are other parts of that continuum. Some critical criminologists have included psychologists amongst the unwitting agents of this invasive process (Groombridge, 2006). Applying Foucault's analysis of the power structures of society, psychology is part of the evolving of 'disciplines' whereby individuals are regulated and properly ordered.

The rest of this chapter is focused on describing the operation of the criminal and penal law today. First, we will survey some broad features of the law's operation, before examining the rationale forwarded for different ways of dealing with offenders. Second, we will take a closer look at some of the details of the criminal justice and sentencing process. Third, we will review such evidence as there is concerning whether or not the various 'disposals' available to the courts achieve their planned objectives. More detail on the operation of those disposals will be given in Chapter 17.

Criminal law concepts

In Chapter 2 we spent some time tackling the knotty issue of how to define crime, and one of the commonest options, and the one most widely taken for granted, is in terms of acts that break and are punishable by the criminal law. We saw that there are problems with such a definition, and reviewed a range of other possible approaches to conceptualising crime. In everyday operation, however, the definitions codified in the statutes of the criminal law are the ones that prevail, and for all practical purposes the ones that demand our time and attention. Within them, however, there are also subtleties of definition.

Criminal law takes different forms in different parts of the world. That is to be expected, given the numerous other variations that exist across nations and cultures with distinct traditions and histories. Legal systems have been classified in several ways by scholars in the field, though most agree that this is a fraught process, given the numerous dimensions along which such systems vary (Glenn, 2006). Some experts reject the idea that *any* classificatory system can be satisfactory. Nevertheless, a number of attempts have been made at producing one, with most revolving around the view that the majority of judicial systems can be grouped into major 'legal families' under one of three broad headings: civil law, common law and religious law. Other types of law exist, though the numbers of people subject to them are small compared to the number subject to the principal three. More importantly, there are also various kinds of hybrids of the three dominant systems, with some countries' laws (e.g. those of Scotland) combining influences from several directions as a function of their histories.

» In **civil law** traditions – the principal ethos in the majority (over 150) of the world's countries – the fundamental framework of law relies on a formalised written code as the primary source in the design of specific statutes. The origins of this are traced to Roman law, and examples include France's *Napoleonic Code*, the German *Criminal Code*, or Scandinavian law, hence this family is also sometimes loosely called the 'Continental European' model. Judges interpret the code in individual cases, but do not formulate decisions in a way that then becomes binding on later cases.

» By contrast, the *common law* family could be described as more pragmatic in that it places greater reliance on the evolution of law through the accumulation of decisions made in relation to individual cases (*case law*, sometimes called *judge-made law*). Judges make decisions in cases that come before them, which then become the rule to be applied in subsequent cases, a practice known as 'legal precedent'. This is the prevailing system in approximately 80 jurisdictions, including England, the United States and many members of the Commonwealth of Nations from Australia to Zambia.

» In a third group, the law is based on religious belief and practice. This group includes *Islamic* or *Sharia* law, which is the system in operation in 30 countries including Egypt, Saudi Arabia, Indonesia and other predominantly Muslim countries. This law is derived directly from the *Qur'an* and the *Hadith* and thus from the teachings of the prophet Muhammad. Other belief systems (e.g. the Jewish *halakha*) are applied in everyday matters or in dispute resolution in some countries but do not constitute a framework for the laws of any state.

In contrast to this, Mattei (1997) considered that a division like the one above is 'Western-centric', and proposed a different tripartite taxonomy for legal systems, dividing them into three broad categories: the rule of professional law, the rule of political law, and the rule of traditional law (sometimes called 'customary law'). Each is predominant in a different part of the world, and each maps onto a leading system of social organisation or 'social constraint'.

Notwithstanding these differences, there are also problems that are common to *all* jurisdictions, and there is today progressively more sharing and a greater exchange of ideas between legal practitioners in different countries. There is also steady growth in cooperation between police forces, including some supranational police organisations (such as Interpol, with 190 member countries, and Europol, with 27); extradition arrangements have been agreed between many governments; and a body of international criminal law has been developed collaboratively. Perhaps the pinnacle of such international cooperation to date was the establishment, in 2002 in The Hague, of the International Criminal Court (ICC). This was set up for the purpose of pursuing prosecutions against those charged with war crimes, genocide and crimes against humanity. However, although 122 countries have fully signed up to membership of the ICC, a significant number of others have signed but not ratified it in their own legal systems. Several more, including China, India and the United States, the world's three most populous countries, declined to become signatories.

Routes through the criminal justice process

Once someone suspected of having committed an offence is arrested by the police, a process of investigation commences, with numerous facets and stages (as described in Chapters 12 and 13), including decisions regarding whether or not to charge the individual, and whether or not to grant police bail. In England and Wales, the next stage of decision-making is in the hands of the Crown Prosecution Service (CPS), which was set up by the Prosecution of Offences Act 1985. (The post of Director of Public Prosecutions originally dates back to 1880, but the DPP dealt only with the most difficult cases.) The role of the CPS is to determine whether cases will be prosecuted; and if so, to select the appropriate charge, to prepare cases and present them in court, and to provide assistance to victims and witnesses. If the CPS considers that sufficient evidence is available to obtain a conviction, the case proceeds to the law courts. The point at which the case is dealt with – assuming, as we do here, that the defendant is found guilty – will be a function of a number of factors, the most significant being the seriousness of the offence of which the individual has been convicted.

In England and Wales, offences are divided into two categories according to their gravity: *summary offences* and *indictable offences*. Summary offences can be tried in a Magistrates' Court only. These are less serious types of crime, and include, for example, most motoring offences (e.g. driving while intoxicated), vehicle taking, and more minor assaults. The maximum penalty for a summary offence is a prison sentence of six months, though it may also result in the imposition of a fine, set within one of five levels according to crime seriousness, with the actual amounts adjustable to take account of inflation over time (Davies *et al.*, 2010). Offences that are 'indictable only' are far more serious and are tried in the Crown Court, presided over by a judge. They include all those offences likely to result in longer terms of imprisonment (up to and including life sentences). This group includes murder, serious assault, kidnapping, rape and robbery. For many such offences, maximum penalties are set by statute.

However, there are also many offences which are classed as *triable either way*. This means they may be either summary or indictable offences, depending on the circumstances, their level of seriousness, and other details (Ashworth and Redmayne, 2010). 'Theft', for example, can vary from minor shoplifting to a major jewel robbery; 'criminal damage' might range from an offence of cracking a window with a football to an offence of arson causing massive destruction. Attempts have been made to reduce the proportions of offences that are triable either way as the need for additional decision-making (arising from their variation in seriousness) can increase court costs (Davies *et al.*, 2010).

The resultant system of decision-making and the routes through it are very complex and can be difficult to track, but flowcharts published by the Ministry of Justice are very helpful in representing the process. On the basis of these, Figure 16.2 displays a simplified version of 'flows' through the criminal justice system for the 12 months up to June 2016 (Ministry of Justice, 2016). This shows clearly the directions taken by the roughly 1.85 million defendants who passed through the court system in that year. It is not uncommon for defendants appearing in court to be charged with more than one offence. Where that occurs, the *principal offence* is designated as the one amongst them that would attract the most severe sentence; in turn the *principal sentence* is the penalty that results. Thus, borrowing examples given in the criminal statistics guide (Ministry of Justice, 2016), if a person is charged with two offences but found guilty of only one, that will be his or her principal offence. If found guilty of two or more offences, the principal offence will be the one for which the heaviest sentence is imposed. If the same disposal is used for two or more offences, the principal sentence is the one which according to statute carries the most severe fixed maximum penalty.

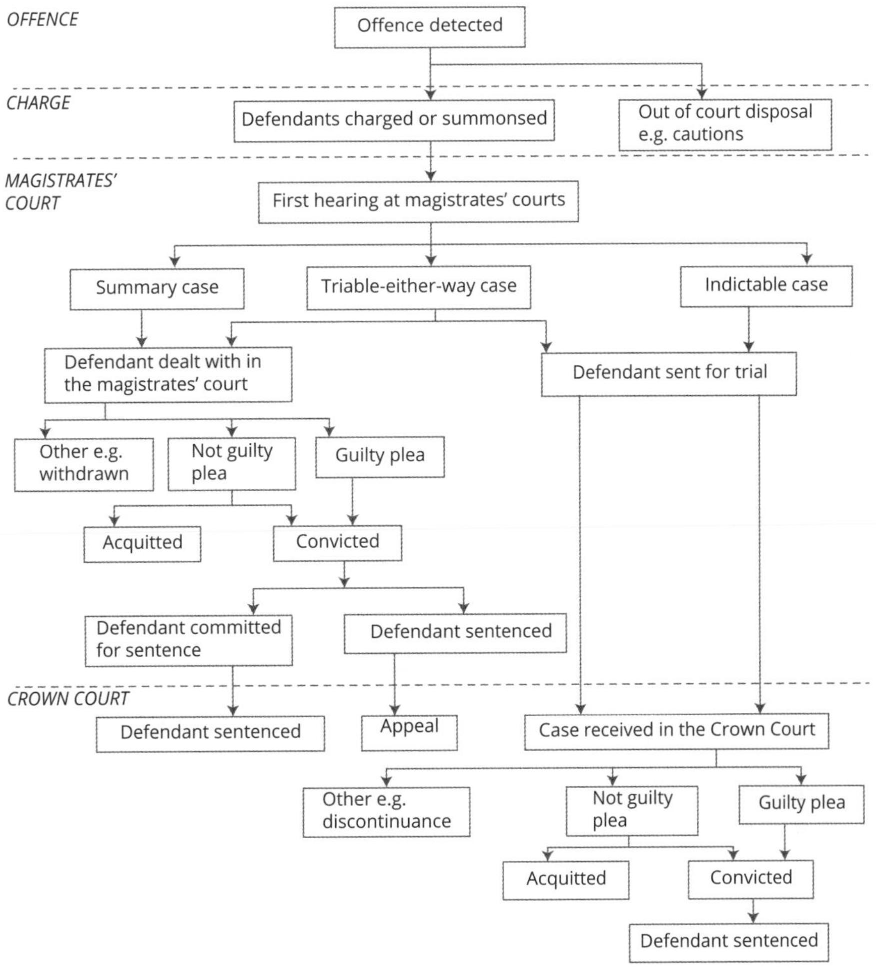
OFFENCE
Offence detected
CHARGE
Defendants charged or summonsed
Out of court disposal e.g. cautions
MAGISTRATES' COURT
First hearing at magistrates' courts
Summary case
Triable-either-way case
Indictable case
Defendant dealt with in the magistrates' court
Defendant sent for trial
Other e.g. withdrawn
Not guilty plea
Guilty plea
Acquitted
Convicted
Defendant committed for sentence
Defendant sentenced
CROWN COURT
Defendant sentenced
Appeal
Case received in the Crown Court
Other e.g. discontinuance
Not guilty plea
Guilty plea
Acquitted
Convicted
Defendant sentenced

Figure 16.2
The main court processes for criminal cases in England and Wales.

Source: Ministry of Justice (2016) © Crown copyright 2016. Contains public sector information licensed under the Open Government Licence v3.0: http://www.nationalarchives.gov.uk/doc/open-government-licence/version/3

By the end of this sequence of decisions, taking the 12 months to June 2017 as an example, 1.43 million defendants were prosecuted in England and Wales. The most common sentence was a fine, in 74.0 per cent of cases. A total of 40,897 people were given prison sentences and 131,508 were made subject to court orders which included community sentences (probation, unpaid work), or suspended or deferred prison sentences (Ministry of Justice and Office for National Statistics, 2017a, 2017b, 2017c). Other types of decision included issuing orders for pre-release supervision of prisoners. In the next section, we examine the rationale that is given for what happens during sentencing. In the section following that, we consider the extent to which the stated objectives of the process are in fact achieved.

16

The sentence of the court

The brief historical sketch that began this chapter underlines one of the most deeply ingrained conventions in the entire field of criminal justice: that *crime* and *punishment* are intimately and inextricably connected. The standard way of addressing the former is by administering a dose of the latter. Citizens expect that this issue is one that will be addressed by the criminal courts. The appointed core task of the courts is to implement the provisions of the criminal law and to penalise people who have been found guilty of violating it.

Penology is that branch of law and of criminology that focuses on the study of legal punishment and how it is administered. When a person is found guilty of committing a crime, the sentence imposed upon him or her may be designed to achieve a number of separate but interrelated legal purposes. Whilst there are variations between different countries with respect to this, textbooks on penology in the English-speaking world typically list six broad aims of sentencing: *retribution*, *denunciation*, *incapacitation*, *deterrence*, *rehabilitation* and *restoration* (Ashworth, 2015; Davies *et al.*, 2010). The first two of these, retribution and denunciation, are sometimes called *non-consequentialist* models of delivering justice, as they are complete processes in themselves and not expected to have specific effects on the individuals made subject to them. By contrast, the four other ideas that inform sentencing decisions – *incapacitation*, *deterrence*, *rehabilitation* and *restoration* – are intended to lead to observable effects, and for this reason are sometimes grouped together as *consequentialist* (or 'utilitarian') objectives. Let us look at what each of these involves.

Retribution

The concept of **retribution** is grounded in an approach to ethics known as *deontology*. Within this approach, philosophers seek to establish a set of principles that are thought to be fundamental to the way human beings should relate to each other. The approach is derived from the work of the German philosopher Immanuel Kant (1724–1804), who sought to define a set of irreducible principles – the 'categorical imperative' – which were the basis of all moral action. The Kantian or deontological approach to crime and justice advocates a principle whereby judicial punishment rectifies an imbalance in the socio-moral framework caused by the offender having committed the crime. By doing so, he or she has gained an unfair advantage over other members of society, and the inequity or imbalance so created must be remedied by taking something away from the perpetrator, or causing him or her some commensurate disadvantage.

Note that retribution is wholly distinct from the idea of *revenge*. The latter may well be a feeling or urge that people such as victims or families experience, but it is not generally considered a basis of sound judicial practice.

Once the offender has been appropriately punished, the retributive process has run its course and is complete in itself. There would be no particular value in examining its effects beyond that point, therefore it has done its work, as it were, by being carried out.

Denunciation

This function of punishment is centred on the role of criminal justice in expressing disapproval or condemnation of the guilty person's conduct in having committed the crime. The word 'sentence' derives (via Middle English and Old French) from the Latin word *sententia*, meaning a feeling or opinion communicated by someone to others. This captures the idea that sentencing is also intended to serve an *expressive* function: it conveys to everyone involved, and to observers, the public's reaction to the criminal offence. The public nature of this denunciation is an important aspect of the process. By *censuring* the individual, the court is not only punishing that person but also issuing a statement regarding what the community as a whole regards as unacceptable behaviour, and thereby reasserting its 'moral boundaries' (Davies *et al.*, 2010, p. 354). Judges' summaries at the time of sentencing often contain statements that reflect this function, and in some cases, where there has been a high level of public interest or media attention, the judge's remarks may be directly quoted in the news coverage of the trial.

Some sociologists who have analysed the penal process suggest that it is precisely society's desire for retribution and denunciation (rather than reform and rehabilitation, for example) that provides the rationale for the continuing use of punishment. As sentencing objectives, neither retribution nor denunciation has, nor are they intended to have, any measurable outcomes. Retribution achieves its effects by simply being carried out; there is no expectation of behaviour change as such and, as McGuire (2017a) remarks, it is a kind of 'closed loop'. The damage done to society is remedied by the rearranging of advantages and disadvantages that results from punishment. Alongside this, society reasserts its boundaries, and the identity and sense of belonging of those who *uphold* the law is validated by the fact that they can observe punitive sanctioning against those who do not. Indeed, some sociologists consider it naive to think of punishment 'solely in crime control terms' (Garland, 1990, p. 20). It is not the purpose of sentencing to *change* anything: its role is primarily, if not purely, symbolic. On the other hand, as the philosopher Ted Honderich (2006) has suggested, from the realisation that punishment fails to achieve its supposed purpose it does not follow that it must serve some other purpose which can only be discovered through historical or contextual analysis.

Incapacitation

Incapacitation, conceptually the simplest of penal strategies, is an approach to crime prevention that entails removing convicted persons from the circumstances in which they are likely to commit further crimes. In the past this might have been done by banishment or exile, as happened in traditional societies, or by transportation to other continents, as practised in Europe from the 17th to the 19th centuries. The most stringent method of doing this today is by imprisonment. However, there are also several other measures that can limit individuals' opportunities to reoffend in particular ways, perhaps the most common being *disqualification* (from driving, from holding other kinds of licences, or from being a company director). Incapacitation can also be accomplished by measures such as night-time **curfews** (requiring some individuals, especially young offenders, to be at home and indoors by specified times), by *Restraining Orders* (which designate exclusion areas that the individuals are forbidden to enter, usually places where they have committed offences previously), or by *tagging* (electronically monitored home confinement). In a sense, these measures are the current equivalents of the medieval ball and chain in impeding movement.

Deterrence

The idea of **deterrence** may be the most widely assumed objective of sentencing, and is basically encapsulated in the idea of trying to persuade would-be offenders not to break the law by convincing them of the adverse consequences that await them if they do. This fundamental notion, sometimes referred to as *deterrence theory* (at other times *deterrence doctrine*), is considered to have two interrelated components. One is that of *general deterrence*: the expectation that the public visibility of punishment and the threat of being subjected to it will deter prospective law-breakers, and indeed will bring about a broad suppressant effect in reducing crime in the community as a whole. The other is *specific deterrence*: the expectation that the personal experience of imprisonment or of other punishments will reduce the likelihood of future criminal acts by those who have been punished for past acts.

Like the idea of incapacitation, deterrence theory has a consequentialist or future-oriented emphasis. It presumes that because of the risk of fines, compulsory unpaid work, imprisonment, or other restrictions on liberty, offenders will want to avoid breaking the law. In accordance with the classical theory of criminology from which it is derived (see Chapter 4), the underlying rationale of deterrence is that increasing the *cost* of crime will persuade the individual – who, it is assumed, will weigh up these factors beforehand – that it is not in his or her interests to commit the crime. The desired effects are therefore twofold: reductions in the likelihood that the punished offender will reoffend (specific deterrence), and increased public safety through a widespread lowering of the rate of both reoffending and of first-time offending (general deterrence).

Rehabilitation

For many years, it was commonly believed to be a natural by-product of the other purposes of sentencing (such as retribution and deterrence) that individuals would also benefit in terms of personal change and reform (Gaes, 1998). By contrast, **rehabilitation** is more often viewed today as a separate objective of sentencing: one that is likely to be achieved through education, training, counselling, therapy, behavioural management, or other procedures, all of these being designed to implant in the individual, and to help that individual develop, new patterns of attitudes or skills. Rehabilitation is dealt with only briefly here, as Chapter 19 will survey in greater depth the role that psychological approaches have taken in pursuing this aim. While rehabilitative components have been included within sentences for a long time, rehabilitation in its present form is a comparatively recent development and one that as yet, although widely endorsed in principle, still has only a tenuous hold inside some parts of the penal system.

Restoration

In **restoration**, the fundamental principle is the repair of the damage done by a criminal offence to its victim or victims and to the wider community. This kind of approach has long been established in some non-Western societies (with 'traditional' legal systems, as classified earlier), but over the last thirty years or so it has also taken hold in the penal systems of some highly industrialised nations. *Restorative justice* can entail several elements, including the acknowledgement by an offender of his or her responsibility for the offence, the offering of an apology to victims and their families, the making of direct restitution through compensation payments, or the performance of reparative work. Restoration is distinct from retribution as it applies different concepts, though in some respects it could be seen as correcting an imbalance in relationships. It is also distinct from rehabilitation, but is thought to contribute to similar effects by inducing offenders to become more aware of their responsibilities to others.

The effectiveness of sentencing

The question of whether or not any of these interventions achieves its designated goals, and succeeds in reducing criminal reoffending amongst those who have repeatedly broken the law, has been a subject of regular debate in the interconnected fields of criminology, penology and psychology, as well as in the news media. Over approximately the last forty or fifty years, there has been a steadily accumulating quantity of research related to this question, which – borrowing the title of a much-cited paper by Martinson (1974) – is sometimes termed the issue of 'what works'. In this chapter, we will review the evidence for the outcomes of sentencing, with particular emphasis on the question of the effectiveness of punitive sanctions as a strategy. Later, in Chapter 19, we will turn our attention more fully to the value of explicitly rehabilitative approaches.

Penal policy and practice

Almost certainly, strategies of sentencing based on retribution and deterrence continue to be the mainstay of penal policy and practice in most jurisdictions around the world. That general observation, however, conceals wide variations. Those may become most speedily apparent by examining the extent to which imprisonment is used in different countries. Figure 16.3 shows a selection of prison rates for different countries to illustrate the variation that can be found (Walmsley, 2016). Rates of usage of imprisonment are of course influenced by many factors, including how crimes are defined, public attitudes to those crimes, police detection rates, and not least the costs of custody itself; although the condition of prisons in some parts of the world suggests that they have not been on the receiving end of especially large amounts of investment.

Ideas concerning how society should respond when someone commits a crime have also evolved, but in addition they have moved in divergent directions in different

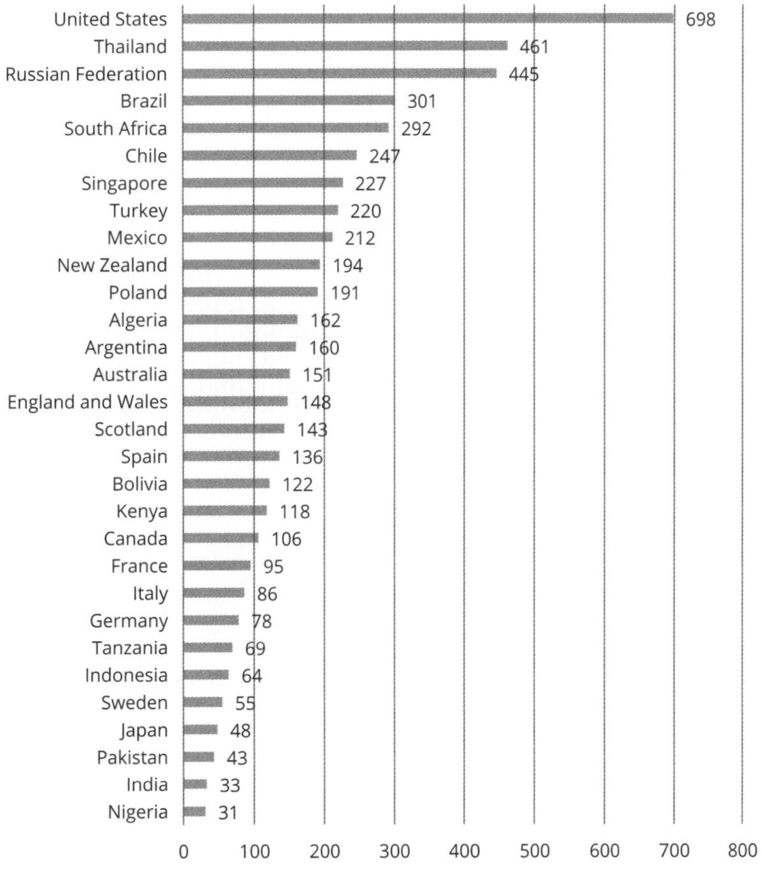

United States 698
Thailand 461
Russian Federation 445
Brazil 301
South Africa 292
Chile 247
Singapore 227
Turkey 220
Mexico 212
New Zealand 194
Poland 191
Algeria 162
Argentina 160
Australia 151
England and Wales 148
Scotland 143
Spain 136
Bolivia 122
Kenya 118
Canada 106
France 95
Italy 86
Germany 78
Tanzania 69
Indonesia 64
Sweden 55
Japan 48
Pakistan 43
India 33
Nigeria 31
0 100 200 300 400 500 600 700 800

Figure 16.3

Rates of imprisonment per 100,000 population in selected jurisdictions, October 2015. The 'world average' was then 144 per 100,000. Figures include remand and sentenced prisoners. China is not shown, as figures were available for sentenced prisoners only.

Source: World Prison Brief, Institute for Criminal Policy Research, Birkbeck, University of London.

16

legal systems. We might expect that the size of the prison population in a country would correspond in some orderly way with the rate of crime in that country. Many analyses have been conducted in efforts to discover such a relationship, but to no avail (Zimring and Hawkins, 1995). The extent of imprisonment appears to be influenced by numerous other factors related to how crime is perceived, the prevailing rhetoric concerning crime, and the impact of high-profile cases and perceived public reactions to them. For example, Figure 16.4 shows the historical trajectory of the prison population in England and Wales over the period 1900–2016. It is difficult to explain this upward trend, and particularly the spectacular recent rise, by reference to crime rates. Those rates have in general been falling since approximately 1995; but that fall cannot be attributed to the growth in prison numbers, as it has also been occurring in other countries where the prison population has hardly changed at all, and has in some cases declined (Byrne, Pattavina and Taxman, 2015).

Most criminal justice systems have two or three levels of courts (Ashworth and Roberts, 2012). In England and Wales there are two main levels, Magistrates' Courts and Crown Courts. The former deals with by far the larger share of cases, the summary cases (94 per cent in the 12 months to March 2016). Most consist of a 'bench' of three lay magistrates (also known as Justices of the Peace), from a national total of over 21,000, advised by a legally qualified clerk. A small number of Magistrates' Courts involve a district judge who sits alone. The Crown

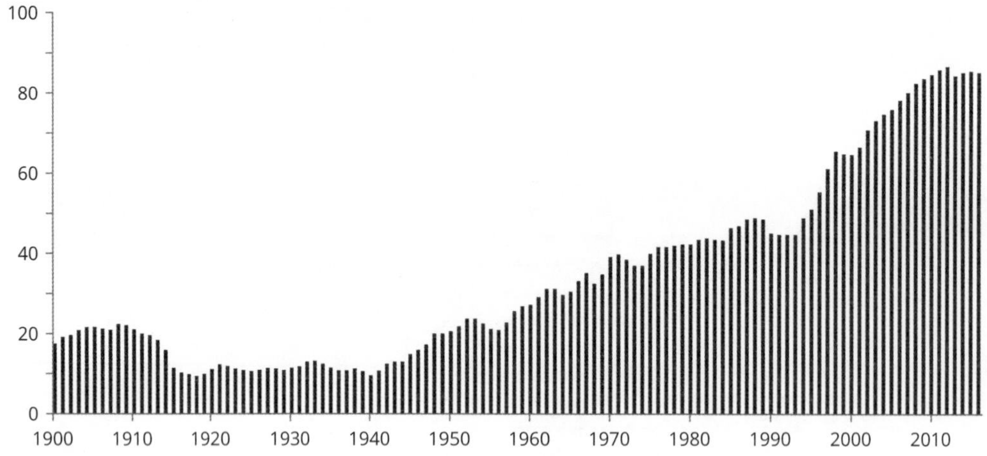
100
80
60
40
20
0
1900
1910
1920
1930
1940
1950
1960
1970
1980
1990
2000
2010

Figure 16.4
Prison population (thousands) in England and Wales, 1900–2016. The data are based on Ministry of Justice Offender Management Statistics 1900–2013 and updated using the Offender Management Statistics Quarterly until 2016.

Source: Allen, G. & Watson, C. (2017). UK Prison Population Statistics. London: House of Commons Library. Contains Parliamentary information licensed under the Open Parliament Licence v3.0: http://www.parliament.uk/site-information/copyright-parliament/open-parliament-licence

Courts, presided over by a judge, deal with the remaining cases: the indictable offences, which are more serious and come directly to the Crown Court, and a few other serious cases passed to the Crown Courts by magistrates. In roughly two-thirds of Crown Court cases, defendants plead guilty and no trial is required; but the remainder of cases are tried by a jury (consisting of members of the public). At a later stage, should it be suspected that a miscarriage of justice has occurred, a case may be assessed by an independent body, the *Criminal Cases Review Commission*, which may then refer the case to the Court of Appeal. Similarly, where convicted persons appeal against sentences, the case is heard by a higher court, the Court of Appeal, which is accountable ultimately to the Lord Chief Justice.

Sentences are grouped into three 'tiers' (Ashworth and Roberts, 2012). The first, for relatively minor offences, consists of absolute and conditional *discharges* (for the latter, the defendant has to fulfil some requirement set by the court) and *fines*. The second tier consists of *community sentences*, which are intended for use as alternatives to shorter custodial sentences, and which, since the Criminal Justice Act 2003, can incorporate one or more of twelve requirements specified by the court (such as unpaid work, probation supervision, or attendance at an offending behaviour programme: Raynor, 2012). The third tier consists of *custodial sentences*, which may be suspended (and can have added to them any of the twelve elements of a community sentence) or immediate (the offender then being taken directly to prison).

Apart from fines, the main punitive sanction common to most sentences is some degree of restriction of liberty. Community sentences vary in how exacting they are – for example, in the requirements imposed, the amount of time specified for unpaid work, or in the duration of supervision orders – and in the demands they place on an individual's time. Thus most sentences contain a mixture of activities tailored to the court's appointed purposes, and in the majority of cases they entail a combination of the different ingredients described earlier. In deciding which sentence to apply, courts make use of a range of structured explanatory materials, developed by a specially established advisory body, the **Sentencing Council**. (This was originally established as the Sentencing Guidelines Council by the Criminal Justice Act 2003, but was re-established in its present form in 2010.)

Prison sentences vary considerably in length, from a matter of days to a full lifetime, and the type of regime to which a prisoner is allocated can place varying degrees of restriction on activities and daily movement – although often that may be a matter of resource and staff availability, rather than of prisoner management as such. At the time of writing, there are 139 prison establishments in England and Wales, 16 in Scotland and 4 in Northern Ireland. They perform a variety of functions. Some are *local prisons*, which hold those on remand awaiting court appearances, or convicted prisoners serving short-term sentences. *Training prisons* hold those serving longer sentences and include facilities for work and for vocational training of various kinds; in some cases they also provide specialised therapeutic services. *Higher security prisons* hold those who are thought to present a serious risk to the public, or to pose a risk of escape, or both. They are organised in a 'dispersal system' to allow speedy transfers in the event of prison disturbances. The next 'Focus on ...' box shows Ministry of Justice information on the way prisoners and prisons are classified.

FOCUS ON ...

Categories of prisons and prisoners

The Ministry of Justice (England and Wales) divides adult prisoners into security categories, as shown below. There are separate prison arrangements for male and female prisoners (Ministry of Justice, 2017b).

Prisoner categories

Categories for prisoners are based on a combination of the type of crime committed, the length of the sentence, the likelihood of escape, and the danger to the public if the offender escaped. For adult male prisoners the four categories are:

- *Category A* Prisoners whose escape would be highly dangerous to the public or to national security.
- *Category B* Prisoners who do not require maximum security, but for whom escape needs to be made very difficult.
- *Category C* Prisoners who cannot be trusted in open conditions, but who are unlikely to try to escape.
- *Category D* Prisoners who present a low risk; who can reasonably be trusted not to try to escape, and for whom open conditions are appropriate.

For female prisoners the categories are different and comprise:

- *Category A* Prisoners whose escape would be highly dangerous to the public or to national security and for whom escape must be made impossible.
- *Restricted status* Any female, young person or young adult whose escape would present a serious risk to the public and who requires to be held in designated secure accommodation.
- *Closed conditions* Prisoners who do not require the highest security but present too high a risk for open conditions.
- *Open conditions* Prisoners who present a low risk, can be trusted in open conditions and for whom such conditions are appropriate.

Prison categories

Prisons differ somewhat in their function according to the main categories of prisoners they hold:

- *High security prisons* These hold Category A and Category B prisoners. Category A prisoners are managed by a process of 'dispersal' in a number of designated prisons and can be moved between them if needs be. For Category B prisoners, these prisons provide a regime similar to that provided by a Category B prison. The Category B prisoners held in a high security prison are not necessarily any more dangerous or difficult to manage than those in Category B prisons.
- *Category B and Category C prisons* These hold sentenced prisoners of the corresponding categories (see above), including life-sentenced prisoners. The regime focuses on programmes that address

16

offending behaviour and provide education, vocational training and purposeful work for prisoners, who will normally spend several years in one prison.

- *Local prisons* These serve courts in the adjoining area. Historically, their main function was to hold prisoners on remand or awaiting sentence and, once a prisoner had been sentenced, to allocate them to a Category B, C or D prison, as appropriate, to serve their sentence. However, pressure on places means that many shorter-term prisoners serve their entire sentence in a local prison, while some longer-term prisoners also complete some offending behaviour and training programmes there before moving on to lower-security conditions. All local prisons operate to Category B security standards.
- *Open prisons* These have much lower levels of physical security and only hold Category D prisoners. Many prisoners in open prisons are allowed to go out of the prison on a daily basis to take part in voluntary or paid work in the community, in preparation for their approaching release.

Reference

- Adapted from Ministry of Justice (2017b), © Crown copyright 2017. Contains public sector information licensed under the Open Government Licence v3.0: http://www.nationalarchives.gov.uk/doc/open-government-licence/version/3

Most prison terms are fixed at the time of sentencing, but there are various provisions for 'early release', whereby the actual time served can be reduced. A fraction of the sentence (usually one-third) may be automatically remitted, though portions of this may be lost in response to disciplinary infractions by the prisoner (Padfield, Morgan and Maguire, 2012). Prisoners serving determinate sentences of 12 months or more may also apply for **parole**. Decisions regarding this are made by members of the Parole Board, whose decision-making takes account of psychologists' reports, amongst other sources of information. Some prisons also contain a number of individuals sentenced to **Imprisonment for Public Protection** (IPP) sentences, a possibility created by the Criminal Justice Act 2003 for the management of sentence progression according to assessed risk. In March 2011 there were 13,587 prisoners serving IPP sentences (Padfield *et al.*, 2012). Although this type of sentence was abolished in 2012 and the numbers have been declining since, by mid-2016 there were still 4,000 prisoners serving sentences in this category (Parole Board, 2016). However, it was announced that all those 'over tariff' were to be released by the end of 2017.

Life sentences differ from this, in that judges specify a minimum time to be served after which the prisoner may apply for parole; and even if parole is granted, he or she will remain liable to recall. Finally, as discussed in Chapter 15, a small number of prisoners, those who have committed extremely serious offences – usually multiple homicides, or offences of extreme cruelty or callousness – and who are considered highly dangerous, are subject to a *whole life tariff* and will never be released. It is estimated that there are 35–40 such individuals detained in the prison system of England and Wales, though that number may have risen in recent years. *Young Offender Institutions* (YOIs) are designed for juvenile offenders aged 15–17 and young adults aged 18–20 years. As of late 2016, there were eight YOIs for males and three dedicated young person units for females.

Do deterrent sentences work?

As already noted, some sentencing purposes (retribution and denunciation) do not offer the prospect of any specific outcomes, so they are not amenable to measurement of their effects. Other approaches are 'consequentialist' and are intended to have discernible, even measurable effects, so presumably the approaches can be evaluated with reference to those effects. It is reasonable then to ask: are those effects obtained?

Specific deterrence

In what follows, we will consider evidence concerning the impact of punitive sanctions – of penal decisions that are made, based on the expectation of producing deterrent effects. Several kinds of evidence can be employed to evaluate the specific deterrent effectiveness of prison and other punitive sanctions. They include official criminal statistics; comparisons between different lengths or types of sentence; the effects of more demanding regimes; and the impact of 'three strikes' laws.

Official statistics

Official statistics show that there is a relatively high rate of reoffending following most punitive sentences. For example, in the United States, the Bureau of Justice Statistics tracked a group of 272,111 prisoners released from prisons in fifteen states over a three-year period from 1994. By that point, just over two-thirds (67.5 per cent) had been rearrested, and 51.8 per cent had returned to prison (Bureau of Justice Statistics, 2002). In the United Kingdom, the headline measure of 'proven reoffending' is defined as any offence committed in a one-year follow-up period that receives a court conviction, a caution, a reprimand or a warning. For those adults released from custody during the year ended March 2015, this figure was 44.7 per cent (Ministry of Justice, 2017a). By the time *two* years had passed, the figures had generally risen above 60 per cent.

In addition to these raw figures, a more searching analysis comes from examining different types of sentence that we would expect to produce different effects. Figure 16.5 shows the relationship between predicted and actual rates of reconviction over two years for large samples of offenders monitored by the UK Home Office during the 1990s (Lloyd, Mair and Hough, 1994). The predicted rates were obtained using a specially developed risk assessment, the *Offender Group Reconviction Scale* (OGRS-2; since replaced by a revised version, OGRS-3). This uses criminal history data to estimate individuals' likelihood of further offending over a projected two-year period. The striking aspect of this chart is not the comparison between the three types of sentence, but rather the fact that within each type the predicted and actual rates are very close, indeed almost identical. There is no evidence of a 'suppressant' effect of imprisonment over community sentences: the rates at which individuals reoffend are the rates that were predicted, regardless of the court decision that was then made concerning them. Similar results to these were obtained over successive years, as found in later studies by Home Office researchers (Kershaw, 1999; Kershaw, Goodman and White, 1999).

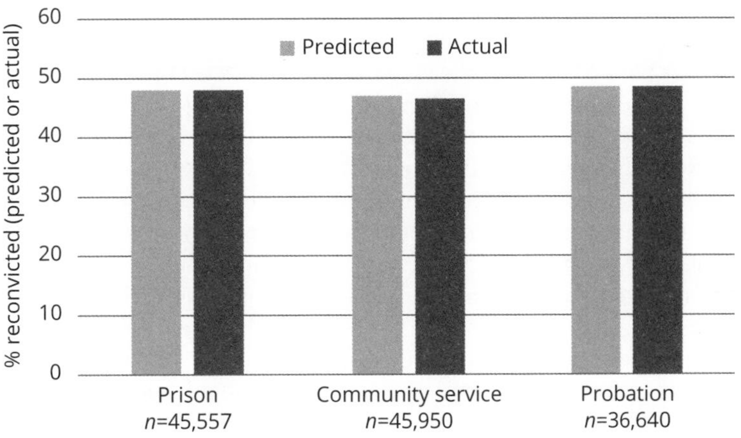
% reconvicted (predicted or actual)
60
50
40
30
20
10
0
Predicted
Actual
Prison
n=45,557
Community service
n=45,950
Probation
n=36,640

Figure 16.5
Two-year predicted and actual rates of reconviction following prison, community service and probation sentences.

Source: Home Office. © Crown copyright 1994. Contains public sector information licensed under the Open Government Licence v3.0: http://www.nationalarchives.gov.uk/doc/open-government-licence/version/3

16

Results similar to these were obtained from a systematic review by Villetaz, Killias and Zoder (2006) of studies comparing the effects of custodial and non-custodial sentences. Of 27 comparisons made, 14 showed no difference, whereas 11 found non-custodial sanctions, and 2 found custodial sanctions, to have superior effects (i.e. lower reoffending). Moreover, in a large-scale study of 4,246 offenders conducted in the Netherlands, with an eight-year follow-up and with a range of factors including criminal history variables controlled, there was a significantly lower recidivism rate amongst those sentenced to community service (unpaid work) than to a short sentence of imprisonment (Wermink *et al.*, 2010). That pattern also emerged in a similar study in Denmark (Klement, 2015). Indeed, at least for those who would otherwise be sent to prison for short periods (less than 12 months), suspended sentences proved to be as effective as custody itself. This has been found in studies in both Spain (Cid, 2009) and Australia (Trevena and Weatherburn, 2015).

We might expect that for individuals placed on probation, or for prisoners granted parole, the possibility of custody or of a return to it would have clear deterrent effects. In the United States, high rates of revocation or 'breach' of probation or parole conditions led to jail being increasingly used as a punitive sanction in these circumstances. However, a study by Wodahl, Boman and Garland (2015) suggests that this does not have the desired effects. Examining 800 instances of probation or parole violation, the study compared the effect of recall to jail with the use of 'graduated sanctions' imposed as part of community sentences. The latter measures can include, for example, the imposition of a period of unpaid work as a consequence of missing a supervision appointment. Analysis showed that the use of jail sanctions was no more or less effective than community-based sanctions, with respect to the time till the next violation, the number of subsequent violations, or the likelihood of completion of community supervision.

On the basis of an extensive literature search, Perry (2016) reported an overview of 12 systematic reviews of sentencing and four of deterrence. Firm conclusions proved difficult to draw as the evidence base concerning outcome effects was found to be quite limited. One type of sentence, the use of *drug courts*, in which individuals with significant substance use problems are offered supervised treatment as an alternative to judicial sentencing, was found to have positive support with adult, but not with younger offenders (Mitchell, Wilson, Eggers and MacKenzie, 2012). But deterrent sanctions yielded either no evidence of any effect, or a harmful effect.

Sentence length

If punitive sentences had deterrent effects, we might expect that the longer someone spends in prison, the less likely he or she will be to reoffend following eventual release. Puzzlingly, however, international data contradict that. Gendreau, Goggin and Cullen (1999) systematically reviewed this area in a report for the Solicitor General of Canada. They combined a set of 23 studies, producing 222 comparisons of groups of offenders (total sample size: 68,248) who spent longer versus shorter periods in prison (respective averages of 30 as compared to 17 months). The groups were similar on a series of five risk factors. Contrary to what would be predicted by deterrence theory, offenders who served longer sentences showed slight increases in recidivism of between 2 and 3 per cent; there was a small positive correlation between sentence length and subsequent rates of reconviction. More recent reviews too have found that on balance imprisonment has a criminogenic rather than a preventive effect (Durlauf and Nagin, 2011; Nagin, Cullen and Jonson, 2009). There appears to be a possible additional crime-related effect of placement in higher security levels. Gaes and Camp (2009) found that when prisoners assessed as requiring high security were allocated at random to higher or lower security levels, the post-release recidivism rate of those allotted to higher levels was 31 per cent higher than for those allotted to the lower level.

Questions about the place of prison as the central feature of penal policy have been asked for a long time. What is perhaps remarkable is that even within a few years of its inception, on the basis of what we would now call 'evaluation research' by the authorities in France, prison was considered to have been a not very successful idea. Judging by reports published in the 1820s and 1830s, 'the prison, in its reality and visible effects, was denounced at once as the great failure of penal justice' (Foucault, 1979, p. 264). The rate of recidivism following release was considered unacceptable, though it was far lower than the equivalent figures found today. It was readily seen that prisons 'do not diminish' the crime rate but rather increase it; that 'detention causes recidivism'; that institutions were replete with repressive measures, and induced those made subject to them to feel sorry for themselves, and to see their punishment as unjust. Prisoners thereby experienced prison as an abuse of power, and so became more rather than less hostile to society; the net effect being, as Foucault expresses it, 'he accuses justice itself' (1979, p. 266). Furthermore, prison facilitated the placing together of those with antisocial tendencies, what has been called a 'behavioural contagion' effect; it caused the families of those imprisoned to become destitute; and it created conditions that made a return to law-abiding life following release next to impossible. These observations were made, and these conclusions drawn, two hundred years ago.

Tougher regimes

It is said to be a popularly held belief that sentences fail because they are just not harsh enough: prison is not sufficiently punishing. What we need, some argue, are tougher, more physically demanding regimes inside penal institutions. This idea is however at odds with the available evidence. First, such an approach has been tested several times. One example was the British 'short sharp shock' experiment of the 1980s. Another was the larger-scale 'boot camp' initiative in the United States in the 1990s. Neither of these produced any positive backing for the idea of 'getting tough': outcome studies showed those changes made no difference to subsequent rates of reoffending (MacKenzie, Wilson and Kider, 2001; Thornton, Grayson, Curran and Holloway, 1984). Second, investigation of the relationship between adverse prison conditions and reoffending after release shows that results are the reverse of popular expectations: worsening prison environments are associated with increases in recidivism rates. This is based on studies in the United States (Chen and Shapiro, 2007; Listwan *et al.*, 2013) and in Italy (Drago, Galbiati and Vertova, 2011). The effects of such conditions become apparent even before release. Where prison conditions are deliberately made harder by adding further restrictions or deprivations, prisoners' behaviour while detained usually deteriorates (Bierie, 2012).

An attempt to parallel this approach in the community consisted of sentences designed as intermediate between imprisonment and probation, which involved various permutations of intensive supervision and surveillance. These became known in the penal folklore of the time as 'smart sentencing', based on the hope that these innovations would also reduce criminal justice costs. However, findings from these innovations were also uniformly disappointing (Petersilia and Turner, 1993), a trend confirmed in a subsequent meta-analysis of 136 studies (Gendreau, Goggin, Cullen and Andrews, 2001). Similarly discouraging results emerged from the evaluations of outdoor pursuit or 'wilderness challenge' programmes, where young offenders were taken on wagon trains or other ventures (Wilson and Lipsey, 2000); and from so-called 'scared straight' programmes in which young offenders were confronted with dire warnings from older counterparts who had led a life of crime and who expressed their regret at having done so (Petrosino, Turpin-Petrosino and Finckenauer, 2000). Curfews, though probably more a form of incapacitation than deterrence, could reasonably be expected also to have some deterrent effects, but two systematic reviews have failed to find any (Adams, 2003; Wilson, Olaghere and Gill, 2016).

Three strikes

One of the most punitive departures of all was the 'three strikes and you're out' policy implemented in some American states from 1994 onwards. The application of this law can be illustrated by the case of Curtis Wilkerson, who was imprisoned for life at the age of 33 after stealing a pair of socks worth $2.50. Mr Wilkerson became liable for this penalty because he had two previous offences on record, for abetting robbery when he was aged 19 (Kristof, 2009). Evaluation of this policy in California, where it was zealously pursued, found effects that were the direct opposite of what had been hoped for. Between 1994 and 2008, approximately 41,500 offenders were sentenced under the 'three strikes' law in the Golden State. But there were large variations in the extent of its use between different counties, some using it up to six times more often than others. However, follow-up analysis of crime data in the counties which applied the legislation *least* showed that they experienced a slightly *greater* decline in violent crime than those counties which used it most (Males, 2011). These data offer a particularly dispiriting example of the belief that the core problem with the penal system is that it is not hard enough: that it does not mete out punishment sufficiently gruelling to persuade offenders to mend their ways.

California, however, is just one example. Twenty-five American states implemented 'three strikes' policies. Kovandzic, Sloan and Vieraitis (2004) analysed the possible effects of such changes across the twenty-one of them where data were available, looking at the impact on 188 cities with a population of 100,000 or more over a total period of 20 years. They examined the impact on seven types of offence: homicide, rape, robbery, aggravated assault, burglary, larceny and car theft, yielding a total of 147 comparisons. Within this, 72 of the 147 tests indicated that 'three strikes' laws did reduce crime, with 29 of them reaching statistical significance; while 31 indicated a statistically significant *increase* in crime. Overall, there was a ratio of one crime increase for every one crime decrease. Eight states showed an increase in homicide, only one showed a decrease, and the remainder showed no change.

General deterrence: capital punishment

The above research pertains to the effectiveness (or lack of it) of *specific* deterrence. Corresponding tests of the idea of *general* deterrence often centre on the most severe punishment of all, the death penalty. The continued existence of this kind of sentence is a highly emotive issue. For those who oppose it and who press for it to be abolished, 'any discussion of its effectiveness as a deterrent is irrelevant' (Hood and Hoyle, 2015, p. 8). For those who advocate its use, the rationale for applying capital punishment is very substantially based on its supposed deterrent effects.

The number of countries where capital punishment is still used has been gradually falling over recent decades. Nevertheless, as of April 2014 there were still 39 countries where the possibility of using it remained in force and where it had been exercised at some point in the previous ten years. According to Hood and Hoyle (2015, p. 8), who conducted a global survey of its use on behalf of the United Nations, the case for retaining capital punishment 'usually rests not only on retributive sentiments but also on assumptions about its unique deterrent effects as compared with alternative lesser punishments'. Hood and Hoyle (2015) tracked countries according to their pattern of use of capital punishment over a 50-year period. Some countries or states retained the use of the sentence throughout that period. Others had either not used it during that time or had at some point formally abolished its use. This allowed comparisons to be made between countries, and within countries over time, to test whether there is a relationship between capital punishment and rates of the crimes subject to that penalty.

Studies of these kinds have not found that the availability of the death penalty as a sentencing option has any clear suppressant effect on rates of capital crimes such as homicide. Of particular interest in this analysis, the United States had a nine-year interlude (1967–1976) when execution was not permitted, as a result of a moratorium and subsequent rulings by the Supreme Court. Following that, its use was resumed in 37 of the 50 states. Without wishing to sound too gruesome, this constituted a 'natural experiment' which allowed researchers to evaluate its possible effects. Sorensen, Wrinkle, Brewer and Marquart (1999) analysed crime statistics for the period 1984–1997 in Texas, the state with the most active use of the death penalty, but found no discernible relationship between the execution rate and the murder rate. Indeed, a comparison of homicide rates in California, New York and Texas over an even longer period (35 years) found that they showed very similar trends and changes of direction over time; the figures follow each other 'in close unison for the entire 1974–2009 period' (Nagin and Pepper, 2012, p. 40). Yet during those years 447 people were executed in Texas, 13 in California, and none in New York.

Some econometric studies, using multiple regression or time-series analysis, have reported finding deterrent effects. Among the most widely cited are those of Ehrlich (1975), who claimed that each execution saved on average seven or eight lives; and a later study by Dezhbakhsh, Rubin and Shepherd (2003), which claimed that each execution saved as many as 18 lives. The latter led come commentators to argue that capital punishment was therefore 'morally obligatory' (quoted in Hood and Hoyle, 2015, p. 392). However, these studies have been heavily criticised for methodological flaws, for their underlying assumption of Rational Crime Theory (which does not fit an especially large proportion of homicides), and for assuming that where an association is found between increased use of the death penalty and declining numbers of murders the former is the cause of the latter. A more recent meta-analytic review, by Yang and Lester (2008), concurs with the conclusion that the death penalty had some deterrent effect. Whether or not this effect appeared, however, depended on the type of methodology employed, with other analyses finding no effect, and still others suggesting that the death penalty had a brutalising rather than a deterrent effect (i.e. the murder rate increased). A later study, possibly the most thorough analysis of data comparing American states, covered executions in the period 1977–2006: this found no positive 'death penalty effect' (Kovandzic, Vieraitis and Boots, 2009). Similarly, re-analyses of the data of Dezhbakhsh *et al.* (2003) by Donohue and Wolfers (2004, 2006) could not obtain the same results and revealed major flaws in their method. It is extremely difficult to sustain claims that there is a causal link between executions and reduced homicide rates.

Using a different methodological approach, some particularly compelling evidence was found by Zimring, Fagan and Johnson (2010) in what they called a present-day 'tale of two cities'. These authors undertook a side-by-side comparison for the period 1973–2007 between Singapore and Hong Kong. In many respects these densely populated Asian cities have a great deal in common. They are populated mainly by people of Chinese origin: in Hong Kong 95 per cent; in Singapore, 75 per cent, Singapore also having a sizeable proportion of people of Malay (13 per cent) and Indian (9 per cent) origin. They are both highly successful economies, with industrial, trading and financial service sectors. They have low unemployment, and roughly equivalent *per capita* annual incomes.

In terms of some aspects of criminal justice policy, however, they are diametrically opposed. From 1967 onwards Hong Kong had no executions, and the death penalty was formally abolished in 1993. In sharp contrast Singapore's execution rate rose steeply from 1991–1992 onwards and at one point was the highest in the world, though it steadily declined thereafter. Despite this very marked dissimilarity, the two cities had remarkably similar, almost parallel rates of homicide throughout the entire period studied. The findings of Zimring and his colleagues (2010) are shown graphically in Figure 16.6 on the next page.

Prison, as well as execution, has also been researched in relation to its anticipated general deterrent effects. Most people almost certainly fear the idea of being imprisoned, so it is widely taken for granted that in addition to specific deterrent effects, discussed earlier, it will also have general deterrent effects. However it difficult to discern whether prison is actually effective in this way as a crime control strategy. Searching for a relationship between the number of people imprisoned and the level of crime in a society cannot adequately test for deterrent effects because a proportion of any association that is found could be due to incapacitation. There is also a possibility that prison is in some respects *criminogenic*, due to the assimilation of antisocial attitudes

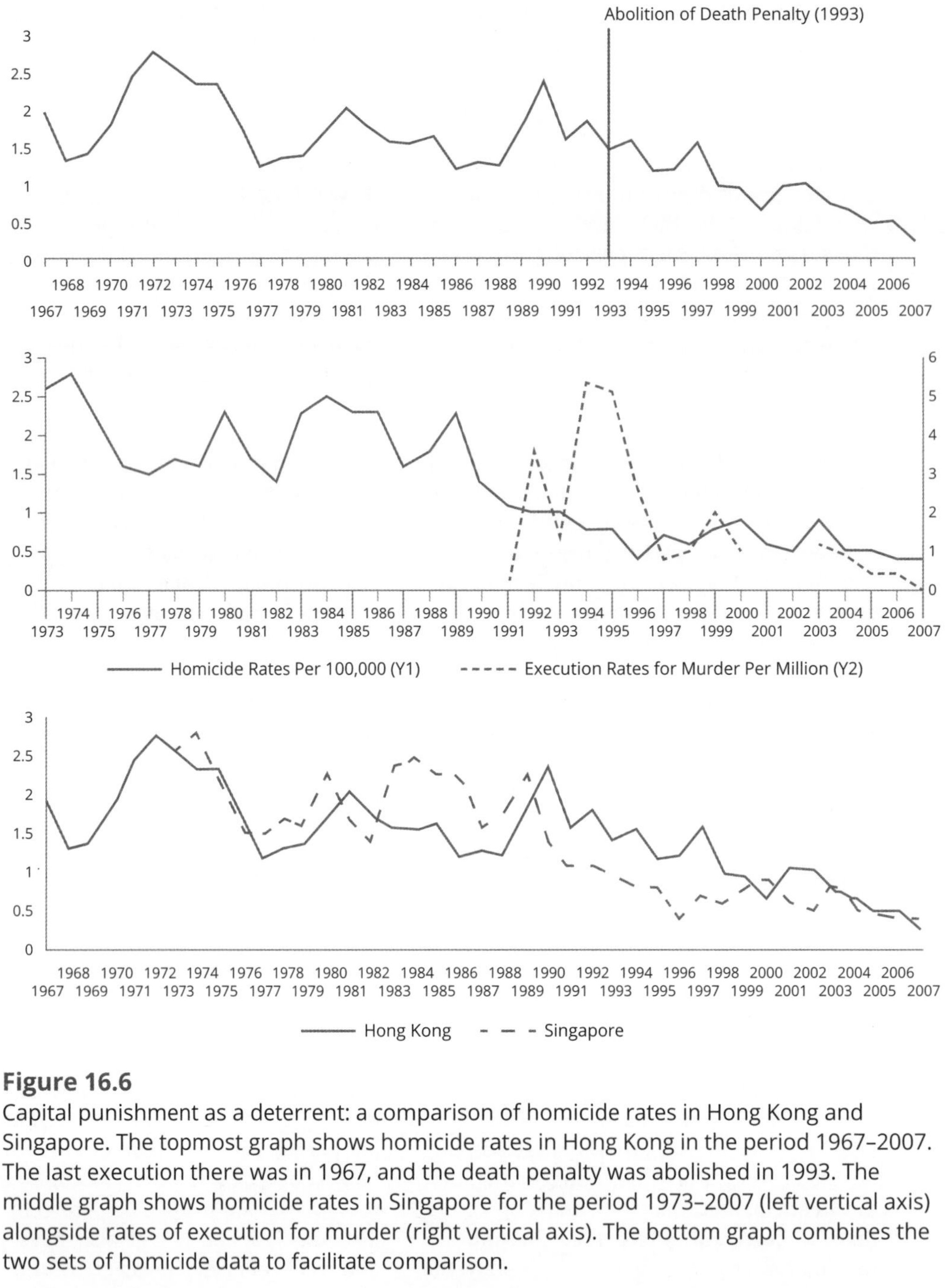
Abolition of Death Penalty (1993)
3
2.5
2
1.5
1
0.5
0
1968 1970 1972 1974 1976 1978 1980 1982 1984 1986 1988 1990 1992 1994 1996 1998 2000 2002 2004 2006
1967 1969 1971 1973 1975 1977 1979 1981 1983 1985 1987 1989 1991 1993 1995 1997 1999 2001 2003 2005 2007
3
2.5
2
1.5
1
0.5
0
6
5
4
3
2
1
0
1974 1976 1978 1980 1982 1984 1986 1988 1990 1992 1994 1996 1998 2000 2002 2004 2006
1973 1975 1977 1979 1981 1983 1985 1987 1989 1991 1993 1995 1997 1999 2001 2003 2005 2007
Homicide Rates Per 100,000 (Y1)
Execution Rates for Murder Per Million (Y2)
3
2.5
2
1.5
1
0.5
0
1968 1970 1972 1974 1976 1978 1980 1982 1984 1986 1988 1990 1992 1994 1996 1998 2000 2002 2004 2006
1967 1969 1971 1973 1975 1977 1979 1981 1983 1985 1987 1989 1991 1993 1995 1997 1999 2001 2003 2005 2007
Hong Kong
Singapore

Figure 16.6

Capital punishment as a deterrent: a comparison of homicide rates in Hong Kong and Singapore. The topmost graph shows homicide rates in Hong Kong in the period 1967–2007. The last execution there was in 1967, and the death penalty was abolished in 1993. The middle graph shows homicide rates in Singapore for the period 1973–2007 (left vertical axis) alongside rates of execution for murder (right vertical axis). The bottom graph combines the two sets of homicide data to facilitate comparison.

Source: Figures 1, 4 & 5. From Zimring, F. E., Fagan, J. & Johnson, D. T. (2010). Executions, Deterrence, and Homicide: A Tale of Two Cities. Journal of Empirical Legal Studies, 7(1), 1-29, John Wiley & Sons Ltd. Copyright © 2010 by John Wiley & Sons, Inc. All rights reserved. DOI: 10.1111/j.1740-1461.2009.01168.x

and other influences. Tahamont and Chalfin (2016) review research studies where attempts were made to differentiate the relative strengths of these effects. Overall, they could only conclude that 'aggregate crime rates are not very sensitive to marginal changes in the severity of a prison sentence' (2016, p. 22). Despite the centrality of prison as a general deterrent, findings in relation to this remain inconclusive.

The catalogue of findings just presented contains very little if any evidence that punitive sentences of any sort achieve their appointed aims. The totality of the findings raises fundamental questions over the principle of deterrence as a basis for sentencing policy and practice. Yet the use of punishment/incarceration for the purpose of deterrence continues ubiquitously, perhaps because many people accept at face value the idea that suffering unpleasant consequences as a result of offending will lead offenders to think twice and forgo future criminal activity. However, the parameters of *effective* punishment, defined as an attempt to reduce a pattern of behaviour by making its consequences more aversive, are well researched and understood, and it is difficult to envisage how they can be made to work properly in the criminal justice system (McGuire, 2004a; Miethe and Lu, 2005). Some features of punishment are considered in the accompanying 'Focus on ...' box.

FOCUS ON ...

Parameters of punishment

In penology, official punishment is often described in terms of three parameters:

- *Certainty* The likelihood of legal punishment as a result of committing a crime.
- *Celerity* The amount of time that lapses between an offence being committed and an official sanction being imposed.
- *Severity* The magnitude of a punishment or the estimated amount of distress or discomfort a convicted person would experience.

These features can be measured *objectively* – certainty, for example, can be measured as the proportion of crimes of a specific type that result in formal punishment, while severity can be measured as the amount of a fine or the length of a prison sentence. They can also be measured *subjectively* or *perceptually*, reflecting individuals' personal estimates of the chances of being caught, or of just how bad it would be for them if they were. From the perspective of attempting to reduce crime, it has been argued that subjective or perceptual features are more important (Gibbs, 1986).

There are numerous studies with a direct bearing on the question of which methods work best for changing behaviour. Gendreau (1996) estimated that, cumulatively, the pertinent research literature runs to more than 25,000 source references. This corpus of work establishes firmly that *positive reinforcement* is a more effective method of behaviour change than *punishment*. The latter may nevertheless be effective in some cases, but only when certain conditions prevail will it achieve its optimum effects (Axelrod and Apsche 1983; Cooper, Heron and Heward, 2007).

Echoing the list above, psychological research has shown that punishment achieves its maximum effectiveness when all of the following conditions are met:

- It is inevitable or unavoidable (the chances of escape are very remote).
- It is applied early in the problem behaviour sequence.
- It is administered without delay following each instance of the problem behaviour.
- It is applied at higher rather than lower levels of severity.
- There are alternative behaviours an organism (a person) can pursue to obtain a desired goal.

In practice, it is extraordinarily difficult, indeed probably impossible, to fulfil all of these conditions in the complex everyday environment of the criminal justice system.

First, only a very small fraction of criminal behaviours result in significant loss of liberty. The chances of being arrested, convicted and punished for a crime are surprisingly low. With reference to the UK, government figures have suggested that on average only 2 per cent of all offences committed (taking official statistics and victim surveys into account) result in a conviction. Following conviction, only one in seven of indictable offences leads to a custodial sentence (Home Office, 1993b). This yields an approximate probability of being sent to prison for a crime of 1 in 300.

Second, when punitive sanctions are administered, this usually occurs after a gap – weeks or months after the offence occurred. During that period, people engage in many other activities. There is no possibility of isolating a selected behaviour (the crime) and connecting it through a learning or behaviour change process to the punishment that is designed to be its consequence (Blackman, 1996).

Third, court sentences are graded on a loose scale of severity known colloquially as the 'tariff'. However, this bears a rather uneven relationship to the *seriousness* of crimes (Fitzmaurice and Pease, 1986). Although we often hear that penalties are too lenient, many citizens would have reservations about the continual use of exclusively severe sanctions.

Fourth, given the goal-directed nature of much acquisitive crime and the limited personal resources, lifestyles and circumstances of those who commit the majority of acquisitive crime, it is often the case that desirable alternatives – such as a meaningful, well-paid job – are limited or out of reach. Similarly, given the impulsive nature of some other crimes, it is clear that people do not stop before committing them to consider possible alternatives or likely consequences. In the absence of other possible means of reaching a goal, even behaviour that is punished will not necessarily be eradicated (or in behavioural terminology, 'extinguished').

There is evidence of deterrence being effective in particular circumstances, when it fulfils some of the criteria described in the 'Focus on...' box: for example in being linked to immediate and certain consequences, and combined with the possibility of alternative courses of action. This is illustrated in studies of *focused deterrence* that have been used to reduce gang violence in some US cities. The strategy within this, loosely called 'Pulling levers', was first tried in *Operation Ceasefire*, a problem-oriented policing initiative concerning gang-related retaliatory gun homicides amongst youth (<24 years) in Boston (Braga, Kennedy, Waring and Piehl, 2001). Police communicated directly with offender groups and conveyed plans for swift and massive responses to shootings. This included disrupting gangs' other illegal activities, with added enforcement consequences including stiffer plea bargains and sentences; but also making more community services available to targetted offenders. The approach was subsequently tested in several US cities. A meta-analysis found a medium-to-large mean effect size of 0.604 across 10 studies, representing a significant drop in key target outcomes, including homicide rates (Braga and Weisburd, 2015).

The suggestion that punishment does not work especially well and that it can in fact be counterproductive might sound puzzling and be difficult to accept. Surely everyone knows that if we do something and then suffer for it, we will avoid doing it again? This is a point on which psychology can make a significant contribution to criminal justice. As the 'Focus on ...' box suggests, official punishment departs markedly from the required parameters, in behavioural terms, of an efficient *aversive conditioner*. Research in criminology suggests that changing the *certainty* factor by increasing the perceived likelihood of being arrested is a better strategy than changing the *severity* factor by making punishments harsher (von Hirsch, Bottoms, Burney and Wikström, 1999).

Yet the commoner scenario is for governments to respond to public concerns about crime with 'get tough' rhetoric, which when acted upon has repeatedly proved ineffectual. Dwelling on the theme of punishment may in any case miss the pivotal point about conformity to the law. There is strong evidence that citizens' general compliance with the law is more likely to be a function of their endorsement of it, and their respect for it, than of their fear of official sanction should they break it (Tyler, 2006).

Criminal responsibility and culpability

The classical concept of criminal action propounded by Beccaria (discussed in Chapter 4) is still widely influential today as an underlying explanation of a great deal of crime. This asserts that crime is based on rational calculation. Acting on the basis of self-interest, individuals weigh the likely *benefits* of committing an offence against the possible *risks* of doing so, and make a decision accordingly (Becker, 1968). The normative model is thus one of individual responsibility for criminal action, and this assumption plays a pivotal part in decisions made by criminal courts. It also fits with dominant models of citizens as economic agents, making choices as consumers or in other spheres of their activity.

However, most judicial systems also recognise that there are some circumstances under which offences may *not* have been a product of such careful calculation, and may even have happened without conscious decisions or any willingness to commit them on the part of the people involved. In other words, there are instances in which even if it is shown that the individual *committed* an offence (the *actus reus* element is present), he or she, as a result of other factors, may not be fully *responsible* for it (the *mens rea* element is absent).

Criminal liability

For criminal liability or culpability to be demonstrated, some conditions have to be fulfilled. As described by Lacey and Zedner (2012), they include four requirements or *normative elements*, as follows.

Capacity

To be considered capable of committing crimes and thereby 'regarded as legitimate subjects of criminal law', individuals must have 'basic cognitive and volitional capacities' (Lacey and Zedner, 2012, p. 170). Without those attributes they cannot properly be considered as fully responsible for crimes they might commit. This sets a general exclusionary principle for criminal liability. The most obvious example of this is the doctrine of *doli incapax* (literally, 'incapable of crime') applied to children or, at least, to individuals below a designated age. As noted by Maher (2005), there is a very wide variation in the age of **criminal responsibility** in different jurisdictions. It ranges from 7 to 18, and is typically higher in countries that operate within a civil law tradition (as described earlier). It is 7 in Ireland, 10 in England and Wales and in most Australian states, 12 in the Netherlands and Canada, 13 in France, 14 in Germany, 15 in Scandinavian countries, 16 or 18 in most American states, and 18 in Belgium. As this is a general principle, it is distinct from the idea that someone might lack capacity because of a temporary mental state, which has to be assessed on an individual basis.

Conduct

Similar to the definitional or 'fair labelling' requirement (described in Chapter 2), individuals can only be held criminally accountable when their actual *behaviour* has transgressed a stated legal boundary (Herring, 2016). We cannot be criminally liable for our thoughts. Nor should we be liable as a result of some aspect of our status or identity (e.g. our religion or sexuality), or for omitting to do something we were not under any duty to do.

Responsibility (fault)

Criminal liability is a function of having had a causal role in the event that constituted the crime. Individuals are not held responsible for genuine accidents, and it is incumbent upon the prosecuting authorities to demonstrate the operation of intention, negligence, recklessness, or some other culpable state of mind (*mens rea*). However, as we noted in Chapter 2 there are also crimes that come under the legal category of *strict liability*, for which the prosecution need not prove a direct element of responsibility. If we are caught driving a car on the wrong side of the road, we are automatically liable to a finding of guilt, and that will remain so whatever our state of mind regarding our behaviour.

16

Defences

Even if the above requirements are met, it is still possible for an individual to argue that he or she was not fully responsible for a crime, and to escape some degree of criminal liability by forwarding a *defence*. This would consist of evidence concerning some aspect of the circumstances surrounding the offence or of the defendant's beliefs at the time. For example, the defendant might claim to have acted in self-defence, or to have been gravely threatened by others if she or he did not commit the crime, or for some reason to have been unable to control her or his own actions. Cases of this kind are of particular interest to psychologists as court authorities will require an assessment of individuals' mental states or perceptions of the situations in which they find themselves. Such cases are also often linked with concepts of mental disorder, as discussed in Chapter 11 and later in this chapter. The net outcome of these legal arguments, if successful, is to permit a defendant to show that he or she should not be held fully accountable for a crime.

The above concepts of criminal liability apply in *common law* systems and do not map very tidily onto corresponding concepts in *civil law* systems. However, Dubber (2006) suggests that the two can be unified into a cohesive form. Lacey and Zedner's (2012) approach to this was based on a consideration of normative requirements, as set out above. Approaching the problem from more pragmatic direction, Dubber's analysis would entail stating that a person is criminally liable if he or she 'engages in (1) conduct that (2) inflicts or threatens (3) substantial harm to individual or public interests (4) without justification and (5) without excuse' (Dubber, 2006, p. 1318).

The essence of these requirements, however they are framed, is that they allow an individual who has committed an offence to mount a defence against the prosecution's case that he or she was fully responsible for the behaviour that constituted the offence. There are both *general* defences, which are applicable across a broad range of crimes, and *specific* defences, which are applicable only to the most serious crimes, notably murder. The main categories of legal defence under the law of England and Wales are illustrated in the next 'Focus on ...' box.

FOCUS ON ...

Legal defences reducing culpability

Defences are legal arguments that can be used by an accused person, who admits to having broken the law, in attempts to establish that he or she was not fully responsible for the crime with which he or she is charged. We discussed one major category of defence, *diminished responsibility*, in Chapter 15. The following are further examples of defences available in English law.

Herring (2016) divides defences into three categories: (a) those based on a finding that what the defendant did was actually permissible; (b) those based on showing that pressure was exerted on the defendant by another person; and (c) those that are based on a finding about the defendant's mental condition.

Duress

Duress is a possible defence for almost all crimes, with the exception of murder, attempted murder and treason. The defendant has to show that he or she committed the offence because he or she was threatened with death or grievous bodily harm (nothing less will suffice), and that a reasonable person would have acted as the defendant did in the circumstances.

Loss of control

Like the defence of diminished responsibility, the defence of *loss of control* is applicable only to murder. This defence was defined in the Coroners and Justice Act 2009 and replaced the defence of 'provocation'. It allows the charge of murder to be reduced to manslaughter, but is distinct from the stipulation of abnormality of mental functioning defined in the Homicide Act 1957.

In these cases, it has to be established that the defendant lost self-control as a result of a 'qualifying trigger'. The latter can be fear of serious violence, or being seriously wronged by an extremely provocative act or circumstances of an extremely grave character, or a combination of the two.

Automatism

The rarely used defence of *automatism* involves claiming that the offender's mind was disengaged from the actions he or she took – that because of some external factor they were not the result of willed decisions. It therefore amounts to a denial of the *actus reus*.

Examples of automatism have included offences committed during or close to an epileptic seizure (the defendant's action being shown to be a result of a reflex); while affected by a state such as hypoglycaemia (linked to diabetes); or as a result of *night terror* (an uncommon mental condition entailing a particularly vivid and powerful nightmare).

Necessity

The defence of *necessity* has been applied in cases where defendants have sought to show that in committing an offence they were avoiding something worse – that is, that they chose 'the lesser of two evils'.

Even if this is shown, however, necessity is not available as a general defence (meaning it would be applicable to a wide range of crimes and not to just one specific crime) and it may not lead to an acquittal. In one case, a drunk man fell asleep in the back of his car. He woke to find the car moving down a hill, but managed to control the car and to steer it to safety without anyone being injured. He was nevertheless convicted of drink-driving.

Insanity

The possibility of being found not guilty of a crime on the grounds of *insanity* came into English law after an incident in 1843 in London, in which Daniel M'Naghten shot Edward Drummond, Private Secretary to the Prime Minister, Sir Robert Peel, believing Mr Drummond to be the PM. Mr M'Naghten had reportedly been suffering from delusions to the effect that the government was persecuting him (though historic evidence disputes whether he actually was: Mackay, 2010).

In subsequent debates, the House of Lords formulated what became known as the *M'Naghten Rules*, which became the basis for insanity decisions in many countries. For a defence of insanity, it must be proved that at the time of committing an offence the defendant was labouring under a 'defect of reason, from disease of the mind, so as not to know the nature of the act that he was doing, or if he did know, did not know that what he was doing was wrong'. This still applies in the Criminal Procedure (Insanity and Unfitness to Plead) Act 1991. It is separate from mental health law discussed in the main text, but decisions taken on the basis of the 1991 Act are likely to be put into effect using the Mental Health Act 2007. That is, the defendant will probably be found to be suffering from a mental disorder and detained under the Mental Health Act.

There are also other circumstances in which a person could be found not to have been in possession of the *mens rea* for an offence which are not technically defences. They include *involuntary intoxication* and having made a genuine *mistake*, but any such case would be considered carefully to establish whether the conditions did negate *mens rea*. 'Mistaken belief' means being genuinely wrong about the facts of a situation. That should not be confused with mistaken belief about the law: that argument is unlikely to succeed unless a new law had just been passed but most people had not yet heard of it.

Some types of offence have been explicitly defined in recognition of the role an individual's mental state might play in reducing his or her capacity for rational deliberation. One example of this is the offence of *infanticide*, defined in the Infanticide Act 1938. This Act allows that a mother who kills her child within the first 12 months after its birth is not necessarily guilty of murder. This defence may be invoked if it has been established that the woman had not fully recovered from the effect of giving birth, most commonly as a result of post-natal depression. Infanticide, described by Herring (2016) as 'unusual' in that it is the name both of an offence and of a defence, is by virtue of this provision a lesser crime than murder. It draws a less severe penalty, equivalent to that for manslaughter (potentially up to life imprisonment), but often resulting only in a Probation Order.

Mental health legislation

Probably the reason why individuals are most frequently considered not to be wholly culpable for their actions is that they have been found to be suffering from a mental disorder. The importance of this situation is such that it is governed by a separate framework of legal statutes. These govern society's response to individuals who are thought to pose a risk to themselves or to others, and meet criteria for diagnosis of some of the disorders we discussed in Chapter 11. Some form of mental health legislation has been in use for a long period of time.

Fennell (2010) describes the history of mental health legislation since the Middle Ages in England. The world's oldest psychiatric hospital is the hospital of St Mary of Bethlehem (Bethlem: the origin of the word *bedlam*). It first admitted people with mental disorders in 1377. There was mental health law already in force even before then. In medieval times, under the *De Prerogativa Regis* (1324), people who lost their sanity had their lands held by the Crown, but any proceeds and profits generated by that land were returned to the family when the afflicted individual recovered or died. During the 17th and 18th centuries there were numerous private 'madhouses', but they were reputedly places where people were confined against their will and subjected to abuse. The Vagrancy Act of 1744 was the first piece of legislation designed to restrain those in the community whose actions suggested that they were 'dangerous to be permitted to go abroad' – that is, to remain at liberty (Fennell, 2010, p. 6). Where it was thought necessary, such persons could be put in chains. The Madhouses Act of 1774, of which there were new versions in 1828 and 1832, was designed to regulate establishments so named.

The County Asylums Act of 1808 gave local magistrates powers to detain disturbed people in specially built institutions, but even then many 'lunatics' were taken to prison instead. A larger change came from 1845 onwards with the Lunatics Act and the creation of a national network of public asylums. This was followed by the Lunacy Act 1890, the Mental Deficiency Act 1913, and the Mental Treatment Act 1930, illustrating a long-standing differentiation between those with intellectual disabilities and those with mental disorder, which still applies in the present day. The contemporary framework of law in this field, however, stems from the Mental Health Acts of 1959 and 1983. The latter was amended in 2007 and became fully operational from November 2008. Shortly preceding this, the Mental Capacity Act 2005 was introduced, which, together with its accompanying documents and regulations, provides 'a complete legislative framework of decision-making for mentally incapacitated adults' (Fennell, 2010, p. 60). Although none of the currently prevailing Acts stipulates legal requirements for the psychology profession as such, the statutes contained within them have important implications for the work that applied psychologists are expected to do.

Under the Mental Health Act 2007, individuals who are assessed as suffering from some forms of mental disorder can be detained in hospital. The Act defines circumstances in which that can happen under civil law, and in those circumstances no court hearing is required. Admission can be undertaken informally (that is, on a voluntary basis), or requested by relatives, or initiated by medical personnel. In most cases detention must be authorised by two psychiatrists. Under other sections of the Act, on the order of the court individuals can be admitted for fixed periods for assessment, and, if it is thought necessary, can be detained in hospital for treatment (*Hospital Order*), with no time specified for the period of stay; and if needs be with added powers such that the Ministry of Justice must consent before they can be discharged (*Restriction Order*). Grounds for detention must be regularly reviewed, and detained patients can apply to have their cases heard by the **Mental Health Tribunal**, part of the government's Courts and Tribunals Service. The Tribunal is a legal body which works independently of secure hospitals and which evaluates evidence both from detaining authorities and from external witnesses concerning the legal grounds for a patient's detention. *Discharge* can be granted on the basis that an individual no longer suffers from a mental disorder of a nature or degree that requires treatment in hospital, or no longer poses a risk to self or to others. Conversely, for detention to *continue*, the Tribunal must be satisfied that appropriate treatment is available in hospital to ameliorate the person's mental condition. Alternatively, patients can be managed outside hospital using a **Community Treatment Order**.

While this is highly unlikely to have any immediate or even short-term implications, it is worth noting that the present legal framework in the United Kingdom and other countries that have separate mental health laws is at odds with the United Nations Convention on the Rights of Persons with Disabilities, adopted by the UN in 2006 and made operational in 2008. Fennell (2010) notes that it contravenes the Convention for a country to have discrete laws that can authorise the detention of a person on the grounds of mental disability: such a procedure is discriminatory and should be abolished. That is not to say that such persons cannot be detained, but that the grounds for doing so should be 'de-linked from the disability and neutrally defined' (Fennell, 2010, p. 69).

Conclusion

Penal codes, or sets of laws designed to regulate societies by forbidding certain acts and by specifying punishments for those acts, go back to ancient times. The system of laws and the interconnected apparatus of police, courts, prisons and community agencies that deal with crime has developed over a shorter but still sizeable period. The result is a very complex set of arrangements which reflects the impact of a wide range of sometimes contradictory pressures, for example between protecting the public and also recognising individual rights.

Thus while there are firm principles that underpin the legal and penal systems, the ways in which those principles apply in individual cases continue to generate situations and problems that may never have occurred before. Forensic psychologists need an understanding of those principles, and of the basic processes that influence the principal 'routes through the system' that the majority of individuals take. At the same time, it is also important to recognise that periodically previously unforeseen and unique issues and cases will arise, requiring an open-minded, flexible and adaptive approach.

Chapter summary

This chapter has focused on two of the key decision points that will be encountered on virtually all journeys through the system, in which an individual who has been prosecuted for a crime appears in court and a decision is made about innocence or guilt; and then, if the latter, a sentence is imposed. The effects of this sentence may be potentially far-reaching, not only on the individual's life but also on the lives of others, including any victims and their families, the offender's family, and sometimes whole communities.

- After a brief glimpse into the history of penal law, we reviewed differences between the frameworks that apply in the different legal systems that have emerged in different parts of the world.
- Sentencing has been justified on several different grounds, each of which can lead to quite different expectations about the effects of sentencing and what it can achieve. We considered the various basic principles on which sentencing is founded, mainly within one legal system, and how they relate to each other in practical decisions made by the courts today.
- We also examined the routes that are taken towards the sentencing decision and then following it, an area we examine further in Chapter 17.
- The question of whether sentencing does indeed have particular outcomes has varying degrees of relevance, depending on what were considered to be the grounds for choosing a particular sentence. The chapter reviewed evidence from criminology, penology and psychology on whether sentencing achieves its proposed effects, and explanations as to why it may not reliably succeed in doing so. We examined the effectiveness of sentencing as a proposed deterrent to criminal activity, focusing in part on capital punishment as it raises fundamental issues about the power of the law.

Further reading

Large numbers of books deal with sentencing from a legal standpoint, and all cover the ground of explaining basic elements of penal law and process. Fewer of them, however, set sentencing in a wider context, and the following are recommended because they take a broader approach.

» Andrew Ashworth (2015). *Sentencing and Criminal Justice*, 6th edition (Oxford: Oxford University Press). This provides a clear exposition of the ideas behind sentencing, alongside information on how it has evolved and how it operates in practice.

» Paul Cavadino, James Dignan and George Mair (2013). *The Penal System: An Introduction*, 5th edition (London: Sage). This is a very helpful overview of the system in England and Wales, placing greater emphasis on a criminological perspective (as compared to the legal focus of the book by Ashworth).

» Terence D. Miethe and Hong Lu (2005). *Punishment: A Comparative Historical Perspective* (Cambridge: Cambridge University Press). This discusses the history and philosophy of punishment from an international perspective. For a discussion of philosophical aspects of punishment, see the thought-provoking book by Ted Honderich (2006). *Punishment, the Supposed Justifications Revisited* (London: Pluto Press).

» James Bonta and Don A. Andrews (2017). *The Psychology of Criminal Conduct*, 6th edition (London and New York: Routledge). This provides detailed evidence concerning the failure of penal sanctions.

» Sentencing practice changes over time, and books cannot always keep pace. For details of the principles that underpin sentencing in the courts of England and Wales, and the frameworks used for sentencing decisions, visit the website of the Sentencing Council: https://www.sentencingcouncil.org.uk

» Another useful source is the UK government's criminal justice website, which is also linked to the Office for National Statistics and makes information available on a continually updated basis about the operation of all segments of the criminal justice system: https://www.justice.gov.uk

» If you are working with individuals detained under the Mental Health Act, it is important that you consult the *Code of Practice* which accompanies the Act, which specifies many details of its operation (there are both full and 'easy read' versions): https://www.gov.uk/government/publications/code-of-practice-mental-health-act-1983

After Sentencing: Follow-up Services

This chapter is concerned with sentencing and with the aftermath of sentencing, which we can understand as being the punishment that a convicted offender will receive once they have been found guilty. It is important to understand that a prison sentence is only one form of sentence, and in many situations it might be considered the least helpful from the perspective of trying to reduce recidivism and to protect society. For some individuals, it is the case that they will receive a prison sentence and, having served it, they will be released. However, the various structures of the legal system are far more complex for individuals who are considered to be dangerous, or for whom at least an element of their sentence was to bring about change (i.e. reducing their risk of reoffending). We set out below an overview of some of the most important of these structures, and how they can impact upon how individuals might move through the legal system once they have been sentenced. We will also consider the various roles that a forensic psychologist might play as a result of the sentence imposed upon an offender. It is important to have a sense of these issues because they impact upon the people with whom a forensic psychologist might come into contact at various stages of the offender's journey.

Chapter objectives

- To develop an understanding of the factors that may impact on sentencing decisions.
- To have an overview of the different kinds of sentences that are typically available.
- To start to consider how the imposed sentence may play a role in an offender's path through the judicial system.
- To develop a sense of how sentencing may impact on the role that a forensic psychologist may play in an offender's journey.

The purposes of sentencing

In principle, punishment for criminal behaviour comes to an end (except, potentially, in the case of the whole life sentence imposed for murder in the UK, which is a sentence with no predetermined release date). This is in line with the idea that society requires that individuals are meaningfully punished for their antisocial behaviour, and that meaningful punishment is possible (although the role of punishment as individual and social deterrent and its politicisation is much debated – see Alschuler, 2003). The 'Where do you stand?' box on the next page also highlights various viewpoints.

Presumably the idea of meaningful punishment is that individuals learn the negative consequences of their actions and will therefore be less likely to act in antisocial ways in the future, thereby reducing crime and protecting the public (see Joyce, 2009). It also assumes that individuals are capable of change; and that given enough time and appropriate support, this can be a change from offending to non-offending behaviour, whether this is through therapeutic intervention, such as attending sex-offender treatment programmes, or through some kind of deterrence, as might occur by the risk of having one's liberty reduced (for a critique of whether prison works, see Burnett and Maruna, 2004). The fact that there are sentencing guidelines in the UK suggests that decisions have been made concerning what constitutes sufficient or appropriate punishment, taking into consideration human rights, and how long it might take for a person to change. (For serious crimes, the US also has guidelines, set out by the United

WHERE DO YOU STAND?

Punishment

In legal terms, punishment is a consequence of committing and being convicted of an offence, and is imposed by the system of laws of a particular jurisdiction with the idea that the consequence results in some form of inconvenience or suffering. At its most basic, we might see punishment as being a deterrent for others; as teaching offenders a lesson, so that they do not behave in the same way again (as Scott (2008) describes it, deterring the rational offender requires the pain of punishment to outweigh the pleasures derived from the crime); or as a signal that society believes that the behaviour is particularly wrong, as might be the case in life sentences or death sentences. Broadly we can think of these three positions as *deterrence*, *rehabilitation* and *retribution*, but in all cases punishment is acting as a form of *communication* (see Duff, 2003).

These differing views of punishment are likely to stem from different philosophical positions – for example, the rehabilitative approach must assume that change is possible and that the explanations for antisocial behaviour can be identified. A retributionist approach is based on the idea that people deserve punishment if they commit a crime. The approaches may also have different outcomes. Whereas a deterrence or rehabilitation model seeks as its principal goal to change behaviour away from crime, the same is not necessarily true for retribution. Retribution is not necessarily about teaching someone a lesson: it may simply be about giving people what they 'deserve'.

Perhaps the clearest example of a retributionist approach is the use of the death penalty. One might argue that it also has a deterrent aspect, as Ehrlich has (1975), but there is ongoing debate as to the deterrent nature of the death penalty; Radelet and Lacock (2009) suggest that there is clear empirical evidence that it does not have a deterrent effect. It is likely that the picture is more complex than a simple relationship, depending not just on the existence of the death penalty in a particular jurisdiction, but also on how frequently it is used, how it is reported, and the circumstances under which it is applied.

Where do you stand on this issue?

1 Which of the three approaches – deterrence, rehabilitation and retribution – best describes your own opinion of punishment?
2 Does your view fit with the way in which you understand the system of punishment in your own country or state?
3 Even if one were to take a retributionist view of punishment, are there arguments that would allow this position yet prevent the use of the death penalty?

States Sentencing Commission, but they are considered as only advisory, as are the individual state sentencing guidelines.)

The Criminal Justice Act 2003 sets out the five purposes of sentencing, and judges are required to take these into account when deciding a sentence. They are:

- the punishment of offenders
- the reduction of crime (including its reduction by deterrence)
- the reform and rehabilitation of offenders
- the protection of the public
- the making of reparation by offenders to persons affected by their offences.

These play an important role in determining sentencing.

Factors that impact on sentencing

Before an individual must deal with more subtle forms of restriction, such as those that might occur on release (see below), there are a number of ways in which society determines whether that person is appropriate for release. These are dependent on the sentence or Hospital Order that the offender received, and then how he or she might be managed or monitored after release (for example, through probation or the Multi-Agency Public Protection Arrangements (MAPPA) process). The most obvious example of this is that once individuals have served the minimum required portion of their sentence (known as the *tariff* or *minimum term*) – which, depending on circumstances such as admitting the offence before the trial, is often less than the full sentence – they will be released.

The Sentencing Council, a part of the Ministry of Justice, is responsible for setting guidelines for sentencing in England and Wales, and its offence-specific guidelines can be downloaded from its website. As an example, let us consider the crime of *manslaughter on the basis of provocation*. First, the requirements for an act of murder having taken place have to be proven; and then the fact that although it was murder, there is evidence to prove that this murder was in response to *provocation*, and that the person who had committed the offence had lost control – usually on the basis of things said or done by the victim. Additionally, it must be proven that this loss of control was '*reasonable*' in the circumstances; and also that the loss of control was *excusable* (in the sense that the offence can therefore be considered manslaughter rather than murder). Once this has been established, the judge is required to consider the degree and duration of the provocation, the time delay between the provocation and the offence, the individual's behaviour after the killing (e.g. attempts to evade detection versus providing medical assistance or calling the authorities), and whether or not a weapon was used.

With this information, the judge determines what the starting point for a sentence will be (based on the degree of provocation: 12 years for low provocation, 3 years for high provocation), and then considers the mitigating and aggravating factors to determine the available sentencing range (for example, for low provocation the range would be from 10 years' custody to life in prison; and for high provocation it would be custody for up to 4 years).

The point at which an individual confesses a crime also plays a role in the sentence that he or she receives. For example, early confession results in a reduced sentence, whereas although a last-minute confession may have some impact, that impact will be much smaller. This implies that a confession has some kind of meaning about the individual's risk or, less helpfully from a psychological perspective, that the person is being rewarded for using less of the court's time. An interesting study from Canada has looked at the factors that impact on the decision to confess (see Deslauriers-Varin, Lussier and St-Yves, 2011; see the 'Focus on ...' box), and demonstrated that confession is influenced by a range of criminological factors (e.g. the seriousness of the crime), situational factors (e.g. the use of legal advice), and individual factors (e.g. guilt). It is not clear to what extent these factors relate to reduced reoffending. For example, individuals who confess are less likely to have sought legal representation, but

FOCUS ON ...

Decisions to confess

As suggested in the text, there are factors that might impact upon an individual's decision to confess to a crime. For example, in England, to the offender's benefit, an early confession may result in a reduced sentence. Of course, *pleading* 'not guilty' and subsequently being *found* 'not guilty' would result in no sentence at all, and an offender may believe that the police do not have enough evidence to prosecute a case, and so it will never get to trial – the decision-making process can be quite complex.

Experience shows that some people do confess and some do not, and it would be useful to *understand* that decision-making process because, if the factors are within our control, increasing the number of valid confessions (i.e. not an increase of confessions for crimes that a person did not commit) would result in fewer trials, thereby saving resources for the legal system. However, previous studies have either produced contradictory results or identified factors that are *not* within our control. A study by St-Yves (2002) showed that sex offenders are more likely to confess if at the time of their interview they were single. A study by Deslauriers-Varin, Lussier and St-Yves (2011) identified factors that influence decisions to confess to crimes: 221 adult males participated in the study, all imprisoned in a Canadian federal prison, and data were collected from a variety of sources such as their prison files, police reports and self-report data. Comparing men who confessed with those who did not, the researchers found that age, ethnicity, education, marital status and parental status did not differentiate between the two groups, and nor did the number of previous convictions or offence type. Those who confessed were more likely to have committed more serious crimes, to report feeling greater guilt, and to feel that the evidence against them was strong; and did not employ the services of a lawyer during their interviews.

One conclusion from this study is that there are factors that can be manipulated during police interviews that could lead to more confessions, and it would be beneficial to be aware of these as some might be unethical (e.g. persuading offenders that they don't require a lawyer) and may allow for a later appeal.

Questions

1 Should a confession lead to any form of sentencing benefit?

2 From a forensic perspective, is it likely that a person who confesses will be more amenable to change, or might this be evidence rather of an individual who is manipulative?

there is as yet no research looking at a possible link between using legal representation and reductions in reoffending.

Once all the factors that could impact on a tariff have been considered, the five purposes noted in the Criminal Justice Act, which we saw above, come into play in order for the judge to decide the actual tariff, or sentence, that must be served.

Later, once the tariff has been served, the individual will usually be released. However, when there is no determined tariff, or if for some reason the individual is detained longer than the tariff, the individual may appeal to the Parole Board in an attempt to be released.

Parole Boards

When individuals are taken into custody, it is possible that they may remain within the criminal justice system for longer than their original sentence, for example through receiving discretionary life sentences or extended sentences (both of which are discussed in the following section) imposed under Section 44 of the Criminal Justice Act 1991 (now Section 85 of the Powers of the Criminal Courts (Sentencing) Act 2000). It is the task of the Parole Board to determine whether individuals who have received any of these types of life sentence, or an Imprisonment for Public Protection (IPP) sentence, have served their sentence – as, at sentencing, a life sentence does not necessarily mean for 'life' – and should be released. The basic principle of release concerns whether the individual poses a threat to the public, particularly with regard to those individuals on an IPP sentence. The evidence that might be used by the Parole Board will include the person's behaviour whilst incarcerated, how he or she has addressed his or her offending behaviour through various forms of intervention, and the extent to which any identified risk factors, such as drug use and mental health issues, have been addressed.

However, there are also a number of other important considerations for individuals who have been separated from society for a lengthy period of time. Firstly, by definition, 'lifers' and individuals with IPPs will have spent an extended period of time in prison, and may have become institutionalised (see Sapsford, 1978, for an early study and overview of work concerned with this issue). Secondly, again by the nature of being lifers and IPP prisoners, these individuals are considered complex and potentially dangerous, and it is suggested (see Padfield,

2000) that community services may not be sufficiently trained to offer the necessary support and monitoring that these individuals are considered to need in order for them to desist from offending.

It may seem that it is relatively easy to become imprisoned, yet somewhat harder to be released; and although this may raise concerns, it should not come as a surprise, given that the legal system is attempting to balance the rights of the individual who has committed an offence, and who is therefore considered at risk of doing so again, and the rights of society to be protected from such individuals and such behaviour. A famous study by Rosenhan (1973) perhaps demonstrates why it should not necessarily be more straightforward to be released from prison. In this study, individuals who had committed offences pretended to be hearing voices, so that they would be removed from prison and admitted to mental health facilities, but on admission they ceased to report any symptoms, behaved normally, and kept notes of the events that they experienced whilst still detained. In some cases the note-taking was interpreted as part of the mental health issue that had been diagnosed. We might wonder from this to what extent some behaviour in prison may be considered to be linked to criminality when actually it is not, and what behaviour might be overlooked when it might actually be a useful identifier of ongoing risk (referred to as 'offence-paralleling behaviour' (see Daffern *et al.*, 2007).

Parole Board hearings

Parole Boards meet three years before the end of an individual's minimum term, in the first instance, to determine whether an individual should be released. The meetings can take one of two forms, either oral or paper-based. Oral hearings typically take place where an indeterminate sentence is being considered, or if an individual is making an appeal against a recall to prison. Paper hearings are typical for determinate sentences. Parole Board panels also took on an additional role – as a result of a ruling by the European Court of Human Rights in 1992 – of independently and regularly reviewing post-tariff lifers' and IPP prisoners' circumstances and making decisions as to whether they should be released or detained for a further period.

The panel consists of three members, led by a judge or a member of the Parole Board, and the process is similar to a court hearing. Witnesses may be called, the individual can be legally represented, and the decision is made as to whether the person should be released, moved to a prison with a lower level of security, or continue to be detained (see Padfield, Liebling and Arnold, 2000). A victim, or one of his or her relatives, may attend and present a Victim Personal Statement outlining how the crime has impacted on the victim's life and making recommendations for conditions the victim believes should be imposed if the prisoner is to be released.

In principle, if individuals are consistently unable to persuade the panel that they are no longer a risk, they may remain in prison for the whole of their natural lives. There are a variety of reasons why it may be difficult to persuade a panel, other than individuals being unwilling to engage in interventions or because of their behaviour in prison. For example, given the finite resources of the Prison Service it may not be possible for all individuals to have access to programmes that they are considered to need in order to reduce their risk. Similarly, individuals with learning disabilities or mental health issues may not be found to be suitable for such programmes.

Sentences assessed by Parole Boards

As we saw in the Rosenhan case above, the importance of ensuring the appropriateness of individuals' release is extremely important. It is therefore particularly important for Parole Boards to make sure that individuals who have served IPPs or different types of life sentences, and who are therefore seen to pose the greatest risk to society, are ready to be released. Below we outline these different types of indeterminate sentences: mandatory life sentences, discretionary life sentences, automatic life sentences, individuals detained at Her Majesty's Pleasure and determinate sentences.

In the UK, the development of our current law has a long and complicated past, particularly in the case of crimes of murder. Until 1964 it was possible in the UK to receive the death penalty for murder, and the last two hangings took place on 13 August 1964, one in London and one in Liverpool. In effect the death penalty was abolished in 1965 for murder, although it was still a possible sentence in Northern Ireland until 1973, and it was as late as 1998 that the death penalty was abolished for military offences (such as mutiny). Currently there are a number of different responses to serious crimes in the UK, which may be understood as an evolution of sentencing after the death penalty had been abolished – for example, whole life sentences, mandatory life sentences and discretionary life sentences, as described earlier. Whole life sentences are a response to particularly serious murders (e.g. the abduction and murder of a child): no minimum term is provided and, except in exceptional circumstances, this sentence does equate to life imprisonment.

Adding to the complexity of how offenders are managed or dealt with after they have served their minimum sentence, which is in part the responsibility of the Parole Board, are the debates and decisions regarding responses to crime that are not solely legal but social and political too. These reflect the ideology of the political party in power, society's views, and concerns regarding crime, for example (see Padfield, 1996).

Mandatory life sentences

A *mandatory life sentence* does not equate to 'life' in the UK. It is the only sentence that can be passed for murder, which can be imposed on anyone over the age of 21. (The same sentence for anyone convicted of murder between the ages of 18 and 21 is referred to as 'sentence for life'; while for individuals between the ages of 10 and 18 it is referred to as 'Detention during Her Majesty's Pleasure'.) However, the judge may use discretion, considering mitigating factors and sentencing guidelines, with a range of different 'starting points' of 15, 25 or 30 years. From these starting points, the minimum term is then determined by the judge. Where a judge decides that the murder is particularly grave (e.g. the abduction and murder of a child) an individual may receive a 'whole life order', for which no minimum term is set.

Her Majesty's Pleasure

As above, when an individual commits a murder and is over 10 years of age and under the age of 18, he or she will receive a sentence of detention at **Her Majesty's Pleasure**. This sentence may have a minimum term before which an individual may not be considered for release, and once this tariff has been served the individual's case will be regularly reviewed by the Parole Board. If released, the individual will be subject to supervision for an indefinite period (Youth Justice Board, 2011).

Discretionary life sentences

A *discretionary life sentence* may be imposed for offences other than murder that may receive a life sentence (e.g. attempted murder, rape, or armed robbery) and if the court considers that the individual, who must be over the age of 21, is a danger to the public. This sentence is referred to as 'custody for life' when the individual is between the ages of 18 and 21 when convicted, and as 'detention for life' for a person between the ages of 10 and 18. At the time of sentencing, the judge will have reached the decision that no estimation can be reliably made as to the length of time during which that person may remain dangerous.

In response to a decision by the European Court of Human Rights, which considered that discretionary lifers should regularly receive reviews as to the legality of their continued detention, the Parole Board holds Discretionary Lifer Panels (since 1992). Currently regulations dictate that a review should take place every two years, the first taking place once the minimum sentence has been served. Padfield, Liebling and Arnold (2000) provide a comprehensive overview of the work of Discretionary Lifer Panels, including an observational study of the process of decision-making.

Automatic life sentences

A person can receive an *automatic life sentence* if over 18 and convicted of a second offence that is defined as 'serious' (which would include murder, rape and carrying a firearm with criminal intent), provided that the offence occurred before 4 April 2005 (when this ruling was repealed). This sentence has now been replaced by the IPP, but there are individuals in UK prisons who have received this sentence.

Determinate sentences

Offenders with *determinate sentences* include individuals who are on *Discretionary Release* (those who are serving more than four years and who are eligible for release halfway through their sentence), and individuals who receive an extended sentence for public protection. Additionally, if an individual with a determinate sentence has been released and has then breached the conditions of that release, and as a consequence is back in prison, they may be referred to the Parole Board to consider re-release.

Mental Health Review Tribunals

The Parole Board has responsibility for making decisions regarding individuals who have been imprisoned. In cases where an individual has been detained on the grounds of mental health concerns, this responsibility falls to a **Mental Health Tribunal**, which again consists of three people: one medical, one legal and one layperson. There are separate Mental Health Review Tribunals for England, Scotland and Wales. Their remit is to consider the evidence for the person's detention under the Mental Health Act and to determine whether the person should be further detained (due to risk – either risk to others or risk due to their own vulnerability or incapacity – or because of a need for further treatment), or whether they might be released under a range of different options (for example, a *conditional release*, whereby an individual is released but with requirements if they are to remain at liberty, such as engaging in some form of intervention, reporting to a probation officer, living at a particular address, or having a **curfew**). This is the case for all patients who are not referred to as 'restricted', where *restriction* means in the UK that the Ministry of Justice must agree to any plans for leave, transfer, or discharge, because those patients are considered to pose a high level of risk. The tribunals consider a range of information during their decision-making, for example an individual's need for medical treatment, based on the patient's diagnosis, the protection of the public, and the best interests of the patient (which may not include their release in some circumstances). The tribunals can also recommend that an individual be transferred to another hospital, that he or she be allowed leave, or that a Community Treatment Order might be appropriate.

Freckelton (2003) provides an interesting overview of why, in many cases, Mental Health Review Tribunals are likely to be compromised, due to the nature of the review process and the information that the tribunal will be using to make its decision. Freckelton suggests that an understanding of this process may result in a fairer review of an individual's current circumstances and mental health. For example, if an individual believes that a tribunal is likely to be biased, this might prevent the patient from communicating effectively, which may be interpreted mistakenly by the board as being indicative of poor mental health. Similarly, some people who attend tribunals may be taking medication that influences their mood or their alertness, and this can play a role in the proceedings of the tribunal and may impact on the views of the board members, their responses to the patient, and how the patient then responds. Tait (2003) provides a similar overview, along with some recommendations as to how tribunals might be more usefully managed to result in a more valid outcome.

Criminal Cases Review Commission

One of the underlying assumptions throughout this chapter, and indeed the entire book, is that the people we have referred to as 'offenders' are *guilty* of an offence; and that as a result of that guilt, along with other factors, their route through the legal system can be charted and understood, as can the consequences of that route. In the above material, all the issues concerned with tribunals and boards have suggested that release from incarceration, of whatever kind, is dependent on the calculated level of *risk* that these individuals pose and the amount of change that they are able to demonstrate.

However, there are also situations where innocent individuals are in fact victims of *miscarriages of justice*, and such cases come within the purview of the **Criminal Cases Review Commission**, an independent public body whose role is to determine whether there has been a miscarriage of justice and, if so, whether an individual should be recommended for release or a change in sentence. In UK legal case history there are a number of cases where previous convictions that have resulted in long terms of incarceration have later been overturned. This may happen for a variety of reasons, for example because new evidence suggests that confessions had been unfairly obtained or because new scientific evidence (e.g. using DNA) demonstrates that a convicted person could not have been involved in the crime. Kyle (2004) provides a number of examples, including that of the Maguire Seven, who were convicted in 1976 of being involved in bombings in London through evidence suggesting that they were in possession of the explosive nitroglycerine, which was subsequently used by the Irish Republican Army (IRA). Later evidence suggested that their contamination could have been entirely innocent, but six of the seven people had by that time served their sentences (ranging from 4 years to 14 years) and been released, while the seventh had died in prison.

It was cases such as these that led to the setting up of the Criminal Cases Review Commission (established in March 1997 by the Criminal Appeal Act 1995) in order to review Crown Court and Magistrates' Court cases if an appeal was made. Importantly, the Commission does not have the authority to release prisoners or to alter their tariff, but it can refer a case either to the Court of Appeal or back to the Crown Court in order that new information can be considered, which would usually be either new evidence or a point of law that had not previously been considered. The belief that a judge or jury simply came to the wrong conclusion is not enough for the Commission to refer a case back to the courts. Up to the end of July 2016, the Commission had received a total of 21,311 applications, of which 20,259 had been completed; and of those, 603 had been heard by the Court of Appeal. The most up-to-date information is available on the Criminal Cases Review Commission website.

Multi-Agency Public Protection Arrangements

Multi-Agency Public Protection Arrangements (MAPPA) is a multi-agency approach to managing the risk posed by violent and sexual offenders who have been released into the community, through collaboration between the National Probation Service, the Prison Service and the police. Additionally, a number of other agencies have a duty to cooperate with MAPPA, for example job centres, health trusts, social services and landlords providing social housing. Introduced in 2001, the process has been assessed on a number of occasions, and interestingly one of the regularly occurring issues that has been identified is the difficulty in ensuring that psychological input is available (e.g. Kemshall *et al.*, 2005). One of the many possible roles in which forensic psychologists can impact on an offender's route through the criminal justice system is by providing information to other professional bodies; and indeed in many cases, if psychologists are involved in the assessment and intervention of an offender, they will be invited to attend MAPPA meetings. There are specific categories of offenders who may fall under the scrutiny of MAPPA, known as Category 1, 2 and 3 offenders and three other categories of offenders (see Table 17.1).

The role of MAPPA is to provide a structure for information-sharing between agencies, with the aim of preventing offending. Initially this focused primarily on monitoring, but gradually behaviour change, risk management and treatment needs also became a part of MAPPA, and psychologists and psychiatrists were therefore invited to attend meetings concerning clients whom they had assessed or with whom they had been working. The meetings are intended to develop individualised risk management

Offence category	Offence type
Category 1	Registered sexual offenders
Category 2	Violent or sexual offenders who have received a sentence of 12 months or more
Category 3	Offenders who are considered to pose a risk of serious harm to the public, and: (a) it is complex to manage them, or management requires specific commitment of resources; or (b) cases that may lead to high levels of media or public scrutiny
'Potentially dangerous'	People who have not been convicted or cautioned, but who are believed to be likely to cause serious harm
Terrorists	Convicted of an offence under any terrorist legislation
Domestic extremists	For example, animal rights extremists

Table 17.1 Multi-Agency Public Protection Arrangements (MAPPA): categories of offenders.

plans before individuals are released, and then to monitor those individuals after release. For a detailed account of MAPPA systems and processes, see Kemshall and Wood (2007).

Community sentences

According to Solomon and Silvestri (2008), in 2007 there were more than 111,000 individuals serving community sentences and nearly 80,000 in custody in the UK. *Community sentences* became available to the courts with the setting up of the Probation Service in 1907, yet despite their longevity and the large numbers of people who receive a *Community Order*, there has been little research into how they might work to facilitate change and mitigate risk.

Community sentences are typically a response to lesser crimes, such as benefit fraud and car theft, but they may also be seen as a response to the overcrowding in UK prisons, whereby individuals considered to pose less of a risk may not be detained but may instead be supervised in the community. Typically we imagine community sentences to consist of picking up litter or helping to clean urban areas, but in fact they may also consist of other elements such as undergoing some form of education or intervention. In addition to treatment (including treatment for drug and alcohol issues), conditions may be attached to a Community Order: for example, there may be a requirement that the individual receive basic education, provide reparation to victims, or be restricted in their movements (e.g. being banned from football matches) and in the times when they can be outside their residence; and to monitor such restrictions they may be *electronically tagged*. In 2007, 32 per cent of those individuals who had received a Community Order were required to undertake unpaid work (Solomon and Silvestri, 2008).

One of the concerns raised by community sentencing is that it may be viewed by the public as a 'soft' option, with only a small punitive element. Smith (1984) suggested that the public tend to view Community Orders as suitable for those individuals who do not require punishment or control, and that offenders who are deemed dangerous do not fall into this category. This creates a dilemma, as the public (and the media) are less welcoming of Community Orders, and may respond in ways that might trigger the further offences they so fear. Despite concerns regarding the effectiveness of community treatment programmes, however, a 2007 study by Palmer and colleagues has demonstrated that each of three intervention programmes – Enhanced Thinking Skills, Think First, and Reasoning and Rehabilitation – carried out in the community resulted in reduced reconviction rates for individuals who completed such a programme, in comparison to individuals who either did not complete one of these programmes or were not given the option of such a programme. In the same year, a study by Levenson, Brannon, Fortney and Baker (2007) suggested that 65 per cent of a sample of 193 people from Florida believed that treatment in the community was effective in reducing sexual offending. Clearly, this is in contrast to the previously mentioned work by Smith, and also contradicts other data from the Levenson *et al.* study, which indicated that the majority of respondents thought that sexual offenders require 99 years in prison. The explanation provided by the authors for the high rate of support for community treatment is that respondents were not perceiving community treatment as the only source of protection, but recognised that this would also include restrictions of movement, public notification, and other responses from professionals. A series of meta-analyses conducted by Marsh, Fox and Sarmah (2009) concluded that prison on its own was not particularly effective in preventing reoffending, and that some aspects of community sentencing were more so. A qualitative study conducted by Rex (1999), which involved interviewing individuals on probation, suggested that the majority of probationers thought that probation *did* work to prevent reoffending, both with a direct effect on offending behaviour and an indirect effect in relation to known triggers (for example, drug use and alcohol use).

Probation services

The National Probation Service (NPS) is part of Her Majesty's Prison and Probation Service and supervises approximately 30,000 higher risk offenders per year. Those assessed as medium and lower risk are managed by 21 Community Rehabilitation Companies (CRCs), though the different agencies work in partnership. The stated aims of the National Probation Service are: 'protecting the public, reducing reoffending, the proper punishment of offenders in the community, ensuring victims' awareness on the part of the offender and the rehabilitation of offenders' (Nellis, 2002, p. 62). Probation services become involved *prior* to an individual receiving a sentence as they also work with offenders in order to produce pre-sentence reports, which may be used by judges and magistrates in reaching their sentencing decisions. The probation service therefore plays an important role in the assessment of offenders pre-sentence and in supporting them post-sentence. Pre-sentence reports consist of an assessment of the offender (e.g. mental and physical health, current employment, support in the community, regret for their actions, and the likelihood that they will engage with probation and other services); and also notes any extenuating circumstances, any need for treatment, and any other factors that might help the judge make an informed decision as how best to sentence that offender. Post-sentence, probation services provide and manage approved premises for offenders who have received a residence requirement as part of their sentence or licence, and they also provide a range of intervention programmes (such as sex-offender treatment programmes) for individuals.

Assessing risk

As we have suggested, subsequent to serving their time, whether that be simply their minimum sentence or after a successful Parole Board or Mental Health Tribunal hearing, individual offenders should, in principle, be allowed to reintegrate with society. However, there are a number of reasons why individuals may *not* be released after serving their sentences, and primarily this is a reflection of the level of risk that those individuals are thought to pose. It may seem contradictory that someone would be released who is still considered by professionals to pose a risk, but for legal and ethical reasons it is not possible to simply continue to detain people indefinitely on the grounds that they *might* present a level of risk to society (see Henham, 1997). Indeed, the whole concept of 'risk' implies a degree of uncertainty as to how an individual may behave in the future, and as this is a dynamic concept it is difficult to predict how the level of risk may change across a range of situations.

Research has attempted to identify the factors that impact on risk – those that increase it and reduce it – in order to develop tools that can be predictive of the likelihood that an individual would reoffend if released (that is, the risk of **recidivism**). Level of risk

WHERE DO YOU STAND?

Risk

In the case of the criminal justice system, risk is typically concerned with the likelihood of someone reoffending. (There are other areas of risk that might be important to consider, such as the likelihood of *initial* offending, and the likelihood of harming self.) The likelier that person is to reoffend and the greater the severity of that offence, the greater the risk from that individual is considered to be.

Research has sought to identify *risk factors*, which are linked with recidivism, and *protective factors*, which are related to desistance from offending. Risk factors are commonly split into two categories: *static* or *historical* risk factors, which cannot be changed (e.g. the age at the time of the first offence; having been a victim of sexual abuse); and *dynamic* risk factors that are amenable to change (e.g. the use of drugs; the current age; a pro-criminal lifestyle). In principle, a concern of forensic psychology is to help reduce individuals' level of risk so that they may be reintegrated back into society or, if that is not possible, to make them manageable within the service where they live (as might be the case for someone with a severe mental illness).

Risk is measured using a variety of tools, such as the HCR-20, the Static-99 and the SAVRY, and decisions are made about individuals on the basis of these results. However, it is not surprising to find that risk prediction is not perfect – indeed, a systematic review and meta-analysis involving 24,827 people suggested that risk-assessment tools for assessing violence have only low-to-moderate levels of prediction of reoffending (see Fazel, Singh, Doll and Grann, 2012). It is not surprising because it is unlikely that we currently have, or perhaps ever will have, a complete definition of the risk and protective factors for all offenders and all crime types. That being the case, we may have to accept that however long someone stays in prison, and however many interventions they receive, in some cases there will remain areas of risk that have not been identified.

Suppose we consider risk to be simply the likelihood that a particular kind of person who has offended in a particular manner will reoffend in the next five years. What level of risk would you be prepared to accept to allow someone to be released from prison? A 20 per cent chance that someone like that would reoffend within five years? (That is: out of 100 people who have offended in that manner, it is expected that over five years 20 of them will reoffend.) Or a 10 per cent chance?

Where do you stand on this issue?

1 Does your view depend on the nature of the offence that someone might commit, if we assume that thereafter she or he may also commit the same kind of offence again?

2 If we accept that risk is difficult to predict and that measuring it accurately is complex, how else might a person's risk be managed beyond the reductions that can be produced through psychological and medical interventions?

is important from a therapeutic perspective, too, given that studies have suggested that treating low-risk offenders produces a small reduction in recidivism (3 per cent), whereas in high-risk offenders the effect is larger (a 10 per cent reduction in recidivism: see Andrews and Dowden, 2006). This is the basis of the **Risk–Needs–Responsivity principle** (RNR: Andrews, Bonta and Hoge, 1990), which suggests that the *level of intervention* provided to an offender should be in proportion to the *level of risk* of reoffending that they pose.

Two broad categories of **risk factors** have been identified: those referred to as *static* (historical and unchangeable, e.g. the age of an individual's first offence) and those referred to as *dynamic* (potentially changeable, e.g. an individual's level of victim empathy or impulsivity), and efforts have been made to understand how these may impact upon future outcomes. For sexual offending, long-term recidivism appears to be best predicted by static factors (Hanson and Bussière, 1998), because those identify established characteristics of an individual. In contrast, reoffending can be prevented only by considering the factors that can be changed: the dynamic factors (Beech, Friendship, Erikson and Hanson, 2002). What makes the issue of risk complex is identifying which factors are important for a particular individual. Research has demonstrated that this is dependent on a variety of other elements, such as the presence or absence of mental health issues, and the specific offences that the person commits (e.g. Coid, Hickey, Kahtan and Zhang, 2007). For this reason, risk is always an *estimate* rather than a precise measure, which means that some individuals who are likely to commit new offences are released, whilst others who are unlikely to do so may nevertheless remain in detention. It is through research that psychology and psychiatry aim to reduce these errors. For example, a study by Swinburne Romine and colleagues (2012) in the US analysed the offending behaviour over a period of 30 years of 744 sexual offenders who had attended an outpatient sex-offender treatment programme. They found that the overall reoffence rate for contact sexual offenders was 10 per cent (75 individuals) and for non-contact sexual offenders it was 4 per cent (29 individuals). Within these data, the individuals' age at the start of treatment was linked to recidivism (over the age of 45 there was a marked reduction in recidivism), and the number of years back in the community impacted upon recidivism (the riskiest time being between 5 and 10 years in the community). They also discovered that failure to complete treatment *per se* did not increase risk, but failure to complete treatment because the individual had been discharged from the group *did* increase risk. This study demonstrates a number of areas that are linked to reoffending, but as the levels of reoffending for contact and noncontact sexual offences are relatively low, it is likely that a range of other factors are protective. The authors state that the two most important risk factors are 'general antisocial characteristics' for contact reoffending and 'greater sexual deviancy' for non-contact reoffending (both risk factors measured by the Static-99R test).

Given that risk assessments are estimates, forensic professionals have to accept both that they can be inaccurate, in that the individual may go on to reoffend, and also that there is a time factor, in that risk may change over years, either increasing or decreasing (as demonstrated by the findings of Swinburne Romine and colleagues, 2012). Clearly, as *estimates* risk assessments can also be accurate, but unfortunately the media focus on the times when decisions to release individuals result in further offences or when offenders are not released when perhaps their risk is low. (For example, in 2009 the Great Train Robber, Ronnie Biggs, unable to speak or move, was considered by a Parole Board to still pose a risk.) Of course there are some individuals who are likely never to be released, presumably because they are considered to pose enough of a threat that they might offend again: for example, Ian Brady (infamous for several child murders in the 1960s, who died in prison in 2017, as did his accomplice, Myra Hindley), and Peter Sutcliffe (the 'Yorkshire Ripper', who killed women in the 1970s, who in 2017 was moved from a high security hospital to a prison). Indeed there are a number of murderers who probably won't be released (according to Hansard (2009), there are 24 males and fewer than 5 females who are whole-term lifers). Interestingly, among this group is Charlie Bronson (real name Michael Gordon Peterson, now known as Charles Salvador) who has not killed but who has proven to be difficult to manage in the prison system (because of hostage-taking and fighting). Are these individuals a risk to society, or are there other reasons why the decision-making process leads to their continued detention? Is it possible that there is a recognition that the public would struggle with the release of someone convicted of 13 murders (e.g. Peter Sutcliffe), and that it is rather that the individual may himself, or herself, be at risk of harm from others? It cannot be denied that there are processes other than risk estimates that are a part of the decision-making with regard to the level of risk that is tolerable and the possible consequences if someone were to offend again – processes that include politics and societal pressures (more on this below in relation to sex offenders). As an example, *The Sun*, a UK newspaper, discovered that David McGreavy, a man who had killed three children, was being detained, 23 years later, in a low security prison, and reported this with the headline: 'How can they think of letting such a beast go free' (*The Sun*, 2 January 2006). Shortly after this, McGreavy was moved from open conditions to a prison with greater levels of security, apparently at his own request, as again reported by *The Sun* ('Child Killer is Caged': 27 July 2007). At about the same time, the BBC reported that the then Home Secretary, John Reid, had informed the Parole Board of his view that McGreavy should not be released ('Reid opposed child killer release': BBC, 23 April 2007). Referring back to the Criminal Justice Act's (2003) five purposes, it may be felt that in some of these cases reparation to individuals and society could never be achieved.

Other factors that limit an individual's freedom

As we have considered, there are a number of ways in which an individual's freedom may be affected other than through a prison term. A more concrete example would be a custodial sentence and time on the Sex Offender Register for men who have sexually offended against children. The **Sex Offender Register**, implemented in 1997, has been described as 'a measure aimed at helping to protect the community from sex offenders not an additional penalty' (Home Office/Scottish Executive 2001, p. 11). It is based on the idea that 'if convicted offenders knew that an effective tracking system was in operation they may be deterred' (Hughes, Parker and Gallagher, 1996, p. 34). Thus, on release from prison the individual will still be required to register with the police on a regular basis and to inform the police if they move or if they leave home for more than seven days. If an offender has also received a **Sexual Offences Prevention Order** (SOPO) there may be other restrictions, such as where that person may live and work, and whether they may have access to certain internet functions, if such restrictions are considered necessary to protect the public or particular individuals. Additionally, foreign travel can be banned; individuals must provide the police with their National Insurance number; and they may be required to provide photographs and fingerprints (Sexual Offences Act 2003).

In the UK, certain professionals (such as headteachers) may be informed of the movements of sexual offenders; whereas in the US under certain circumstances, due to **Megan's Law** (see Montana, 1995), communities may have access to information about these individuals – for example, a photograph, a description of the offence, and the offender's licence plate (see Sabin, 1996). Megan's Law is named after a seven-year-old girl, Megan Kanka, who was raped and murdered in New Jersey in 1994 by a known sex offender, Jesse Timmedequas. Her parents sought a change in the law to allow local communities to be informed about sexual offenders in the area. This was not intended to be a further punishment, but to help communities be more aware of issues of risk. The State of California Department of Justice has an internet site allowing for searches by name, address, city, county and zip code.

Research (Lasher and McGrath, 2012) has looked at the impact of Megan's Law by reviewing studies concerned with the reintegration of sexual offenders into the community, showing both the positive and negative consequences of this approach. For example, of the 1,503 offenders covered by the eight studies reviewed, 8 per cent reported having been personally attacked and 20 per cent had been harassed or threatened by neighbours. More positively, 74 per cent of the offenders suggested that community notification resulted in them being more motivated to desist from offending. For an overview of how the UK deals with released sexual offenders, see Petrunik and Deutschmann (2008); and for the US approach, see Beauregard and Lieb (2010). In the UK the separate police forces share information concerning registered sexual offenders in order to maximise the value of the register for detecting new offences, and there is an enhanced Criminal Records Bureau check which would prevent a job applicant on the register from working in risky areas, such as looking after children or having access to vulnerable adults.

Just as the law accepts that for most individuals who are detained there is a point at which they must be released, so too it accepts that sex offenders who are on the Sex Offender Register cannot be kept on it for life without the right to appeal; in the UK, a Supreme Court ruling stated that this would be against the individual's human rights. The register is one of the methods used to monitor individuals convicted of a sexual offence, and the length of time that one is kept on the register depends on the prison sentence received. Those given a jail sentence of more than 30 months for sexual offending are placed on the register indefinitely. Individuals imprisoned for between 6 and 30 months remain on the register for ten years, or for five years if they are under 18. Individuals sentenced for 6 months or less remain on the register for seven years, or for three and a half years if under 18. Individuals cautioned for a sexual offence are put on the register for two years, or for one year if under 18. The differences here are interesting: we might consider that time on the register links back to the concept of risk, but although that might be true there are some important inconsistencies. Firstly, we must recognise the inconsistencies in the legal process such that individuals who have committed the same offence may not receive the same sentence, and this may impact on their time on the register. Secondly, individuals who have spent more than thirty months in prison are more likely to have had the opportunity to attend a sex-offender treatment programme, which might have decreased their risk, whereas those on shorter sentences are unlikely to be able to participate in treatment.

A Sex Offender Register is an example of a legally recognised approach to restricting the freedom of sexual offenders. More subtle is the reaction of society to sexual offenders, which we touched on above. Certain newspapers in the UK are well known for their use of emotionally laden terms when referring to sexual offenders (such as 'pervert', 'monster', and so forth); and as Pollak and Kubrin (2007) wrote, the language used in news reports has a great effect on how the public perceive crime and criminals. A study by Gavin (2005) indicated that the source that participants most often cited as being responsible for their views concerning sexual offenders was newspapers. Additionally, clinical experience suggests that offenders themselves have experience of, and beliefs about, society's reaction to them. Clinical experience indicates that it is fairly frequent for sexual offenders to report that they have been threatened or had their property damaged after being released from prison, and many describe society's view of them as being 'scum' or 'dirt', and feel that society seems unable to forgive them, despite their having served time and worked to improve themselves and to reduce the risk they pose. Social services may restrict offenders' access to their children, either not allowing them to see them at all or only when supervised by a professional; and in some rare cases, if the mother is considered unable to protect the child from the father – because she is too vulnerable, for example, to disregard his requests for contact – the child might be fostered. All of these responses further the experience of offenders in relation to the legal system, their offending and society.

We are not advocating any particular position in relation to this, but it is important to consider how offenders may experience the world post-release, and how this might impact on their post-release behaviour and their risk of reoffending (see Walton and Duff, 2017). For example, if a male sexual offender feels constantly harassed and persecuted after release, it is possible that he might feel that, as everyone believes that he is still a danger, he has nothing to lose. Such an idea has been suggested by Freeman-Longo (1996): that the marginalisation of offenders may reproduce the triggers that led to sexual offending in the first place. This is supported by the work of Levenson and Cotter (2005), who provide evidence that offenders do report increased levels of stress, isolation and hopelessness in response to community notification legislation (see also Winick, 1998). It is possible that the public have a different understanding of this issue than policy-makers, as demonstrated by the work of Levenson *et al.* (2007), who describe a UK-based newspaper poll which showed that, of the 558 people surveyed, only 16 per cent believed that sex offenders could safely live in the community. Additionally, another study reported that offenders believed that notification laws do very little to reduce offending (Brannon, Levenson, Fortney and Baker, 2007), although this is contradicted by the later work of Lasher and McGrath (2012; see above).

Conclusion

This chapter has outlined a number of issues concerned with sentencing, such as the purposes of sentences and what might be involved in that decision-making process, and the aftermath of sentencing, both from the point of view of what may happen post-release and what processes might be involved when an individual's release is not determined by the minimum sentence set by the judge. The complexity of these issues partially reflects the way in which the English legal system has developed over time, taking into consideration our greater understanding of risk, of treatment and of human rights, along with the need to protect the public and, perhaps cynically, the need *to be seen* to be protecting the public.

There are a variety of decision-making stages and, as we have outlined, some of these are outwith the legal system and involve pressure from the public and the media. As a forensic psychologist it is important to be aware of these issues because they are likely to impact on your work and your understanding of the individuals with whom you work, such as their frustration and anger with the legal system, the conditions within which they are working (such as restricted access to their family), and the continuing struggles they face in reintegrating into society. It is also important to consider the impact of risk assessment in this process. Forensic psychologists provide assessments of risk, yet the prediction of risk is not faultless and may result in errors, either further incarcerating or limiting individuals who pose little risk, or releasing those with high levels of risk. For these reasons, our work can have a serious and long-lasting effect both on individuals and on society.

Chapter summary

There are a variety of sentences that a person can receive for a given crime. The purpose of a sentence, along with the nature of the crime, will determine what the actual sentence will be, and it will not always include a period in prison.

If a person does receive a prison sentence, release may be dependent on the decisions of a Parole Board, whose job is to determine whether the offender continues to pose a risk to society, and, if so, what else might be done to address this risk.

On release, an offender may be required to continue to liaise with professional bodies, such as probation services, and release may be conditional on certain restrictions or requirements (such as receiving treatment in the community). The offender's post-release behaviour and circumstances may be monitored by various bodies, including the police, social services, psychologists and housing authorities, through the MAPPA process.

Many of these decisions are based on risk, and risk assessment is a complex process which remains imperfect.

Even in situations where a person has been released and is not subject to restrictions concerning where they can live or the need for treatment, they may still be required to inform bodies of their whereabouts, as with the Sex Offender Register in the UK.

Ultimately, these various provisions are intended to protect society, but they do so by continuing to impact on the complete freedoms of the offender, and in this way they may also impact on how easily that offender may be able to reintegrate into society.

Further reading

It would be useful to access the websites of the various relevant bodies, for example:

» the Ministry of Justice

» the Parole Board

» HM Prison Service

» the Sentencing Council.

These will provide the specifics of each of these bodies in the UK, and also their respective guidelines.

In the US, the websites for the following organisations will provide useful information, although for specific states you might need to access their individual bodies (e.g. Florida Department of Law Enforcement; the Ohio Department of Rehabilitation and Correction):

» the US Department of Justice

» the US Probation Service (USPO)

» the Federal Bureau of Prisons.

For a general introduction, Jacqueline Martin's (2014) book, *The English Legal System* (Abingdon: Routledge), would be a good start as it provides a broad overview of the English legal system.

For more in-depth coverage of prisons, a comprehensive book is that edited by Yvonne Jewkes, Ben Crewe, and Jamie Bennett (2016). *Handbook on Prisons*. 2nd edition. Abingdon: Routledge.

Forensic Psychology: Activities, Standards and Skills

Forensic psychologists' work is important not only for offenders but also for those affected by their offending behaviour or at risk in the future. Part 4 considers psychologists' role in assessing offenders and reducing reoffending; it also considers some ethical issues they may face, and the training and professionalism needed to work competently within the criminal justice system.

18 Professional Roles: Assessing Offenders

Chapter 18 discusses forensic psychologists' role in assessing offenders. In seeking to understand their behaviour, in assessing the risk they may pose, and in reporting clearly and accurately to courts and allied services, forensic psychologists may influence offenders' routes through the criminal justice system and support their desistance from further offending.

19 Professional Roles: Reducing Reoffending

Chapter 19 considers the balance to be struck between punishment and rehabilitation, and the role and effectiveness of interventions designed to reduce criminal recidivism and to facilitate reintegration into the community. What works? Can all offenders benefit, or are some beyond help?

20 Professional Roles: Ethical Issues in Practice

Chapter 20 considers the ethical principles that inform the work of forensic psychologists, its consequences for others, and dilemmas that may arise. Ethical thinking evolves over time: while attending to the guidelines of professional bodies, professionals must also take personal responsibility for their own integrity and safety and for the welfare of their clients. Supervision and record-keeping are crucial.

21 Professional Training, Competence and Expertise

Chapter 21 describes the steps towards professional qualification in forensic psychology in the UK. The profession itself is still developing and forensic psychologists must be up to date in their knowledge, their competence and their awareness of ethical and philosophical issues. They must also exercise responsibility in their dealings with clients and fellow professionals.

Professional Roles: Assessing Offenders

Chapter 18 is concerned with the assessment of individuals who have come into contact with the legal system as a result of having broken the law. Our aim here is to provide you with an overview of the reasons why assessment is important in understanding offenders and their behaviour and, ultimately, in providing them with the necessary support that could help them desist from further offending. We will consider a range of different approaches available for assessing individuals, and some of the issues that are raised by the process of assessment.

Chapter objectives

- To describe a range of methods used in assessment in forensic psychology, and discuss their respective advantages and disadvantages.
- To explain the basic principles of risk assessment and to examine key issues that arise within it.
- To outline the possible role of case formulation in forensic psychology.
- To analyse the structure of psychological reports and the nature of the report-writing process.

Assessment of individuals for legal purposes, to inform the decisions that will be made concerning them, is one of the core tasks of forensic psychology. It can occur at a variety of places within an individual's journey through the system – for example, there may be a pre-trial assessment; or an assessment may be required by a judge prior to sentencing; or convicted prisoners or detained patients may be assessed for allocation decisions, for appraisal of risks and needs, or to review their progress. Within these areas, there are many specific objectives for which assessments might be conducted.

The purposes of assessment

Assessment is not therefore something that is done as an end in itself. It is designed to serve a purpose, and will usually result in a report, either verbal or written, prepared for a specified recipient or audience, in order to provide information that will in turn be entered into a decision the recipient is required to make. (Were that not the case, the recipient would be unlikely to have requested or commissioned the report.) In trying to understand assessment, therefore, a first useful realisation is that almost always it is an activity that is embedded in a series of other activities. Within that context, assessment itself can also be viewed as a *process*, with a sequence of steps to be taken in order to carry it out thoroughly. This involves having an overall strategy driven by the *objective* of the assessment – what it is for, who has requested it, and what it is intended to tell them. In forensic psychology, however, the parameters within which we conduct assessments differ somewhat from other areas of applied psychology. Thus a second useful realisation is that in most assessment and report-writing, there are, as it were, two potential consumers of the findings we generate, and their respective interests may be markedly different. There is a balance to be struck between the need for safety in society and the rights of the individual who may be a threat to it. Considering how to address that can be a major concern in many individual cases. It is invaluable to consider these facets of an assessment before embarking on it, as doing so will greatly facilitate the remainder of the task and will enable us to clarify the various choices we need to make in order to do the best job possible.

Essentially therefore, assessments are carried out to inform someone – such as a judge, a barrister, a criminal justice team, a forensic mental health team, or an agency – in order to help that person or organisation to make a decision about the individual we have assessed. Thus the output from assessment has to be communicated, usually in the form of a psychological report. The chapter will conclude, therefore, with an examination of the nature of those reports and the processes involved in producing them.

In what follows we will focus on the assessment of individuals once they have had a judgment made against them. We will consider some of the issues with which the forensic psychologist needs to be conversant. The assessment of an individual within a forensic context is intended to allow the psychologist and other professionals to develop an understanding of that individual, but with two very specific aims in mind: to understand what that person's current *needs* are and to understand the current level of *risk* he or she *poses*. This is a relatively new approach to assessment, as previously the focus was on predicting the likelihood that an individual might reoffend, which is in itself quite complex. It is also the case that previously there was a sense in which prediction was considered to be stable across time, whereas levels of risk are now known to be dependent on changes in the factors that have been assessed. So, for example, changes in an individual's social environment, use of drugs, or relationship status, if shown through research as being likely to impact on the types and levels of risk that person is thought to present, can now be taken into account so that the risk assessment responds dynamically to those changes.

Such an approach makes sound sense. Consider the following example. A man imprisoned for sexual offences against children is likely to be less of a risk whilst in prison, because while there he has no access to children. On release, even having undergone some form of intervention, estimates of the risk he poses will increase, simply due to the fact that there are now potential victims in his environment. The risk may increase to the point of reoffending if the intervention was not particularly effective or if other needs are not being met. An individual's needs may involve specific intervention, for example an anger-management treatment programme, or a range of more socially oriented needs such as adequate housing, a job, and opportunities to access education. If the needs of an individual can be met through prosocial avenues, then it is anticipated that antisocial behaviour will reduce (see Bonta and Andrews, 2017). This ties in well with an approach to working with sexual offenders which sees offending as evidence that an individual developed antisocial strategies as a way of dealing with stress (see Stinson and Becker, 2013). Individuals with criminal convictions will still have to deal with stress, of course, but if their strategies can be appropriately developed then their responses can become prosocial.

The process of assessment

Following Wright (2011), we can conceptualise the process of conducting assessments as comprising six consecutive and interrelated steps. In common with many others who have written on this topic, Wright advocates use of a *hypothesis-testing framework* when planning and conducting assessments. That means – because no assessment method in psychological science is perfectly error-free, and because no one we ever assess is likely to possess perfect self-knowledge – that it is advisable to proceed in a cautious, incremental manner, using the information we collect to build up a picture gradually and to check the accuracy of what we are finding as we go forward. The six steps listed by Wright (2011, p. 4) are as follows:

1. Conducting a psychological assessment interview;
2. Selecting psychological tests;
3. Administering, scoring, and interpreting the tests;
4. Integration of data from the above and other information sources;

5 Writing a psychological assessment report;

6 Providing feedback to the person assessed and to the source of the referral.

Hypothesis testing means that as we proceed, based on the progressive accumulation of new information, we accept some ideas about the individual's functioning and reject others. While in the early stages this will necessarily be tentative and exploratory, as information mounts we can become more focused in terms of the questions we ask and the information we seek to collect. Throughout the process, we should regularly review the information gathered and ask ourselves why we believe some things about the individual and not others; that is, we should evaluate the basis for our beliefs concerning him or her. This also helps to uncover gaps in the information, which we can return to in a later session.

Assessment strategies

Assessment interviews

Direct, face-to-face discussion with an individual is seen by most practitioners as an essential component of any thorough assessment process, and is advisable if at all possible. However, in forensic psychology there are situations in which interviews cannot be conducted because individuals are unwilling or unable to participate in them. This may be a function of security considerations, of the individuals' refusal to cooperate, or of their mental state. As we are interested in individuals' subjective viewpoints and personal accounts of events, hearing them describe these in their own words is often pivotal to any other work that is done. Initial interviews are designed to allow individuals to describe those experiences, to provide personal histories, to express opinions, and to report directly on their thoughts, feelings and behaviour.

Conceptually, assessment interviews can be approached from three directions. First, they can be regarded as a form of social interaction and exchange. Obviously they involve interpersonal communication – asking questions, receiving replies, making responses to those replies, and exploring the meanings and implications of the entire exchange. At intermediate points, the interviewer might provide short summaries of the ground covered so far, before embarking on a new area of discussion. Within the encounter there may be an intricate interactional process and complex interpersonal dynamics, and, in some cases, a high level of emotional intensity.

Second, an interview requires an exercise of complex cognitive skills of several kinds, both in terms of the immediate processing of the information that is generated, and the accompanying analysis and synthesis that are needed in order to make sense of it. Alongside these, the interviewer needs to steer the social interaction process, to communicate receptiveness, and to relate things that are said at one moment to others that were said earlier or may be mentioned some time later. This involves a range of basic or generic competences (such as knowing how to ask questions clearly and how to respond appropriately to avoidance or defensiveness), and higher-level or meta-competences (such as integrating the information into an emergent model of the individual's functioning).

Third, some interviews, primarily those that involve a high level of structure, can be approached as a type of psychometric instrument. That is, we can compute statistics for their reliability, validity and related features, just as we might do with self-report questionnaires, personality inventories, or other kinds of quantitatively based assessment tool. As more variants of this type of interview have been devised and evaluated, there has been a generally upward trend in the reliability and validity of assessment interviews.

Assessment interviews can take a variety of formats and can be placed on a continuum according to the level of structure they entail. For example, some mental health interviews have been developed for diagnostic purposes: that is, the information obtained will be fed into a diagnostic procedure such as those that underpin the DSM or ICD systems (described in Chapter 11). In these systems there is a prearranged set of key questions to be asked, corresponding to the criteria for the disorder from which the individual is thought to be suffering. Some questions may be supplemented by probes which invite individuals to expand on their answers or to provide more detail on the nature of their experiences or mental states. Examples of this approach include a number of highly *structured* diagnostic interviews employed within psychiatry. Other interviews are focused very specifically on assessment of a particular type of clinical problem. For many interviews of this type, specific training is needed. Segal and Hersen (2010) provide a valuable source concerning structured interview assessments of this kind.

For many other purposes, however, initial interviews generally adopt a *semi-structured* format. That is, practitioners decide in advance to examine certain areas, and in relation to these they may select some standard assessment questions. In other respects, though, the interview will be primarily an attempt to enable individuals to talk freely and to describe their personal history, their offences or other problems, and the effects these are having on their lives; and in general to tell the story of their difficulties as they see it. Some approaches to assessment involve even less structure, and may take the minimal format known as an *interview guide* – though generally speaking this format is more frequently used in the context of qualitative research than in assessment interviewing.

Communication during interviews needs to be managed carefully, but without making the encounter seem too contrived or stage-managed. The forms of questions that are used can have a significant impact on how much an individual talks and particularly on how much personally sensitive information he or she is willing to divulge, and some textbooks on interviews discuss these aspects of the process (Ivey, Ivey and Zalaquett, 2014; Segal and Hersen, 2010). Just as important are the non-verbal responses that the interviewer makes, as these can communicate whether or not you are listening and the extent to which you are interested, receptive and engaged. Those features in turn will influence the interviewee's level of reciprocity; and research shows that fuller involvement in the interview, more open expressiveness, a developing sense of being understood, and similar factors all have important effects on whether or not the process as a whole is beneficial with respect to the relationship between interviewer and interviewee (Crits-Cristoph, Gibbons and Mukherjee, 2013; Orlinsky, Rønnestad and Willutzki, 2004).

These dimensions of assessment interviewing, and the psychologist's awareness of them, take on an elevated importance when an interview involves working with someone from a culture other than one's own. Additional thought and attention needs to be given to the process of communication, with reference not simply to its linguistic aspects – and the possible need, in some circumstances, to work with the aid of an interpreter – but also to cultural values and to issues such as the appropriateness of exploration or disclosure of certain areas of personal or family life (Ivey, Ivey and Zalaquett, 2014; Suzuki and Ponterotto, 2009).

Psychometric scales

Historically, as described in Chapter 1, the development of **psychometric assessment** was viewed as a cornerstone of psychology, although psychologists themselves have continued to debate whether the constructs of interest to them can meaningfully be measured (Borsboom, 2005). But where it can be achieved, the use of structured, quantitative methods to compare individuals with one another (a *nomothetic* objective) can add valuable information to the assessment process. This advantage derives from the process of *standardisation* which involves administering the measure to a large number of respondents, on the basis of which there will be population *norms*, showing typical score patterns for the population as a whole or for selected subgroups relevant to the purposes of the measure. For any measure used, the psychologist must make an informed choice about its usefulness and appropriateness, from the perspectives both of whether it focuses on an issue relevant to the assessment and whether it is suitable for the individual to be assessed. For example, some scales may have been developed purely on the basis of research with adult males, people from the UK, people without learning disabilities, and so on, and if the person you are assessing does not reasonably match the population with whom that test was standardised, your results may not provide an accurate reflection of that person. Beside these requirements, the two principal criteria used to judge a psychometric instrument are its *reliability* and *validity*.

Reliability refers to the extent to which any psychometric assessment is consistent in its capacity to measure a characteristic or attribute. For example, are two individuals who obtain different scores on a measure genuinely different? Should someone completing a measure at one point in time obtain a similar result at a later point in time? If that does not happen, will we be able to explain why? Psychological tests are for the most part carefully designed to ensure that they possess this property, and the manuals that accompany them will report statistics concerning it, known as *reliability coefficients*. These indicate the extent to which, for example, items composing the measure are correlated with each other (*internal consistency reliability*); the extent to which scores are consistent over time (*test-retest reliability*); or, for measures where different assessors provide ratings of someone, the extent to which their scores tend to agree with one another (*inter-rater reliability*). There are several statistical formulae for computing all of the foregoing coefficients (Gregory, 2011).

Validity is defined as the extent to which a psychometric assessment can be said to do what it was designed to do, such that 'inferences made from it are appropriate, meaningful, and useful' (Gregory, 2011, p. 110). The items that the measure contains should be representative of the category of behaviour or other functioning that it is designed to assess. Put another way, the results of a psychometric assessment constitute a small sample of the individual's behaviour with respect to the variable being assessed. This feature is described as the *content validity* of an assessment. There are several other types of validity. They include *face validity*, which simply describes whether or not an assessment appears credible to users as covering the ground it is believed to be focused upon. A second type is *criterion-related validity*, which refers to the extent to which scores on the measure correlate with some other indicators of the individual's performance in the selected area of interest. This is sometimes analysed further into *concurrent validity*, which reflects the measure's scores relative to other assessments of the same variable, and *predictive validity*, which is the extent to which scores on the measure will reliably forecast an individual's behaviour or self-reports on some other variable at a later date. A final, and possibly the most crucial, aspect of validity is known as *construct validity*, which refers to whether or not a measure successfully and accurately assesses the psychological attribute it was meant to capture. Achieving this can pose major challenges in psychology, given that the constructs we believe we are measuring by means of psychometric methods are in fact hypothetical – that is, they are used by us to explain the characteristics we observe, but they are not directly observable in themselves.

All of the foregoing comments apply within a specific model of the construction of psychometric assessments known as *classical test theory*. As its name implies, this was the original conceptual model in psychometrics, and it has been the traditional basis for the development of psychological tests. It is grounded in the assumption that any specific test score reflects two underlying components, the *true score* and the *error score*, the latter comprising a number of sources of error (which can in principle be identified and their relative contributions apportioned). In contemporary applied psychology, this model is gradually being replaced with more advanced concepts in psychometrics, such as *item response* or *latent trait* theory. This and other approaches involve some seismic shifts in the basic concepts of what we consider we are measuring when we use psychometric assessments (Borsboom, 2011; Gregory, 2011).

The use of the best established psychometric assessments is now highly regulated. This includes requirements for those using them to have an appropriate level of training (a first degree, a testing certificate, or verified attendance at a specialised training event). It involves adherence to commercial contracts regarding permission for use and for the purchase of tests, and it requires test users to act in accordance with laws that forbid photocopying, reproducing or distributing the test materials. It also involves adherence to ethical principles and standards of test use, which include obtaining *informed consent* from those asked to complete a test, and principles governing the provision of feedback. It is the responsibility of practitioners using any of these methods to ensure they have the competence to do so, and to act in accordance with professional ethical codes in relation to test usage, alongside other aspects of their practice.

Although attempts to measure psychological attributes are often familiarly referred to as psychological 'tests', as we have been doing here, only a small proportion of psychometric assessments are genuinely *tests* in the sense that they compare individuals with some criterion of optimal performance or assess their proficiency in a specified task. The most widely used methods in this respect are *intelligence scales, assessments of specific abilities or aptitudes* and *neuropsychological assessments*.

What are widely called *personality tests* are designed to assess an individual's typical functioning as he or she describes it; in other words, they are based mainly, and often entirely, on self-report. More elaborate personality and mental health assessment inventories are designed in order to allow comparisons to be made between the individual being assessed and relevant sectors of the population (such as *normative comparison samples* or *criterion reference groups*). Considerable effort has been expended in developing and evaluating standardised psychometric instruments that can be used for assessment of a wide range of specific psychological problems. In addition to broad-ranging inventories, there are also numerous well-established scales for addressing specific problems – for example, assessments of alcohol or drug dependence, anger, hostility, depression, antisocial attitudes, criminal sentiments, self-esteem, or techniques of neutralisation. It is probably impossible to keep up to date with the pace of production of new psychologically based measurement tools. The most comprehensive source for discovering what is currently available is the *Mental Measurement Yearbook*, originally compiled under the editorship of Edward Buros in 1938. This has been published at regular intervals over many years and includes reviews of new psychometric assessments, or revised editions of existing ones as they appear (Carlson, Geisinger and Jonson, 2017). The Buros Center for Testing, where this work is done, also produces a retrospective index of available tests and scales (Anderson, Schlueter, Carlson and Geisinger, 2016).

Other assessment methods

In forensic psychology there is a range of assessment methods available that can be used to supplement and support interviews and psychometric scales, or used in their own right. They cover different aspects of antisocial behaviour, mental health, personality, attitudes, and so on. This chapter is not designed to go into detail about each of these; our hope is rather to provide an outline of some of the basic processes and methods of these other forms of assessment, and that this outline will allow you to structure and tailor any individual assessment to the specific needs it raises, based on your preliminary knowledge of your client and the goals of the assessment. However, it is important to note that not all assessment methods are interview methods, nor are they all based on psychometric testing. For example, a number of physiological techniques have been developed to assist in the assessment of offenders, including those who have committed sexual offences.

Assessing sexual interest: plethysmography

Plethysmography is based on the proposal that an individual's sexual interests or preferences can be investigated using physiological sexual arousal as a proxy. This is done by measuring blood flow to the sexual organs. There are forms of this for males and females respectively. *Penile plethysmography* (PPG), also called *phallometry*, involves monitoring the volume or the circumference of the penis during erection. *Vaginal photoplethysmography* (VPG) involves a tampon-shaped device which emits light and records the amount reflected back, also as an indicator of changes in blood flow. As males commit the majority of sexual offences, PPG is used considerably more often than VPG in forensic contexts (VPG is more likely to be used in treatment of sexual problems amongst women who have been sexually victimised). In PPG assessment, individuals are shown a planned sequence of neutral and erotic images of varying types as stimuli, and changes in arousal are recorded in response to each.

It seems plausible to expect that the measurement of changes in blood-flow in the penis or vagina would correlate with sexual arousal, and would therefore provide an accurate measure of the latter. PPG has therefore been suggested as being suitable for assessing the sexual interest of offenders and for evaluating, for example, the extent to which men who have offended against children and have completed intervention programmes are still sexually aroused by images of children. In principle, information from the PPG could then be used to inform decision-making in relation to that individual's treatment or containment (whether or not to move the individual to a different level of security), and so forth.

However, there are uncertainties with PPG. For example, Seto, Murphy, Page and Ennis (2003) showed that when assessed by PPG only 30 per cent of their sample of adolescent sexual offenders produced strong responses to child stimuli. It is possible that for the remaining 70 per cent the underlying drives for the offences were not sexual; but if that is the case, then such a possibility alone implies that the PPG may not be a dependable form of assessment for sexual offenders. Earlier research had demonstrated the opposite effect, in fact: that non-offending adult heterosexual males show an arousal response to female children (e.g. Freund, 1976). This finding is complemented by responses to an anonymous questionnaire administered by Briere and Runtz (1989) to 193 male college students. A proportion (21 per cent) acknowledged sexual thoughts about children. Some said they masturbated to these fantasies, and 7 per cent thought that they would act on their fantasies if they could be sure of remaining undiscovered. So PPG may not be able to accurately discriminate between offenders and non-offenders, which would include former non-offenders who might go on to offend, and former offenders who would *not* go on to offend. For these and other reasons, the validity of the PPG has been called into doubt; Merdian and Jones (2011) review several of the difficulties. There is also concern that an arousal response could be controlled, so that post-treatment, an individual might *appear* less sexually aroused by children than when tested pre-treatment, even if this were not actually the case. For example, a simple physical strategy to produce a reduced response to otherwise arousing stimuli would be to masturbate several times before the test.

Further questions regarding the usefulness of PPG in assessment have been raised by studies such as that of Adams, Wright and Lohr (1996). They set out to examine the responses of heterosexual homophobic and heterosexual non-homophobic men to homosexual stimuli, using PPG. They found that only homophobic men reacted in an aroused manner to the homosexual stimuli. This could be interpreted as suggesting that homophobic men are repressing their own homosexual interests (i.e. homophobia is a result of having homosexual thoughts and feelings but being distressed by them), which would support early psychoanalytic thinking regarding homophobia (for example see West, 1977). However, the authors suggested that their results might not necessarily be an indication that homophobic heterosexual men are sexually aroused by homosexual stimuli. It might instead be that such stimuli make them anxious, as anxiety has been shown to increase PPG-measured arousal. If the latter explanation is correct, then PPG may be picking up anxiety – related to the stimuli used in the test, or about being tested in this manner – rather than identifying sexual interest (Hale and Strassberg, 1990). Anxiety regarding being tested through genital plethysmography is not unlikely given the intrusive and intimate nature of the method (see Odeshoo, 2004, for an overview of PPG and legal issues that it raises).

Viewing time and gaze pattern. Plethysmography is not the only approach in seeking to assess sexual interests; several *non-physiological* methods have also been developed (Kalmus and Beech, 2005). They include, for example, the *Abel Assessment for Sexual Interest* (AASI: Abel *et al.*, 2001), which it is claimed is less intrusive, less obvious, and can be used with both genders. This test requires that individuals first look at images of people, chosen to depict a varied combination of ages and gender, and then rate how sexually attracted they are to each image. Participants typically suppose that their ratings are the data of interest. In fact, however, the system is recording the *viewing time* of each image, and it is these timings that provide the data used to determine sexual attraction. A computerised version of such a measure, called *Affinity*, has been developed using different stimuli, but its discriminant validity (power to identify sexual interest in children) was fairly low (Mokros *et al.*, 2012). Exploring another possibility, researchers have suggested that the *gaze pattern* – that is, exactly what we look at when viewing an image – can be used to identify sexual interest (see Hall, Hogue and Guo, 2011). It is thought that these more subtle approaches to measurement may provide more reliable methods of identifying sexual attraction, although it is possible that anxious responses to stimuli might again be involved, and further research is necessary.

Polygraphy

The **polygraph** is often popularly referred to as a 'lie detector'. But, as Grubin (2010) points out, there is as yet no identifiable physiological response that relates directly to the act of lying, so this is a misnomer. Polygraphs actually respond to *changes in arousal* in an individual, which may be produced by the stress of lying; this is based on the 'conflict theory' of Davis (1961), which states that lying when a task demands one to be truthful produces a physiological response. However, arousal level could also change due to other factors. An analysis by Bell and Grubin (2010) suggested that even within the brain there is no specific response to lying. It is only through an examiner's careful questioning and control of the environment that other possibilities are ruled out, so that response fluctuations are most likely to be due to some element of deception. For example, if a person moves whilst answering a question this might alter the response; if their attention is drawn to something unexpected in the room, such as a spider, a response may change; or if the respondent is generally anxious about the testing procedure the results may be less easy to interpret. This is not to suggest that a polygraph is unable to detect changes that might correlate with honest or dishonest answers, but it is important to ensure that there are as few extraneous variables as possible during testing.

One common method to generate differential responses to questions used within a polygraph test is known as the *Comparison Question Test* (CQT; see Ben-Shakhar, 2002), which assumes that innocent interviewees will respond more freely to a comparison question about their own past misdeeds than to the topic under investigation, whereas a guilty interviewee will show a greater response to questions related to the investigation than to a comparison question. Another approach, the *Guilty Knowledge Test* (GKT; e.g. Staunton and Hammond, 2011), is based on the idea that a guilty person will show a greater level of reaction when responding to items that only they could know (as the guilty party) as compared to an innocent person responding to the same item. For instance, if the details of an assault have not been made public, the basis of the GKT is that on being asked a question about the crime – such as 'Was the professor hit with a hammer, a lampshade, or a spoon?' – the perpetrator will respond to a greater degree than will someone who had no involvement in the incident. Despite these and other efforts to refine polygraphy, however, Grubin (2010) suggests that the accuracy of the polygraph is only between 81 per cent and 91 per cent. That is unlikely to be accurate enough for its results to be admitted as evidence in UK courts, and its use has been rejected in most jurisdictions. However in some American states the results of polygraphy are admissible in court, despite the conclusion of a report of the US National Research Council (2003) that evidence in support of it was very weak.

One of the arguments for the use of polygraphy is the claim that the threat of deception being revealed leads to offenders being more honest in their descriptions of the number of offences they have committed and their behaviours during offences. If true this would have obvious implications for treatment and risk assessment (see Grubin, 2008). However, in some studies (e.g. Emerick and Dutton, 1993) it is not clear that the polygraph is acting as anything more than an implied threat – in other words, the polygraph is not a more precise assessment technique in and of itself, but rather it is individuals' beliefs that their dishonesty will be detected, and that this will result in further negative consequences for them, that produces the sharing of more information. Moreover, the fact that people might report more offences and a greater offending repertoire does not necessarily mean that they are being more honest, and it is not clear in all cases how one would check the veracity of new information disclosed under a polygraphic assessment. Grubin (2008) suggested that the polygraph could be a useful tool for developing a more complete risk assessment of an individual; and this claim was supported to some extent by other authors (e.g. Gannon, Beech and Ward, 2008), although they suggested that it is impossible to test polygraphy experimentally in this context because of other factors that might be linked to increased disclosure.

In the UK the Offender Management Act 2007 allows for the assessment of individuals post-conviction using the polygraph. Proposals were made for sexual offenders to be *compelled* to be assessed in this way (Wilcox, 2009). However, while research suggested that probation staff found some disclosures made during testing to be useful, studies have not found any reliable association between such disclosures and subsequent sexual recidivism (Gannon *et al.*, 2013; Konopasek, 2015). The suggestion that the polygraph could be used in a way that was analogous to urine testing with substance-abusing offenders has not been supported by research (Meijer, Verschuere, Merckelbach and Crombez, 2008).

Brain-based lie detection. One strand of the spectacular growth of interest in neuroscience in recent years has consisted of research on whether the act of lying is detectable from changes in activity in different areas of the brain. Attempts to do this have entailed the use of *electroencephalography* (EEG) and more recently brain scanning by means of *functional magnetic resonance imaging* (fMRI). These possibilities have generated considerable interest, but results of studies have not shown sufficient consistency to meet evidential criteria for admissibility in court, such as the Daubert Standard discussed in Chapter 15 (Pardo and Patterson, 2014). But in any case, such studies usually entail a task in which participants are asked to *simulate* dishonesty under controlled conditions. There is a large gap between this and lying to conceal one's guilt in the course of a criminal investigation.

Functional analysis

In addition to the approaches described above, Beech, Fisher and Thornton (2003) suggest that a **functional analysis** should be carried out to identify the *antecedents, behaviours and consequences* (ABCs) involved in an offence. Beech *et al.* addressed this to sexual offending but it can be applied to any kind of offence, and it is incorporated in some intervention programmes. Functional analysis rests on the assumption that all behaviour serves some kind of function, and that particular setting conditions or triggers (the antecedents), or the likelihood of particular outcomes (the consequences) result in that function becoming more salient or more valued at a particular time. Where that occurs, the specific behaviour is more likely to be carried out in order to achieve that function (or consequence). To the extent that the ABCs can be sufficiently mapped, it then becomes possible to identify which contingencies are maintaining the behaviour. That in turn makes it possible to ascertain ways in which more appropriate behaviour could be elicited or acquired, and could, over time, replace the offence-supporting behaviour with more prosocial alternatives.

At each stage it is important to identify the thoughts and feelings that are associated with these aspects of the offending process in order to understand what an individual is trying to *accomplish* through that behaviour, and how each step changes the person's thinking, feeling and decision-making. Exploring these motivations for offending can provide useful information both for the assessment of risk and in making decisions regarding the intervention best suited to the individual's needs. For example, Ward, Hudson and France (1993) analysed descriptions of sexual abuse by offenders and suggested that they were able to identify a number of initial motives for their behaviour, the most prominent being sexual reasons, desire for intimacy and negative affect – but there were slight changes across the offence process. For a more in-depth description of functional analysis, see Follette and Bonow (2009). An illustration of the use of functional analysis with groups of prisoners, enabling them to acquire skills in behavioural self-management, is given by Sample, Wakai, Trestman and Keeney (2008).

Idiographic assessment

Several methods of assessment are based on the *idiographic* approach which we briefly discussed in Chapter 1, and information gained from this type of assessment can play a vital role in functional analysis. The objective here is not, as in many psychometric assessments, to use test norms to compare an individual's scores with those of others, but to explore specific aspects of an individual's thoughts, feelings or behaviour, in relation to other information we have about him or her, and about the situation in which he or she acted. Use of ABC analysis as described above is one example of idiographic assessment; there are many other assessments of this type.

Applied to analysis of criminal offences, they include the *timeline* method, used by Zamble and Quinsey (1997) for the analysis of offence patterns in reconvicted Canadian prisoners. One form of this method is an extended recounting of the events leading up to an offence, as shown in the upper part of Figure 18.1. This is based on the idea that 'psychological time', or recall of the period preceding crucial events, has an almost logarithmic shape, with experience being analysed in finer detail the closer we move towards the event itself. In a second version, shown in the lower part of Figure 18.1, parallel information is elicited, alongside behavioural events, on internal reactions such as feelings and thoughts recalled by the perpetrator of an offence, using a diagrammatic record that extends up to one month before it. In a sense, this involves what Weist (1981)

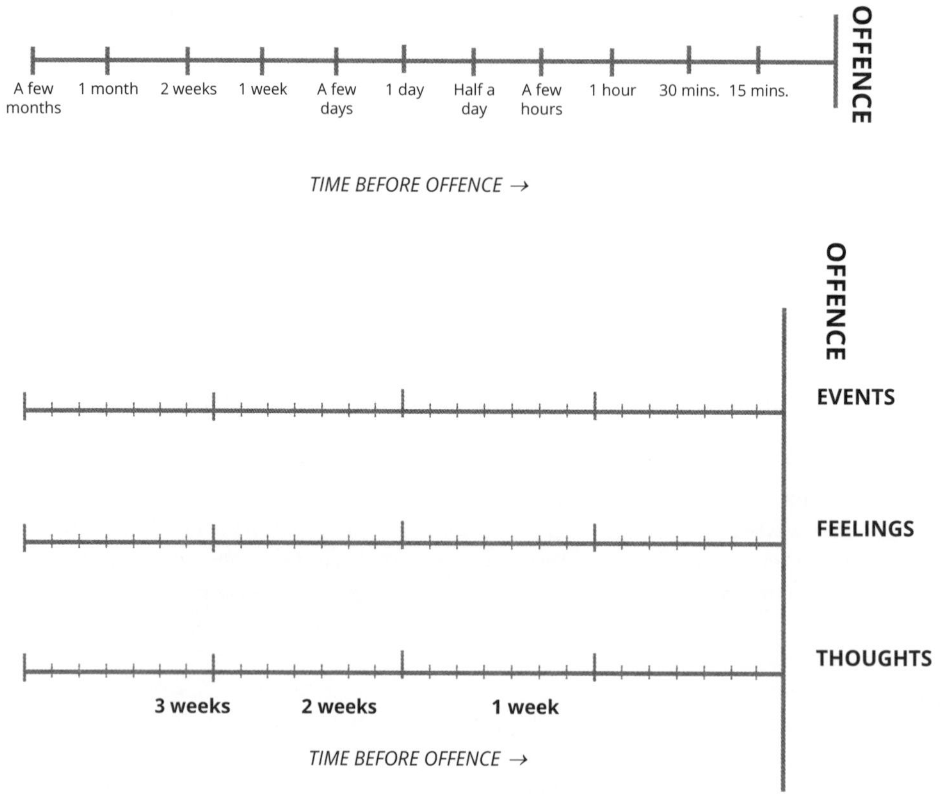
A few months
1 month
2 weeks
1 week
A few days
1 day
Half a day
A few hours
1 hour
30 mins.
15 mins.
OFFENCE
TIME BEFORE OFFENCE →
OFFENCE
EVENTS
FEELINGS
THOUGHTS
3 weeks
2 weeks
1 week
TIME BEFORE OFFENCE →

Figure 18.1
Analysis of offence patterns: timeline assessments.

Source: Figure 2.1 The "timelines" used in the interview. From Zamble, E. & Quinsey, V. L. (1997). The Criminal Recidivism Process. New York: Cambridge University Press. Copyright ©1997 Cambridge University Press.

called a 'walk-through' of the crime event, an approach whose application she illustrated in relation to some violent and sexual crimes. Zamble and Quinsey (1997) obtained rich data on the relationship between criminal acts and other events in individuals' lives.

The timescale covered by such analyses can be enlarged as illustrated by other techniques such as Agnew's (2006b) *storyline* concept, in which an individual recounts what he or she regards as the principal formative events influencing the adoption of a criminal lifestyle. Agnew distinguished this approach from the standard preoccupations of criminologists with background or situational factors. (We ourselves might add it could also help to loosen the standard preoccupations of some forensic psychologists with personality and dispositional factors.) This idea is illustrated in Figure 18.2. A storyline is 'a temporally limited, interrelated set of events and conditions that increases the likelihood that individuals will engage in a crime or a series of related crimes'. Storylines include 'those "objective" events and conditions that increase the likelihood of a crime or a series of related crimes (e.g. a physical assault by another, a period of unemployment). They also include the individual's perception of and reaction to these events and conditions (e.g. increased anger, a desperate need for money)' (Agnew, 2006b, p. 121). There are some 'major storylines' that become stock accounts of circumstances conducive to crime, and Agnew isolates a number of these narratives. Note that such self-narratives may also be an important element in understanding not only participation in crime, but also eventual *desistance* from it, powerfully illustrated in the work of Maruna (2001). West and Greenall (2011) have re-emphasised the value of index offence analysis in forensic assessment, and provide a format for undertaking it that combines the offender's own account of the sequence of events with information obtained from other sources, including forensic crime-scene analysis. All of these kinds of assessment can provide key information to be incorporated in a *case formulation*, to be discussed below.

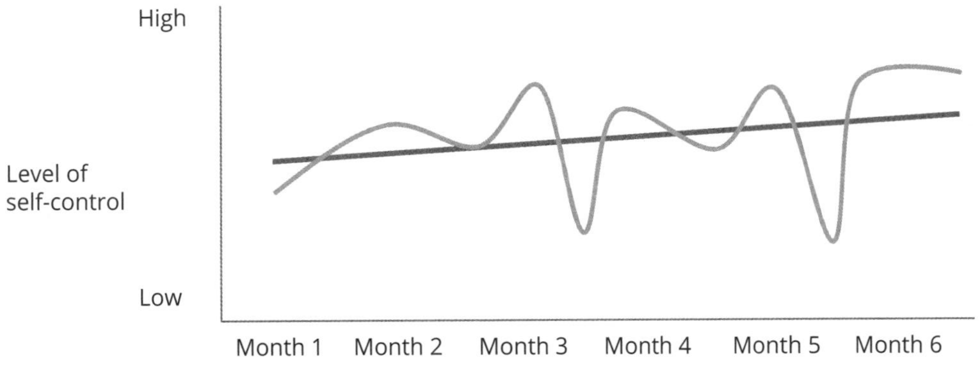
High
Level of
self-control
Low
Month 1
Month 2
Month 3
Month 4
Month 5
Month 6

Figure 18.2
The concept of a 'storyline' in assessing the likelihood that individuals will engage in a crime. 'Level of self-control' is a key operative concept in many theories of crime, and is seen as a variable that is relatively stable or that alters only very slowly over time. This is conceptually represented by the straight thick line in the figure. The account of events given by any individual, however, is likely to include a story of shifting or oscillating self-control. This is represented by the thin line, which indicates deviations around the mean level of self-control, influenced by many factors that will be part of the individual's narrative.

Source: Figure 1. From Agnew, R. (2006b). Storylines As a Neglected Cause of Crime. Journal of Research in Crime and Delinquency, 43 (2), 119–147. Copyright © 2006 Sage Publications. DOI: 10.1177/0022427805280052

18

File reviews and reports

In addition to direct assessment of the individual who is being assessed, if that individual has had previous contact with criminal justice, mental health or other types of services, and particularly if that contact has extended over a lengthy period of time, it will be important to obtain access to and to review the contents of the case file. This will usually contain background, historical and possibly developmental information, and copies of previous reports; and it might potentially include notes from earlier interviews by other staff. (In some locations reception interviews will be done routinely, whereas in others individuals may have freedom to choose whether or not to consent to them.) An enormous range of information may be available on file, including court reports going back for many years, judges' summing-up statements and directions to juries, previous psychometric and risk assessments, disciplinary records, work records, and a variety of other material. In certain circumstances additional collateral information may also be accessible, such as depositions (sworn evidence statements), and other supplementary information. This information will be essential for some purposes, for example in crime-scene and offence analysis as described by West and Greenall (2011), or in completion of other assessments such as the *Psychopathy Checklist* (discussed in Chapter 11).

However, file contents, including previous reports, need to be used with caution and discretion. While they are often a source of crucial and invaluable information, it is not uncommon to find attributions made within them on the basis of what, when traced backwards in time, amounts to hearsay. Nor is it unusual in clinical services to find that the offender's number of convictions, relationship status or even date of birth differ between reports. Also, it often happens that errors are carried over from one report to the next when reproduced by consecutive authors without critical evaluation, so that what began as mere speculation at one point in the past evolves with the passage of time into taken-for-granted fact.

Risk assessment within a forensic context

In forensic psychology, one of the most frequent uses of assessment is to estimate an individual's level of risk of reoffending and of causing further harm, with the intention of using that information to inform decisions concerning the management of him or her. In different environments the risk that is being assessed may vary, and the issues that need to be managed will also differ. For example, once imprisoned, the risk a sexual offender poses to children would be low; whereas there may be concerns about men who offend against adults, who are violent, or who self-harm. In the community, the potential risks are broader in scope and, in the case just mentioned, would include a sexual risk to children; so decisions need to be made about the conditions set for such a person being supervised in the community. In relation to individuals whose circumstances are not going to change in the near future, measures of risk are concerned with what should be done to best support that person. Where the circumstances might be changing – for example, if an individual is moving to a lower level of security, or has applied for parole – part of the risk assessment concerns whether they should be *permitted* to move on and how the likely changes might impact on that person's risk of reoffending. It is thought that with appropriate planning and management, risk of further offending can be significantly reduced.

Risk assessment is not an exact science, partly because human behaviour is too complex for all of the factors that might increase or decrease risk to be definitively identified, or for the specific contribution of different risk factors to be quantified. The second issue is that 'risk' is something that is dynamic, despite the fact that many assessments focus on static risk factors. Furthermore, in a critique of risk assessment in forensic contexts, Rogers (2000) noted that despite the fact that a variety of studies have shown the importance of *protective* factors in reducing reoffending (e.g. Plutchik, 1995), the vast majority of research up to that point only considered *risk* factors. As we saw in Chapter 3 there are many factors which although not direct risk factors themselves may impact upon other factors that are. Thus while an individual's employment or relationship status may serve a protective function, the strength of these influences relative to risk-related variables is still not well understood.

Four broad categories of risk factors are identified in the risk assessment literature:

1. *Dispositional factors*, such as antisocial or psychopathic personality characteristics.
2. *Historical factors*, such as adverse developmental events, a prior history of crime

and violence, prior hospitalisation, or poor treatment compliance.

3. *Contextual antecedents*, such as **criminogenic needs** (aspects of a person and his or her situation that, when they change, are associated with changes in criminal behaviour), deviant social networks, or a lack of positive social supports.
4. *Clinical factors*, such as psychiatric diagnosis, a poor level of functioning, or substance abuse.

A comprehensive risk assessment should seek to identify the presence or absence of these risk factors. However, it is important to be aware first, that there is not always agreement on how to categorise individuals in relation to each of these factors. For example, in the USA the typical cut-off for being categorised with psychopathic disorder is a score of 30 on Hare's revised *Psychopathy Checklist* (PCL:R), whereas in the UK it is typically 25. Psychopathy, however identified, is usually considered to be a static risk factor, but there is some evidence to suggest that it may in fact be dynamic; in some studies the risk of violence by an individual diagnosed with psychopathy can change as the individual ages (e.g. Porter, Birt and Boer, 2001). Second, the picture of how the various factors interact differs from one individual to another and cannot be determined from risk assessment alone, underpinning the importance of the process of case formulation to be discussed later in the chapter.

Approaches to risk assessment

For ease of description we can consider that risk assessment follows one of three strategies: *unstructured clinical judgment*; *actuarial assessment*; and *structured professional judgment*. These are sometimes seen as having emerged in sequence and portrayed as successive 'generations' of risk assessment methodologies (McGuire, 2017b).

Unstructured clinical judgment

This describes the use of unaided, clinically informed, but subjective judgment in making decisions and predictions. When engaging in this a practitioner is likely to be drawing principally on his or her professional experience and recollection of past cases. While such judgment still needs to be exercised in a wide range of practical situations, for risk assessment purposes it is over-reliant on the use of professional discretion, lacks transparency and accountability, and does not lend itself to replication. That was the case despite some evidence that clinicians were quite consistent in how they gather information (e.g. Clavelle and Turner, 1980). In an influential study Monahan (1981, p. 60) found that psychologists and psychiatrists using this approach were 'accurate in no more than one out of three predictions of violent behavior over a several year period among institutionalized populations'. Thus the use of assessment in legal contexts was criticised, and its validity and applicability were called into doubt, given that judgments of clinical 'experts' appeared to be no better than those of laypeople (Faust and Ziskin, 1988). As an approach to risk assessment, clinical judgment by itself is no longer viewed as adequate, at least on a standalone basis for making decisions. Nevertheless, several of the more structured forms of risk assessment discussed below do incorporate some forms of clinical judgment, though it is applied in carefully designated ways.

Actuarial risk assessment instruments (ARAIs)

At the opposite end of the continuum of methods, the actuarial approach involves development of an equation, formula, algorithm, table, graph or other formal quantifiable procedure to arrive at a probability estimate (Grove and Meehl, 1996). The distinguishing feature of ARAIs is the use of explicit rules for combining items into a global risk assessment (Bonta, 1996). As far as possible each element of this should be based on empirical research. If this could be done reliably and thoroughly, the actual procedure could be computer-driven. Most actuarial assessments make use of data on static risk factors only, for example the *Offender Group Reconviction Scale* (OGRS-3: Howard, Francis, Soothill and Humphreys, 2009). Others however incorporate some variables that have been based partly on clinical judgments, for example the *Violence Risk Appraisal Guide* (VRAG: Harris, Rice, Quinsey and Cormier, 2015), but it must be converted into a numerical value to be entered into the assessment. The majority of these methods are published in manual form with supporting psychometric evidence and administration guidelines. There is evidence that the advent of an actuarial approach resulted in an impressive increase in predictive accuracy as compared with unstructured clinical judgment. Research demonstrated that actuarial tests were routinely more accurate than clinical assessment (see Dawes, Faust and Meehl, 1989; Gardner, Lidz, Mulvey and Shaw, 1996). Loza (2003) estimated that their use led to an improvement in predicting general recidivism from 60 per cent to 80 per cent, and violent recidivism from 40 per cent to 53 per cent. Hanson and Morton-Bourgon (2009) also found actuarial measures to be unequivocally superior to clinical judgment in the prediction of sexual and violent offending; and Smid, Kamphuis, Wever and van Beek (2013) found they also led to more appropriate decisions concerning allocation to treatment.

Structured professional judgment (SPJ)

Structured professional judgment involves a synthesis of actuarial methodology and some features of clinical judgment. Assessors focus on established risk factors; but in appraising some of them, they draw on professional judgment to do so. That is most likely to apply to the assessment of dynamic risk factors, and the inclusion of these is seen as one of the major advantages of this approach. Thus, this method is empirically based but avoids the possibly restrictive reliance on a formulaic procedure for combining information. The element of judgment within this approach can also be applied in a number of ways. In some methods, clinical judgment can be used to supplement or modify the information gained from actuarial assessments. In others, judgment is exercised in a way that is *anchored* to specified descriptors contained in the assessment process. The inclusion of dynamic factors also means this approach can be employed in risk management, in treatment/intervention planning, and evaluation of progress. To use the majority of these methods, training is usually required, designed and sometimes provided by a scale's authors. Guy, Packer and Warnken (2012) identified a total of 19 SPJ tools then available. Some, such as the *History-Clinical-Risk Management* instrument (HCR-20), have since been issued in revised form (HCR-20-V3: Douglas, Hart, Webster and Belfrage, 2013).

A model for the assessment of sex offenders

Focusing more specifically on those who have committed sexual offences, Beech and Ward (2004) propose a model of assessment, based on current multifactorial models of sexual offending, which they describe as an etiological framework for understanding the risk of further offending. This is a noteworthy development as it was the first example of a theory-led assessment approach, rather than other approaches which are either experientially or empirically led without necessarily being underpinned by a psychology of offending. The authors suggest that they are not trying to develop a new tool or develop a new theory of sexual offending, but rather to bring together two approaches to the assessment of risk, namely the assessment of static, historical factors (e.g. age of first offence) and the assessment of dynamic factors (e.g. factors amenable to change, such as attitudes to women). By doing so this approach may help to reduce some of the various problems that have been highlighted in the assessment of offenders.

Beech and Ward identify four main areas that contribute to an assessment of an individual's level of risk:

1. *Distal factors* These constitute developmental factors, such as experience of abuse and rejection.
2. *Vulnerability factors* These are made up of static historical factors (e.g. the age at which the first offence occurred) and 'stable dynamic' factors (or psychological dispositions), such as the level of interpersonal functioning and offence-supporting cognitions (e.g. 'Children can consent to sex'). These are amenable to change, but do so only slowly over time unless they are addressed in therapeutic work.

3. *Contextual factors* The vulnerability factors mentioned above are moderated by these elements in the individual's environment and behaviour, which include substance abuse, access to victims, and poor social integration.
4. *State factors* These are 'acute dynamic' factors, such as variations in physiological arousal or the intermittent presence of deviant thoughts.

The assessment of these various areas requires the use of both clinical and actuarial skills, potentially benefiting from the fact that the assessments are theory-led and the model fits well with a number of the major theories of sexual offending, such as Ward and Siegert's (2002) *Pathways Model* of child sexual abuse and the *Integrated Theory of Sexual Offending* discussed in Chapter 9. These authors suggest that this model offers considerable benefits through, for example, considering temporal aspects of offending, redefining 'state' or acute dynamic risk factors, and linking early adverse learning events with psychological vulnerability, such as differences in attachment or *theory of mind*. The latter denotes the ability to attribute mental states such as intentions, beliefs or wishes to other people and to recognise they may be different from one's own (see Craissati, McClurg and Browne, 2002; Elsegood and Duff, 2010). Additionally, the reconceptualisation of dynamic risk factors, to take into consideration the existence of dynamic factors that are stable and those that are acute, may allow for a more detailed assessment and formulation of an individual, seen within their current context (or within hypothesised future contexts).

Risk assessments with sex offenders can also be misinterpreted: Studer, Aylwin, Sribney and Reddon (2011) point out potential difficulties. For example, if, as a result of having developed trust in therapists, an individual admits to more offences, that will lead to an increased risk score (despite indicating positive change) and potentially have a counterproductive effect of transfer to higher security. Repeating risk assessments that consist solely of static factors will not produce any new information and is a waste of time.

The risk of risk assessment

Risk assessment is not without controversy; not so much from its potential utility, but rather from whether it is being carried out in the best way. This reflects the complexity of making predictions about human behaviour and identifying the salient factors that might make those predictions both possible and accurate enough to be useful. When considering a risk assessment, whether that is for a current report or when making a plan to carry one out, the following issues are worthy of consideration.

Base rates

One issue for statistically based risk assessments – measures designed, for example, to predict risk of sexual reoffending – is the *base rate* of that type of offending: that is, how frequently sexual offending occurs within the population. The **base rate** interacts with a test's ability to accurately identify sexual offenders who are going to offend again (known as *true positives* – those who are predicted to reoffend and who do go on to do so), and its *in*ability to accurately identify sexual offenders who are *not* going to reoffend (known as *false positives* or *Type I Errors* – those predicted to be reoffenders but who do *not* reoffend). The relationship between these variables is such that the greater the base rate, the better a test is able to yield accurate predictions. If the base rate is low, the 'paradox of the false positive' comes into play: essentially, when a base rate or 'incidence' of anything is low, prediction is more difficult and the false positive rate can become very high (see Szmuckler, 2003, for a brief and readable account of the base-rate issue).

Predictive accuracy is of course a crucial attribute for a test, as it plays a decisive role in how an individual is dealt with by the legal system and what restrictions are put on that person if he or she is released from prison. The challenge is that the base rates for all crimes are low, and this results in the utility of tests being low too. Evaluating a test's predictive accuracy entails the use of some specialised terminology, as set out in Figure 18.3. This shows a 2 × 2 matrix or contingency table representing the possible combinations of predicted outcomes (reoffence versus no reoffence) cross-tabulated with actual outcomes (again, reoffence versus no reoffence). The resultant four subdivisions of the table include the *true positives*, those who were forecast to commit a new offence and went on to do so; and *true negatives*, those forecast not to reoffend who actually did not, and so also confirmed predictions. In the two other quadrants are *false positives*: predicted to reoffend but not doing so; and *false negatives*, the nightmare dread of all practitioners, predicted not to reoffend but actually doing so.

		Actual outcome	
		Reoffence	*No reoffence*
Predicted outcome	*Reoffence*	**A** True positives	**B** False positives
	No reoffence	**C** False negatives	**D** True negatives

Sensitivity = the rate of true positives (A/A+C)
Specificity = the rate of true negatives (D/B+D)

Figure 18.3
Basic terms used in studying predictive accuracy.

Various kinds of comparative statistics can be computed on this basis, depending on the distribution of outcomes in a given study population. The *sensitivity* of a predictor is the proportion of the actually violent who are correctly predicted; conversely, the *specificity* is the proportion of the non-violent who are correctly predicted. For any given predictive test or tool, the information generated from using it can be converted into an overall index of its accuracy using the model of **Receiver Operating Characteristics** (ROC; Mossman, 1994). The ROC is a plot of the true positive rate (the sensitivity of a test) against its false positive rate (calculated as 1 minus the specificity of the test)

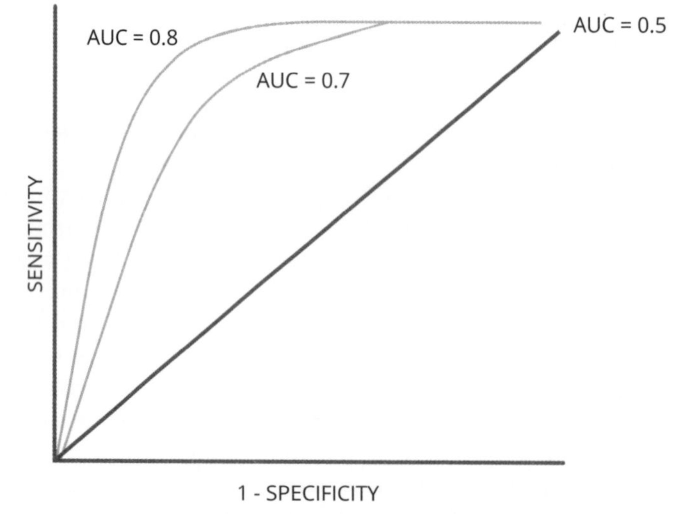
AUC = 0.8
AUC = 0.7
AUC = 0.5
SENSITIVITY
1 - SPECIFICITY

Figure 18.4
Receiver Operating Characteristics (ROC) analysis and illustrative values for the *'area under the curve'* (AUC).

for different test cut-off scores. (The cut-off score is the point at which the test would imply that an individual with a score any higher would be likely to offend again.) This produces a plot in which the measured area below the line, called the **area under the curve** (AUC), is a measure of the test's ability to make an accurate prediction – in this case, of sexual recidivism. The larger the AUC, the better the test (see Rice and Harris, 1995), and the more immune it is to changes in the base rate.

As shown in Figure 18.4, if a test were perfectly accurate, then the area under the curve would be 1.0 (i.e. the test would have a perfect true positive rate and a 0 false positive rate), so it would be able to discriminate perfectly between people who will reoffend and those who will not. An area under the curve of 0.5 would mean that there is a 50 per cent chance that a person will be correctly categorised by the test: this is no better than guessing. Tests that return an AUC of between 0.90 and 1.0 are considered excellent at prediction; those returning a value of 0.60–0.70 are considered poor at prediction. Given the importance of this prediction for an individual, it is plain to see why the requirements for test AUCs are so stringent. It might seem that looking at a test's ROC and AUC should be crucial in determining which tests might be best used in a given setting; but as Rice and Harris (1995) make clear, the use of ROCs should not be seen as a panacea, as they are not without their limitations.

Several reviews have been published comparing the predictive accuracy of the numerous risk assessments scales that are now available, often using the AUC as a principal benchmark. Some studies of this dealt with risk assessment of offenders in prisons or on probation (Campbell, French and Gendreau, 2009; Farrington, Jolliffe and Johnstone, 2008), while others focused on those with mental disorders detained in secure units (Fazel, Singh, Doll and Grann, 2012; Singh and Fazel, 2010; Singh, Grann and Fazel, 2011; Whittington *et al*., 2013; Yang, Wong and Coid, 2010). One focused specifically on sexual offending (Tully, Chou and Browne, 2013) and another on risk assessment in relation to partner violence (Nicholls, Pritchard, Reeves and Hilterman, 2013).

Some key trends emerge from these reviews. Assessments of this kind are valuable in enabling practitioners to systematise the information they collect on individuals, and the risk factors so identified are often the focus of intervention efforts. On average, the scales in current use are helpful in that they yield levels of predictive accuracy that represent significant improvements above chance. No single scale emerges as consistently superior to others, and the variation within the findings is such that the same scale may be found to have performed well in one set of studies but less well in another. Most scales produce AUCs in the region of 0.70–0.75 over follow-up periods of a few years. Some report longer follow-ups: in relation to sexual offending for example, see the comparative study by Smid, Kamphuis, Wever and Van Beek (2014). A small number of studies report predictive accuracy greater than this, but they are typically based on much shorter timescales. Thus despite improvements in our ability to predict recidivism including serious crimes, there is still considerable room for error in current risk assessment instruments (Rossegger *et al*, 2013). Given, as noted earlier, that the scales are constructed and tested using aggregate group scores, there is a potentially large margin of error when they are applied to individuals. Some researchers have expressed marked concerns over this (Hart, Michie and Cooke, 2007; Szmuckler and Rose, 2013). To address this problem, Conroy and Murrie (2007) outlined steps that can be taken to bridge the gap between risk scores based on studies with large samples and assessment in the individual case.

The reviews just mentioned, and several tragic cases, demonstrate that risk assessment is not foolproof. There are various examples of individuals who have been considered safe enough to be discharged back into the community, but have then gone on to commit further very serious offences (e.g. in the UK, Christopher Clunis, Derek Field, John Straffen). As a result of confidentiality standards only those directly involved can know the details of how assessments were conducted and decisions made in those and other cases. While offences committed in these circumstances are often the subject of considerable media attention, full accounts from within the organisations will not be made public unless there are formal inquiries. However, analysis of a series of 28 independent reports into homicides committed by offenders with mental disorders who were released from detention in the 1990s found that issues associated with risk assessment and communication of information emerged as significant problems in a proportion of cases (Reith, 1998).

Mediators and moderators

There are other important, sometimes critical factors that might influence the variables that make up a risk assessment, and as such they should be carefully considered. A *moderator* is a categorical or continuous variable that affects the direction or the strength of the relationship between the independent (predictor) and dependent (outcome) variables. Gender and race often operate in this way; these are both examples of moderators which can impact on the strength and direction of the relationship between a predictor and risk. A study concerned with the ability of the PCL:SV to predict violence suggested that the relationship between psychopathy and violence was dependent on ethnicity (Hicks, Rogers and Cashel, 2000). Similarly, gender has been shown to alter this relationship (e.g. Salekin, Rogers and Sewell, 1996). A *mediator* is a variable that accounts for (a portion of) the relationship between the independent and dependent variable, and might be part of the explanation of it. Research concerned with mediators has demonstrated that having observed parental violence as a child does not directly predict spousal abuse, but that observing parental violence impacts on one's ability to deal with conflict, which in turn impacts on the level of distress in one's marriage. Both poor conflict-resolution skills and marital conflict predict spousal abuse (Choice, Lamke and Pittman, 1995). Thus, although there is no *direct* effect from observing parental violence, and it might therefore not be considered within a risk assessment, the finding that it is related to other factors that do directly link with spousal abuse suggests that it may nevertheless be important from the perspectives of risk and treatment. The roles of moderators and mediators further demonstrate the challenge to psychology in developing accurate methods to predict future behaviour, and thus to providing assessments of risk in forensic contexts.

Communicating risk estimates

A key issue, alluded to at the start of this chapter, is the need for assessments to be usable by the host of non-psychological professionals who may make use of them. This is worth restating because the miscommunication of the results of risk assessment can have major consequences for individuals. Although it is the 'least studied' aspect of the process, accurate communication is considered to be so important as to be deemed by some authors as *essential* to its effectiveness (e.g. Mills, Kroner and Morgan, 2011).

It is likely that you have come across risk assessments, either in your work or through what you have been taught, and that you have come across labels for individuals such as 'medium risk of reoffending' or 'low risk of reoffending', or perhaps a percentage has been used. With the use of labels there is an inherent issue: different assessors may not agree on what constitutes 'medium risk', and it may not be clear what 'medium' actually means. Similarly with the use of percentages. If we see that an individual is described as having 'a 70 per cent risk of reoffending', what are we referring to? Do we mean the risk of reoffending in the same way as previously, the risk of offending in a new way, or something else? Is this meaning shared by all of the professionals who may need to make use of that information?

In order to reduce this confusion, various assessment methods have been developed to provide a definition. The *Offender Assessment System* (OASys), used by the National Probation Service and HM Prison Service in the UK, defines an individual who represents a 'medium risk' as demonstrating 'identifiable indicators of risk of harm. The offender has the potential to cause harm but is unlikely to do so unless there is a change in circumstances, for example, failure to take medication, loss of accommodation, relationship breakdown, drug or alcohol misuse' (HM Prison Service, 2005, p. 16). Although this definition is helpful, it is notable that a degree of individual decision-making is still involved regarding whether there are 'identifiable indicators', what 'potential to cause harm' means, and what the specific 'change in circumstance' might be. The use of percentages does not immediately remedy this situation. If an individual is rated as presenting 'a 70 per cent risk of reoffending', what that actually means is that, referring to a database of relevant information, out of 10 people who share the same important characteristics, 7 of them went on to reoffend and 3 did not. Thus the estimate is not based on that specific individual, but on the kinds of people that she or he most closely matches with respect to empirically established risk factors. As research findings accumulate, the factors that are considered in the matching process should gradually become more accurate, but it is unlikely that it will ever become possible to identify and take into account *all* of the risk factors and the protective factors (defined below), so risk assessments including those based on percentages will always be estimates at best.

WHERE DO YOU STAND?

Risk assessment and communication

As outlined in the main text, there is a potential issue with communicating 'level of risk' between different professionals.

As an example, forensic service staff are frequently asked to liaise with social services in order to assist in making decisions about whether an individual should be allowed back into the family home. If this person's previous offences had been against young girls who were not related to him, what risk are we assessing, and how can we go about that?

- Are we concerned with an *overall* risk of offending against children or with a *specific* risk to his own children? Is this a concern only if his children are girls?
- How might the risk change from having contact *outside* the family home, overseen by his partner, to contact *within* the home, still overseen by his partner?
- What related factors might change to become more protective? What might change and increase the risk?

Currently, it is unlikely that a single label or percentage can encapsulate all of the possibilities, because the antecedents to behaviour are complex and interdependent. Part of the issue is also that social services have a specific remit in relation to this man and his family, whereas a forensic service will be thinking more broadly, so the goals of the services may not always be the same.

One possible way around this issue would be to have a more comprehensive method for assigning levels of risk that provides a more inclusive measure, thereby incorporating all potential victim types and circumstances. Imagine for a moment that this is actually possible, and suppose that a mean percentage risk of 70 per cent indicates that 7 out of 10 men, similar to the particular individual of concern, would reoffend in any of these situations and against any of these victim types. If that were possible, perhaps we would have a more reliable and meaningful method for sharing levels of risk. This might be considered a *universal* category system, and as such would be more risk-averse and so more likely to protect potential victims.

One potential problem with this approach is that a grand mean such as this may underestimate risk, because it is also taking into account *low* levels of risk for specific victim types and circumstances. (Or could we factor out these areas with some certainty? That is another issue to consider. Could this be done, and reliably?) Another potential problem is that our offender may acquire a risk label related to offences that he has never committed and may never commit, with all the potential consequences that go along with labels, such as limiting access to jobs, housing or relationships.

Where do you stand on this issue?

Comprehensive and meaningful risk assessment and communication are complex issues, but they are crucial for the safety of potential victims and the reasonable treatment of people who have offended.

1. Can you think of ways in which risk could be more effectively calculated and communicated, based on either a very specific focus or a more global perspective?
2. What are the pros and cons for the accuracy of your approach, the potential risk to potential victims, and the consequences for offenders that your approach (or approaches) imply?

Assessment of risk allows individuals to be provided with the most suitable support and helps to protect them and the public from potential future offending. Thus it is concerned with addressing the necessary balance between the need for safety in society and the rights of the individual who may be a threat to that safety. It also plays an important role in determining the courses of action that legal and therapeutic processes will take, because precise and reliable assessments can inform those processes for a particular individual. For that reason, one of the most important aspects of producing a good assessment is that it is clear, and comprehensible to non-specialists, so that the various statutory bodies, which may not always include psychologists, are able to make the best use of the information in their decision-making processes. Those bodies include the courts, probation service, Parole Board, Mental Health Tribunals, MAPPA meetings, and so on. Indeed, Mills, Kroner and Morgan (2011), in listing four elements of risk assessment – (a) determining the individual's level of risk (risk estimation); (b) identifying the salient risk factors that contribute to that risk; (c) the identification of strategies to manage or minimise the risk; and (d) communicating the risk information to decision-makers – are unambiguous in stating that communication is a crucial element of the process.

However, given that determining an individual's level of risk is not simple, clear communication is not without its challenges. Janus and Meehl (1997) cite the work of Alexander Brooks, an American law professor who forwarded one of the earliest analyses of 'dangerousness'. Brooks suggested that it consisted of four elements: the *magnitude* of harm; the *probability* that harm will occur; the *frequency* with which harm will occur; and the *imminence* of the harm. Grubin (2004) translated these elements into types of risk to be considered when assessing sex offenders, that is: likelihood of offending; imminence of offending; consequences of offending; and frequency of offending. It is not clear whether there is an empirical basis for these suggestions but they do appear to have face validity and they provide us with a sense that not only is risk dynamic, as suggested earlier, but that it is also multifaceted and complex. For example, consider two individuals: one is considered likely to offend imminently and often; the other is thought unlikely to offend soon, but were he or she to do so the consequences for the victim (i.e. in terms of the intensity of the violence) would probably be considerable. Would we be required to work differently with them?

How should the various bodies that work with offenders, such as the police, prison and probation service, or forensic mental health teams, take account of such differences, and indeed is it possible to accurately predict these kinds of details? As Grubin (2004) stated, we need to be specific regarding what behaviour the risk assessment is concerned with. Conroy and Murrie (2007) endorsed the same point in stating that all risk is 'domain-specific' and we should have a clear objective regarding the nature, severity and timescale of the risk we are trying to assess.

Rogers (2000) wrote: 'Psychologists can't prevent the rest of the world from being venal or stupid. If jurors or judges misuse accurately-stated probabilistic information, that's not the psychologist's fault' (p. 602). However, the fact that assessments may be used with profound consequences – such that, for example, a man might lose contact with his children or remain in highly secure services – poses an ethical dilemma for the psychologist. Despite your best efforts to be up to date, accurate, impartial and professional, your report may still be misrepresented, misused, or misunderstood. Perhaps the best that assessors can do is to ensure that they produce the best assessments possible, which will require that they are knowledgeable about the theory of risk assessment and the appropriateness of various scales (and their limitations), that they are suitably trained and experienced in using and interpreting those tests, and that the ways in which the data are reported provides the clearest picture of what the assessment indicates.

Further complications

Overall, what makes risk assessment complex, other than in cases where theory-led decisions have been made *a priori*, is that at the outset one cannot know with any certainty what specific concerns need to be included in one's assessment. However, research has demonstrated that there are some variables that are related to risk regardless of the specific offence. For example, meta-analyses have demonstrated that certain variables – including offender age, number of previous convictions, pro-criminal attitudes and associations, and measures of antisocial personality – predict general recidivism amongst, for example, juvenile delinquents (Lipsey and Derzon, 1998), adult sex offenders (Hanson and Bussière, 1998), adult offenders (Gendreau, Little and Goggin, 1996), and offenders with mentally disorders (Bonta, Law and Hanson, 1998).

Despite this generalisability of some variables, it is only really through the initial meeting with the client that one can begin to map which areas need to receive special attention and what special tools might be required in order to do this. Although there may well be material provided by referrers, such as the police or the probation service, and although these may act as a useful initial guide for the assessment, as we noted earlier it is important to keep in mind that some of these reports may be relatively old, may have been prepared for other purposes, and may contain inaccuracies. Additionally, as people and circumstances change over time, earlier reports may no longer be relevant, and some factors that are found to have changed may not be particularly valuable predictively (see Gottfredson and Moriarty, 2006, for this and other criticisms of the process of assembling information for risk assessment purposes).

Also, for certain groups of people the assessment process may require further consideration. For example, in the case of an individual with intellectual difficulties, the choice of assessment process will need to take into account the extent to which a given approach may affect that person's ability to fully express himself or herself, the reliability of the individual's memory, and any tendency he or she may have towards suggestibility (Clare, 1993). Similarly, in the assessment of female sexual offenders, it is important to keep in mind the possibility that the accused woman may have been coerced into offending and that this might impact upon the assessment (see Gannon, Rose and Ward, 2008). Indeed, risk assessment has been criticised for being both 'gendered' and 'racialised' as it is perceived by some not to have taken these issues into account, with the result that women and minority groups (it is suggested) are neither appropriately classified nor appropriately treated (Hannah-Moffat, 1999).

Case formulation

Several researchers and practitioners have proposed that the most useful way of drawing together the results of forensic assessment is in the form of a **case formulation**. This can incorporate and synthesise the findings of interview, psychometric, psychophysiological, case file, idiographic and other assessments, together with those obtained from structured risk assessments using the standard scales designed and validated for that purpose.

A *case formulation*, sometimes called *case conceptualisation*, is a working model or a set of hypotheses that constitutes an attempt to explain *why* someone has acted or is acting in certain ways, or is experiencing the distress that led to seeking help (and which may be the driver of his or her antisocial behaviour). Amounting to what is in essence an individualised theory, a formulation involves specifying the functional or cause–effect relationships amongst the various manifest behaviours of an individual, and developing an account of the aetiology of a problem, which represents the 'best-fit' explanation of why he or she acts, thinks or feels in that manner. Its usefulness can be re-appraised and evaluated as assessment proceeds, extending the hypothesis-testing concept suggested by Wright (2011) for assessment itself. Thus case formulations are open to revision as further information emerges. The practitioner's primary task is to construct a theory which can make sense of all the information gathered about an individual person; that is, of the pattern of problems reported by that individual or his or her recorded pattern of behaviour (Haynes, O'Brien and Kaholokula, 2011). In forensic psychology, a core element of that will be the individual's principal offence and criminal history.

Case formulation was extensively developed in clinical psychology but in recent years there has been a strong emerging consensus on its usefulness in forensic psychology. For example, reviewing risk factors for sexual offending, a key recommendation of Mann, Hanson and Thornton (2010) was the adoption of a case conceptualisation framework as being likely to provide a clearer understanding of why an offence was committed. This affords a far more helpful picture than a compilation of risk factors alone, as it focuses on the nature of the mechanism(s) at work in influencing an individual's behaviour. Similar points are made and amplified by other authors (Hart, Sturmey, Logan and McMurran, 2011; Ireland and Craig, 2011). Vess (2008) describes combining the results of actuarial measures with information from case formulation in risk assessment with sex offenders. With reference to personality disorder, given that the causal paths linking it to violence are not well understood, again in place of a simple listing of risk factors case formulation can be valuable in translating what emerges from risk assessment into risk management (Logan and Johnstone, 2010; Logan, Nathan and Brown, 2011; Sturmey and Lindsay, 2017).

Drawing on relevant research and on explanations of offending behaviour, such as those described in earlier chapters of this book, can provide a context for understanding the actions of the person we are assessing. By doing this, we connect the relevant *nomothetic* knowledge base to the *idiographic* information concerning the client.

The case formulation approach is not without difficulties however. When different practitioners attempt formulation with the same individual case, there may be large differences between the conclusions they draw. Expressed in psychometric terms, the reliability of formulations is often poor, and that in turn draws into question the validity of the exercise. This might be a result of divergent professional or theoretical 'allegiances'. That can be partly overcome by the development of formulations using multiple perspectives, or within teams, but for practical reasons those options may not often be feasible.

Report-writing in forensic psychology

Psychological assessment generates large amounts of information, and as we noted at the outset that work is undertaken for a purpose. It usually has to be conveyed to a third party and the standard means of achieving that is in the form of a written psychological report. When learning how to prepare psychological reports, usually one of the first things we want to know is how they should be organised. Most reports are divided into sections, and we need to plan what each section contains and how they should be ordered in relation to each other.

Suggested general structures or formats of reports usually consist of something such as the following:

- Identifying information (name and date of birth) of the subject of the report.
- The reason for and the context of the referral.
- The basis of the report (a list of the sources of information used).
- Details of the background or developmental history of the individual about whom the report is written.
- Analysis of offending behaviour and other problems.
- A brief overview of the assessment methods employed.
- Results of the assessments, and an explanation of their significance.
- A case formulation, where possible.
- Specific findings pertaining to the referral questions that were asked.
- General conclusions and any recommendations.

Often there will also need to be details supplied about the report's author, to establish his or her expertise in relation to the forum where the report will be used.

This general scheme relates to assessment reports; other types of report might include additional sections on intervention and evaluation or other material, as appropriate to the report's objectives, the nature of the work, and the context in which it has been prepared. Ackerman (2006) presents an overview of several other issues to be considered in the process of preparing forensic reports, including standards of evidence, intended audience, report structure, and ethical considerations.

Theory of report-writing: the Expository Process Model

The familiar structure just outlined is however only one aspect of report-writing, and Ownby (1997) drew attention to some more fundamental attributes of good psychological reports. The 'overriding purpose' of reports, according to Ownby, should be to influence the way in which the report's reader (the 'third party' mentioned above) deals with the person who is the subject of the report: to alter the reader's beliefs about and behaviours toward that person. According to this viewpoint, reports should provide statements that are both *credible* (in order to change beliefs) and *persuasive* (in order to change behaviours). Ownby (p. 31) listed specific purposes of reports as follows:

1 to answer referral questions as explicitly as possible, depending on how well defined the questions are;

2 to provide the referring agent with additional information when it is relevant to his or her work with the client and when it is appropriate for the use to which the report will be put (this includes providing a general description of the client);

3 to make a record of the assessment activities for future use; and

4 to recommend a specific course of action for the recipient of the report to follow in his or her work with the client.

Ownby further suggested that reports can be described in terms of three ingredients. First, there are *structural variables*, meaning the sentences, paragraphs and sections of the report; second, there are *organisational variables*, such as models, formats and styles that reflect the type of report it is designed to be; and third, there are *contextual variables*, such as the referral agent, the referral problem and the referral environment, within which the report is prepared.

This leads to a theory of report structure, which Ownby called the **Expository Process Model** (EPM), to the effect that while the second two of these ingredients will inevitably vary (almost by definition), the first of them should be *invariant*. Ownby's thesis was that the best type of sentence, paragraph or section remains the same, regardless of the other features of the reporting such as organisational and contextual variables. Reports must of necessity be tailored to their contexts, but certain structural features of them should remain invariant.

This then leads to a proposal about how the structural ingredients should be assembled, and to empirical testing of the foregoing proposal. Ownby has shown that 'model-based' statements in reports are consistently perceived as more credible than statements that have not been developed in this way. The 'model' referred to here is an attempt to articulate how best to link together the data or information generated in an assessment and its conclusions. One of the commonest problems in psychological reports is the absence of a clear link between the two. The EPM represents a kind of discipline for ensuring that your report succeeds in making that link.

The model revolves around the use of what are known as *middle-level constructs* – terms that are mid-way between the concrete information obtained in an assessment or other clinical work, and the higher-level, more abstract theory that probably drives the psychologist's activity in general terms (which could be a product of his or her theoretical orientation). The EPM specifies a procedure to go through in order to ensure cohesiveness between the data on which your report is based (for example, the information you have gained from an assessment), the middle-level constructs you are using to make sense of it, your testing of hypotheses in regard to these, and how this testing logically drives your conclusions and in turn your recommendations.

Middle-level constructs will probably serve their purpose better if the psychologist clarifies certain assumptions, such as his or her theoretical orientation in making use of certain constructs and not others.

Paragraph structure

Writing a report using the Expository Process Model is most easily accomplished if the paragraphs within it follow a specific structure. The model proposes that paragraphs should consist of three elements:

1. A *topic sentence* that includes a 'given-new sequence'. This unusual term refers to a way of presenting information in which we first re-state a piece of information the reader is presumed to know already, but then add a new piece of information to it, at this stage phrased generally and requiring substantiation.
2. Several *given-new sequences* then follow that provide substantiation of the new information in the topic sentence. As Karson and Nadkarni (2013, p. 147) remark, within each paragraph of a report you are answering the question: 'How do I know that?'
3. A *final statement* summarises the paragraph, relates its meaning to the referral question, and leads into the next paragraph – or some combination of these.

In a study conducted some time ago, Petrella and Poythress (1983) carried out a systematic comparison of psychiatric, psychological and social work reports. The reports were rated 'blind' by independent legal personnel, who concluded that the latter two were of superior quality on a range of measurable characteristics. In preparing reports psychologists and social workers consulted with a wider range of sources of information, and were more methodical in linking the evidence they had gathered to the conclusions drawn and the recommendations made.

Of course, the price of maintaining this standard is, so to speak, eternal vigilance regarding the quality of the reports we write. As part of sound professional practice, Ownby (1997) also proposed a scheme whereby practitioners could evaluate their own reports and presented criteria for doing so. Having completed a report, therefore, we should build in time for a final review and ask ourselves some self-reflective questions about it, as suggested in the next 'Focus on ...' box.

FOCUS ON ...

Self-evaluation of reports

Building on his theory of report-writing and the Expository Process Model (discussed in the main text), Ownby (1997) also suggested reviewing our own reports as if we were their recipients, and that we use the following questions as a way of reviewing the quality of the reports we have written.

The questions below are adapted from his framework and applied to forensic psychology report-writing:

1 Did the report answer the referral question?

2 Did the report give you new information about the person referred?

3 Did the report help you develop new ideas for working with him or her?

4 Was the discussion about what causes this person's difficulties helpful?

5 Were the recommendations (about legal decisions, therapy, etc.) helpful?

6 Did the recommendations show that the author of the report understood the limitations within which you must work?

7 Overall, how useful is this report?

8 What information should have been included but was not?

9 What terms were unclear, or seemed to be jargon, or were not adequately explained?

10 What suggestions would you make for improving this report?

Armed with this self-reflective inventory, and although it is difficult to be a wholly independent judge of our own work, we might be better able to be self-critical than we would otherwise.

Reference

- Adapted from Evaluation Form for Psychological Reports. From Ownby, R. L. (1997). *Psychological Reports: A Guide to Report Writing in Professional Psychology*. 3rd edition. New York, NY: John Wiley & Sons, Inc.

Chapter summary

This chapter has considered a number of issues in relation to the assessment of individuals, highlighting various principles that would be helpful in developing an appropriate assessment approach. It has considered the different methods of assessment used by many applied psychologists, including interviews, psychometrics, psychophysiological measures, idiographic methods, and obtaining information from case files. Added to these, and of major importance in forensic psychology, it has examined the process and methods of risk assessment and different approaches to it. Finally, we considered the tasks of drawing information together and of communicating it in reports to other professionals or agencies.

Although assessment is continually evolving and models of assessment are being developed to strengthen the conclusions that can be reached based on findings, the forensic psychologist must recognise that no assessment approach will replace the need for careful thought and planning in order to represent an individual fairly. It is not possible to be prescriptive about what questions should be asked and what tests should be used. These are decisions that are informed by experience, the specifics of the setting and the individual being assessed, and support from suitably qualified and experienced colleagues.

Further reading

For texts specifically aimed at understanding assessments and related areas covered in this chapter, the following are valuable sources.

» Kevin D, Browne, Anthony R. Beech, Leam A. Craig and Shihning Chou (eds) (2017). *Assessments in Forensic Practice: A Handbook.* (Chichester: Wiley-Blackwell). Contains chapters on many aspects of assessment and also on its use in particular contexts and with specific populations.

» Corine de Ruiter and Nancy Kaser-Boyd (2015). *Forensic Psychological Assessment in Practice: Case Studies.* (New York and London: Routledge). Provides accounts of assessments in specific cases illustrating a wide range of issues, based on the authors' experience working in the Netherlands and in the United States.

» Marc Nesca and J. Thomas Dalby (2013). *Forensic Interviewing in Criminal Court Matters: A Guide for Clinicians.* (Springfield, Il: Charles C. Thomas). A wide-ranging introduction to forensic interviewing and key aspects of what is involved.

» Ira K. Packer (2009). *Evaluation of Criminal Responsibility.* (New York: Oxford University Press). Focuses on the specific issue of this specialised purpose of assessment in the context of the US insanity defence.

» Eric Y. Drogin, Frank M. Dattilio, Robert L. Sadoff and Thomas G. Gutheil (eds) (2011). *Handbook of Forensic Assessment: Psychological and Psychiatric Perspectives.* (New York: Wiley). Provides frameworks and practical advice related to forensic assessment and report-writing for a wide range of purposes in both criminal and civil proceedings, focused in a North American context.

» Peter Sturmey and Mary McMurran (eds) (2011). *Forensic Case Formulation.* (Chichester: Wiley). Includes detailed accounts of the process of developing case formulations, explaining different models and approaches, reviewing relevant research, and giving illustrations in relation to violence, sexual offending and work with specific populations.

» Michael Karson and Lavita Nadkarni (2013), *Principles of Forensic Report Writing* (Washington DC: American Psychological Association). Provides valuable guidance on how to prepare reports;

though set in a US context the principles discussed are applicable anywhere.

» Risk assessment has become a fairly crowded field and there are many books to choose from. The following cover different parts of this area:

For an overview of concepts and issues in practice, Jeremy F. Mills, Daryl G. Kroner and Robert D. Morgan (2011), *Clinician's Guide to Violence Risk Assessment* (New York, NY: Guilford Press).

On risk of sexual offending: Leam A. Craig, Kevin D. Browne and Anthony R. Beech (2008). *Assessing Risk in Sex Offenders: A Practitioner's Guide* (Chichester: Wiley).

For a review of tools for assessment of violent offending, Randy K. Otto and Kevin S. Douglas (eds) (2010), *Handbook of Violence Risk Assessment* (New York, NY: Routledge).

For a framework for guiding the process of carrying out risk assessments in individual cases, see Mary A. Conroy and Daniel C. Murrie (2007). *Forensic Assessment of Violence Risk: A Guide for Risk Assessment and Risk Management* (Hoboken, NJ: John Wiley & Sons).

Professional Roles: Reducing Reoffending

Sentencing achieves the purpose of signalling society's disapproval of offending (denunciation, retribution), and it can reduce crime opportunities, at least for fixed periods (incapacitation). But there is much less evidence that sentencing on its own secures deterrent or rehabilitative effects. By contrast, there are now substantial amounts of evidence that rehabilitation, including better reintegration into the community and reductions in criminal recidivism, can be secured by more constructive approaches drawing on psychological research and the evidence gained from that research concerning effective ways of working. This chapter focuses on that set of issues, often referred to as the area of 'what works'.

Chapter objectives

- To survey studies that evaluated interventions designed to reduce criminal recidivism.
- To summarise key issues in debates on the relationship between punishment and rehabilitation of those who have broken the law.
- To identify trends and to draw conclusions concerning the features of successful interventions.

Policy and practice in criminal justice are influenced by many kinds of factors. They include the law itself, and the framework it sets for sentencing; the prevailing ethos in society regarding how crime is perceived, usually reflected in dominant media narratives; and the availability of empirical evidence on what effects might be obtained by pursuing different courses of action. There is a view, perhaps fairly cynical, that the last of these is least likely to play a meaningful part. The course of criminal justice and of social attitudes to punishment over time is sometimes likened to a pendulum, swinging between what are thought to be more punitive policies on the one hand, and more liberal ones on the other.

This chapter reviews the evidence that is available on how to reduce the likelihood of reoffending amongst those who have been convicted of offences and sentenced by the courts. That evidence poses a major challenge for the view that the best way to reduce the behaviour of 'known criminals' is by punishing them more severely, whether by means of longer sentences, more physically demanding prison regimes, or more austere institutional environments.

In Chapter 16 (Figure 16.4) we saw the extent of growth of the prison population of England and Wales over the period up to 2016. One of the reasons for the rapid rise in use of imprisonment, not only in England and Wales but in other countries also, was a widespread belief that other attempts to alter criminal behaviour had failed. Such beliefs are often traced to a journal article by Martinson (1974) which is widely regarded as having precipitated a period of what one writer has called penal 'pan-pessimism' (Walters, 2005, p. 50). If it is true that offender rehabilitation is mere wishful thinking, judges and others passing sentence may well feel they have little option but to send people to prison. Similarly, legislators may consider that the more punitive options should be strengthened within the available framework of sentencing 'disposals'. While it is difficult to chart a clear cause-and-effect relationship here, many writers on the subject attribute the steady rise of prison populations in the USA and in the UK at least partly to the pronouncements of Martinson and others who adopted a similar stance. McGuire (2013) provides an overview of the debates that surrounded this issue, and of the process by which the steady flow of new evidence concerning the effectiveness of other, non-punitive interventions led to more extensive use of such interventions within criminal justice systems.

Approaches to crime prevention and reduction

The penal system offers one possibility of initiating change for those who have repeatedly broken the law. It is useful, however, to place this in the context of other possible ways of achieving the same result.

A three-way distinction offered by Guerra, Tolan and Hammond (1994) can be helpful as a means of classifying attempts to reduce amounts or rates of antisocial and criminal behaviour. These authors distinguished crime-prevention efforts in terms of three levels of activity: primary, secondary and tertiary.

» *Primary prevention* refers to efforts to decrease the likelihood that crime will occur in the first place. Achieving this requires community-wide initiatives and there are many approaches amongst them, which we can group under two main headings. One set consists of forms of *situational prevention* designed to reduce the total volume of crime in society; these are generally the domain of the police and the security industry. They include familiar measures such as locks and alarms on buildings or vehicles, physical protection, provision of good street lighting, architectural and environmental design, installation of CCTV cameras, neighbourhood watch schemes, and other commonly used measures. (Some findings in this area were discussed in the 'Where do you stand? Situational crime prevention' box in Chapter 4.) The other set of approaches comprise *long-term developmental prevention*, which has been the focus of a number of specially designed experiments in high-crime neighbourhoods, neighbourhoods usually characterised by high levels of socioeconomic deprivation. Probably the best known is the Perry Preschool Prevention project, a randomised experiment focused on young children carried out in Ypsilanti, Michigan. Extra resources, including welfare provision, family support and parent training were allocated to the experimental group, and this group showed a positive impact – reduced rates of delinquency, unemployment, mental disorder, suicide attempts and other social problems – up to 15 years later (Schweinhart, Barnes and Weikart, 1993). In a longer-term follow-up, by which time participants had reached the age of 40, these advantages were maintained (Schweinhart, 2013). This project was also highly cost-effective, yielding a benefit–cost ratio (dollars saved to dollars spent) of 7 to 1.

» *Secondary prevention* refers to work with groups who may be at risk of involvement in delinquency, such as children who are bullying others at school, children in residential care, or those experimenting with substances under the influence of older peers. For example, Goldstein (2002) summarised the rationale, methods and results of addressing low-level aggression in schools through the use of systemic anti-bullying programmes, which simultaneously addressed the problem at the individual, classroom and school-wide level. There is a limited amount of evidence that secondary prevention can have longer-term pay-offs in terms of reduced rates of delinquency (Gill, 2016; although note that Gill uses terms slightly differently, and classes this type of work as 'person-based primary prevention'). The example of secondary prevention that has the most empirical support is the use of *mentoring* with 'at risk' adolescents (Tolan *et al.*, 2013).

» *Tertiary prevention* refers to direct work with adjudicated offenders: those already convicted by the courts. This work takes place in the penal system, in prisons, in secure units, or during probation or youth justice supervision, and is designed to reduce the subsequent criminal conduct of those who have been sentenced. This is a key area of activity for forensic psychologists, and is the prime focus of interest in the present chapter.

In the research we describe below, the outcome variable of principal interest in most studies is the rate or level of criminal recidivism. If two or more groups are being compared, researchers will report their respective *recidivism rates*, over a fixed period after their date of sentence or after they have taken part in some designated activity. **Recidivism** is a rather general term and can be defined in several ways. It might be based on individuals' self-reports, their rates of arrest, or their rates of reconviction in court. The seriousness of any reoffending might be gauged by use of a proxy (indirect) measure, for example the type of sentence then imposed – usually, whether or not they are imprisoned. In some research, intermediate variables such as measures of attitude change, skill acquisition, or other psychometrics are recorded; and perhaps also other outcomes, such as rates of gaining and holding onto jobs, rates of enrolling in education, rates of substance use and so on, depending on the selected participant group and the objectives of the intervention being evaluated.

Reviewing outcome research

Large-scale 'treatment-outcome' research contradicts the view that nothing constructive can be done to alter offending behaviour. While success can never be guaranteed, steps can certainly be taken to maximise the chances of a positive outcome. Some of those steps are now fairly well known. Others are yet to be clarified and are in need of further research.

The systematic study of criminal sentencing and of the treatment of offenders has been powerfully shaped over the last three decades by the appearance of literature reviews that employed the approach known as *statistical review* or *meta-analysis*. As we saw in Chapter 3, this is a method of integrating the findings from separate basic (primary) research studies. In cross-sectional or longitudinal studies in which researchers are testing hypotheses about the relationships between variables, effect sizes are most frequently reported in terms of correlation coefficients (or *beta* coefficients in the case of regression analyses). Both these and other statistics are also used in reporting meta-analyses of outcome research.

In most primary intervention-evaluation or treatment-outcome studies, the standard way of reporting results is in terms of *statistical significance* tests. For example, did the intervention group have a lower rate of discipline problems or post-release offences than the comparison group, and if it did, was it statistically significant? An alternative way of analysing results is in terms of *effect size*: what was the *extent* of any such difference that was found? Outcomes can be represented in various ways, but in this context the function in each case is the same: to provide a measure of the magnitude of any difference between experimental and control conditions following an intervention. In meta-analysis, this statistic is calculated for each dependent variable of interest in each study in the review. For some studies, more than one effect size may be extracted, as the authors may report more than one category of variables (e.g. psychometric test scores, observational data and recidivism rates). The findings are then computed across studies. The principal outcome of interest then is known as the *mean effect size*. An outline of different approaches to calculating and reporting effect sizes is given in the 'Focus on ...' box in Chapter 3.

Since its initial use in the field of criminal justice by Garrett (1985), who evaluated the effects of residential treatment on young offenders, meta-analysis has been employed in a large number of reviews of treatment-outcome studies with offenders (Wilson, 2001). By late 2012, over 100 meta-analyses of different aspects of tertiary-level offender treatment had been published (see McGuire, 2013). MacKenzie and Farrington (2015) reviewed meta-analyses and controlled trials published in the period from 2005 onwards. More broadly, in a wide-ranging 'review of reviews', Weisburd, Farrington and Gill (2016; see also Weisburd *et al.*, 2017) synthesised evidence concerning different approaches from across the 'known territory' of crime prevention and rehabilitation. Their review covered a total of 118 meta-analyses or systematic reviews from seven areas of evaluation research: developmental and social prevention; community interventions; situational prevention; policing; sentencing and use of deterrence; drug treatment; and correctional interventions. We focus here mainly on the last of these, as that is the one most closely linked to the work of forensic psychologists.

Results concerning correctional interventions are of considerable interest to many psychologists, in part because they themselves have carried out a large proportion of the research in this field. More importantly, many of the effective methods that have been validated by the available research have been based on the application of psychological theory and psychologically based methods of engendering change.

Systematic reviews and meta-analyses: coverage

The majority of the reviews that have been conducted, and the preponderance of the primary research on which they are based, originate from the USA and Canada. However, data from many countries are incorporated within some of them. Most studies are published in the English language, but for the largest review conducted so far (the CDATE review, briefly described in the next paragraph), contacts were made with 14 non-English-speaking countries, and more than 300 reports were obtained in languages other than English. There are also integrative reviews and meta-analyses of correctional interventions in Germany and other European countries (Egg, Pearson, Cleland and Lipton, 2000; Lösel and Koferl, 1989; Redondo, Sánchez-Meca and Garrido, 2002).

As just mentioned, the largest single review of this kind so far attempted was the *Correctional Drug Abuse Treatment Evaluation* (CDATE) project (Lipton, Pearson, Cleland and Yee, 2002a, 2002b). It was carried out by National Development and Research Institutes (NDRI) in the USA. This project ran for a four-year period, and during that time reports were collected from many countries. Altogether, researchers assembled more than 10,000 documents, including 1,600 that were reports of intervention experiments with recidivism as an outcome measure. Regrettably, the accumulated materials from this review have never been published in full. They were stored in the NDRI headquarters in the World Trade Center in New York City. In the aerial attacks on the twin towers on 11 September 2001, in what can be no more than a footnote given the scale of those tragic events, the entire collection was 'irretrievably lost' (Lipton *et al.*, 2002b, p. 93).

Not surprisingly, since most crimes are committed by men, the overwhelming majority of the primary studies in this field deal with male offenders. In one of the largest published meta-analyses, carried out by Lipsey (1995), only 3 per cent of the available studies focused exclusively on samples of female offenders. With regard to age, most reviews focus on interventions with adolescent or young adult offenders in the age range of 14–21 years. This covers the peak age for officially recorded delinquency in most countries. The remaining studies are either concerned exclusively with adults or include offenders across a wide range of ages. Concerning ethnicity, while many primary studies provide data on the proportions of offenders from different ethnic groups, the pattern of this is variable: ethnicity is not uniformly reported. However, given the over-representation of minority communities under criminal justice jurisdiction in many countries, many of the findings are based on populations containing a broad mixture in terms of ethnicity.

Several reviews have focused on selected types of offence or offender classifications. The largest single group has been concerned with interventions to reduce sexual offending, and cover work with both adolescents and adults (Alexander, 1999; Bilby, Brooks-Gordon and Wells, 2006; Brooks-Gordon, Bilby and Wells, 2006; Dennis *et al.*, 2012; Gallagher *et al.*, 1999; Hall, 1995; Hanson *et al.*, 2002; Kim, Benekos and Merlo, 2016; Långström *et al.*, 2013; Polizzi, MacKenzie and Hickman, 1999; Reitzel and Carbonell, 2006; Schmucker and Lösel, 2015, 2017). However, the quality of research available in this area has given rise to some scepticism regarding what conclusions can be drawn, and Eher and Pfäfflin (2011) have advised caution when interpreting the reviews. Only those interventions adhering to RNR principles (see below) have been reliably found to have a significant treatment effect.

There are numerous meta-analyses on different aspects of violent offending (see McGuire, 2008, 2017c). Some focus on violence in general (Dowden and Andrews, 2000; Jolliffe and Farrington, 2007), and others specifically on the relationship between anger and violence (Henwood, Chou and Browne, 2015; Saini, 2009). Ali, Hall, Blickwedel and Hassiotis (2015), in an update to an earlier review, located six studies on the reduction of outwardly directed aggressive behaviour amongst people with intellectual disabilities. There are also several reviews that deal with domestic violence by males against a female partner (Babcock, Green and Robie, 2004; Feder, Wilson and Austin, 2008; Miller, Drake and Nafziger, 2013).

Several other reviews have been published that focus on specific types of offences. Two are concerned with interventions for drink-driving offenders (Miller *et al.*, 2015; Wells-Parker, Bangert-Drowns, McMillen and Williams, 1995). Several reviews have dealt with the impact of treatment for substance-abuse problems on subsequent criminal recidivism (Mitchell, Wilson and MacKenzie, 2006; Pearson and Lipton, 1999; Prendergast, Podus and Chang, 2000; Prendergast, Podus, Chang and Urada, 2002). However, many evaluations in the latter area have been conducted within healthcare settings, where the main outcomes of interest are health status and reduced drug misuse rather than criminal conduct. Thus the field of drug treatment has often been reviewed separately from that of criminal justice interventions (Holloway and Bennett, 2016). On a related question, another review was focused on the effectiveness of relapse prevention, a model initially developed in the addictions field, but also utilised in offender treatment (Dowden, Antonowicz and Andrews, 2003). As we will see later, there are also reviews focused on offenders categorised as suffering from psychopathy, in the sense defined by Hare (1996).

A few meta-analyses have focused solely on different types of punitive sanctions, such as 'intermediate punishment' (intensive community-based surveillance, at first colloquially called 'smart sentencing' in the United States: Gendreau, Goggin, Cullen and Andrews, 2001); and allied types of interventions such as 'scared straight' (Petrosino, Turpin-Petrosino and Finckenauer, 2000), correctional 'boot camps' (MacKenzie, Wilson and Kider, 2001), and outdoor-pursuit, 'wilderness challenge' schemes (Wilson and Lipsey, 2000). Some of these reviews are concerned mainly with young offenders. But we should also note that several of the broader meta-analyses included studies evaluating different kinds of punitive sanctions, alongside studies of other more 'constructive' types of intervention (Perry, 2016). On a related although somewhat different note, there is also a review of the extent to which coercion into treatment produces better or worse effects than when participation is voluntary (Parhar, Wormith, Derkzen and Beauregard, 2008).

Some reviewers have dealt more exclusively with the more constructive, non-punitive methods and have evaluated whether selected approaches to working with offenders secure the desired result of reduced reoffending. There are several meta-analyses of educational and vocational programmes for adults (Wilson, 2016; Wilson, Gallagher and MacKenzie, 2000; Visher, Winterfield and Coggeshall, 2005). There is one review of the impact of specially designed socio-therapeutic prison regimes in Germany (Lösel and Koferl, 1989), and another of therapeutic communities defined in wider-ranging terms (Lipton, Pearson, Cleland and Yee, 2002a). There are several integrative reviews of the effectiveness of structured, 'manualised' cognitive-behavioural programmes (Allen, MacKenzie and Hickman, 2001; Lipton, Pearson, Cleland and Yee, 2002b; Wilson, Bouffard and MacKenzie, 2005), and there is also a dedicated meta-analytic review on the outcomes obtained for the single most widely used programme of this type, *Reasoning and Rehabilitation* (Tong and Farrington, 2006). However, a particularly thorough review of these interventions was reported by Lipsey, Landenberger and Wilson (2007), and this will be described more fully below. Meta-analysis has also been used to synthesise findings from evaluations of restorative justice (Andrews and Bonta, 2010; Latimer, Dowden and Muise, 2005) and victim–offender mediation (Nugent, Williams and Umbreit, 2004).

Other meta-analyses have been carried out to examine the effects of what are classed as 'moderator' variables, such as gender and ethnicity. One review was undertaken in order to test whether similar patterns of effects would be observed with females as have been found with males (Dowden and Andrews, 1999), while another explicitly tested whether 'mainstream' forms of intervention used with white offenders are equally effective with ethnic minorities (Wilson, Lipsey and Soydan, 2003). While the latter review concentrated on studies with young people, a review of studies of cognitive-behavioural programmes with *adult* offenders found that interventions led to significant effects regardless of ethnicity, with differences between ethnic groups not significant (Usher and Stewart, 2014).

Finally, after an initial period in which these issues were neglected (Gendreau, Goggin and Smith, 1999), researchers turned attention to the question of the implementation of interventions. A central question within this was whether contextual or other aspects of service delivery had an impact on outcomes. Dowden and Andrews (2004) reviewed the relationship between different staff skills and agency practices in delivering programmes, and the resultant impact on recidivism. Lowenkamp, Latessa and Holsinger (2006) reviewed evidence on the *risk principle*, the predicted relationship between assessed likelihood of future offending and actual outcomes. Andrews and Dowden (2005) and Lowenkamp, Latessa and Smith (2006) surveyed research on the importance of treatment integrity and on quality of delivery, as factors influencing the relative success (or failure) of criminal justice programmes. Andrews (2011) summarised progress in this field and described a framework for synthesising what is known about programmes themselves with what is known about organisational environments and other 'nonprogrammatic' factors.

Challenges of research and review

Clearly, meta-analysis has become a widely applied method in the process of research review, but some researchers, on a variety of grounds, have been sceptical about its use:

- *Poor original research* If the quality of the original research is poor – and unfortunately a proportion of it is – it will not really be sensible to draw any firm conclusions, even from the most carefully conducted review of that research. This awkward scenario is sometimes captured in the phrase 'garbage in, garbage out'.
- *Weak study design* Given the circumstances in which most research of this kind takes place, the design of some evaluation studies is very weak. It can be difficult to employ random allocation to experimental and comparison samples; and the members of different samples are often not well matched, as researchers may have little control over who is placed under what conditions. As this activity takes place in the 'real world' of the criminal justice system, neatly designed experimental trials are often difficult to carry out. Uncontrolled variables can make it difficult to interpret the outcome data and conclusions may be far from robust (Lipsey, 1999).
- *Not comparing like with like* Research studies, even in the same area, often differ remarkably from each other. They may vary in design, in the size and composition of participant samples, in the measures used, and in how the data are analysed. In a review, this so-called 'apples and pears' problem can preclude the drawing of conclusions as it may be impossible to find any clear pattern. Some outcomes emerge quite consistently, but there is often a large degree of heterogeneity in study findings. This area, like some other parts of psychology, also suffers from an insufficient amount of research replication (Lösel, 2017).
- *Inadequate follow-up* The follow-up period in many studies is often quite short: six to nine months is not uncommon. However, there are also studies with one-year or two-year follow-ups, and a few where data have been collected for as long as five years and, in a small number of cases, even longer.
- *Small sample sizes* Sample sizes in some studies are small at the outset. If there is a further loss due to attrition, which is a frequent occurrence in criminal justice research, it may be difficult to draw

sound conclusions. This can add the further obstacle that, when attempting to review studies, anything other than the most 'broad brush' conclusions may be difficult to draw (Lipsey, 1995). Although the volume of research output in this field is fairly large, involving many hundreds of primary studies, when we look more closely the number in any chosen category of interest can be disappointingly small (Lösel, 2001).

One problem that meta-analysts acknowledge and take steps to control is that of *publication bias*. It is well known that research studies with statistically non-significant findings are less likely to be submitted to journals because researchers believe they are less likely to be published. There is a possibility, therefore, that those studies that are publicly available are unrepresentative of the research actually done, and therefore that they do not accurately represent the 'real' pattern of intervention effects. If so, resting our conclusions on published work alone could give a distorted picture.

In response, meta-analysts say that many of the above shortcomings can be corrected, or at least taken into account. For example, studies with larger samples can be given more weight, and well-designed and poorly designed experiments can be evaluated separately to see if they yield broadly similar effects. Although publication bias is unlikely to be eradicated, it can be minimised by making every possible effort to locate unpublished studies. Alternatively, its effects can be estimated by computing what is known as the *file-drawer number*. This is the number of unpublished studies with zero or negative effect sizes that would be needed to overturn a positive effect found in a set of published studies. Procedures for addressing all of these difficulties are now incorporated in most meta-analyses.

Regarding the quality of research, however, there is little reviewers can do, other than to argue for more and better-designed studies (Lum and Yang, 2005). While it would be beneficial if there were more randomised controlled trials conducted in criminal justice, evaluations using 'non-equivalent' designs can still provide indicators of effectiveness in practical settings. Although samples may not be perfectly matched, it may be easier in those circumstances to test the value of an intervention in routine practice (Hollin, 2008).

General impact of interventions

Careful reviewers of the meta-analyses that are now available have drawn the conclusion that when the literature is examined, even taking the above concerns into account, a convincing picture nevertheless emerges of positive outcome effects for some interventions. Only a few decades ago it was argued that criminal behaviour was not amenable to change. The overall finding from meta-analyses summarised here strongly contradicts that negative conclusion (Lipsey and Cullen, 2007; McGuire, 2013; Wilson, 2016). The impact of intervention on criminal recidivism is on average positive and statistically significant. It is associated with a net reduction in reoffending rates in experimental relative to comparison samples. That conclusion is accompanied by a second conclusion, which some may find disconcerting: the observed effects achieved from psychological interventions are consistently better than those obtained from the use of punitive or deterrent measures. Despite that finding, punitive or deterrent measures remain the normative approach to the dispensation of criminal justice throughout the world (Lipsey and Cullen, 2007; MacKenzie and Farrington, 2015).

That being said, the average effect taken across a broad spectrum of different types of treatment or intervention, in the region of 5–10 per cent, is not especially large. That figure may not be intuitively easy to interpret as it stands and it may be useful to translate it into different terms. Imagine that on average, across all the datasets available on punishment or treatment of offenders, the mean recidivism rate at follow-up was 50 per cent. Using that as a benchmark, the average finding obtained from the meta-analyses would correspond to recidivism rates of 45 per cent for experimental groups, and 55 per cent for control groups, respectively.

Does this finding tell us anything meaningful in practical or policy terms? One way of putting this question in perspective is to consider the distinction between what Rosenthal (1994) has called 'statistical significance' and 'practical significance'. The mean effect just described, although fairly modest, is statistically significant, and is comparable with the size of effects that in other fields are used to justify changes in practice. For example, some healthcare interventions that are generally regarded as producing worthwhile benefits have similar, and sometimes lower, mean treatment effects. McGuire (2002), drawing partly on Rosenthal (1994), composed a list of relevant comparisons with findings obtained from research on healthcare interventions. For example, the mean effect size of aspirin in reducing myocardial infarctions (heart attacks) was 0.04; of chemotherapy for breast cancer it was 0.08–0.11; and of heart bypass surgery in reducing coronary thrombosis it was 0.15. Set against that background, an average effect size of 0.10 does not look so bad.

But like all averages, the single figure just discussed simplifies the picture. Between the various subsets of the studies that have been reviewed, there are quite large differences in outcomes. Some interventions yield zero and others negative effects, so when a meta-analysis encompasses studies of such approaches their results lower the overall mean effect, and the figure quoted above reflects this. Moreover, given the complexity of the research we are discussing here, there are numerous factors at work and it can be difficult to separate the effects of treatment from other types of influence. The extent of observed effects is often moderated by several categories of variables.

One trend noted in some meta-analyses is that effect sizes for property offences (theft, burglary and robbery) or for drug-related offences are typically lower than those obtained for personal (violent and sexual) offences (Redondo *et al.*, 2002). The number of studies where this kind of comparison can be made is fairly small, but it is illustrated in a study of a prison-based programme in England and Wales, Enhanced Thinking Skills (ETS). Travers, Mann and Hollin (2014) found that the programme was associated with large reductions in reconvictions over a two-year period for violent and sexual offending, but it appeared to have had little impact on acquisitive offending and a slightly negative effect in relation to robbery. There is not enough evidence to confirm this speculation, but the variation in effectiveness may be partly a function of the potentially larger role played by economic, social and environmental factors in the occurrence of acquisitive crimes.

Results also differ between settings. Whilst the prison is often accorded central place in the dispensation of justice, and certainly consumes the largest share of penal budgets, several of the reviews indicate that, on balance, community-based interventions have larger effect sizes than those delivered in institutions (Andrews *et al.*, 1990; Lipsey and Cullen, 2007; Lipsey and Wilson, 1998; Redondo *et al.*, 2002). Where the relevant comparisons have been made, the ratio of relative effect sizes obtained has ranged from approximately 1.33/1 to as high as 1.75/1.

There are also some complex interactions between settings where interventions are provided, the types of methods used, and the 'quality of delivery' – the way in which the work is done. The best-designed services have their optimal benefit when provided in a non-custodial setting. By contrast, badly designed, inappropriate forms of intervention emerge as ineffective whatever the context (prison or community). Furthermore, even well-designed programmes can have zero effect, or even counterproductive effects, if they are poorly delivered.

Factors influencing differential outcomes

When selecting and planning interventions that will have the best chance of achieving good outcomes, these and other types of variation are if anything more important than the *average* effect. There is now a widespread consensus that it is possible to maximise effect sizes by combining a number of elements in offender programmes (Andrews, 2001). Effective interventions are thought to possess certain common features, which Andrews *et al.* (1990), in an early and highly influential review, called 'human service principles'. When Andrews and his associates pinpointed those features that contributed separately to enhancing effect size, and computed effects for the 39 studies that possessed those features, they found that in combination the features produced an additive effect, corresponding to an average reduction in recidivism rates of 53 per cent. So although the mean effect size across all studies quoted above may not be particularly remarkable in itself, when interventions are appropriately designed and delivered, and include combinations of features, it is possible to secure far larger gains. The idea of 'human service principles' developed from these results has continued to be tested and is now consolidated by a steadily expanding body of evidence. This has progressively evolved into what is now called the Risk–Needs–Responsivity (RNR) model (Andrews, Bonta and Wormith, 2006; Bonta and Andrews, 2017).

One of the most widely disseminated innovations flowing from the above findings has been the compilation of methods and materials into a number of prearranged formats known as *programmes*. Some practitioners express hesitation on hearing this word as it may suggest images of a rigid and impersonal method of working that is somehow detached from the need for direct interaction between offenders and criminal justice personnel. Strictly defined, however, a 'programme' consists simply of a planned sequence of learning opportunities that can be reproduced on successive occasions (McGuire, 2001). Used in criminal justice settings, its general objective is to reduce participants' subsequent criminal recidivism. Within that context, the typical programme is a prearranged set of activities. It has clearly stated objectives, and comprises a number of elements which are interconnected according to a planned design. This is usually recorded in a specially designed manual which specifies in detail how a programme should be delivered. Manuals themselves also vary in how prescriptive they are, with some allowing considerable scope for practitioners to adapt aspects of the materials for different groups with whom they are working (McMurran and Duggan, 2005).

Expert reviewers, then, agree that there are certain features of criminal justice interventions that maximise the likelihood of securing a practical, meaningful impact in terms of reduced reoffending. The major findings on which there is now general agreement include the following:

- *Theory and evidence base* Intervention efforts are more likely to succeed if they are based on a theory of criminal behaviour that is conceptually sound and that has firm empirical support. This provides a rationale for the methods that are used and the method of change believed to be at work when an individual participates. For example, if the expectation is that he or she will desist from offending, will this be accomplished by learning new skills, by changing attitudes, by an improving ability to communicate, by increasing self-knowledge, by solving problems, by learning to work through bad feelings, or by some permutation from within these components? Most of the manual-driven programmes currently employed in criminal justice services use methods derived from Cognitive Social Learning Theory (*cognitive-behavioural* interventions). Whilst this approach is by no means the only theoretical option available, to date it has the most consistent record in yielding positive outcomes.
- *Risk level* It is generally regarded as good practice to assess the risk of future offending and to allocate individuals to different levels of service accordingly. Risk assessment is usually based on information about an individual's criminal history, such as the age at which he or she was first convicted and the total number of convictions to date. The most intensive types of intervention should be reserved for those individuals assessed as posing the highest risk of reoffending, and this is an integral part of the RNR model (Andrews and Bonta, 2010). The volume of evidence concerning its importance is now fairly substantial (Andrews, Bonta and Wormith, 2006; Lowenkamp, Latessa and Holsinger, 2006).
- *Risk factors as targets of change* Research on the emergence of delinquency suggests that certain patterns of social interaction, egocentric attitudes, poor social or cognitive skills, and other factors are associated with its onset and maintenance. If work with offenders is to make a difference to their prospects of reoffending, those same factors should inform its outcome targets. They are therefore called **dynamic risk factors**, and there are clear reasons for prioritising them in rehabilitation services. These factors have sometimes alternatively been called 'criminogenic needs',

which has given rise to debate concerning the relationship between these factors and broader frameworks of human motivation and needs analysis (Ward and Stewart, 2003). That in turn has led to the development of a conceptual framework proposed as an alternative to RNR, the Good Lives Model (GLM: Ward and Maruna, 2007).

» *Multiple targets* Given the multiplicity of factors known to contribute to criminal activity, there is virtual unanimity amongst researchers that more effective interventions will comprise a number of ingredients, addressing a mixture of the aforementioned risks. Interventions that successfully do this are termed **multimodal**. For example, working with a group of persistent offenders might involve training them in cognitive and social skills, helping them to acquire self-control of impulses, and providing support for these changes through supervision or mentoring. Equally, that training might be accompanied by giving assistance with accommodation, employment and other everyday practical problems – although remedying 'welfare' problems alone has not been found to have a significant impact on rates of reconviction.

» *Responsivity* There are certain methods or approaches that have a superior record in engaging and motivating participants in criminal justice interventions and helping them to change (Andrews, 2001; Andrews, Bonta and Wormith, 2006). There are two aspects to this. First, the concept of *general responsivity* signifies that rehabilitative efforts will work better if participants have clear, concrete objectives, if contents are structured, and if there is a focus on activity and the acquisition of skills. Personnel involved in providing this should possess high-quality interpersonal skills and be able to foster supportive, collaborative relationships within clearly explained boundaries. Second, the concept of *specific responsivity* signifies that it is vital to adapt intervention strategies to accommodate diversity amongst participants with respect to age, gender, ethnicity, sexuality, language and learning styles.

» *Treatment integrity* Lipsey (1995) and other meta-analysts have noted that intervention services appear to work better when they are being actively monitored and evaluated by a researcher. Regular collection of data on how an intervention is delivered sustains its clarity of purpose, and also its adherence to the theory and the methods it was intended to deploy. This feature of an intervention is called its *treatment integrity* or *fidelity* (Bernfeld, 2001; Hollin, 1995), and in the best intervention services it is measured and checked routinely.

To provide the most favourable conditions for the delivery of the above kinds of services, many other ingredients need to be in place. All of the assessments carried out, and procedures for integrating their results, should be founded on the best-validated methods currently available. This applies equally to processes for recording **programme integrity** and evaluating outcomes. It applies also at a strategic level, in the management and co-ordination of the portfolio of programmes and allied services within a criminal justice agency or ministry (Andrews, 2001).

To ensure that this happens, some countries have developed systems for *accreditation* of intervention programmes. This entails producing an agreed set of criteria or standards against which proposals for working with offenders (whether in prisons or in the community) can be judged. Only approaches that meet the criteria are approved for implementation. This is then supported by a system of monitoring or audit, in an attempt to maintain standards of delivery; a form of quality-assurance process. Aspects of this will be described in more detail below, with reference to the United Kingdom.

Ineffective approaches

In contrast to the findings just described, several approaches receive little or no support as methods of working in criminal justice. Indeed, the meta-analytic reviews reveal that some approaches to working with offenders have not only zero but actually negative effects. That is, they are associated either with no change or with actual *increases* in offending behaviour. As noted earlier, they drag down the mean effect across all interventions found in some of the largest meta-analyses. For example, vocational training activities that do not lead to genuine prospects of employment fail to have any measurable impact on reoffending rates (Lipsey, 1995). Also, there is very little evidence that interventions that are based on psychodynamic approaches or allied models, on unstructured counselling, or on milieu therapy, or that employ other methods based on the assumed promotion of 'insight', lead to positive effects in the reduction of reoffending (Bonta and Andrews, 2017; Wilson, 2016).

Recalling the evidence that was reviewed in Chapter 16, the consistently poorest outcomes are obtained from the use of punishment. This nevertheless remains the predominant method of dealing with offenders across the globe. These findings raise critical questions about the ubiquitous reliance on deterrence as the principal *modus operandi* of the penal system. Even if punishment is used for reasons such as retribution, rather than for any observable effects on crime, we might expect that evidence concerning the absence of effects would outweigh the retributive rationale; but that does not seem to be the case.

Positive outcomes

Returning to more positive outcomes, the most soundly based approaches to reducing reoffending involve structured cognitive-behavioural programmes focused on risk factors for criminal recidivism (McGuire, 2013). Variants of this approach have been well supported, primarily for individuals with mixed patterns of offending that may include property, violent and substance-related crimes (Hollin, 2001; McMurran and McGuire, 2005; Motiuk and Serin, 2001). The largest available review of these interventions, by Lipsey, Landenberger and Wilson (2007) located 58 studies published between 1980 and 2004. The majority were quasi-experimental designs, with only 33 per cent using randomisation, and an average follow-up period of 12 months. Lipsey and his colleagues found that 84 per cent of the reviewed studies reported positive outcomes, although the mean effect size in some was not significantly different from zero. Overall, however, meta-analysis yielded a mean odds ratio of 1.53, equivalent to a 25 per cent reduction in recidivism, from an average of 40 per cent in control groups to 30 per cent in experimental groups. The authors noted significant heterogeneity in outcomes with a Q value of 214.02. Contrary to what has been found in reviews of some other areas, however, there were no significant differences between randomised and non-randomised designs.

Checks were made to ensure that the results obtained were unlikely to be a function of publication bias, and a number of analyses were run to examine the role of moderator variables. The two variables that emerged most prominently were the risk level of the participants and the quality of implementation of the programmes that were employed. Studies with identified 'best practice' features (a strong design, zero attrition, an intent-to-treat analysis, recidivism defined as arrest, and a high quality of delivery) yielded a mean odds ratio of 2.86, corresponding to a 52 per cent decrease in recidivism, which represents a reduction from a control groups mean of 40 per cent to an experimental groups mean of 19 per cent. The 'Focus on ...' box outlines the theoretical framework of cognitive-behavioural methods, which provides the conceptual basis for the typical ingredients found in many structured offending behaviour programmes.

19

FOCUS ON ...

Cognitive-behavioural methods

Cognitive-behavioural therapy (CBT) is a theoretically driven, psychologically based approach to the amelioration of a broad spectrum of individual and family problems, covering the whole lifespan. The approach is widely used in mental health and other services, and to date it remains the best researched and most firmly 'evidence-based' of the different treatment models available in those fields. Variants of it have been adapted for use in criminal justice services.

The behavioural components of the approach draw on the fundamental principles of learning theory, and the application of classical and instrumental conditioning to therapeutic change. But the earlier radical behaviourism of B.F. Skinner and other researchers was modified to incorporate concepts such as modelling and internal representation. One landmark in this was the formulation by Bandura (1977, 1997) of Social Learning Theory. The cognitive components focused on the relationship between automatic and controlled processing of information, thought to lead to habitual patterns in the ways individuals perceive themselves and others, think about difficulties they are facing (or avoid doing so), and solve problems (or allow them to accumulate).

The initial development of CBT grew from recognising the importance of the precept that 'not infrequently, whether relevant or irrelevant, the things people say to themselves determine the rest of the things they do' (Farber, 1963, p. 196). As practised today, however, CBT evolved from a synthesis of behavioural learning theory with findings from cognitive and clinical psychology during the 1970s. There was then a convergence of concepts and findings from these formerly quite disparate areas, usually traced to the work of Mahoney (1974), Meichenbaum (1977) and others.

The central tenet of CBT is the realisation that cognition (thoughts), emotion (feelings) and behaviour (actions), three apparently distinct domains of activity and experience, are in fact interdependent and in a constant state of interplay and exchange. Furthermore, there is also a causal (bidirectional) interplay between them and environmental events, a model Bandura (1977) called reciprocal determinism. Another way of describing this is to say that individual behaviour and experience are a function of *person–situation interactions* (Mischel, 1973, 2004, see Chapter 5).

Some psychologists define CBT fairly narrowly, with reference specifically to cognitive therapy for depression. Others see it as a family of interventions, rather than as a single approach, and include these approaches:

- **Behaviour modification** This applies a model based on operant conditioning; the environmental contingencies of behaviour regulate its patterning over time; functional analysis enables individuals to identify and modify patterns within this.
- **Behaviour therapy** This is based on classical conditioning, and the view that problems arise from inappropriate associations (e.g. irrational fears, which may have distant roots in people's lives) that can be unlearned.
- *Social skills training* A set of procedures to enable individuals to improve their abilities and their effectiveness in interactions with others.
- *Self-instructional training* A set of methods for identifying and remedying patterns of thinking that have become dysfunctional.
- *Problem-solving therapy* Building on the two previous methods, this is focused on helping individuals to learn more elaborate, higher-order skills for overcoming personal difficulties.
- *Cognitive therapy* A therapeutic approach focused on the identification of dysfunctional thoughts and their replacement with others that are less likely to induce negative feelings.
- *Schema-focused therapy* An approach that emphasises exploration of fundamental or core beliefs, held outside normal awareness, that result in repeated distress or harm in people's lives.

Specially designed programmes with additional components have been developed for adults who have committed violent offences. These may include a focus on anger control, modulation of moods, and recognition and self-management of risk (Bush, 1995; Henning and Frueh, 1996). In one study of an anger-management programme, Dowden, Blanchette and Serin (1999) reported a three-year follow-up of 110 participants and matched controls. For lower-risk cases, there was no impact on levels of reoffending. For high-risk cases, on the other hand, there was a 69 per cent reduction in general (non-violent) reoffending, and an 86 per cent reduction in violent reoffending.

Not all the evaluations of this method have demonstrated successful outcomes, however; and in other instances treatment gains have been very small. Howells and Day (2003) have drawn attention to the importance of assessing 'readiness for change' in assigning prisoners to anger control sessions. Still larger questions arise with reference to the distinction between *expressive/ emotional* and *instrumental* aggression. To date, as we have already noted offences involving instrumental aggression are less thoroughly researched than angry aggression, and there is comparatively little evidence available concerning which interventions are effective.

Jolliffe and Farrington (2007) analysed data from a series of 11 studies of interventions with adult male violent offenders. The methods that were tested included anger-control training, intensive self-management training, a mulitmodal skills programme (*Aggression Replacement Training*), electronic monitoring, and other specially devised prevention approaches. The average effect size obtained was a reduction in recidivism of between 8 per cent and 11 per cent, equivalent to a reduction from 50 per cent reconvicted in comparison groups to between 39 and 42 per cent reconvicted in treatment groups. Use of cognitive skills training, role-play and relapse-prevention methods were found, in combination, to yield the largest outcome effects.

For men who have committed offences of domestic violence, research suggests that in order to achieve successful outcomes additional sessions must be included: sessions that examine perceptions of male and female roles, beliefs concerning responsibility for actions, and concepts of masculinity (Babcock, Green and Robie, 2004; Dobash and Dobash, 2000; Feder and Wilson, 2005; Russell, 2002).

For offences against property, available research is rather limited in scope and design, and what has been published focuses mainly on young offenders (see McGuire, 2003, for an overview). Since the majority of such offenders have committed more than one type of offence, acquisitive or property-related offences are usually subsumed alongside other types of offence in **multimodal programmes**.

It has frequently been found that a sizeable proportion of those who have repeatedly broken the law also have substance-abuse problems, and for this reason many criminal justice agencies include programmes designed to address such problems within their treatment provision. This type of treatment is of course offered more widely in healthcare services, as the problem of substance misuse is experienced by many members of the population without their having broken the law, and such misuse can lead to major health problems. Many interventions within this field are also informed primarily by the cognitive-social learning model, and the background to some programmes of this type is outlined in the 'Focus on ...' box on page 442.

Still further ingredients are added in work with individuals who have committed sexual offences, the vast majority of whom are male. In addition to cognitive and social skills training and similar activities, these interventions sometimes also include a focus on deviant sexual arousal, cognitive distortions, and other sessions designed to address the established risk factors for this kind of offence. As we saw in Chapter 9, the picture of the risk factors that operate in this respect has evolved over the years as more research has accumulated. Some areas that were previously thought to be important have been called into question by more recent evidence (Mann, Hanson and Thornton, 2010). The precise contents of programmes may vary further according to specific types of offence, differentiated mainly by whether victims are children or adult women (Marshall, Fernandez, Marshall and Serran, 2006).

In relation to sexual offending, there have been some difficulties in translating the results of treatment-outcome research into practice. Controversies have arisen over the prison-based sex-offender treatment programme (SOTP) provided in England and Wales. The initial evaluation of this produced somewhat ambiguous results. The programme did not demonstrate a significant effect in reducing sexual reconviction *per se*, but a significant difference was found between treated and comparison groups when sexual and violent reconvictions were combined (Friendship, Mann and Beech, 2003). Some authors expressed concerns over the lack of sound outcome evidence for the SOTP (Ho and Ross, 2012). Greater

FOCUS ON …

Treatment of substance abuse and of drug-related offending

Given the severe health risks posed by high levels of alcohol or other substance use, many attempts are made to manage or eliminate problematic levels of use are provided in healthcare settings such as addiction clinics. Some models of intervention for chronic substance abuse and dependence are almost exclusively medical in their approach. They include medically assisted *detoxification* (removal of the toxic substance from the body), supported by palliative medication to facilitate withdrawal, and other forms of pharmacological treatment designed to counter the physiological damage caused by harmful drugs.

Psychological interventions generally adopt a learning-based approach in which substance dependence or addiction is conceptualised as the result of a gradual learning process and the emphasis in treatment is on breaking the connection between the substance and the changes in mood or emotion associated with it. There are several approaches within this. Both the National Institute of Health and Care Excellence (NICE; 2007, 2011b) in the United Kingdom and the National Institute on Drug Abuse (NIDA, 2009) in the United States have reviewed the research in this field and have made treatment recommendations.

Behavioural therapies and *cognitive-behavioural therapies* have been shown to be effective in the reduction of substance dependence. Research suggests that there are favourable outcomes in relation both to alcohol (Raistrick, Heather and Godfrey, 2006) and to other substances (Holloway, Bennett and Farrington, 2005). Large-scale studies such as the National Treatment Outcome Research Study (NTORS), a clinical trial conducted across 54 sites, have shown the possibility of reducing criminal recidivism through substance-abuse treatment (Gossop, Trakada, Stewart and Witton, 2005). Springer, McNeece and Arnold (2003) describe how treatment programmes are best adapted within criminal justice settings.

Given the difficulties that can arise in securing the engagement of individuals in seeking change, many treatment approaches are linked with *motivational enhancement* strategies, and even relatively brief interventions of this type have been shown to have a beneficial effect.

Relapse prevention refers to an interconnected series of methods, again derived from a cognitive-social learning model, designed to help individuals to identify high-risk situations – situations that might prompt them to return to substance misuse – and to acquire skills in coping with those situations. This involves both the acquisition and practice of new forms of self-management, together with a more broad-based effort at establishing a substance-free lifestyle. The relapse prevention model has been shown to have positive effects in reducing rates of reoffending, especially where it involves planning and rehearsal for the offender to prepare for risk situations, and the training of significant others (Dowden, Antonowicz and Andrews, 2003).

Another set of approaches is based on a 'disease model', in which some individuals are thought to be genetically vulnerable to the effects of a given substance and thus more susceptible to becoming addicted to it. On this view, the only effective remedy is complete *abstinence* from the noxious substance. This approach had its origins in the approach to the treatment of alcohol practised by Alcoholics Anonymous (AA), the worldwide self-help movement. The core idea has been widened to address addiction problems more generally; and because of their format, the resultant approaches are sometimes referred to as 'twelve-step models'. While these programmes are not amongst the recommendations made by NICE or NIDA, there is a consensus that the individual's own objectives and treatment preferences are an important element in success.

concern followed as a subsequent, larger-scale study with a mean follow-up period of 8.2 years found that treated sex offenders committed significantly more sexual reoffences than members of the comparison group (Mews, Di Bella and Purver, 2017).

Notwithstanding the very disturbing results of this study, the overall trend of findings is towards positive and significant effects of sex-offender treatment in general. Schmucker and Lösel (2015, 2017) reported a meta-analysis of 29 comparisons with an aggregate sample of 4,939 treated and 5,488 untreated sex offenders. They found a mean odds ratio of 1.41, which is statistically significant and corresponds to an average reduction in recidivism for treated as compared to untreated groups of 26.3 per cent. For the most part interventions yielded better results in the community than in prisons (a result also obtained in the review by Kim *et al.*, 2016); and there was evidence that individual treatment was superior to group-based treatment. In other respects there was considerable heterogeneity in the findings. As the authors noted, the 'magnitude of treatment effects vary substantially' (p. 599), and they concluded that there were too few high-quality studies to demonstrate treatment effectiveness unequivocally. Other features associated with better outcomes were largely in accordance with what would be predicted by the RNR model, and there has been recognition that sex-offender treatment is more likely to be effective if it adheres to the RNR approach (Hanson, Bourgon, Helmus and Hodgson, 2009; Harkins and Beech, 2007).

In contrast, other reviews have not obtained positive findings (e.g. Långström *et al.*, 2013) and the weakness of most research studies in this area suggests that it is difficult to draw firm conclusions regarding treatment outcomes. We should also note that large effects have been reported from the use of medical procedures with sexual offenders. These include hormonal treatment, and surgical castration (bilateral orchiectomy) which has been carried out in a number of countries. The latter has been found to virtually eradicate reoffending, but the number of reported cases is very low and outcome studies here too are very poor (Lösel and Schmucker, 2005; Sreenivasan and Weinberger, 2016). In addition there are confounding factors that make results difficult to attribute to the surgery alone, notably very high motivation to be released from long-term imprisonment. With regard to anti-libidinal medication, there is evidence that this is likely to be helpful for some offenders, notably those where high levels of sexual preoccupation are a primary risk factor (Nair, 2016). But it can also have serious unwanted side-effects. While some reviewers of this area have remained sceptical regarding positive treatment effects (Hoberman, 2016), others have considered 'that CBT is the preferable treatment modality' (Kim *et al.*, 2016, p. 114).

Structured programmes applying cognitive-behavioural methods are not, however, the only types of intervention that have been found to yield positive results in reducing offence recidivism. For individuals with lengthy histories of substance abuse linked to their offending, **therapeutic communities** have been shown to be beneficial. These may be located in institutions or in the wider community, and there are several different models on which they can be based (Lipton, Pearson, Cleland and Yee 2002a). Therapeutic community models also emerged as effective from a review of research on interventions for 'persistent' or 'prolific' offenders, defined as those with six or more previous criminal convictions (Perry *et al.*, 2009). This review employed a method of *Rapid Evidence Assessment*, and the conclusions drawn were unfortunately limited by the relatively poor design quality of most of the studies that were located. The 'Focus on ...' box on page 444 describes the approach and methods employed in therapeutic communities, which can take a variety of forms.

Education and vocational training are also associated with positive outcomes. Wilson, Gallagher and MacKenzie (2000; see also Visher, Winterfield and Coggeshall, 2005) reported a meta-analysis of 33 studies, which yielded 53 tests of the impact of education, vocational training and allied programmes with adult offenders. The mean effect size corresponded to recidivism rates for comparison and intervention groups of 50 per cent and 37 per cent respectively.

The net end-product of comparing the results of different types of interventions is a

FOCUS ON ...

Therapeutic communities

Like several other intervention methods used in criminal justice, the concept of a therapeutic community (TC) has its origins in mental health services. In the UK what became regarded as a 'movement' within social psychiatry was set in motion by the work of Maxwell Jones, who pioneered such clinics in a number of British psychiatric hospitals in the 1940s and 1950s. The client group comprised emotionally very damaged individuals, often with traumatic histories, who experienced chronic problems of living. Attending therapy for weekly sessions was seen as insufficient to address the extent and depth of their difficulties. It was thought that recovery could be achieved only through a process of gradual resocialisation, developing clearer self-understanding, and acquiring new skills, which together would alter an individual's entire outlook. The ethos within such communities was democratic: that is, it was intended to abolish the power differential between staff and service users.

With reference to criminal justice, TCs have been established both in prisons and in community-based settings. Probably the best-known example in the United Kingdom is Grendon prison, which has operated a TC wing since 1962. However, TCs differ in the particular model on which they are based, with some (generally originating in the UK) placing more emphasis on democratic processes, and others (generally originating in the USA) more traditionally hierarchical in their structure, and described as 'concept-based' (Vandevelde, Broekaert, Yates and Kooyman, 2004).

Therapeutic communities for offenders have been developed most extensively primarily with two somewhat loosely identified user groups: (a) offenders with lengthy histories of substance abuse; and (b) offenders assessed as 'high risk', who have typically been convicted of serious crimes and who are serving lengthy sentences. For individuals with entrenched substance-abuse problems, a number of well-designed studies have shown positive effects of prison-based TCs both on subsequent substance abuse and on criminal recidivism (MacKenzie, 2006). Benefits are further enhanced by continuation of treatment and support efforts when the offender returns to the community. Outcome evidence for Grendon suggests that those who remain in treatment in the TC for at least 18 months show significant benefits and a reduction of 10 per cent in their rate of reoffending, though the significance of these data is difficult to estimate, given that those who seem not to be benefiting are transferred elsewhere.

Using studies from the CDATE meta-analysis described earlier, Lipton *et al*. (2002a; Pearson and Lipton 1999) conducted a meta-analytic review of 42 TC interventions with offenders; 35 with adults and 7 with juveniles. The effect sizes obtained were positive, although not large (10–18 per cent reduction in recidivism). As a context for these modest effects, we should bear in mind that services of this kind are directed almost exclusively towards persistent, high-risk offenders with concomitant substance-abuse problems, a group whose difficulties many people regard as intractable and who often do not respond to other interventions.

Shuker and Sullivan (2010) provided an overview of many aspects of therapeutic communities, their history, development and application, and their theoretical principles; and also reviewed studies reporting evaluations of progress and outcomes.

spread of effect sizes. Some methods will be found to have worked slightly better or far better than others, while some will have made no difference, and a few may have made matters worse. This is a richer and potentially far more informative pattern of results than the mean effect size alone. Figure 19.1 illustrates a range of effects from a selection of meta-analytic reviews and other large-scale datasets. It shows the stark disparity between the poor or negative effects obtained from more punitive approaches (discussed briefly earlier,

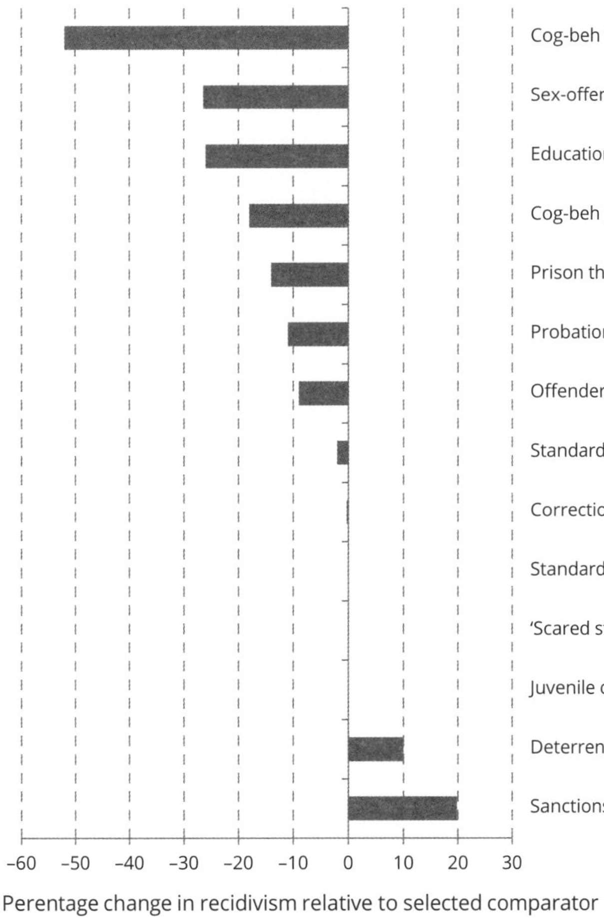
Cog-beh 'best practice' programmes
Sex-offender treatment
Educational / vocational programmes
Cog-beh programmes mean effect
Prison therapeutic communities
Probation programmes predicted vs. actual
Offenders with mental disorders
Standard probation supervision
Correctional 'boot camps'
Standard imprisonment predicted vs. actual
'Scared straight' programmes
Juvenile curfews
Deterrence-based sanctions (youth)
Sanctions/deterrence (adults)
-60 -50 -40 -30 -20 -10 0 10 20 30
Perentage change in recidivism relative to selected comparator

Figure 19.1
Reducing reoffending: effectiveness of different interventions. Illustrative variations in effect sizes from meta-analyses of outcome studies. Bars extending to the left of the zero-effect line represent reductions in recidivism amongst experimental samples relative to control groups or differences between actual and predicted rates of recidivism. Bars extending to the right represent increases in recidivism amongst experimental samples relative to comparison groups. In both cases the horizontal axis shows relative effect size. The upper part of the graph shows effect sizes on subsequent recidivism rates from a number of reviews of cognitive-behavioural and employment programmes. The lower part of the graph shows effect sizes for a number of criminal justice interventions.

and more fully in Chapter 16) and the effects obtained from the interventions just outlined. This disparity is vividly underlined by a series of results obtained from a survey of intensive supervision programmes in a Midwestern state of the USA. Lowenkamp *et al.* (2010) collected data from 58 such programmes, involving follow-up of a total of 11,020 offenders who had been assigned to them. The programmes were first divided into two broad categories, according to whether they operated primarily in terms of a sanctions- or deterrence-based philosophy (16 sites), or with one based on 'human service principles', now more familiarly known as the RNR model (42 sites). The two categories were then subdivided according to the extent to which programmes exhibited features of treatment integrity, using a specially prepared measure, and were graded as 'high', 'medium' or 'low'. When their relative effect sizes in relation to criminal recidivism were then compared, the results were as shown in Figure 19.2.

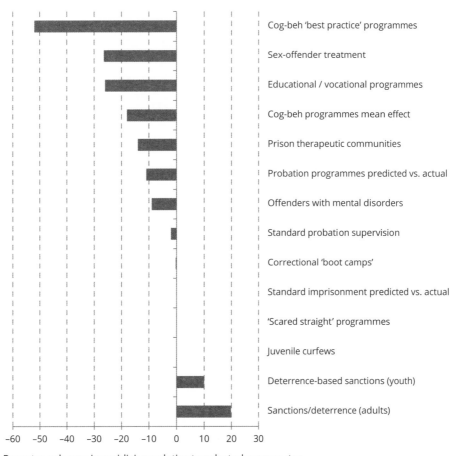

In addition to evaluating interventions with respect their impact on recidivism, and comparing the relative effects of different

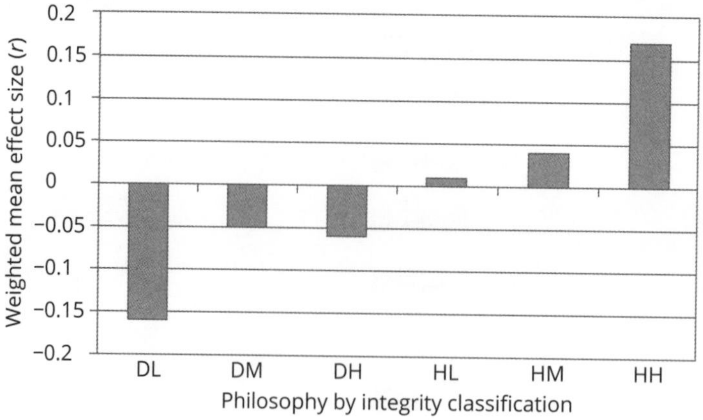

Weighted mean effect size (r)
0.2
0.15
0.1
0.05
0
−0.05
−0.1
−0.15
−0.2
DL
DM
DH
HL
HM
HH
Philosophy by integrity classification

Figure 19.2

Reducing reoffending: treatment philosophy and levels of integrity of services. Bar chart showing relative effect sizes when comparing two 'treatment philosophies' (deterrence v. human service/RNR) at three levels of treatment integrity ('low', 'medium', and 'high'). Key: DL = deterrence, low integrity; DM = deterrence, medium integrity; DH = deterrence, high integrity; HL = human service, low integrity; HM = human service, medium integrity; HH = human service, high integrity.

Source: reprinted from Journal of Criminal Justice, 38 (4), Lowenkamp, C. T., Flores, A. W., Holsinger, A. M., Makarios, M. D., Latessa, E. J., Intensive supervision programs: Does program philosophy and the principles of effective intervention matter?, p. 374. Copyright 2010, with permission from Elsevier. DOI: https://doi.org/10.1016/j.jcrimjus.2010.04.004

methods or programmes, it is also possible to compare such programmes with respect to the costs involved in setting them up and delivering them over time (set-up costs and running costs). This has led to the expansion of another approach to evaluation, which has become more widely used in recent years, broadly called *economic evaluation*. This approach is described in more detail in the 'Focus on ...' box below.

FOCUS ON ...

Cost–benefit analysis

Apart from their impact on recidivism or related indicators, another way to evaluate criminal justice interventions is in terms of how expensive they are to run and how that investment compares with any sums saved by preventing further crimes. The outcome variable used to measure this is called the *cost–benefit ratio* (or the *benefit–cost ratio:* this is simply a matter of which way round the figures are presented).

In criminal justice this ratio reflects the balance between costs and savings. First, there are costs involved in delivering the intervention, such as an **offending behaviour programme**. Delivering such a programme in a probation setting, for example, will entail staff salaries; direct costs of premises, furniture, heating and lighting, computer and camcorder equipment, manuals and transport; and indirect costs such as insurance.

Second, there are the savings. If a person commits a crime there are the costs of policing, court hearings, legal personnel, hospital treatment of victims, counselling, and property repairs: and penal costs such as those of subsequent incarceration or supervision. Computing these sums is an elaborate and highly skilled accounting exercise. The totals obtained can then be divided by the numbers of people involved; the effectiveness of the intervention (its impact on reoffending) is then factored in. The result is expressed as a ratio per person of the amount of money saved to the amount of money spent.

The first attempt at calculating a cost–benefit ratio in relation to offender treatment was made by Prentky and Burgess (1990), who carried out an exercise of the above kind in relation to a high security institution, the Massachusetts Treatment Center (MTC), which specialised in working with men who had committed sexual offences. Follow-up studies showed that the group discharged from the MTC had a reoffence rate 15 per cent below that of a comparable group released from prison. Prentky and Burgess showed that for each man sent to the MTC as compared to prison, the State of Massachusetts saved $68,000.

A number of reviews of economic outcomes have since concluded that there are sizeable financial savings to be made from investment in direct interventions across both youth and adult correctional services. Since 2001, a series of comparisons between the benefit–cost ratios of different interventions has been produced by the Washington State Institute for Public Policy (Lee, Aos and Pennucci, 2015). They identified several that achieved a 'win–win' outcome: they lowered crime *and* they reduced costs. Monetary savings could be made even when reductions in crime were quite small. While the savings from some programmes were modest, several others emerged very positively. They include, for example, *Aggression Replacement Training* (Goldstein, Nensén, Daleflod and Kalt, 2004). When used with young offenders in institutions, this yielded a benefit–cost ratio of US $27.40 for every $1.00 spent; a remarkable return on investment. A follow-up study of the treatment of high-risk young offenders at the Mendota Youth Treatment Center, Wisconsin, showed that members of the treatment group were six times less likely than controls to be reconvicted of a violent offence. Economic analysis of the intervention showed a cost–benefit ratio of 1:7 (Caldwell, Vitacco and Van Rybroek, 2006). Other economic analyses of criminal justice interventions have reported a range of benefit–cost ratios (McDougall, Cohen, Swaray and Perry, 2003; Welsh and Farrington, 2000). Findings in this area have recently been reviewed by Mallender and Tierney (2016).

There is striking evidence of superior benefit–cost quotients for community-based treatment of drug-related offending as compared with imprisonment. Several reports illustrate the marked advantage on almost all outcome indicators, including recidivism, subjective well-being and the costs of community-based treatment relative to incarceration. For example, here are the respective yearly costs of the two approaches in two US states: in Maryland $4,000 and $20,000; and in California, $4,500 and $27,000 (McVay, Schiraldi and Ziedenberg, 2004). For Illinois, which in 2005 had a prison population of 64,800 and 90,000 people under probation supervision, Braude, Heaps, Rodriguez and Whitney (2007) estimated that providing community-based treatment instead of incarceration for 10,000 persons, plus treatment for 15,000 probationers, would yield savings for the state of $223.3 million.

Finally, Weisburd, Lum and Yang (2003) note that even if a programme evaluation does not produce statistically significant findings in the orthodox sense, that does not necessarily mean that it has not 'worked'. Even a small change might be enough for the intervention to have paid for itself, and this might be taken as the marker of a 'bottom line' in judging its contribution.

Can treatment work for everyone?

Given the sometimes quite impressive results that have emerged from the research just described, one question inevitably arises: will psychologically based treatment work for everyone? It is vital to avoid making exaggerated claims, as to do so can undermine a profession's credibility. It would be naive to think that one could make any generalisation about the effectiveness of interventions that would not be subject to some limits. The largest effect sizes found still leave a sizeable proportion of experimental samples untouched. There will always be people who are unresponsive or who are actively resistant to treatment, and in criminal justice there will also be a proportion who will not participate, making the process of testing interventions more challenging.

Expectations of positive effects appear to be lowest when attention turns to the subgroup of offenders designated as 'psychopathic'. There is a widely shared view not only that treatment is ineffective with this population, but that it can even make them worse. This idea seems to have gained wide acceptance mainly because it has so often been repeated. The conclusion is often traced to a study by Rice, Harris and Cormier (1992), which was a follow-up of patients discharged from Oak Ridge, the maximum security division of Penetanguishene Mental Health Centre in Ontario, Canada. Rice and her colleagues compared rates of violent recidivism amongst psychopaths and non-psychopaths over a period of ten years after discharge from the institution. Their conclusions have often been interpreted as showing that those denoted as psychopaths are inherently 'untreatable'.

In the Oak Ridge study, amongst non-psychopaths there was a significant difference (expressed as percentage reoffending) between treated and untreated groups for both general (44 per cent v. 58 per cent) and violent (22 per cent v. 39 per cent) recidivism. By contrast, for 'psychopaths' while there was no significant difference between treated and untreated groups for general recidivism (87 per cent v. 90 per cent), the *treated* group later committed more violent offences (77 per cent v. 55 per cent). Without doubt, the sparseness of research on this topic, combined with the thinness of positive outcome evidence, has led to a firm impression that with this group treatment gains are unlikely. This has been called *therapeutic pessimism* and even *nihilism* (Salekin, 2002). When we examine closely the frequently heard claim that 'treatment makes psychopaths worse', however, it appears to be based on the single finding just mentioned.

Closer inspection suggests that the conclusion was actually misplaced. The value of the treatment at Oak Ridge was highly questionable. Many aspects of it would not, and on ethical grounds almost certainly *could* not, be implemented today. Treatment was conducted in the Social Therapy Unit, a therapeutic community (TC). However, in the Oak Ridge regime the basic model of this treatment was adapted in some fundamental and pervasive ways, and departed considerably from the original TC concept. Assignment to the unit was non-voluntary. Contact with staff was kept to a low level; and participants, wearing no clothes, spent up to 11 days in small groups in what was called a 'Total Encounter Capsule' (Barker and McLaughlin 1977). The researchers themselves later published some misgivings about the approach (Harris, Rice and Cormier, 1994). Since then, other authors have concluded that there is no firm evidence that treatment makes psychopaths worse (D'Silva, Duggan and McCarthy, 2004).

For many reasons, research studies on treatment of psychopaths are extremely difficult to do, and it is perhaps not surprising to find that there are no well-designed outcome trials in this area. Nevertheless, in the period since the Rice *et al.* (1992) study, several researchers have sought other evidence of treatment responsiveness in psychopathic offenders. In a meta-analysis by Salekin (2002), 42 studies were located. However, only eight entailed comparisons between treated and untreated samples, and the dependent variables were intermediate measures rather than recidivism outcomes. Five studies used behavioural, cognitive, personal construct or interpersonal therapy (with a combined sample size of 246). Results showed high effect sizes on mediating variables. Salekin (2002, p. 93) concluded that therapies 'addressed patients' thoughts about themselves, others and society ... they tended to treat some psychopathic traits'.

It may be that views concerning the possibility of securing positive outcomes with this group have been changing, with, for example, Reidy, Kearns and DeGue (2013, p. 536) suggesting that 'a specifically and carefully crafted intervention may be effective in reducing violence by psychopathic individuals', while Polaschek and Daly (2013) identified a developing consensus that such an intervention can be devised. Evidence supporting that contention remains tentative, however, and derives mainly from research with high-risk sexual offenders rather than with those convicted of other types of violence (Doren and Yates, 2008; Olver and Wong, 2013; Wong *et al.*, 2012). If a meaningful impact is to be secured with this group, preliminary indications from sites where such work is being done suggest that successful interventions need to be both intensive in their format and to extend over lengthy periods (Saradjian, Murphy and McVey, 2013; Wilson and Tamatea, 2013).

Several reviews have lent support to the possibility of positive treatment effects with offenders who are also diagnosed with major mental disorders, including those with features classified as 'psychopathic'. Several reviews have examined the developing literature on the possibility of reducing violent reoffending and aggressive behaviour amongst people who have been convicted of assault and have also been diagnosed with mental disorders, and either imprisoned or detained in secure mental health facilities. Understandably, many studies in this area focus on treatment services designed to reduce symptoms and to improve mental health and personal well-being. However, a proportion also focus on the reduction of adverse incidents within institutions, or on rates of reoffending once individuals have been discharged to the community. With regard to the latter, meta-analytic findings suggest that the variables specified in the RNR model are more closely associated with general and violent recidivism than are clinical variables such as diagnosis (Bonta, Blais and Wilson, 2014).

Martin, Dorken, Wamboldt and Wootten (2012) reported a review of interventions for offenders with major mental illnesses, as previously defined under Axis 1 of the DSM-IV. This excluded studies concerned with substance abuse, intellectual disability or personality disorders. Martin *et al.* calculated 37 outcome effects from a set of 25 studies with a combined sample of 15,678 individuals. The mean effect size on criminal justice outcomes at 0.19 (Cohen's *d*) was positive but comparatively small. Findings included significant effects on arrest, time spent in jail, time to failure and violent crime, although the impact on reconviction fell just short of significance. Morgan *et al.* (2012) carried out a similar review of treatment of offenders, but only four of the studies they located provided data on criminal recidivism, yielding a mean effect size (Cohen's *d*) of 0.11, which is analogous to the average effect sizes reported in the general offender treatment literature. Amongst those four studies, however, there was a wide range of effects. Three reported positive effect sizes, whereas the fourth obtained a pronounced negative result.

Ross, Quayle, Newman and Tansey (2013) carried out a systematic review of ten studies each of which tested interventions to reduce aggressive behaviour in forensic settings. Amongst them two were RCTs, six were pre-post studies (with no comparator sample) and two were small case series. Methodological quality, which was analysed in some detail, varied considerably, and there was also an assortment of outcome variables, which made it difficult to detect trends amongst the results. Eight of these studies reported reductions in physical aggression, although only one, by Polaschek, Wilson, Townsend and Daly (2005), found a drop in violent recidivism at follow-up.

Studies of a specific form of therapy, *dialectical behaviour therapy* (DBT), were reviewed by Frazier and Vela (2014). DBT was designed for and is most widely used with individuals who have been diagnosed with borderline personality disorder, a frequent symptom of which is a marked pattern of emotional dysregulation. These authors analysed twelve studies of the impact of DBT on anger and aggression, seven of which employed a randomised controlled trial (RCT) design, though there was a somewhat varied mixture of comparison groups. No overall effect size was calculated, but ten of the studies reported significant reductions on measures of anger or aggressive behaviour, two of them finding reductions in violent indiscipline in correctional settings.

Research influencing practice

Most of the studies analysed in the reviews summarised above were conducted on a comparatively modest scale, and often, though certainly not always, under reasonably well-controlled conditions. The question therefore arises as to whether similar findings can be secured when interventions of this type are disseminated on a larger scale and assimilated into routine practice. Impressed by the sorts of findings just surveyed, governments of several countries embarked on policy experiments in which specially designed programmes or other services were introduced into prison or probation sentences.

In England and Wales, the experiment took the form of a large-scale policy initiative, the *Crime Reduction Programme*, which was put into practice from 2000 onwards. It entailed the gradual introduction of structured programmes at many prison and probation sites. It was accompanied by an 'accreditation' process to select the programmes most likely to achieve good results, and an elaborate system of monitoring standards of delivery and evaluating outcomes (National Probation Service, 2004). The criteria used in this process (which were revised in 2016) are shown in the 'Focus on ...' box below. The Correctional Services Advisory and Accreditation Panel (CSAAP), part of the Ministry of Justice in England and Wales, evaluates proposals for the introduction of programmes in both prison and probation services. In the course of its work the Panel has approved a total of 42 programmes for use. Amongst them, 18 are for prisons, 14 for probation and 10 for use in both settings (Correctional Services Accreditation Panel, 2010).

FOCUS ON ...

The Correctional Services Advisory and Accreditation Panel (CSAAP)

Criteria for programme accreditation 2016

1) A clear description

There is a clear explanation of what the service or programme involves and who is expected to benefit from it.

2) Rationale for enabling the reduction of reoffending and the promotion of desistance

There is a clear explanation of how the service or programme will deliver its intended outcomes and this rationale is based on an understanding of the evidence on the causes of crime and desistance.

3) Selects participants appropriately

There is a clear explanation of how participants are selected for the service or programme, and how it matches the risk, needs and responsivity characteristics of the people it is delivered to.

4) Addresses factors relevant to the reduction of reoffending and the promotion of desistance

The service addresses risk factors linked to reoffending and/or increases protective factors linked to desistance. (In general, services and programmes that address multiple risk factors are likely to be more effective.)

5) Skills orientated and constructive

The service or programme is structured and develops skills which contribute towards leading a crime free life. (If not, there is a robust justification for using another approach that does not develop skills.)

6) Participant motivation, engagement and retention

The service or programme should engage and retain participants to enable them to complete all aspects.

7) Quality assurance

The service or programme has an effective quality assurance process in place. It pays attention to staff skills and training, and checks that staff deliver the service as intended.

8) Evaluation of impact including that the service does no harm

The service or programme is evaluated to confirm it has the desired effect. There are measures in place to monitor the impact of the service or programme on participants and others and to make revisions in the event of unexpected negative and unwanted consequences.

Programmes need to be accompanied by a considerable quantity of supporting documentation. Each programme requires five manuals:

- Theory Manual: describes the intervention model and evidence supporting it
- Programme Manual: describes the content, exercises and materials used

- Assessment and Evaluation Manual
- Management and Operational Manual
- Staff Training Manual

Each of the eight criteria is then scored as follows: 2 = fully met; 1 = partially met; 0 = not met.

A programme must score at least 14 points to be awarded accredited status. For fuller detail see Correctional Services Accreditation Panel (2016). For a candid history of the Panel's work, see Maguire, Grubin, Lösel and Raynor (2010).

Reference

- Based on Ministry of Justice. © Crown copyright 2016. Contains public sector information licensed under the Open Government Licence v3.0: http://www.nationalarchives.gov.uk/doc/open-government-licence/version/3

The results of these endeavours were, however, rather varied. Some significant reductions in recidivism were reported following participation in prison programmes (Friendship, Blud, Erikson and Travers, 2002), but other evaluations have shown only marginal evidence of positive outcomes (Cann, Falshaw, Nugent and Friendship, 2003).

Results in community settings were generally more positive, though a major issue in such settings was the very high attrition rate amongst those allocated to attend programmes. (Fortunately there was later evidence of significant improvement in completion rates since the initial period.) Evaluations of the probation *Pathfinder* programmes showed that those who completed programmes were significantly less likely to reoffend than the comparison sample *not* allocated to attend (Hollin *et al.*, 2008; Palmer *et al.*, 2007). Whilst the evaluations could not be based on randomised experimental trials, the studies were designed in accordance with the principles of the TREND statement for high-quality quasi-experimental designs (Desjarlais *et al.*, 2004). Further analysis showed that these effects could not be explained solely in terms of prior features of the participants (McGuire *et al.*, 2008); in other words, it is likely that there was indeed a treatment effect.

Official statistics also indicate positive effects resulting from participation in many probation programmes. These statistics are not based on either experimental or quasi-experimental evaluation designs, however, but on comparisons between predicted and actual reoffending rates over a two-year follow-up period (Hollis, 2007). The risk assessment instrument employed for this purpose, the *Offender Group Reconviction Scale* (OGRS), was developed and tested by Copas and Marshall (1998) and has a high level of predictive validity. Analysis of data on over 25,000 offenders by Hollis (2007) showed that there were statistically significant, and sometimes quite large, reductions in reoffending amongst those who had completed probation programmes.

The British government's Crime Reduction Programme remains one of the largest initiatives ever undertaken in applying evidence-based practice to an area of public policy. Whilst many practitioners and researchers welcomed its arrival, it is also true that others had considerable reservations about it. Some people were ideologically opposed from the outset, seeing the programme as soulless, target-driven 'managerialism' which paid little regard to the social circumstances that form the background to a great deal of crime. Others were sceptical from the outset and highlighted the gradually widening gap between what was anticipated and what actually occurred (Stanley, 2009). Even amongst those who in principle supported the departure, the scale and pace of its dissemination took many by surprise. Moreover, the entire process occurred simultaneously alongside a number of other major organisational changes, which may have been a factor in weakening the results (Raynor, 2004). Thus figuratively speaking, the terrain over which the programme was driven was fairly rough, and perhaps not the most favourable for ensuring a straightforward test of its effectiveness.

The successes and failures of transferring what has been found in research to the much larger and less predictable context of everyday practice have produced some valuable lessons for forensic psychologists and others involved in the enterprise. They have drawn attention back to the marginalised issues of implementation and delivery, and to the organisational factors that need to be considered if what have been called 'demonstration' programmes are to be open to rigorous evaluation and constructively translated into 'practical' programmes. The former refers to what are usually researcher-led projects conducted on a fairly limited scale. The latter denotes programmes that are transferred into broader-scale use as an integral part of service provision in criminal justice settings (Lipsey, 1999). Palmer (1995) initially spelt out a framework for managing this process of transfer, and for identifying some of the gaps to be bridged, formulating a distinction between *programmatic* and *nonprogrammatic* aspects of intervention and innovation. The first refers to the design and contents of the intervention programmes themselves. The second denotes contextual, responsivity, organisational and management factors that influence how well the programmes are delivered. Nonprogrammatic issues were revisited in a review by Andrews (2011), who also highlighted the fact that the weaker findings of some programme evaluations might be explicable in terms of the limited attention often paid to the nonprogrammatic factors. A more robust framework is now available for guiding the implementation process and for engaging with evidence-based practice more realistically than before.

Conclusions

It seems justified to conclude that there is more evidence than ever before that it is possible to secure reductions in patterns of criminality amongst persistent offenders. Such a conclusion is supported by a substantial volume of research findings, and analysis of these findings indicates that the observed effects are not due to methodological artefacts or other explanations. This is in sharp contrast with past ideas about treating such offenders. As Weisburd *et al.* (2017, p. 426) have noted, this picture is 'directly at odds with the "nothing works" narrative that dominated thinking in these areas'. Furthermore, as Lipsey and Cullen (2007) have argued, the effects of the interventions are uniformly more positive than those found for penal sanctions, yet the latter retain a pre-eminent and seemingly incontestable position in most justice systems.

It is difficult to anticipate the likely patterns that work in criminal justice might take in different countries in the coming years. National contexts vary enormously, and the balancing of priorities will naturally reflect concerns within each state. It is crucial that there should continue to be a fruitful relationship between research and practice. If criminal justice is to pursue **evidence-based practice**, the approach that has become accepted in other fields – and it appears vital that it *should* do so (Cullen, Myer and Latessa, 2009) – it is possible to identify some principles that should inform research, and which could be common to many countries:

1. Information concerning the success of effective interventions should be disseminated – to criminal justice staff; to judges and court officials; and to government ministries and other providers of funds.
2. The best evidence produced to date suggests that we should select intervention approaches that draw on a psychosocial model of the causes of offending behaviour.
3. It is essential to conduct comprehensive assessments of individuals, using the best validated methods available.
4. It is equally important to make thoughtful use of the information obtained in allocating individuals to intervention programmes.
5. Criminal justice interventions should continue to be quality controlled, and their delivery should be carefully monitored and evaluated.

There have been significant developments in the field of 'tertiary prevention' of criminal conduct in recent years, but a great deal more needs to be done. As regards designing and delivering effective programmes, still more knowledge is needed and vital questions remain:

- Do we need to develop new programmes or do different types of service need to be developed to address specific types of offending behaviour?
- If so what they would look like?
- Perhaps there is already enough variety in the programmes available. If so, do they need greater refinement or a change of emphasis to produce better results?
- What influences attrition from offending behaviour programmes? How could we reduce such attrition?
- Can we develop better strategies for engaging individuals in intervention programmes (McMurran, 2002)?
- How important is the working alliance in this context?
- Is the timing of delivery of a programme during a sentence a significant factor in its effectiveness?
- Are interventions more effective if delivered during prison sentences or during periods of community supervision?
- How can interventions can be adapted to accommodate diversity amongst participants in terms of gender, culture, ethnicity, age, sexuality and other variations?
- How do contextual and organisational factors affect implementation of services, and what strategies can we develop for making this process more effective?

Chapter summary

A major theme running through this chapter has been the contrast between the findings reviewed here and those discussed in Chapter 16. We briefly examined the history of efforts to carry out rehabilitation and *tertiary* prevention in criminal justice settings, comparing that with what have respectively been called *primary* and *secondary* prevention. The bulk of the chapter then focused on evidence pertaining to the outcomes of evaluation research in the area of 'tertiary prevention'.

- We considered the principal method, meta-analysis (originally discussed in Chapter 3), which has been used to synthesise the findings from large numbers of studies in this area, together with some criticisms of this method and reservations concerning its usage.
- This led to an overview of the findings obtained through meta-analysis of interventions designed to reduce criminal offending. We identified and summarised the general features that are associated with the more consistently effective interventions. This summary included discussion of the *Risk–Needs–Responsivity* (RNR) model, which has received wide support from the results of outcome research.
- This was followed by a more detailed examination of the approaches that have been found to 'work' with adult offenders and young offenders. Where possible, findings were also reviewed in relation to different types of offence; and we noted that the application of interventions was moderated by other 'nonprogrammatic' factors, such as settings, the level of organisational support, and the quality of delivery.
- This in turn was followed by a discussion of what has often been a contentious issue: whether individuals assessed as having personality disorders associated with severe antisocial conduct (and with 'psychopathic' features) could be induced to change their behaviour and to desist from reoffending.
- Finally, we described some of the policy changes that have occurred because of the findings reviewed earlier, and the wider impact of these findings; and the dissemination of structured rehabilitation programmes in various parts of the criminal justice system, both in the United Kingdom and some other countries.

Further reading

- For the most comprehensive review to date of the research literature relevant to the ground covered in this chapter, see the book edited by David Weisburd, David P. Farrington and Charlotte Gill (2016): *What Works in Crime Prevention and Rehabilitation: Lessons from Systematic Reviews* (New York, NY: Springer).
- The volume by Leam Craig, Theresa A. Gannon and Louise Dixon (2013), *What Works in Offender Rehabilitation: An Evidence-Based Approach to Assessment and Treatment* (Chichester: Wiley-Blackwell), provides a set of overviews of research on specific types of offence.
- The more polemical book edited by Joel A. Dvoskin, Jennifer L. Skeem, Ray W. Novaco and Kevin S. Douglas (2012), *Using Social Science to Reduce Violent Offending* (New York, NY: Oxford University Press), questions why the available evidence is not acted upon and applied more systematically and extensively.
- There are many books examining treatment or rehabilitative work related to specific types of offence.
- On sexual offending, Douglas P. Boer (ed., 2016): *The Wiley Handbook on the Theories, Assessment and Treatment of Sexual Offending* (Chichester: Wiley-Blackwell).
- On substance-related crime, the wide-ranging book by Carl Leukefeld, Thomas P. Gullotta and John Gregrich (eds, 2011): *Handbook of Evidence-Based Substance Abuse Treatment in Criminal Justice Settings* (New York, NY: Springer).
- The three-volume *Wiley Handbook of Violence and Aggression*, edited by Peter Sturmey (2017; New York, NY: Wiley-Blackwell), has chapters on many aspects of theory, research, assessment and treatment of aggression and violent offending.
- For a volume focusing more specifically on applying the methods of cognitive-behavioural intervention in forensic settings, see Raymond Chip Tafrate and Damon Mitchell (2014). *Forensic CBT: A Handbook for Clinical Practice* (Chichester: Wiley).
- For discussions of the development of structured programmes, see the edited volume by Clive R. Hollin and Emma J. Palmer (2006), *Offending Behaviour Programmes: Development, Application and Controversies* (Chichester: Wiley)

Professional Roles: Ethical Issues in Practice

Ethics, in practical terms, are principles that are put in place to provide boundaries on our behaviour so that we behave within an accepted standard. For example, you will probably have come across the idea of 'research ethics', and you may have considered issues such as 'informed consent' (such that research participants, for example, understand what they are volunteering for), data confidentiality, and the appropriate reporting of data. As society changes, so accepted standards of behaviour change, and ethical principles change also. More broadly, ethics is an area of philosophy that is concerned with questions such as the rightness and wrongness of actions, and it may be applied to consideration of criminal behaviour, justice, military intervention, or medical practice – indeed, in all aspects of human endeavour.

Chapter objectives

- To become aware of the issue of ethics within psychology.
- To become familiar with some of the dilemmas, specific and general, that have existed in psychology.
- To examine early examples of work in psychology that would now raise ethical concerns, and to see these as indicative of the evolution of ethical thinking.
- To consider the possibility that good intentions may not always result in ethical outcomes.
- To become familiar with some of the ethical issues that relate directly to forensic practice.

This chapter is concerned with ethics in general, and more specifically with the issue of ethics for the forensic psychologist. Now that forensic psychology is a regulated profession, there is a much greater focus on the behaviour of its professionals, especially as they may be working with particularly vulnerable members of society. The content of this chapter will help you consider where your own views and behaviour stand in relation to ethics, and to form a basic model for thinking about dilemmas in practice.

What do we mean by 'ethics'?

At its most basic, *ethics* is concerned with the process of making choices, be those choices about whether or not to drink **Fair Trade** tea, or whether a nation should include the death penalty in its legal system. The process of ethical decision-making involves evaluating the pros and cons that are important to us so that we can make an informed choice bearing in mind the benefits and losses to ourselves and – if we are to behave ethically – to others. In the case of choosing tea, the pros and cons might involve the *price* of the tea, what proportion of that money goes to the producers, whether or not the land is used sustainably, and – depending on what factors influence how we conceptualise the world and ourselves – how we wish others to see us. Ethical thinking can clearly be individual and difficult to generalise, and it is for this reason that, over time, various professional bodies have developed ethical guidelines so that members of those professions have a common basis for decision-making. If we were to rely on the opinions and attitudes of individuals to determine behaviour within a profession, we would have to tolerate a great degree of uncertainty and variability.

A set of ethical guidelines that may be familiar to most people is the **Hippocratic Oath**, which is still the basis for ethical conduct in medicine. It originates from approximately 400 BC, and contains guidelines such as 'whatever houses I may visit, I will come for the benefit of the sick, remaining free of all intentional injustice, of all mischief and in particular of sexual relations with both female and male persons, be they free or slaves' (Edelstein, 1943). Pre-dating this by about 1600 years was the *Code of Hammurabi*, a Babylonian code of laws, which included this declaration: 'If conspirators meet in the house of a tavern-keeper, and these conspirators are not captured and delivered to the court, the tavern-keeper shall be put to death' (King, 1915). Wecht (2005) notes that the Code of Hammurabi also deals with aspects of medical practice.

Each code attempted to describe the most suitable ways to deal with situations

WHERE DO YOU STAND?

Treatment at any cost

Treatment, as defined by the change in someone's behaviour, is complex. Consider your own efforts at, for example, giving up smoking, doing more exercise, or sticking to resolutions like avoiding alcohol. For most of us this kind of change is not easy. How then might we think about the process of changing more complex behaviours, such as sexual behaviour?

In a paper by Blakemore *et al.* (1963), a procedure is described in an attempt to deter an adult male from **Transvestism**. The patient was a 33-year-old coal miner who voluntarily sought treatment in order to be 'rid of his perversion' (p. 30). The treatment consisted of aversion conditioning, whereby during approximately half of 400 trials when he was allowed to dress in his favourite female outfit, he received electrical shocks through the soles of his feet. The authors reported that six months after treatment the man claimed no interest in cross-dressing.

A report by Maletzky and George (1973) described a process of using covert desensitisation (imagining unpleasant experiences, feelings or responses such as vomiting) and a noxious smell to treat men who had been referred to them for 'treatment for homosexuality' (p. 655). Based on the mean data from 10 men, the authors reported that the treatment was successful, based on self-reported levels of homosexual and heterosexual thoughts and behaviours. A study with the same goal was described by Thorpe, Schmidt and Castell (1963), but using electric shocks; and a decade later by Tanner (1973). Thorpe *et al.* reported that their intervention was ultimately 'unsuccessful', and it is not clear from Tanner's work whether the intervention was 'successful' in changing homosexual thinking or behaviour.

In most of these cases the people undergoing the intervention were volunteers (one in the Tanner study was not), but given the views society held at that time towards transvestism and homosexuality, the 'treatment' may not have been 'voluntary' in the same sense as we might consider it now. However, in each of these cases, and in many similar ones, the participants underwent the experience of painful or unpleasant stimuli with the goal of effecting change.

Where do you stand on this issue?

1 To what extent do you think that ethical decision-making regarding treatment should be based on the *outcome* of the treatment or on the experience of the individual *during* treatment?

2 Is it reasonable to traumatise people if there is some identified potential positive outcome and how could you argue this position?

3 If it *is* reasonable, does it make a difference whether people are volunteers or not? If they are *not* volunteers, what kinds of behaviours would you consider justified in using unpleasant experiences to change?

in which people might find themselves, presumably to result in the greatest benefits for that society in that time period. Over time, new codes have developed for new professions, and to take account of societal and technological changes. For example, with the abolition of slavery, an ethical code need no longer note that both slaves and free people should be treated equally; and the availability of new medical treatments requires that we continually consider the benefits and costs to individuals and society of providing certain treatments when paid for by the NHS. However, ethical reasoning is now considered to be based on five principles, as presented in Table 20.1 (see also Haas and Malouf, 1995).

Ethical principle	Definition
Non-maleficence	Doing no harm
Fidelity	Being trustworthy
Beneficence	Promoting the welfare of others
Justice	Treating everyone equally well
Autonomy	Allowing others to make decisions for themselves

Table 20.1 Principles of ethical reasoning.

Source: inspired by information in Haas & Malouf (1995).

Even such relatively simple principles are, under the surface, more complex. For example, treating everyone equally *well* must take into account the circumstances of each person – considering their age, gender, ethnicity and so on. It is not simply a matter of treating everybody the *same*. Similarly, promoting the welfare of others may involve a professional causing extreme discomfort to another person, with the possibility of lasting harm or even death. Such is the case with surgery, and to a lesser extent with dentistry. It is not hard to think of examples where psychology also could result in extreme discomfort to another, such as working with someone to help them understand unpleasant experiences. This might be the case, for example, in working with the female non-offending partner of a man who has sexually abused children (see Cahalane, Duff and Parker, 2013); or in supporting an individual in not engaging in a preferred sexual practice, such as having sex with children, by means of some form of sexual offender treatment programme. One could also consider some of the earlier practices for behaviour change described in the 'Where do you stand? ... Treatment at any cost' box.

Ethics and psychology

Psychology, like other sciences, is awash with ethical dilemmas, though perhaps this is unsurprising given that psychology focuses on, and frequently carries out research on, human participants, and also treats people. For examples of ethical dilemmas, see the 'Focus on ...' box, which considers the issues regarding the famous studies of Milgram (1963) and Zimbardo (see Haney, Banks and Zimbardo, 1973), and the impact these had.

FOCUS ON ...

Ethical dilemmas in psychology

There are a variety of studies that could be used to think about ethical principles in psychology, and the two studies considered here have been chosen because they are usually considered early in psychological careers, not necessarily because they are the best examples or the worst cases. However, each of the two studies did set out to investigate important issues.

Zimbardo's work

Zimbardo's work was concerned with what the authors refer to as 'interpersonal dynamics in a prison environment' (Haney, Banks and

Zimbardo, 1973, p. 69), as determined by the social forces of the roles the participants took on and by the setting. Understanding how the social roles play out in a prison is important in understanding, for example, times when prison officers might break boundaries or rules, or where inmates might become more likely to assault officers or to riot.

The participants, all carefully screened, were randomly assigned to being either prison guards or prisoners, and acted out their roles within a fake prison. The descriptions of the roles were left quite open, although physical punishment and aggression were banned. Once the two groups had been identified, the 'guards' were called to a briefing the day before the experiment took place; and the 'prisoners' (who did not know that they had been selected to act as prisoners) were arrested at their homes, by real police officers and without prior warning (though they had been told to stay at home on that particular day). Once in the prison they were stripped of personal belongings and clothing, left to stand alone naked for a period of time, and then required to wear muslin smocks, rubber sandals, a chain and lock on one ankle, a nylon stocking as a cap, and no underwear. The guards were provided with military-style uniforms, reflective sunglasses and wooden batons, and were permitted to wear underwear.

Questions

The original paper does require reading to fully understand the impact of this experiment on both sets of participants; for our aims we can consider just the information given above.

1 Despite the fact that the research could provide some important information in our understanding of the dynamics within prisons, was it ethical to arrest people at home (their arrests may have been seen by neighbours and friends), to strip them, and to deny them underwear?

2 Even if there are no ethical issues, to what extent might the dynamics that ensued be due to the guard/prisoner interactions and to what extent might they be due to these other considerations?

Milgram's work

Milgram's (1963) work – the original of which is worth reading, and is accessible via Columbia University – was concerned with examining what Milgram referred to as 'destructive obedience', which is obedience in carrying out actions that are harmful to others. His paper makes clear that at least one of the motivations was to try to understand acts of atrocity carried out during World War II.

Milgram's participants were asked to act as the teacher in a learning experiment in which they provided punishment if the 'learner' failed in the learning task (participants were always the teacher, as the selection for that role was rigged). Gradually they were asked to punish the learner with increasing levels of electric shock, using a machine with markings such as 'Danger: Severe shock'. The learner was a confederate and in fact received no shocks, but was instructed to respond to the supposed shocks at a certain level by pounding from the next door room where the 'learner' was seated, and as the shocks continue to rise eventually the pounding ceases. The idea was to see how far people would go in administering punishment to a stranger, even when they were receiving information that the punishment was harmful, and even when their role was to participate in a study (as such there was an element of authority with them being volunteers for the study run by the white-coated researchers).

Questions

Given the motivation for Milgram's study, experiments that might outline the limits of obedience and how these could be manipulated could be important.

1 To what extent does this study raise ethical concerns?

2 It is not uncommon to omit details of a study (here that the learner is a confederate and is not being shocked) in order that the participants respond to a situation that they believe to be real. Is it ethical to place people in a situation where they feel compelled to harm another?

3 If we do that, how should we support participants after they have taken part?

In Milgram's paper there is no description of how participants were managed post-experiment, yet this description is given of one of them:

> I observed a mature and initially poised businessman enter the laboratory smiling and confident. Within 20 minutes he was reduced to a twitching, stuttering wreck, who was rapidly approaching a point of nervous collapse. He constantly pulled on his earlobe, and twisted his hands. At one point he pushed his fist into his forehead and muttered: 'Oh God, let's stop it.' And yet he continued to respond to every word of the experimenter, and obeyed to the end. (p. 377)

Given the state of regulations and ethics at the time of these studies, this is not an exercise in condemning previous research but rather in considering how our understanding of ethics may have changed over time, and what aspects of previous work would now be considered to be inappropriate or dangerous. One could undertake a similar analysis with other research, both new and old, to understand how ethical decision-making has been applied.

4 Do you think that ethical considerations should prevent important psychological concepts from being investigated and how can you construct an argument to support your position?

Even things that we take for granted now – things that are now standard practice within the profession – may still, if we look closely, have the potential to produce a negative impact on others. For example, currently in most psychological research we describe a finding as statistically significant if the likelihood of it happening by chance is 5 per cent. Depending on what that finding is, however, 5 per cent might be too big a chance. For example, if a piece of research showed that **electroconvulsive therapy** (ECT) had a greater impact on depression than cognitive-behavioural therapy (CBT), we might expect, on statistical grounds, that ECT would become the treatment of preference for depression. But would we feel ethically secure in exposing people to ECT knowing that the evidence suggests any positive benefits of the treatment have a 5 per cent likelihood of happening by chance, not because ECT actually is more effective than CBT? Even if the positive effect really was a result of the ECT, how could we weigh the pros and cons of the efficacy of the treatment against its potential side-effects and, at its most basic, the procedure of the therapy, which you might find interesting to find out more about?

In a 2003 paper, Iodice and colleagues suggested that the majority of patients (53 per cent) who have received ECT would choose it again if they became unwell. They did not focus on the fact that over a two-week period the numbers of those 'likely' to choose ECT fell slightly (from 53 per cent to 52 per cent) or that those 'unlikely' to choose increased slightly (from 20 per cent to 27 per cent), nor did they show that there is a statistical difference between 'likely' and 'unlikely'. This does not suggest there is an ethical issue with ECT, but are patients making this decision purely on the perceived efficacy of the treatment – or is there something about it that they don't like? Stevens and Harper (2007) provided a qualitative analysis of how professionals discuss ECT, and considered the fact that their interviewees tended to undermine any criticisms of it. Again, this does not bring into question if the practice of ECT is ethical *per se*, but it may suggest that we would want to ask more questions before making our treatment decision. For an interesting, non-ECT case study, regarding the use of electric shocks with an individual who was distressed by his transvestism, see Blakemore *et al.* (1963; and briefly described in the 'Where do you stand?' box on page 456). What are the ethical issues of treating an individual in this way, despite the fact that he himself wishes to change, and believes this to be possible? Similar debates may be had concerning the use of what is referred to as 'conversion therapy' to 'cure' homosexuality (see Spitzer, 2003).

In addition to the *quantitative* statistical issue mentioned above (as to whether a 5 per cent chance effect might raise ethical concerns in some cases), Haverkamp (2005) discusses ethical dilemmas that may arise in *qualitative* research, where the issue of statistical significance is not relevant. The researcher might consider that interviewing a participant is relatively benign, but what might be the potential longer-term issues if someone were asked to discuss their experiences of physical abuse, for example, or their own offending behaviour? Might they develop a new and potentially healthier understanding of their experience, and as a consequence become more resilient? Or might people who had been abused perceive their victimhood as their own fault; or people who had offended become paralysed by guilt and self-disgust about their earlier behaviour? How might the *form* of the interview impact on these outcomes? To some extent there are not, and cannot be, clear-cut answers, and that makes the area of ethics both fascinating and complex. However, our goal here is simply to suggest that there are many circumstances in which further thought might be useful.

Considering interventions within the forensic domain, what are the ethical dilemmas if we were to use masturbatory reconditioning so that an individual finds pictures of naked children less arousing than before but now finds pictures of naked adult women more arousing? Are we simply shifting the potential victims (at worst) or encouraging a man to objectify women? How might exposure to these stimuli impact on attitudes regarding violence against women (Hald, Malamuth and Yuen, 2010)? Is it appropriate to use **shame aversion therapy** (Serber, 1970), with its clear impact upon the recipient, if doing so might prevent further victims of indecent exposure? Are there dangers to *therapists* in shaming their clients?

More broadly, are decisions concerning the very focus of research themselves ethically problematic? For example, should we be concerned with exploring what might work with a prison population to prevent them reoffending, or would it serve society better if we focused instead on discovering the factors that reduce initial offending? These are the kinds of issues in research, and also in assessment, in treatment, and in our dealings with clients and other professional agencies, that we need to consider if we are to behave effectively and appropriately as forensic psychologists.

Forensic psychology and ethics

Due to the nature of the forum within which it focuses, forensic psychology has its own range of ethical issues, just as counselling or clinical psychology have their own particular areas of concern. Throughout the following discussion, it is important to keep in mind that these issues are *in addition to* the more general issues that psychology has already come to terms with or still wrestles with. It is important to be aware of the **code of conduct** for your particular professional society or association, such as the British Psychological Society (BPS) or the American Psychological Association (APA). In the UK the regulatory body, the Health and Care Professions Council (HCPC), has set out *proficiency standards* for all psychologists, and separate standards for differing practitioner groups within psychology.

It is useful to be aware that codes evolve to keep pace with changes in society and technology, as mentioned above in relation to the Code of Hammurabi. Forty years ago, for example, homosexuality was considered illegal, yet now there is a Gay and Lesbian Section of the BPS. Similarly, with the development of the internet there are new kinds of offences, new ways of offending, and new ways of tackling offending and offenders. One of the most fundamental issues, perhaps, which is quite specific to the forensic psychologist, is the fact that our work involves close contact with individuals who may have behaved in incredibly violent or sexually deviant ways, and naturally this may produce a negative reaction in the psychologist. Until one is actually carrying out an assessment, for example, of an individual who has physically, emotionally and sexually assaulted his daughter from the age of 2 and for 10 years thereafter, it is impossible to know what feelings that process might engender in the psychologist. Whatever one's response, it is likely to impact upon the assessment process, and maybe more so if that response is revulsion and anger. It is therefore ethically essential for the professional to monitor this and to determine whether these feelings might bias assessment or treatment, and if necessary act accordingly, perhaps by referring the case to another professional. The next 'Focus on' box will consider aspects of bias.

FOCUS ON ...

Bias impacting psychologists

To what extent have you reflected on any biases you have that might impact upon how you work with people? Some studies have identified that psychologists are biased in ways that may influence their work. In some ways this should not come as a surprise, perhaps, as we are all likely to have some biases; but we might expect that people who choose a caring profession and have received training may have learned to manage these biases.

An American study from 1995 by James and Haley provided evidence that when clinical psychologists are presented with a description of a hypothetical patient there is some evidence of an age bias. For example, clients described as older were considered less appropriate for intervention and less likely to have a positive prognosis. Similarly, the health of the hypothetical client impacted upon judgments, such that those described as less physically healthy were judged to have a poorer prognosis, be less appropriate for intervention, and be more likely to commit suicide. If biases such as these exist with real clinicians considering real patients, then it is clear that biases will also impact on the ways in which psychologists work. Other work has demonstrated that professionals may be more patronising and condescending with older adults (e.g. Ryan *et al.*, 2000), and may assume that older adults are cognitively impaired (Ellingson, 2003).

It might seem relatively easy to identify when we think we would *not* be comfortable working with someone even before having done so, but how can we know that we *would* be comfortable before being in that situation? If the offender you had to work with was a rapist, what core beliefs would you have to possess in order to work with that person? Thinking about questions such as these in advance is an important process for two reasons: so that you, as the forensic psychologist, do not find yourself feeling uncomfortable when faced with a particular person or a behaviour by which you are affected; and also so that the person you are working with receives the best from you and is not unfairly disadvantaged by your biases. If people can be biased by age and physical health, is it not likely that people might also be influenced by offence-type (e.g. a sexual offence against a child, as compared with the theft of a vehicle)? We all do have biases, and while being able to identify them does not necessarily mean that they can be changed, by acknowledging them you can make informed, ethical decisions about how you work.

Issues for forensic psychologists

A number of specific ethical guidelines have been identified for practising forensic psychologists, taking into account the kinds of work undertaken and the kinds of people worked with. For example, the HCPC states that forensic psychologists must be aware of and understand the potential power imbalance between themselves and their clients, and must know how to manage this appropriately. Interestingly, for *counselling* psychologists the HCPC includes this standard alongside the need to recognise appropriate boundaries and to understand the dynamics of power: it is not clear why this second guideline would not also be appropriate for *forensic* psychologists. This may demonstrate, perhaps, that ethical codes are not always as expected or immediately commonsensical. However, there is an important issue that arises from this. Forensic psychologists work with many other professionals, each of whom will have their own codes of ethics; yet we see here that even with a *shared* regulatory body there is the potential for different professionals to be required to work with different codes of ethics. This may become even more of an issue for the forensic psychologist if she or he is working subordinately to another professional, with a different set of priorities and a different ethical policy. Also important to recognise is that the *absence* of a standard should not be taken as implying that certain behaviours are legitimate: one of the expectations of a professional is the ability to identify ethically complicated situations and to act appropriately even if the situation is not covered explicitly by a professional standard – or, if one is unsure, to consult with colleagues to ensure that one's professional integrity is not compromised.

As forensic psychologists now work in a wide range of areas, we will highlight some of the main ethical issues that may arise by focusing on some of the tasks that tend to be carried out across these different areas, rather than by looking at specific job roles. If you are at the outset of a career in forensic psychology, one issue worth considering is that it is not always apparent *where* one learns about ethical practice. Authors such Handelsman (1986) have described the typical process whereby professionals in training learn about ethics as occurring by osmosis. Indeed ethics has mostly been left out of teaching. In a survey of higher education establishments, V. Lewis and colleagues (2007) showed that only 10 per cent reported that ethics formed a part of courses on research methods. This is not best practice, by any means, and it would be a distinct advantage to you to become conversant with ethical thinking and ethical guidelines (see 'Further reading' for some suggestions), as well as recent ethical dilemmas within your particular service and field.

Assessment

To some degree the ethical issues concerning assessment may be independent of the issues being assessed, but this will depend on the context in which a person is being assessed. For an individual in the community, an assessment of risk might, for example, result in greater scrutiny by the police and the probation service, and certain restrictions on activities (such as employment or entering schools). For an individual who is being detained, however, an assessment of risk might lengthen their detention. In making assessments we should not be swayed by the potential outcome for the client – we should always be fair and honest – but it is impossible not to be aware of the impact of our work on individuals. More widely, too, it is important to consider how these consequences might moderate our thinking and our decision-making. If the potential consequence of an assessment report were that a man's children might be taken into care and later adopted, might our assessment and report be different than it would be if the consequence were instead that he was only allowed supervised contact with his children? If as professionals we consider that a case is 'serious', or if perhaps there is media attention, are we concerned to do all the work ourselves rather than asking psychology assistants to undertake some of the testing and scoring of the psychometrics? One element of being fair and honest at all times is ensuring that the appropriate tests are used and that whoever carries them out knows how to administer them, that the scorer knows how to score them, and that the results are interpreted by someone with sufficient skill. However, even an appropriate level of skill does not guarantee ethical work. For instance, if you have a driving licence you have been tested and judge to be skilled enough to be allowed to drive, but you should still consider factors that might influence your ability to apply your driving skills on a particular occasion, such as mood, health, tiredness, or the amount of alcohol you have consumed. Similar care should be taken when you are involved in making assessments, as even suffering from a cold might impact on your mood, your thinking and your decision-making (Bucks *et al.*, 2008).

In making an assessment you need to identify appropriate tests. This is not without problems, as there is usually a range of tests to choose from and the tests may differ in subtle ways. Most important from the ethical perspective, perhaps, is that the test has been validated using a comparison population appropriate in relation to the person being assessed. The properties of some psychometric tests have not been investigated in forensic settings, and using those tests might unfairly represent an individual's skills and deficits. Similarly, there may be tests that are appropriate only for specific groups – for males, for intance, or for particular age-groups – and some tests may not have been examined in non-English-speaking environments or where there are differences in ethnicity and culture. As well as these issues, there may be concerns that mental illness, learning disability or literacy might impact on the usefulness of a test. It is also useful to consider the age of a test. Older tests may use phrasing that is no longer common or may ask questions that are no longer socially or contextually relevant. The results from such tests would be likely to include levels of error greater than would be considered acceptable and they might unfairly represent the individual being tested.

Within a forensic context, assessments are usually risk assessments: in essence, how likely is this individual to offend again? Decisions about risk are further complicated by the competing demands of society and the individual's rights to liberty (McGuire, 2004b). Society has a reasonable expectation that it should be protected from harm, whether from people who shoplift or from people who murder – although our demands for accuracy in risk assessments for murderers are likely to be substantially greater than our demands regarding shoplifters. But offenders have rights, too – if someone is highly unlikely to offend again and is seen to have been suitably punished, presumably that person should be released. How though do we resolve these competing claims when predictions of risk cannot be absolutely accurate? Some individuals who in fact would *not* go on to offend may be identified as still posing a risk and detained unnecessarily, just as some who are judged to pose no further risk may be released and go on to reoffend. As McGuire (2004b) makes explicit, the state of the risk assessment profession continues to raise a number of important ethical issues, given the ways in which assessment of risk impacts upon people's lives.

Another potential dilemma in relation to assessment is who should carry it out. One might assume that it would be fairer if testing were carried out by someone who knows the individual, so that there is good rapport and, perhaps, less of a tendency by the person being tested to try to provide socially acceptable responses rather than truthful responses. The potential problem with this is the degree to which the tester may, unknowingly, bias an individual's responses, which is known as the Clever Hans effect (Pfungst, Rahn, Stumpf and Angell, 1911). Clever Hans was a horse that was thought to be able to count, until it became clear that the horse's behaviour was actually being influenced by subtle signals from his owner. Similarly, it is possible that, through unconscious non-verbal behaviour, a tester may influence the person who is taking a test – and this is more likely to happen if the individuals involved have already developed some level of communication. The extent to which a psychologist and an offender know each other may also lead to ethical issues if the psychologist is playing a dual role. An assessor who has also been involved in an individual's treatment may experience a **conflict of interest**, from the point of view both of addressing the individual's needs and also of the service's overall success, for example in clearing its waiting list.

Sometimes, however, such dual roles are unavoidable. One of the authors (SD) manages a community Introductory Sex Offender Programme and is responsible for writing reports on the men's progress. These reports rely, to some extent, on recording changes in their presentation, their engagement with the process, and their reactions to various tasks. The reports would not be as detailed if they were written by someone who was not working directly with the men but instead relying on other reports and psychometrics. However, it is possible that this working relationship may hinder the objectivity of a report. McGuire (1997) considered this issue at some length, comparing the potential conflicts of working as a clinician and as a forensic expert, and focusing on such factors as differences in client motivation, confidentiality and the focus of the service. Some authors have suggested that the conflict between these roles may be irreconcilable (Greenberg and Shuman, 1997, 2007); and in their later article these authors provided an example from the Federal Rules of

Civil Procedure which clarifies why the two roles are different: the professional who has been involved in *treatment* 'has functioned as a direct participant in the events at issue' (Greenberg and Shuman, 2007, p. 130). If the professional who has treated the client is also providing evidence for that client, then that professional is required to evaluate his or her own therapeutic work, and it is not clear that this can happen without bias. Mannarino and Cohen (2001) considered the same ideas from the perspective of a professional working with sexually abused children and their families. Dickie (2008), however, suggested that accepting two assumptions – that forensic psychology and the law have the same goal (namely, to prevent and to manage criminal behaviour), and that the legal system can function in a therapeutic manner – would allow for many of these issues to be reconciled.

Appearing in court

Further along the legal process, the blurring of relationships may also become important when a forensic psychologist is appearing in court. McGuire (1997) refers to this as the dilemma between acting as an *advocate* and acting as an impartial *educator*. If one is hired by one side or the other to provide expert testimony in a case, will that lead to bias in what data are collected, how they are interpreted, and how they are presented to the court? Or will the forensic psychologist be unbiased and provide a more scientific view?

Similarly, there is a potential conflict when the psychologist is involved in research in which one of his or her clients is also a participant in the study. For these kinds of situations Fisher (2003) offers some useful advice: 'psychologists should always consider whether the particular nature of a professional relationship might lead to misperceptions regarding the encounter. If so it may be wise to keep a record of such encounters' (p. 65).

Professional boundaries

In all of the situations above, we must consider other aspects of professional ethics, such as the accurate taking and safe keeping of notes, and taking care with professional boundaries.

Knapp and Slattery (2004) provide some insight into how boundaries may change as psychology develops into a profession offering a wider range of therapeutic contexts, including, for example, working at the client's home. Although this may seem unlikely for the forensic psychologist, there are already forensic services such as Youth Offending Teams who do go out to client's homes, and there are multidisciplinary teams who work with offenders with mental health or learning disability issues who might also find themselves visiting a client's residence.

Barnett and colleagues (2007) provide an overview of more general boundary issues that a psychologist may face, and also consider the issues of the multiple relationships that exist between psychologists and their clients. Their particular focus is on the importance of the *power imbalance* between the professional and the client, and they draw distinctions between respecting, crossing and violating boundaries. *Crossing* a boundary is where a client may be treated differently but where the behaviour is contextually appropriate and does not threaten the therapeutic relationship – for example, having physical contact with clients by shaking their hand or offering some form of comforting gesture for a client who is distressed. This becomes a violation when the action is based on the needs of the *professional* rather than those of the client. Nevertheless, these behaviours may be seen as on a continuum, and the authors point out the importance of remaining conscious of boundary-crossing and considering this thoroughly to ensure that such a step is not part of a process leading towards a less appropriate goal. Having some knowledge of boundaries in forensic psychology, and having given some thought to how best to preserve them, are important; according to the APA's Ethics Committee (2002), issues about infringement of boundaries are the source of most complaints against psychologists in the US.

Confidentiality

An important issue related to assessment and treatment is that of *confidentiality*, and its limits in different circumstances. In principle, the communication between a forensic psychologist and a client is protected, which means that the psychologist should not share, and is not obliged to share, the content of that communication, unless the client has given informed consent (see the BPS's *Generic Professional Practice Guidelines*, 2nd edition, 2008).

Legally, however, confidentiality is not absolute. In the UK and in the US, a client's right to confidentiality can be breached, *without* her or his permission, if this is required by law, or if there are concerns about harm to the client or to members of the public. (In some US states this is discretionary, in others it is mandatory.) 'By law' does not mean simply 'if a court requires it'. For instance, in the UK the law states that if someone discloses information that may be linked to a terrorist act, then this must be reported. The law in this matter is not always entirely clear, as national and international laws frequently compete. For example, the requirement to report an individual for a disclosure related to terrorism might be considered as contrary to Article 8 of the Human Rights Act 1998, which states that everyone has the right to respect for their correspondence. Article 8 contains some conditions where this right can be breached, however, such as in cases of national security, public safety, and for the prevention of crime, but to what extent is this legal judgment independent of ethical thinking?

More directly relevant within forensic psychology, perhaps, would be a situation in which you have been engaged by the defence to provide an assessment of an individual for the court. Despite being engaged by one side rather than the other, your duty is to the court, and your report should therefore be unbiased. If during your assessment the individual confessed to the offence to which in court she or he was pleading 'not guilty', what would be the appropriate ethical and legal course of action for you to take? Would such information from you be admissible in court if it had been gained during a psychological assessment? Would it be ethical to continue with the assessment, to provide the report and to accept payment, if you now knew that the individual was guilty, and as you would know also that your report should not address issues of guilt or innocence? According to Lipsitt (2007), in an evaluation report in an American court, a confession would not be admissible.

Treatment

Some of the issues regarding treatment have been touched on already, including the difficulty in making a decision about the use of an aversive intervention. In such situations there is a conflict between the rights of the individual to be treated reasonably and the rights of society to be kept safe.

Some treatments are clearly aversive, such as the use of electric shocks and unpleasant odours, but more modern approaches may still prove aversive. For example, if an individual who is a sex offender is shown a video interview with a victim of sexual assault who is clearly distressed, this may be important in helping the offender to develop a sense of empathy for the victim. However, the offender too may become distressed, both about the victim's distress and because of personal feelings of guilt, shame and remorse. When working with groups of sex offenders it is quite clear that discussions about such offences – the details of the offending, the motivations for such offending, and the perceived benefits in carrying out the offences – can be distressing to some of the offenders. Some would argue, of course, that it is appropriate that offenders become distressed during their treatment: after what they have done, they deserve it – and if distressing discussions prevent more people from becoming victims, then the offender's distress is an acceptable price. However, it is not the role of the forensic psychologist to become part of the punitive process, and this is partly why there are ethical guidelines for working with offenders. While the psychological process may still be perceived as punitive, that is a side-effect, not its purpose; and the intensity of the process must be thought through and monitored throughout the process of treatment.

In some ways, producing change of any kind in another person may involve distress. One way to deal with the ethical issues that this raises, perhaps, is to consider the quesion of consent (see below). Interestingly, while there is a research literature concerned with the potential impact of therapy on the therapist (e.g., Hernàndez, Engstrom and Gangsei, 2010), to date there does not appear to be similar focus on the potentially aversive impact of therapy for the client.

Consent

As described above, confidentiality can be broken with informed consent, and one of the primary ethical concerns within research projects is that participants know what they are agreeing to participate in. This latter issue was a development from the Nuremberg trials (although it was the Helsinki Declaration of the World Medical Association that formalised it – see Hoeyer, 2009), as it was discovered that experiments had been carried out on inmates in work camps without their consent. Even so, informed consent has not always formed the basis of research in psychology and medicine. For example, in one study concerned with jury deliberations, the court officials were aware that the jurors were being taped, but the jurors were not (Katz, 1972); and in another study, Humphreys (1970) clandestinely collected the vehicle number plates of men who had used a public toilet to engage in sex, so that he could interview them at a later date. Similarly, in Milgram's famous studies (e.g. 1963) the participants were not aware that the person they were 'teaching' was in fact a confederate of the researcher, and was not, as it seemed, receiving ever-increasing electric shocks. (For other interesting examples, see the work of Berkun, Bialek, Kern and Yagi, 1962, who were concerned with stress in army recruits).

In the case of research, informed consent may obviously have a biasing effect on results, and a compromise must be reached between the importance of generating unbiased research findings and the potential for harm to be done to participants. One must consider how such harm would be dealt with, and how participants should be debriefed. With regard to assessment and therapy, although individuals may agree to participate, it may be unlikely that they are fully aware of what they are agreeing to. (Or indeed whether their agreement is truly voluntary – can it be truly consensual if the individual fears that failure to comply might be seen by others either as indicative of mental health issues or as lacking in cooperation, either of which might have consequences for that person's release or for future access to his or her children, for example?) Also, and as mentioned earlier, some therapeutic interventions may entail distress, and yet until the person is actually *receiving* that intervention, the presence and level of the distress might not be apparent.

It is also the case that consent to treatment may not be required in cases where an individual is thought not to have the capacity to give that consent and if there may be serious consequences were they *not* to receive treatment.

Where treatment is given without consent, this is typically under conditions of a *section* of the Mental Health Act 1983. Currently it is the medical profession who have responsibility for sectioning, but under revisions to the Act there has been a suggestion that psychologists might also take on this role (Holmes, 2002). This could pose an ethical dilemma for psychologists, as typically psychology is not a coercive practice: while other institutions may require that an individual see a psychologist – as a condition of probation, for example, or prior to sentencing – psychologists work with their clients without force. The potential dilemma occurs when the psychologist is required to act both as the therapist and as the force demanding that therapy take place. Even when one is not part of the sectioning decision itself, there may still be issues with regard to working with individuals who are being treated against their choice. Should a forensic psychologist be involved in a treatment programme that is thought to be for the individual's best interests, even if there is a suggestion of coercion?

Possibly not, but if we examine the overall situation carefully it is clear that many offenders *do* experience coercion, albeit from the prison system (e.g. the possibility of earlier release), in the context of probation, from families, and so on. Although this is a more subtle form of coercion, many offenders are likely to make treatment decisions based on what they perceive they may gain, rather than because they themselves want to change their behaviour. For some offenders such external influences may be incredibly powerful. For example, a man who has offended sexually against children may have to move out of his family home, may lose his job, may lose access or have only restricted access to his children, and may have further restrictions placed on contact with other children in the family (such as nieces or nephews), and on his movements. Given that treatment may be the only decision that is recognised by social services, for example, as moving towards lowering risk and thereby restoring these aspects of his life, there may be emotional, financial and practical reasons why the man may decide to accept treatment. Without such external pressures, would *you* voluntarily decide to change your sexual behaviour, if you currently find it satisfying?

As forensic psychologists we are required to weigh our ethical duty to the individual against our ethical duty to the wider public – including, and centrally, the protection of children.

Conclusion

As the material in this chapter suggests, there are a variety of areas in which ethical thinking is important, both in terms of the welfare of the forensic clients with whom one is working, and in maintaining the professional's own integrity and safety. The difficulties with ethics are that guidelines change over time and may not be as inclusive or as flexible as would be necessary to fit your particular situation. Although it is crucial to keep abreast of the most recent guidelines for your situation, from supervisory bodies (e.g. the HCPC, the BPS and the APA) and from your employer, it is also important to recognise the value of *supervision*. Senior colleagues may have struggled with similar issues in the past.

Most basic, perhaps, is that you recognise that your actions – and your inaction – may have consequences for you, your colleagues, your profession, and the individuals with whom you work, and that you therefore think through the possible implications. Remember that ethical guidelines are really a starting point for thinking about your particular situation: you need to make an informed decision before you act so that you can provide an explicit rationale for your actions if you are questioned about them later. Think carefully and keep a record of your thinking and decision-making process, especially in novel situations. While this will not guarantee that your actions will be viewed as ethical, the process should help you to identify any areas where there is a lack of clarity, and prompt you to gather any further information you need.

Chapter summary

» Ethical principles provide guidelines to help a variety of professionals make informed decisions that reduce harm to those with whom we work and that promote their well-being.

» Ethical principles have evolved over time, taking account of changes in society, in technology, in the professions, and in our understanding of behaviour, amongst other things. Ethical principles are not fixed, but need to be flexible and adaptable.

» We can examine the development of ethics by considering examples of studies throughout the span of psychological research, including research that is carried out with the public, and also research concerning, and the treatment of, particular groups of people.

» Given that psychology focuses much of its attention on human behaviour, the ethical principles for research and intervention in psychology need to account for a broad range of circumstances, and may not be able to provide guidance for every situation.

» Applied psychologists need to consider carefully how their work may challenge ethical principles. For example, in testing some theories the psychologist might cause harm to the client, and in carrying out some interventions the psychologist might cause the client to experience discomfort.

» Ethical principles from professional bodies should be considered as the *starting point* for ethical thinking, not as definitive guidelines that will provide specific solutions to every possible dilemma. Ethical principles do not replace the need for individual thought.

Further reading

» It would be useful to consider the ethical guidelines of your own professional and regulatory bodies. In the UK, these would be the HCPC and BPS; in the US, the APA. In addition, you should become familiar with any ethical guidelines provided by your employer or place of study.

» To begin thinking about the area of boundary issues in working with clients, potentially in multiple roles, this paper provides a useful introduction:

- Barnett, J. E., Lazarus, A. A., Vasquez, M. J. T., Moorehead-Slaughter, O. and Johnson, W. B. (2007). Boundary issues and multiple relationships: fantasy and reality. *Professional Psychology: Research and Practice*, 38: 401–410.

Similarly, the following paper considers ethics within forensic psychology:

- Dickie, I. (2008). Ethical dilemmas, forensic psychology, and therapeutic jurisprudence. *Thomas Jefferson Law Review*, 30: 455–461.

» For a more general view of ethics in psychology, this book provides a good conceptual overview:

- Kitchener, K. S. and Anderson, S. K. (2011). *Foundations of Ethical Practice, Research, and Teaching in Psychology and Counselling*, 2nd edition (NY: Taylor & Francis).

Professional Training, Competence and Expertise

In the UK, the body that regulates the profession of forensic psychology is the Health and Care Professions Council (HCPC). If you wish to practise under the title of 'forensic psychologist', you must be registered with the HCPC because this is now a 'protected' title, and to claim that one is a registered forensic psychologist when one is not is a criminal offence.

The HCPC sets the standards for the profession, investigates complaints, and provides guidelines for training. It works closely with British Psychological Society (BPS), which acts as the professional body for forensic (and other) psychologists. The BPS represents members, provides continuing professional development, promotes the profession, and is involved with developing and maintaining training standards. It also provides its own guidelines, as for example deciding who may use the title 'consultant'.

As a member of the BPS, one can apply for chartered status, which the BPS describes as being the 'gold standard' in professional standards. This chapter provides a brief outline of the current pathways towards becoming accredited as a chartered and registered forensic psychologist. It then goes on to consider some of the issues that face the practising forensic psychologist.

It is important to be aware that although this chapter sets out to represent the current state of affairs, it is always important to consult directly with the relevant bodies, such as the American Psychological Association, the British Psychological Society and the Health and Care Professions Council, before making any decisions regarding education and qualifications.

Chapter objectives

- To develop an understanding of the route towards professional qualification in the UK.
- To understand what the important knowledge base is for qualification.
- To consider some of the professional issues and roles and relationships with other professionals.
- To consider some of the philosophical issues of the profession.
- To be aware of the continuing development of the profession.

Becoming a chartered and registered forensic psychologist

In the UK, in order to be able to refer to oneself as a forensic psychologist and to work as a forensic psychologist there are a number of requirements, effectively split between the British Psychological Society (BPS) and the Health and Care Professions Council (HCPC). The compulsory element is to be registered with the HCPC, but in order to achieve that it is necessary to meet the required *academic* standards of the BPS and the *practice* standards of the HCPC. Figure 21.1 outlines the various routes to reaching the point of being able to apply to the HCPC for registration.

Undergraduate qualification

The first stage is to achieve Graduate Basis for Chartered Membership (GBC) from the BPS, either by achieving an undergraduate degree in psychology from an accredited BPS course or via a BPS-accredited conversion course. It is worth being aware that the requirement for GBC is a minimum of a lower second-class

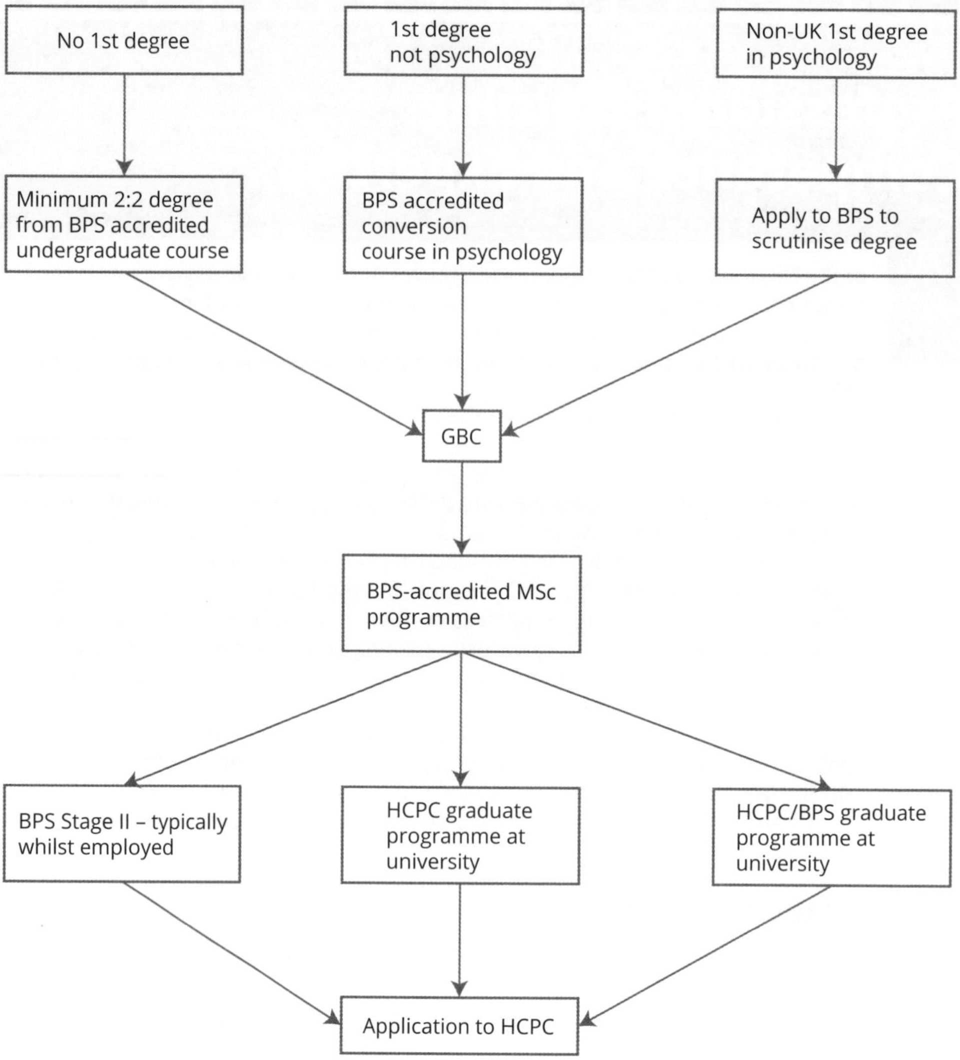
No 1st degree
1st degree not psychology
Non-UK 1st degree in psychology
Minimum 2:2 degree from BPS accredited undergraduate course
BPS accredited conversion course in psychology
Apply to BPS to scrutinise degree
GBC
BPS-accredited MSc programme
BPS Stage II – typically whilst employed
HCPC graduate programme at university
HCPC/BPS graduate programme at university
Application to HCPC

Figure 21.1
Outline of various routes to applying to the HCPC to be registered as a forensic psychologist.

honours degree, whereas to move on to the next stage of the qualification process you may actually require a minimum of an upper second-class degree. This is because as more people wish to join a field of study universities and courses can be more selective in who they recruit. Course-providers may also favour individuals who have demonstrated some understanding of the demands of a given applied profession by having related practical experience. For instance, forensic doctoral programmes may favour those who have worked as assistant psychologists after their undergraduate degree. It would therefore be wise to contact each of the programmes that you are interested in to determine what requirements they may have in addition to particular academic grades.

If your first degree is not in psychology, then a conversion course is a possibility. Different universities have different requirements for entry onto their conversion courses, with some requiring that you have had some university-level education in psychology. One of the most popular methods of converting for GBC is through courses run by The Open University, the UK's largest distance-learning establishment.

For individuals who have not attained their psychology degree from a UK university, the BPS considers each individual case to determine whether that non-UK degree is equivalent to a BPS-accredited UK course. This decision is primarily based on the status of the institution and the level of degree or qualification attained, which must be equivalent to a UK lower second-class honours degree or better. If the first degree is not in psychology, it should have contained at least 50 per cent psychology.

Individuals who cannot meet these criteria have another route available (if they prefer not to attend a UK university to undertake an undergraduate degree or a conversion course), which involves applying for *'Special Case' status* and being assessed according to a number of different criteria. There is still the requirement of having a qualification that maps onto a UK lower second-class honours degree with some coverage in psychology, but in addition candidates taking this route will need to supply evidence of postgraduate courses or experience relevant to psychology, or of journal papers or book chapters that they have authored that are concerned with psychology. Although the BPS guidelines suggest that only one of these areas must be addressed, it is likely that the strength of an application will be much improved by showing evidence of as much coverage as possible. For further details, the BPS website (www.bps.org.uk) is a good source of information.

Postgraduate qualification (MSc/Stage 1)

Having achieved GBC, the next stage is to take an MSc course in forensic psychology that is accredited by the BPS. As forensic psychology has grown in popularity, there are ever more universities developing and offering such programmes, but it is crucial that the course is BPS-accredited if you plan to work as a forensic psychologist. Accredited MSc programmes confer on the individual what the BPS refer to as Stage 1 in forensic training, and this is compulsory to be able to move on to Stage 2, where practical skills are developed. Although the increasing popularity of the topic means that it is being offered more widely, it also means that universities can be more selective in offering places, and it is more and more unusual for anyone with less than an upper second-class honours degree (and GBC) to be offered a place. It is also unusual for places to be funded, unless through a current employer, and all university courses are becoming more expensive. The BPS website provides an up-to-date list of courses that it accredits in psychology, and it would be useful to consult this information whilst considering where to apply. In the latter half of 2016 the BPS list identified 33 accredited postgraduate courses in forensic psychology. Typically an MSc is a year-long programme, although some can be taken part time over two years.

Some universities offer a three-year doctoral programme in which the first year is identical to an MSc, and the second two years are identical to the top-up programmes offered by universities, as will be described in the following section. This first year of study again confers Stage 1 qualification.

Stage 2 qualification

The BPS route

Once successfully through the MSc (which requires both a taught and a research element), the next step towards chartered status, if one is not taking one of the available university routes (see below), is what the BPS refers to as *'Stage 2'*, or the Society's *Qualification in Forensic Psychology*, which is based on supervised practice. This provides the candidate with BPS chartership and the necessary applied skills to apply to the HCPC for registration. The BPS suggests that this requires two years of supervised practice, but realistically, as there are evidence-based requirements, two years should be considered a minimum. Primarily this is because the requirements are achieved whilst the candidate is employed, and even when that employer provides a forensic setting, such as the UK Prison Service, the process is both time-consuming and labour-intensive. The four core competences that are required, and the areas that they consist of, are presented in Table 21.1 on the next page. See also the 'Focus on ...' box, which discusses 'Competences'.

1 Conducting psychological applications and interventions	2 Research	3 Communicating psychological knowledge and advice to other professionals	4 Training other professionals in psychological skills and knowledge
(a) establishing requirements for, and the benefits of, applications/ interventions	(a) designing psychological research activities	(a) promoting awareness of the actual and potential contribution of applied psychological services	(a) identifying and analysing needs to improve or prepare for job performance in specific areas
(b) planning applications/ interventions	(b) conducting research activities	(b) providing psychological advice to assist and inform problem solving and decision-making	(b) planning and designing training and development programmes
(c) establishing, developing and maintaining working relationships	(c) analysing and evaluating psychological research data	(c) providing psychological advice to aid the formulation of policy and its implementation	(c) implementing training and development programmes
(d) implementing applications/ interventions		(d) preparing and presenting evidence in formal settings	(d) planning and implementing assessment procedures for training and development programmes
(e) directing implementation of applications/ interventions carried out by others		(e) responding to informal requests for psychological information	(e) evaluating training and development programmes
(f) evaluating results of applications/ interventions*		(f) providing feedback to clients	

*Here 'psychological applications' refers to the 'application of psychological principles within criminal and civil legal contexts' (Division of Forensic Psychology, dfp.bps.org.uk), thus the idea is that a candidate demonstrates that they have thought through and understood the appropriateness of using psychology, and indeed specific aspects of psychology, in a particular case.

Table 21.1 Four core competences required of a forensic psychologist, and the areas they comprise.

FOCUS ON ...

Competences

The competences for qualification as a forensic psychologist are set by the BPS and the HCPC to ensure that people are suitably trained and prepared for their professional lives, and to ensure a high standard across the profession. This clearly has its advantages for practitioners, services and clients, as standardisation should result in consistency.

There are a number of issues that are worth considering that arise as a consequence of having standards.

Development over time

Standards represent the best thinking at the time they were agreed, and so, as with ethical standards, it needs to be understood that they are likely to change over time. We might consider that standards are a measure of the current *lowest* level of acceptable competence for our profession – we should strive to continue to improve both our practice and our standards.

Changing offences

Competency depends on the current state of affairs. For example, in a pre-digital society there was no need to be competent in understanding the issue of cybercrime. Similarly, we are no longer concerned with the idea of homosexuality being an offence. It is not always possible to predict how society and the law might change, but it is important to remain aware that changes such as these may influence the clients whom we see, the services that develop, and the knowledge we should have.

Conflicts between standards

The standards required of forensic psychologists are also dependent on the setting in which they work. In most cases, the standards and competences that derive from the particular work setting will be *in addition* to those of the BPS and the HCPC – for example, being competent in moving and handling, and or in dealing with specific security issues.

However, it is possible in principle that two sets of standards might come into conflict, and it is therefore essential that the forensic psychologist is able to identify any such conflicts and to find ways in which to manage them professionally. For example, the BPS has a code of ethical conduct for research, but a particular service might not adhere to that code if the research staff are not BPS members. If the guidelines are perceived as overly restrictive and unhelpful, there is the possibility that conflict might arise about how to best carry out the research.

Developing additional competences

The competences of a forensic psychologist should be seen as *in addition* to those required for the Graduate Basis for Chartered Membership (GBC). The research skills that are required for GBC should therefore still be understood as underlying the competences for forensic competencies.

Professional incompetence

It is important for everyone that standards of competence are rigorously maintained. If a forensic psychologist were thought to be behaving in an incompetent manner, therefore, this could result in his or her work being scrutinised by the HCPC, which has the power to place sanctions on professionals (such as requiring that he or she work only under close supervision) or to deregister an individual.

The university route

The final possible route, if one is not doing the BPS Stage 2, is through a programme of study offered by a university, which may be to work towards either HCPC registration or both BPS chartership and HCPC registration, the latter being achieved via a doctorate which some UK universities now offer (e.g. the University of Birmingham, the University of Nottingham, Cardiff Metropolitan University, and the University of Portsmouth). Again, different universities will have different entry criteria for doctoral training, and may offer the doctorate as an extension to an MSc programme or additionally as a top-up for individuals who already possess an MSc (as does the University of Nottingham). The design of these programmes is very similar to that of the doctoral programmes in clinical psychology, where there is a combination of classroom teaching and working in placements. Through that process the doctoral trainee will be exposed to a range of different forensic settings (e.g. community, prison, court and high security) and different client groups (e.g. individuals with mental health issues, individuals with personality difficulties, adolescent offenders and female offenders) to ensure that he or she attains a breadth of knowledge and skills. The same four core roles form the basis of assessing competence.

The only real difference between the courses that offer HCPC-only registration and those that offer both HCPC registration and BPS chartership (the doctoral programmes) is that the doctoral programmes place a greater emphasis on the research component and have been accredited by the BPS. As detailed earlier, it is HCPC registration that is required to work as a forensic psychologist in the UK, although some employers do currently want their employees to have BPS chartership too.

Whereas university qualifications and Stage 2 qualifications are achieved through reaching particular standards of work, HCPC registration is *applied* for (rather than being a qualification) and this is an important difference. Although courses are developed to meet HCPC standards, the HCPC is the final arbiter in determining who will be registered.

Becoming a practising forensic psychologist

On being recognised by the BPS as a chartered forensic psychologist, or when you have completed one of the university HCPC courses (such as Cardiff Metropolitan University), the next step is to register with the HCPC in order to be able to practise psychology using the title of 'forensic psychologist'. The role of the HCPC is to monitor and maintain an individual's **fitness to practise**, which consists of six standards, as presented in Figure 21.2. The specifics of these areas can be explored on the HCPC website (www.hcpc-uk.org).

With the recent shift in responsibility for registering applied psychologists from the BPS to the HCPC, forensic psychology, along with what the HCPC refers to as the 'modalities' of psychology (e.g. clinical psychology, educational psychology and health psychology), has taken on a more overtly professional role in which standards are more closely upheld and monitored. In principle and in practice this is to ensure the protection of the public, as outlined in the Health Professions Order (2001). The HCPC's website provides descriptions of ongoing disciplinary cases across the various professions that it oversees, which may be useful for developing a sense of where professionals err. To ensure that you are working within the approved guidelines, it is vital to keep abreast of the necessary codes of conduct.

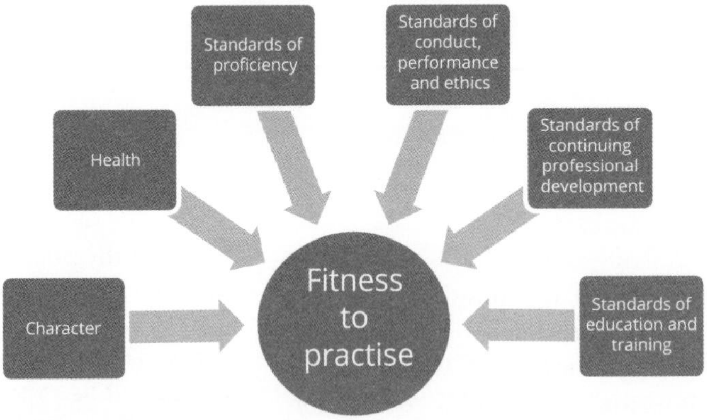
Standards of proficiency
Standards of conduct, performance and ethics
Health
Standards of continuing professional development
Character
Fitness to practise
Standards of education and training

Figure 21.2
Fitness to practise as a forensic psychologist.

Continuing professional development

The various approaches outlined above can bring you to the point of being a chartered psychologist and able to practise as a forensic psychologist, but you should not see this as the end of your training. *Continuing professional development* (CPD) is an essential part of the process of maintaining high standards within forensic psychology. Prior to July 2009, the BPS was responsible for setting out CPD requirements, both in terms of what kinds of learning and experiences would be counted and how much time was required. After July 2009, the HCPC took over this role, and now rather than there being a specific requirement to submit CPD activities on a regular basis, members can be selected for audit.

The HCPC has attempted to be flexible with regard to what counts as CPD, reflecting the fact that as a body it is not just responsible for psychologists. For example, it is open to receiving as CPD evidence business plans, course assignments, evaluations of courses and conferences attended, letters from students, and so on. The idea is that the profile of *your* CPD should reflect *your* role, and can be self-determined. Although this gives the professional the autonomy that is perhaps appropriate, it does require that you know the regulations and requirements and take responsibility for managing some form of CPD record. *The Psychologist*, the monthly publication from the BPS, regularly provides an overview of CPD opportunities – one edition, for example, includes expert witness report-writing, an integral approach to coaching, and maximising interpersonal relationships, amongst others. More details can be accessed via the BPS's dedicated web page: http://www.bps.org.uk/findcpd.

Professional issues and roles

Although the *route* to becoming a forensic psychologist is becoming more clearly defined, this is probably not so true of the *role* of a forensic psychologist. This is partly determined by the working circumstances in which individual forensic psychologists find themselves, and partly due to the evolving nature of the profession.

Originally, psychologists working within forensic systems would have been concerned primarily with issues involved in the legal system, such as eyewitness testimony, jury selection, recruitment of police officers, or interview techniques. Although some forensic psychologists are still working within these areas, they tend now to be academics. It is more than likely that to the lay public the title of 'forensic psychologist' generates an idea akin to a profiler, due to the nature of television dramas and the portrayal of forensic psychology within the media – for recent examples, a search for Paul Britton, David Canter or David Wilson in the popular press will provide examples, although individuals who appear in the media are not necessarily qualified as forensic psychologists. Again, some forensic psychologists may work alongside the police in crime analysis, but most working in this area are again likely to be academics (for example, Julian Boon from the University of Leicester). Where the role *is* somewhat in line with the idea of a profiler, the forensic psychologist may be referred to as a Behavioural Investigative Adviser (BIA). At the time of writing, there are perhaps five individuals whose full-time employment consists of this work; and approximately thirty accredited individuals, often academics, who are brought in on particular cases. The *majority* of forensic psychologists in the UK are to be found working within the prison system, in the assessment and treatment of people who have offended. This is a change that has developed over time, in the same ways that other professional psychological modalities have developed.

The Division of Forensic Psychology (DFP) of the BPS now defines the role of forensic psychology as:

> the application of psychological principles within criminal and civil legal contexts. Forensic Psychologists apply their skills across the domains of assessment, treatment, research, consultancy, training, management and supervision. Client groups include the courts, offenders, victims, and criminal justice personnel such as the police, prison and probation. Forensic Psychologists work across a wide range of settings that include custody, community, health, academic institutions, and the courts, in both public and private practice. Given the central role of transferring scientific methods to practice, Forensic Psychologists will often work across both research and applied roles. (see dfp.bps.org.uk).

In some ways this development makes sense, since forensic psychologists have developed expertise in forensic issues through research and have benefited by working alongside other professionals. However, it has led to a degree of discontent, highlighted some years ago in a short-lived but ill-tempered debate in *The Psychologist*, during which it was suggested that, in comparison with their clinical colleagues, forensic psychologists are not suitably trained to be involved in assessments and intervention, and have a tendency to work outside their sphere of competence. Obviously such generalisations about the professions are ill informed with respect to the current level of training and experience of forensic psychologists, and unhelpful other than in raising the issue of the boundaries or crossovers of the various modalities within psychology. It is not unreasonable to suggest that all professions may suffer from a degree of poor practice, at times; and that through the sharing of knowledge, continued training and a framework of guidelines, individual modalities, and applied psychology more generally, can realise and maintain standards.

Within the forensic area, forensic and clinical psychology share many similar roles and responsibilities, as defined by the competence of each modality, and in principle should complement one another. The same is true for other examples, such as health and education. Working within forensic settings, the forensic psychologist will at times work with individuals who may be dealing with long-term health issues, with dyslexia, and so on, but it is important that professional boundaries, and keeping within one's range of competence, dictate when other professionals are referred to for their expert input. The forensic psychologist should not assume competence in all aspects of psychology that occur within a forensic setting. Instead, it is essential that forensic psychologists see themselves as members of a team, whether within their work setting or more widely: the work will involve close liaison with clinical colleagues and with professionals from other disciplines, such as probation, social work, the police and psychiatry (discussed in more detail in the next section).

Relationship to other professions

Psychology is never individual. Regardless of whether the work is academic or clinical, psychologists work in collaboration with others. This raises some important issues for all psychologists: collaboration implies working towards a common goal, but the reality is that the goals may be subtly different, or the ways of reaching a shared goal may differ from one profession to another.

An example will provide an overview of this issue. Working within a community forensic setting with a man who has sexually offended against children outside his own family, the forensic psychologist has two primary aims: to protect the public from further offending, and to help the individual to understand and control his offending behaviour. In collaboration with other services, such as probation, the police and social services, it might be possible to draw up a plan whereby it is possible to pursue both aims by providing intervention and support for that individual while he resides outside of the family home, perhaps with limited, supervised contact with his own children (who would be considered to be at risk). The police are likely to have a similar overall goal, but they may approach it in a different way: they may decide that the only way to protect the public is to arrest the individual and keep him on remand (i.e. the individual would be kept imprisoned before a trial has taken place and a sentence set) until he can be convicted and sentenced to prison. Social services too may have a similar overall goal, but their approach may be to remove any children from the individual's family home and to take them into care. A psychiatrist may have a similar goal and may decide that the individual's behaviour is due to a mental illness that requires medical treatment, and that the individual must be sectioned in order to be assessed and suitably treated.

In each case the situation is the same, and the professionals are attempting to reach the same goal, yet their approaches may be quite different. This may be partly because of the limits of their roles – for example, a psychologist would not be able to arrest an individual; police do not offer psychological interventions; and a psychiatrist cannot remove children from the family home – and partly because of the underlying *philosophies* of the different roles. Presumably an underlying philosophical belief of psychologists is that behaviour, given the necessary understanding of the antecedents of that behaviour, is malleable using psychological methods (although see Walton and Duff, 2017). That belief does not necessarily preclude a belief in, for example, appropriate use of medication, but as the psychologist has no professional competence in the use of medication and no legal powers to prescribe it, she or he is limited both by philosophy and by profession.

Central requirements in reaching the goal for the individual client is that we are in a position to gather the relevant information for a thorough assessment; that we can develop a complete formulation of the issues of concern (see Sturmey and McMurran, 2011); and, on that basis, that we can construct appropriate support and monitoring. In order to do this we are heavily reliant on the information that other services may have concerning our client, so again the collaboration between services is crucial. Also important is the ability to communicate effectively with these services, from the perspectives both of providing them with information and of untangling the sometimes complex information in reports from a variety of sources. It is unlikely that reports by other services and professionals will follow similar formats to those of psychologists, and they may focus on aspects of the individual and their life in different ways, so good links with these services are essential in order to ensure that clients are represented as fairly and as accurately as possible.

An interesting and major change in recent times is that psychological expertise, in limited form, is no longer the sole domain of the psychologist. The use of approaches such as cognitive-behavioural therapy (CBT) and the IAPT programme (Improving Access to Psychological Therapies; see Cohen, 2008) have allowed other professions, and individuals who are not qualified psychologists (e.g., 'Psychological Wellbeing Practitioners in CBT'), to provide psychological therapies. The roles and levels of intervention are prescribed, however, and CBT therapists, counsellors, nurses, occupational therapists, experienced graduate mental health workers and psychotherapists can undertake this work only when they have been accredited by the British Association of Behavioural and Cognitive Psychotherapies (BABCP). There are financial and efficiency benefits to this approach, but as IAPT is a newcomer to the landscape of psychological intervention, it is not clear how IAPT will work alongside psychology. Initial analysis (North East Public Health Observatory, 2010) demonstrated that IAPT is reaching a number of the set targets (e.g. an appropriate gender split, in line with research) but in other areas it was not proving so successful (e.g. 39 per cent of patients did not receive a provisional diagnosis).

Boundaries of confidentiality with other professions and agencies

As discussed above, different professions may have different underlying philosophies; they may also have different legal demands, remits, ethical principles, and regulations regarding confidentiality (see Chapter 14) that cover other professionals and members of the public and family members. This may be a source of complexity and frustration for the professionals and for the individuals alongside whom they work.

Clearly there are some situations where there is a legal requirement to breach confidentiality, as for example in the case of threatened terrorist activity, or of an individual's stated intention to harm herself or himself or another person. However, there may also be other situations where the various professional boundaries of confidentiality come into conflict. For instance, if you are in conversation with an individual who has offended against children and he confesses to previously undetected offences against other victims, it is likely that other services, such as the police, the National Probation Service and social services, might expect you to inform them. However, the BPS's *Code of Ethics and Conduct* specifically states the following:

> Restrict breaches of confidentiality to those exceptional circumstances under which there appears sufficient evidence to raise serious concern about:
>
> (a) the safety of clients;
>
> (b) the safety of other persons who may be endangered by the client's behaviour; or
>
> (c) the health, welfare or safety of children or vulnerable adults.

In the circumstances outlined above, and given that you do not know the identity of the victim or victims, what is your responsibility? Are you required to breach confidentiality? Should you feel duty-bound to try to *determine* the identities of the other victims, in order that other services can intervene? By not knowing the victim it is not possible for the psychologist to impact on their health, welfare, or safety; and if the individual with whom you are working has already been *convicted* of sexual offences against children, does the existence of additional victims make him more of a current danger, to himself or others? Sometimes guidelines cannot provide specific answers and, as advised by the BPS, it is important to consult with other colleagues about such matters, including other professionals. It is also important that *clients* are aware of the limits of confidentiality and the possible consequences if it needs to be breached.

Importantly, it is not just psychologists who have to deal with the issue of how much information to share. For example, the police too may decide not to disclose the full nature of an individual's offences, either for legal reasons or because they have made a decision that a psychologist does not need to know the detail. Interestingly, in some cases of child pornography there may be an insistence by the police that the psychologist sees some of the material in order to understand the nature of the offences. This may be a cause for concern, as presumably it is illegal for the psychologist to view such images, and there is the issue of the impact that viewing such images may have on the psychologist.

Philosophical issues

There are a number of important philosophical issues that underlie psychology, and they are no less important for forensic psychology. Although we cannot hope to provide a complete overview of the depth and breadth of these issues, they do require some reflection because they underpin much of the work that is done in forensic practice.

Perhaps the most basic philosophical issues for forensic psychology are firstly what determines behaviour, which leads to a brief discussion of how we develop the knowledge that allows us to make informed decisions; and secondly – if we do indeed make decisions, that is – the issue of *free will.* These issues are important to consider within a forensic context as they speak to issues of responsibility. Basically, if one were to take the position that there is no free will, then presumably we would also have to rethink both our current legal system and our ideas about psychological intervention. What is the value of punishing individuals who are not in control of their behaviour? If individuals are not in control of their behaviour, behavioural change could not come about through knowledge, so what value is the value of CBT (cognitive-behavioural therapy), CAT (cognitive analytic therapy) and other talking therapies?

There are no definite answers to these questions, but they raise important points concerning genetics, the environment and learning, amongst others. Working as a forensic psychologist, you may well come face to face with these issues when reflecting on your clients, their behaviour, your practice, and their progress.

Free will

Research has suggested that behaviour is on a continuum, from that which is an *automatic, reflexive response* to environmental circumstances – for example, the knee-jerk reflex, caused by a gentle strike on the patellar tendon, just below the knee, involves no brain function – to behaviours that are *internally generated and selected* (see Brass and Haggard, 2010). If behaviour is not, at least in part, determined by the individual making conscious choices, or being able to intervene consciously in the products of unconscious choices – that is, being able to *choose* not to act, despite the outcome of unconscious processes in response to a given situation, and thereby to inhibit what might otherwise be deemed a 'disposition' to crime (e.g. Clarke, 1980) – then the role of forensic psychology becomes greatly diminished.

Murray (1938) wrote that 'at every moment, an organism is within an environment which largely determines its behaviour' (p. 39), supporting the view that behaviour is strongly influenced by the surroundings in which an individual is situated. We might still argue that forensic psychology could be involved in the *design* of environments, so that they do not 'afford' crime, which is something of an extension of Gibson's original idea of 'affordances' (e.g. Gibson, 1977). Gibson's idea was that the environment provides perceptual information about what is possible within that environment: for example, we can recognise that some trees provide the possibility of being climbed; open windows offer the possibility of entering a building unseen; and unlocked motorcycles offer the possibility of their being stolen. Such an idea has been incorporated successfully to reduce crime in some areas (e.g. Brantingham and Brantingham, 1975; Mayhew, 1979) by designing spaces that, for example, offer no places for concealment (see the 'Focus on ...' box).

FOCUS ON ...

Psychologically Informed Planned Environments (PIPEs)

An understanding of the effects of the physical environment has developed in parallel with an understanding of the effects of the psychological environment, particularly where that environment may play an important therapeutic and prosocial role.

The UK Prison Service and the NHS have carried out research aimed at exploring the impact of psychological environments that have been specifically designed to provide support, both in community settings provided by approved premises – where offenders live, supervised by staff as they are supported in making their transition back into the community – and within more secure settings, such as therapeutic communities. The idea is that staff can be given specific training so that they are able to manage complex individuals more confidently and competently, to improve relationships between staff and clients, and as a result to improve both clients' behaviour (such as reducing recidivism) and their psychological health.

One of the most important aspects of the *Psychologically Informed Planned Environments* (PIPEs) project was the use of collaborative projects both between staff and clients and between clients. The importance of collaboration in undermining the development of 'in' and 'out' groups was established in the late 1970s by Tajfel's *Social Identity Theory* (Tajfel and Turner, 1986). This indicated that collaborative tasks – that is, working towards a common goal – can be helpful in breaking down social categories, and can thereby reduce social exclusion and inter-group tension. It also allows people to feel responsible for aspects of their lives, their local society and their surroundings, and potentially to feel a sense of ownership.

The results of initial studies suggest that these psychologically informed environments do indeed have a positive impact on the relationships between clients and between clients and staff; and also with relationships with those outside that environment, such as family members. Secondly, they seem to have a positive impact on previous constructive changes already brought about by intervention, and staff have reported feeling that they had a greater understanding of why their clients behave as they do.

This is one example in which psychological theory has been implemented within forensic settings and has proven to be beneficial. One could suggest similar explanations of the impact of physical changes, for example that good relationships promote good behaviour (or do not promote bad behaviour). It is important to analyse the features of the psychological environment in order to understand likely outcomes, rather than to assume either that this environment is unimportant or that it is always consistent from setting to setting.

Reference

▶ Tajfel, H. and Turner, J.C. (1986). The social identity theory of intergroup behaviour. In Worchel, S. and Austin, W.G. (eds). *Psychology of Intergroup Relations*, 2nd edition (pp. 7–24). Chicago: Nelson-Hall.

Without free will, is there any need for psychology, and how might abandoning the concept of free will impact upon the legal system? It is a complex philosophical and practical issue. For example, we might suggest that being under the influence of alcohol or drugs leads to *behaviour* that might be considered to be not entirely under the control of free will. However, the *decision* to drink to excess or use drugs *is* under the control of free will (unless one was forced, or the drink was spiked), so would you still be culpable, morally or legally, for your behaviour? Should factors such as alcohol and drugs be seen as mitigating factors?

In the UK, being under the influence of alcohol is not allowed as a defence of diminished responsibility to the charge of manslaughter or other crimes that are referred to as being of 'basic intent' – that is, where the defendant knows, or is reckless to, the consequences of his or her actions. If an individual can be shown to have acted due to a *need* for drink or drugs, this could be seen as resulting in an abnormality of the mind: in this case, the defence of diminished responsibility can be allowed (see *R. v. Sanderson*, 1994). If the law allowed alcohol and drugs to mitigate our responsibility, we would in effect be suggesting that anything else that might make a person behave in a manner that is uncharacteristic could likewise be a mitigating factor. It follows, then, that strong emotions such as anger and hatred might be included too.

However, the admissibility of a plea of diminished responsibility will depend on the specifics of the case. For example, the 4th edition of the *Diagnostic and Statistical Manual of Mental Disorders* (DSM-IV) suggests that 'road rage' may be an example of the recognised mental disorder referred to as 'intermittent explosive disorder', yet in the UK it can be prosecuted under the Public Order Act 1986, and some states in the USA have specific laws against aggressive driving. Depending on the country and the details of the case (see below for the specific case of Jesse Bridgwater), other mitigating factors, as a result of which voluntary control of behaviour is considered to have been lost, include epilepsy, automatism (e.g. sleep walking – although the defence of being asleep whilst committing an offence is not always successful: see Nofzinger and Wettstein, 1995), and, in some US states, hypnosis and post-hypnotic suggestion (Bonnema, 1992–1993).

What about behaviour that is driven by unusual beliefs? If these are the result of mental illness, we may see that as reasonable. For example, research suggests that individuals diagnosed with schizophrenia tend to fail to predict the effects of their actions (e.g. Voss, *et al.*, 2010), which may indicate that their unusual beliefs, over which they have no control, affect their conscious decisions about how to behave. However, what if these unusual beliefs are due to *normal* cognitive processes? As an example, we might consider so-called 'rape myths' – that is, beliefs that are prevalent in men who endorse their own likelihood of sexual assault against women (Malamuth, 1981). We might suppose these to be unusual, yet in one survey 56 per cent of respondents (a random sample of 1,061 people in London aged 18–50, including 349 men, 712 women, 213 aged 18–24, 386 aged 25–34 and 462 aged 35–50, comprising 922 heterosexual, 71 homosexual, 52 bisexual and 16 asexual respondents) expressed the belief that a victim should take some responsibility for a rape (*Opinion Matters*, 2010). In law, however, a man's belief that a woman in a short skirt is 'asking for it' is unlikely to provide a successful defence.

Nonetheless, if our opinions and beliefs are a product of our experience, can we be considered to be in control of them? Or should we be able to control our behaviour *regardless* of our unusual beliefs, given that our beliefs are independent of mental illness? The actions of Anders Breivik (now known as Fjotolf Hansen) in Norway in 2011 may be an example of an individual who is not currently identified as mentally ill but who developed a set of beliefs that resulted in the decision to bomb and shoot (although he was evaluated twice, one evaluation suggested that he was mentally ill, the second that he was not). In his case, free will appears to have led to the belief that, despite his actions being objectively bad, there was no other option available to him and indeed, his defence was that he acted in self-defence.

WHERE DO YOU STAND?

Free will

On 22 July 2011, Anders Behring Breivik exploded a bomb in Oslo and then went on to kill 77 people on a small island off the coast of Norway. At the time of writing, a mental health assessment has not been completed, so although his lawyer has suggested that Anders Breivik is 'probably insane', there is as yet no psychological or psychiatric evidence to support this claim.

Where do you stand on this issue?

1 If there is no evidence of mental illness or personality disorder, should we see these as voluntary actions that can be dealt with by the courts? Or should being under the influence of ideas and beliefs that might result in these actions, no matter how counter-intuitive and antisocial these ideas and beliefs may be, allow Anders Breivik to claim that he acted without true free will? If he did *not* have free will, can he be held morally responsible?

2 Is the idea of free will becoming confounded with social standards? Some people suggest that if an act is antisocial, then that implies a lack of free will and the act requires treatment. Others see such an act as a sign of aberrant free will and believe that the act therefore requires punishment. If I am drunk and sing very loudly, is that the effect of the alcohol? If I am drunk and thump someone, is that free will? Does it matter whether I am morally responsible for singing; does alcohol impact upon free will?

3 Similar questions could be raised about other offences. You are probably aware, for instance, of the concept of 'rape myths': the kinds of ideas and beliefs that people may have that are considered to increase the possibility that they might commit rape – for example, that a woman *wants* to be raped, because being raped is her sexual fantasy; or that a woman who says 'No' is actually just communicating that she needs to be persuaded. If a person genuinely believes that such myths are true, would we consider that to be a mental health issue? (It might be an attitude passed down through the generations in that person's family.) Would we consider that the person's free will is compromised by these beliefs? Or would we take the view that socially agreed standards should always override personal beliefs, and therefore that for an individual to act on personal beliefs rather than according to social standards must necessarily require an exercise of free will?

4 Do these differing views have an impact on people's moral responsibility, and thus the extent to which they might be considered to blame and therefore require punishment?

5 If such a position were considered reasonable and fair, how would we consider offenders who abused children on the basis of a sexual attraction to children? Do you think you have control and can decide to whom you are sexually attracted? Are there elements of your sexual behaviour that are outside the bounds of free will?

Further reading

The interested reader might wish to explore some of these ideas further:

- Chisholm, R. (1967). He could have done otherwise. *Journal of Philosophy* 64: 409–417.
- Fischer, J.M. and Ravizza, M. (1998). *Responsibility and Control: A Theory of Moral Responsibility*. Cambridge: Cambridge University Press.
- Kane, R. (2005). *A Contemporary Introduction to Free Will*. Oxford: Oxford University Press.

In recognition of our greater understanding of the impact of a variety of factors on our behaviour, there is an increasing tendency to use medical evidence in mitigation, for example where there may be evidence of brain damage or epilepsy (Denno, 1988, for an overview; and Raine, 2002). Research (Raine and Yang, 2006) has suggested that damage to particular brain areas involved in moral judgments may be implicated in the behaviour of antisocial individuals and people referred to as 'psychopaths' (Harenski, Harenski, Shane and Kiehl, 2010). Raine and Yang (2006) have suggested that such findings are likely to have a substantial impact on the ways in which the legal system deals with individuals as they imply that free will has been compromised.

Of course, it is not necessarily the case that there needs to be damage in order for behaviour to differ between individuals; small changes in neurotransmitter responsivity in the brain, in the availability of neurotransmitters or differences in cortical development could impact on cognition. This suggests that we can think of behaviour as being influenced at the micro-level, where the paths of particular neurons or the presence or absence of particular molecules could have an important influence on what people do. With that understanding, we might need to reconsider whether individuals are fully responsible for their actions. A case where this was argued, without success, was one concerning Stephen Mobley (Denno, 2006), who was convicted of murder and eventually executed via lethal injection. Although there were possible grounds to suspect that there might have been some form of genetic predisposition towards violence, the court determined that it was an 'unorthodox mitigating defence that attempted to show a possible genetic basis for Mobley's conduct' (Denno, 2006, p. 210). Another case in which medical evidence was used outlines some of the interesting issues of responsibility. In 1999, Jesse Bridgewater was convicted of manslaughter after a car he was driving had hit another car and killed two people. His defence was that he had suffered an epileptic seizure and for that reason was not in control of the car at the time of the accident. If this had been the complete case, then it is likely that Mr Bridgewater would not have been convicted. However, other evidence suggested that he had been warned by his doctor not to drive for a period of time, because of the number of seizures he was having, and that he was also neglecting to take his prescribed medication. Continuing to drive against medical advice and failing to take necessary medication were both acts that *were* under his control (Raspberry, 1999). In law, therefore, it appears that if an individual consciously acts in a way that increases the likelihood that his or her behaviour will be less under voluntary control, then that person is considered still to be responsible for whatever behaviour ensues. This raises an interesting issue, going back to the earlier idea of 'rape myths' and the *Opinion Matters* survey. Of those respondents who believed that the victim should take some of the responsibility if a rape occurred, 64 per cent indicated that they thought that drinking excess alcohol was one such situation in which the victim should take some responsibility; yet many other people would regard this as an example of a '**rape myth**', and would say instead that even if the victim *is* under the influence of alcohol, responsibility for the rape lies entirely with the perpetrator. How do we manage this apparent contradiction: that *perpetrators* are responsible for their behaviour if they have contributed to reducing their own behavioural control, but *victims* are *not* considered responsible for increasing their chances of becoming a victim?

The discussion above is based on the view that we *do* have free will, or at least some degree of free will, rather than our behaviour being wholly determined. The philosophy of free will is complicated as it considers determinism from a number of different perspectives. For example, 'logical determinism' suggests that all statements about the past, present, and future can be reduced to simple *true/false* decisions. However, for the sake of simplicity, and perhaps with greater relevance to the issues under consideration here, we might better consider two other kinds of determinism. *Biological determinism* suggests that our individual biology and environment dictate our behaviour. This is similar to *psychological determinism*, which suggests that it is the processes of cognition – which arise from our neuroanatomy, our neurochemistry and our experiences – that determine beliefs thoughts and personality, and that these in turn determine our behaviour.

These ideas are not new; variations can be found in the work of Galton (1870), who explored the relationship between a person's 'eminence' and his or her family relationships, with the idea that eminence is innate. However, Pratarelli and Mize (2002) have argued that the determinism of biological structure does *not* necessarily imply a determined outcome of cognition, as we are also greatly influenced by many other factors at the time of processing – biology may set limits or potentials for an individual, but it does not 'determine' their future. That is, the genetic element may work probabilistically, resulting in predispositions, but not necessarily the expression of these predispositions. Numerous studies of twins have demonstrated that the environment contributes greatly to the expression of particular behaviours. (For example, it accounts for approximately 45 per cent of the variance in thrill-seeking in twins; see Boomsma, Busjahn and Peltonen, 2002.) Also, determinism assumes that the product of cognition is a single 'result', rather than a set of options and possibilities from which to choose. As Sidgwick (1874) suggested, if one is consciously aware of alternative behaviours being available, then it is difficult to conceive that one cannot choose, for example, the most reasonable course of action, regardless of how often one has previously chosen a different course of action. Indeed, writers such as Bolles (1963) point out that it is just this freedom of choice that was considered to be a defining difference between humans and other animals.

Free will and determinism are the two extremes, and a useful compromise has been suggested by authors such as Baumeister (e.g. 2008), who is following on from the views of Kant (1797). In this compromise position we can think of two systems that regulate behaviour: one that is relatively effortless and automatic, which fits well with ideas of determinism, and a second that requires both effort and energy. As such, the second system is recruited only in response to particular situations. This position perhaps best fits the idea of free will. A flexible position of this sort can account for findings that suggest, intriguingly, that the exercise of self-control or of decision-making both lead to poorer self-control on subsequent tasks (e.g. Vohs *et al.*, 2008). Such a position also fits with a legal system in which accountability is one of the mainstays of sentencing.

Knowledge

As with the above discussion concerning free will, what knowledge consists of and how we accrue it could be thought of as having two extreme positions: the 'empiricist' position and the 'constructivist' position. The *empiricist* position, exemplified by John Locke (who suggested that the fact that children and 'idiots' do not know certain things is proof of there being no such thing as innate knowledge) and David Hume (who argued that our ideas and what links them come directly from the impressions of our senses), suggests in essence that 'knowledge' comes from what we sense around us rather than from what we deduce or infer. This suggests that what we know comes from what we have experienced: the mind is passive, absorbing what is attended to in the environment. This position is in contrast to the idea that some human knowledge is innate. (Originally such knowledge was thought to be the responsibility of God; later theory, known as 'nativism', suggests that such knowledge is genetic, e.g. Pinker, 2002.) The *constructivist* position is that 'meaning' derives from a process whereby we construct our own realities, and that our knowledge is constructed similarly through our interactions with the world (e.g. Chiari and Nuzzo, 1996). Thus there is a focus both on the information that is available and on the possibility of biases within how we actively process it.

From a forensic perspective, these two philosophies, empiricism and constructivism, raise some interesting issues. Both perspectives suggest that there are limits to personal responsibility, as to a large extent we have only *some* control over our experiences and the ways in which information is manipulated in our minds, with the consequence that our understanding of the world and of ourselves is externally mediated. The belief that rape is an appropriate response to certain circumstances may be a product of direct experiences or the peculiarities of a particular individual's construction of meaning and reality. In either case, is that person responsible? It could be argued that knowing that certain environments are risky (i.e. more likely to lead to offending behaviour) might lead the rational person to choose to choose risky environments and to interact with peers who are not offenders. However, this assumes that rationality and free will are linked. Another interesting issue is what forms of intervention might be appropriate to challenge offending behaviour and at what point they might be likely to work. From an empiricist perspective, it is not clear what happens if two experiences contradict one another (e.g. one pro-offending, one anti-offending) and how one is able to make a decision between the two; nor is it clear whether new experiences replace older experiences. A constructivist perspective more easily allows for the impact of psychological input and of other forms of legal intervention, but the input must be appropriate so that it can bring about change and the person's cognitive system must be capable of dealing with the information in the necessary manner.

The future of the profession

We have considered aspects of the profession of forensic psychology as it is, but few professions are static and few professional bodies do not evolve. We now consider how forensic psychology may develop.

Currently, the UK works on the basis of different 'brands' of psychology. After basic undergraduate training, people specialise in their chosen field. The earlier discussion regarding the move towards non-psychologists working in therapeutic roles and the important collaboration between various psychological modalities hints at the idea that the established approach may be outdated.

There has been a move towards a more generic postgraduate approach to psychology, in which individuals become specialised applied psychologists – the underlying competences are the same, but they become specialised through practice. In this way the divisions between clinical, educational and forensic psychologists would likely break down even further, as there would be a greater level of shared experience and knowledge, making it easier to collaborate. Such a change would bring problems, too: there would be greater blurring of boundaries, and thus the potential for changes in job availability and salary structures. Currently, the only funded training courses in the UK are for clinical psychologists, but there is the possibility that this might change with a move towards funding applied psychologists. It is not clear whether this would take the form of funded training courses for other modalities – thereby reducing the funding available for clinical courses – or whether clinical trainees would have to be self-funded or to rely on employers. Although there might seem to be a greater demand for forensic services, the future is thus far uncertain. Since 2011 the NHS has drastically cut costs, and other services constantly have to reduce their provision; the potential knock-on effects for psychological health need to be considered.

As society changes, the definition of 'offending' changes; and this results in changes in the people with whom a forensic psychologist may work. There are some changes that have resulted in important shifts in the profession. Firstly, for example, in the UK it is now many years since homosexuality was considered an offence, so forensic psychologists no longer work with homosexuals solely because of their sexuality. Sexual orientation will be irrelevant in many offences, such as theft and fraud. It may be relevant in other crimes, such as sexual offences, but perhaps not to the extent that one might immediately suppose – after all, to what extent do we consider heterosexuality *per se* as important in sexual offences? Secondly, as laws concerning rape have changed, it is likely that we may see more men being charged with rape who are married to their victims or their current partners. As a final example, with the rise of digital media, forensic psychologists are more likely to work with individuals who have committed offences within this domain, such as internet stalkers, revenge pornographers, those who groom online, and sexual offenders who access and distribute images of children. Changes such as these require that we keep up to date with research and legislation.

A final area of development that will be considered links to that of offence change. The profession must be able to respond to changes in offending, to understand new offences, and to develop ways of intervening both to support victims and to work with offenders to reduce the risk of their reoffending. We may require new models to understand the development and maintenance of offending behaviour, including what the triggers and vulnerabilities might be, and new methods to measure change. The profession is constantly changing, and there will always be new opportunities and challenges.

Chapter summary

This chapter has provided an overview of the process of becoming a forensic psychologist, and has considered the UK qualifications necessary to apply to the HCPC for registration and to become chartered by the BPS. You should ensure that any university courses you plan to follow remain accredited, so that you are able to make progress towards your intended profession.

In order to become qualified, you need to demonstrate competence in four areas, known as the core competences or core roles. The competences are defined by the HCPC and the BPS.

The chapter has looked briefly at the relationship between forensic psychology and other psychological modalities, along with some of the philosophical issues that underlie forensic psychology, including ways in which the profession might develop. In doing so, we hope to have shed light on some of the often hidden complexities of the field, in terms both of joining and of working within it.

All professions provide challenges. It is important to be aware of the most common challenges you may face personally, but also to think about your own circumstances and what opportunities there may be also, and how best to manage these. Forensic psychology also offers a number of important philosophical challenges, including understanding the causes of behaviour and the issue of free will.

Forensic psychology is not a static profession, and the various regulatory bodies are maturing. It is important to remain engaged with developments in the profession, and to be able to think flexibly as these changes impact upon, for example, the clients you see and the interventions that may be most appropriate. It is important that you keep up to date with guidelines published by relevant professional bodies (such as the BPS and the HCPC in the UK, and the APA in the US), as those can change rapidly.

Most importantly, we have emphasised the value of working in collaboration with other professionals for the good of our clients and, more widely, for their families and society.

Further information

Perhaps most important is to keep abreast of the rules and regulations of the bodies that regulate forensic psychology in your country. In the UK, those bodies are the HCPC and the BPS.

For people starting out on the path to becoming qualified as a forensic psychologist, the BPS provide descriptions of accredited courses and the institutions where they are run, and those institutions will give an overview of what the courses include. Not all courses have the same profile, so you would want to ensure that your areas of interest were covered, whether at undergraduate or graduate level.

In addition to reading, it would be useful to speak to people who have recently graduated from particular courses, people on those courses, people who are newly qualified, and long-standing members of the profession. This might be best done through universities or through the specific professional bodies – for example, in the UK the BPS's Division of Forensic Psychology.

Glossary

Actuarial risk assessment instrument (ARAI) One of a set of methods for estimating the likelihood of future offending, in which predictions are made on the basis of a tabulation or dataset showing relationships between independent variables and outcomes on prior occasions, which when analysed yields patterns that can be used for predictive purposes. To date most ARAIs have focused on general reconviction, personal violence, partner violence or sexual reoffending.

Addiction Regular and compelling dependence on use of a substance or repetition of some other experience in order to maintain personal equilibrium, which dominates other aspects of an individual's life and is highly resistant to change.

Actus reus A legal term referring to the behaviour of an individual in committing an offence, defined in statutory terms to clarify the exact nature of any such act.

Admissibility Rules governing the submission of evidence in courts of law, concerning the relevance of the evidence and its likely reliability.

Age-crime curve A graphical representation of the averages from numerous datasets of the relationship between age and likelihood of being convicted of a criminal offence, showing a steep rise during adolescence, a peak in the late teenage years, and a steady decline thereafter.

Aggression The display of anger or apparent intention or preparedness to inflict harm to another, or hypothesised internal state of an individual who acts in that way; usually divided into an *angry, hostile* or *expressive* form and an *instrumental* or *incentive-motivated* form.

Aggressiveness Recurrent readiness to act in an aggressive manner, or a repeated pattern of aggressive behaviour, in a range of different situations.

Anger control training An intervention that combines relaxation with the learning of new self-instructions, applied in provocative situations to reduce levels of angry feelings or behaviour; sometimes called anger management training.

Appeal A formal application for review of a legal decision made by a court, usually submitted to a court in a higher tier in the justice system.

Area under the curve (AUC) A statistic derived from a signal-detection model of quantifying risk which relates proportions of accurate predictions ('hits') to error rates ('false alarms'), providing a measure of the overall predictive validity of a risk assessment instrument.

Assizes These were courts held in the main county towns of England and Wales twice a year, but with a judge from London, that considered serious cases and held trials by jury. They were abolished in 1971 and replaced by Crown Courts.

Automatic thoughts Rapid, almost instantaneous cognitive events or patterns, usually outside awareness, with an important role in the patterning of current behaviour.

Bail A system whereby charged individuals are not held in prisons awaiting their trial. Bail involves conditions, such as having to live at a particular address, surrendering one's passport, or giving a sum of money to the court. If these conditions are breached it is likely that one will be rearrested and then held in prison. Bail is unlikely if you are considered a continuing risk or likely to try to avoid your court hearing.

Base rate The underlying or naturally occurring rate of a selected class of event or reported experience in a population; sometimes called a *prior probability* as it precedes any outside factors or events that might influence it.

Behaviour modification An approach to altering patterns of behaviour based on learning theory, notably on the operant conditioning model of B. F. Skinner and his associates.

Behaviour therapy A psychotherapeutic approach to behavioural and emotional problems employing methods derived from learning theory, based on the classical conditioning model.

Beneficence In practical ethics, a principle of acting in ways that serve to promote the welfare of others.

Biopsychosocial model A conceptual model of human problems based on the proposal that variables from three domains – biological, psychological and social – are all involved in the origins, development and thereby the explanation of them.

Birth cohort study A type of research in which a sample (cohort) usually of children or adolescents is followed prospectively over time and data collected on the subject-matter of interest to facilitate understanding of the temporal and causal patterning of developmental change; a type of *longitudinal study*.

Capital crime In the United States and some other countries, a criminal offence for which the penalty of death can be imposed.

Case formulation An individualised theoretical account, based on information obtained from assessment, of the factors operating in the development and maintenance of a person's psychological distress or dysfunction.

Case law Legal decisions in individual cases that form precedents for guiding subsequent decisions of a similar kind. Sometimes called judge-made law.

Change blindness A recurrently found phenomenon in human attention and perception in which individuals appear not to notice alterations, sometimes even of a quite major kind, in a situation or a pattern of events.

Cholera A bacterial infection that can be fatal through dehydration, and is typically a result of poor hygiene and sanitation. It can be treated and there is a vaccination that is considered to be 85 per cent effective.

Civil law In its broad sense, one of the world's major legal traditions, influencing basic concepts and procedures in the operation of law in a large number of jurisdictions, centred on a codified system of principles as its primary source. In English Law the term also has a more specific meaning as a branch of law concerned with financial, contractual, and other non-criminal legal disputes.

Clever Hans A horse that could accomplish a number of tasks indicative of an ability to understand language. For example, he was able to answer simple mathematical questions and could spell out the name of a painter whose picture he was shown. However, Oscar Pfungst demonstrated that Hans was making use of facial expressions to know when to stop tapping his hoof.

Closing speech The final presentation of a barrister to the jury at the completion of a case and prior to the verdict. Although we might assume that the focus is purely on the factual, barristers take great steps to be engaging and persuasive, so as to sway the jury if they can.

Cluster analysis As used in psychology, a set of statistical methods for examining data on a sample of individuals, to detect the presence of sub-groups of cases within the larger group who have features in common; such as cases that resemble each other with respect to traits, histories, motives, or other variables.

Co-conspirator A person who is involved in the same activity as another person, usually where that activity involves something that is unlawful or might cause harm to others.

Code of conduct A set of rules, derived from basic ethical principles, specifying the expectations of behaviour for the members of a professional association or other formally constituted body, and making explicit the standards for practice.

Coercive family process A cyclical pattern of interaction between parents (or other caregivers) and children first studied at the Oregon Social Learning Center, in which through a sequence of micro-exchanges adults inadvertently increase the likelihood of children acting aggressively in order to achieve goals.

Cognitive-behavioural therapy A form of psychological therapy that emerged from an integration of behavioural and Social Learning Theory with the study of cognitive processes; based on the idea that thinking, emotion, physical sensation, and action are inter-related. There are several varieties of the approach, involving different levels of emphasis on behavioural or cognitive change. It is typically used to address issues with phobias, obsessive compulsive disorders and panic disorders, amongst others, but has also been used with offending behaviour.

Cognitive-Affective Personality System (CAPS) An integrative model of the dynamic relationships between external events, individual appraisals, internal mechanisms, behavioural responses and consequent feedback. The model is used as an explanatory framework in developmental psychology as a means of understanding how stable patterns of person-situation interaction emerge from complex sequences of learning experiences, with reference to both 'normal' and 'dysfunctional' outcomes.

Cognitive distortion Patterns or contents of thinking at odds with expectations or reactions of others with regard to norms for behaviour, particularly in personal relationships. The term is most frequently employed with specific reference to self-serving thoughts or beliefs of offenders concerning sexual activity between adults and children. However, the aetiological significance of such beliefs remains unclear.

Cognitive interview A method of investigative interviewing that draws on psychological research on memory and on strategies for improving information retrieval.

Common law One of the major legal traditions of the world, centred on the accumulation of judicial decisions on individual cases which then become precedents for use in subsequent decisions on similar cases.

Community Treatment Order Under the Mental Health Act in England and Wales, a legal order issued to someone with a diagnosed mental disorder, who has been detained in hospital, permitting them to be discharged and return to the community, but requiring them to comply with specified conditions of supervision and treatment. A similar procedure known as a Compulsory Treatment Order is available in Scotland, and equivalent arrangements are available in many other countries.

Competence In law, an assessment of an accused person's capacity to comprehend, consent to, and cope with the experience of legal procedures, principally with reference to being tried in court but applicable to any phase of the legal process; a term used mainly in the USA.

Compliance A response of acceding to a request, relevant to forensic psychology in circumstances in which during criminal investigations, suspects or witnesses overtly accept or agree to statements with which they do not in fact agree, as a result of pressure or in order to escape from adverse circumstances. This is distinct from *suggestibility* in that individuals are aware of the inconsistency between their beliefs and their actions.

Conflict of interest A situation where one's decision making is possibly compromised because it could be affected by the result. For example, if you were holding interviews and your best friend was a candidate it might be difficult for you to make a decision based entirely on all the candidates' qualities without also considering the future of your friendship.

Consent An agreement voluntarily given by an individual for someone else to carry out an action. In forensic psychology this is of particular significance with reference to sexual offences. Some individuals are not considered capable of consenting to sexual activity. In other cases disputes arise over interpretations of whether consent has been expressed, with more emphasis being given to the need for affirmative and openly communicated consent.

Continuity During development from childhood through adolescence to adulthood, the concept that some features manifest gradual progression in the same generally consistent direction throughout.

Control theory A collection of theories in criminology with the basic premise that individuals will pursue their own self-interest unless constrained either by external social forces (sociological control theory) or internal restraints (psychological control theory).

Correlational research A type of research investigating the degree of linear association between two or more quantitative variables, extensively used in research on variables associated with criminal activity.

Criminal Cases Review Commission Independent organisation in England and Wales established to investigate suspected miscarriages of justice by the criminal courts, in which individuals believe they have been wrongly convicted or sentenced, and to refer cases for appeal where there are considered to be grounds for doing so.

Crime-scene analysis The interpretation of a crime scene, which may be useful in identifying links with other crimes. Proponents of this approach also suggest it is useful for identifying crime-scene motive and offender characteristics.

Criminal responsibility and culpability A fundamental principle in criminal law, that individuals can only be legally culpable for actions for which they were responsible.

Criminogenic needs An alternative term used to describe *dynamic risk factors*, specifying features of individuals that are associated with the risk of involvement in crime but which change over time. They are susceptible to change by direct effort and where that is achieved risks of criminal activity are reduced.

Cross-examination During trials the two sides call witnesses and the process of asking questions of a witness provided by the other side is referred to as cross-examination.

Crossover offending A term used in the study of sexual assault, referring to patterns in which offenders commit offences against victims of both genders, from different age-groups, and in different relationships (contact versus non-contact, inside versus outside families).

Cross-sectional design A type of research in which a sample of interest is studied, and data are collected at a single point in time; sometimes entailing a comparison between two (or more) groups of interest, such as an offending sample and non-offending controls.

Crown Prosecution Service (CPS) The CPS is the principal prosecuting authority in England and Wales. They decide which cases should go to trial, advise on suitable charges, prepare the case and present it at court. Additionally they can provide support to prosecution witnesses and victims.

Curfew A legal order that requires a person is at a specified location during a specified time period. Typically this would be for an individual to be at their home during the night.

Daubert standard In United States courts, a set of criteria applied whereby evidence to be presented in a court of law must be accepted by the relevant scientific community as valid in relation to the subject-matter in question.

Daubert Trilogy A set of three landmark cases (*Daubert, Joiner and Kumho Tire*) that have had a major effect on the requirements set for psychological and other expert evidence in US courts of law.

Deductive profiling Profiling where the basis of the profile is the experience of the profiler(s) rather than through the empirical testing of hypotheses.

Defences Legal arguments which an accused person can forward in seeking to establish that he or she was not fully responsible for the offence with which he or she is charged. Defences may be widely applicable, or only allowed for certain types of offence. Examples are diminished responsibility, duress, necessity, loss of control and automatism.

Desistance Amongst persons who have been involved in offending for some time, a gradual reduction in the frequency or seriousness of, or eventual cessation of, criminal activity.

Deterrence In penology, the doctrine that the costs of committing crimes will have a suppressant effect on the frequency or severity of criminal activity. *General deterrence* refers to the effect of visible punishments on the population as a whole. *Specific deterrence* refers to the impact on the subsequent behaviour of individuals convicted and sentenced. *Restrictive deterrence* refers to an effect in which individuals who do offend limit the seriousness of crimes to avoid more severe penalties.

Diagnosis, diagnostic system In mental healthcare, the identification of the nature and where possible the cause of a mental disorder within a system for classification of such disorders. Two diagnostic systems are currently in widespread use: the World Health Organization's *International Classification of Diseases* (ICD-10), which is currently under revision, and the American Psychiatric Association's *Diagnostic and Statistical Manual of Mental and Behavioural Disorders* (DSM-5).

Differential association An observed pattern in which individuals are influenced by those with whom they most frequently associate, particularly in the process of attitude formation. Thought to be an important process in developing individuals' preparedness to break the law, occurring in groups at all levels of society with the outcome depending on patterns of available opportunities.

Diminished responsibility In law this is one of three defences against murder where it is argued that a person cannot be held fully responsible for their actions (i.e. their criminal liability is reduced). For this defence to succeed there are three conditions; (1) There must be an abnormality of mental functioning, (2) This abnormality of the mind must have been caused by a recognised medical condition, (3) The abnormality of the mind must substantially impair the defendant's mental responsibility. If successful the typical outcome is a charge of 'manslaughter on the grounds of diminished responsibility'.

Discontinuity During development from childhood through adolescence to adulthood, the concept that individuals may show abrupt changes, qualitative shifts, or reversals of direction with reference to some aspects of their development. The changes are sometimes explained using stage-based theories of development.

DNA The acronym for *deoxyribonucleic acid*, which can be understood as the basis of genetic information that determines many aspects of our physical and psychological characteristics. It is present in our cells and for this reason can be found at crime scenes contained in, for example, blood, hair, semen and saliva. As such, if it is possible to extract DNA from a crime scene sample and compare it with a database of DNA from known individuals it is possible, within a good level of accuracy, to identify an individual who would have been present at the crime scene. DNA was first used to solve murders carried out in the UK by Colin Pitchfork.

Dynamic risk factor An aspect of an individual's functioning that is associated with his or her risk of involvement in crime but which fluctuates over time and is also susceptible to change by direct effort. This includes variables such as numbers of criminal associates, antisocial attitudes, impulsiveness, limited social or problem-solving skills, anger or other mood states, and involvement in substance abuse.

Earwitness memory The memory for the recall or identification of heard information, typically voices.

Effect size In a research study, an outcome measure indicating the scale or degree of either (a) the relationship between two variables, or (b) the impact of an intervention. In meta-analysis, statistics of this kind are combined across several studies to produce a *mean effect size*.

Electroconvulsive therapy (ECT) A treatment now given under anaesthetic and muscle relaxants whereby an electric current is passed through the brain in order to treat depression. Currently it is not clear how it works but it is known to change patterns of brain blood flow.

Empathy In psychology, the capacity to experience and resonate with the emotional state of another person, with important consequences for attitudes and behaviour. Used more widely, it can also refer to the ability to project oneself into an 'object of contemplation' such as a work of art.

Equifinality In studies of development, a term referring to the possibility that the same or similar outcomes (e.g. antisocial behaviour) can accrue from disparate origins or risk factors.

Evidence-based practice The proposal, developed originally within medicine, that healthcare interventions should be based upon a methodical scrutiny of the evidence of outcome research regarding which types of intervention (if any) are effective for addressing a given problem; the derivation of principles or guidelines for informing clinical practice on the basis of that evidence.

Evidence Dynamics The process whereby evidence can be altered in some way, intentionally or otherwise. Examples of this include behaviour of an offender after a crime, the actions of animals and insects on a body, the weather, and even the acts of ambulance/medical staff in attempts to resuscitate a victim.

Expert testimony, expert witness Evidence provided to a court by an individual whose education, qualifications, skills or experience, is accepted by a judge as having potential value, enabling the witness to provide a specialised, independent opinion on issues before the court.

Expository Process Model A proposal forwarded by Ownby (1997) concerning the internal structure of psychological reports, that specifies levels of concepts and how they can be be communicated.

Eyewitness memory The memory for the recall or identification of seen information, typically the identity of objects (such as faces, colours of cars) or events.

Fair Trade A social movement aimed at increasing the benefits to the producers of various goods (such as coffee and tea) and to promote sustainable farming.

Fake good A term used to describe a person who is attempting to pretend, either in interview or on psychometric tests, that they are not as troubled as they actually are. Often this is because they fear a negative outcome. The opposite of this is 'fake bad' where a person might pretend that they are experiencing greater troubles than they really are, for example, trauma after a car accident.

FBI The Federal Bureau of Investigation is a national security organisation in the US that works both within law enforcement and intelligence and partners with other law enforcement and intelligence agencies with the mission statement to protect the American people and uphold the Constitution of the United States (see www.fbi.gov).

Fitness to plead The assessed capacity of an individual who is a defendant in a criminal court to understand the nature and implications of the proceedings, and to give instructions to a legal representative; used in all jurisdictions of the UK.

Fitness to practise Evidence of appropriate professional qualifications and performance, demonstrating that an individual possesses the necessary knowledge, skills and personal qualities to work competently as a practitioner psychologist, including adherence to codes of conduct. The requirements of this are specified by professional associations or regulatory bodies and form part of pre-registration training requirements.

Functional analysis Originating in behavioural psychology, a detailed assessment of the patterning of environmental events before and after the occurrences of a behaviour that explain its origins and maintenance, and provided information for enabling individuals to alter it. Drawing at first on analysis of antecedents, behaviour, and consequences (ABC) the approach has been extended to include self-reports of cognition and emotion.

General Theory of Crime (General Control Theory) A highly influential theory in criminology developed by Gottfredson and Hirschi in 1990, locating the principal factor associated with involvement in crime in individual differences in self-control, tracing the origins of those differences to family and parenting experiences in childhood.

Genocide Acts defined in the 1948 UN Convention as being committed with intent to destroy, in whole or in part, a national, ethnic, racial or religious group, including: killing members of the group; causing serious bodily or mental harm to members of the group; deliberately inflicting on the group conditions of life calculated to bring about its physical destruction in whole or in part; imposing measures intended to prevent births within the group; or forcibly transferring children of the group to another group.

Geographical profiling A form of profiling involving analysis of the spatial distribution of locations of offences thought to be connected, which when combined with other evidence from crime scenes and police databases, can enable detectives to narrow the area of search covered by a criminal investigation.

Glazier Someone skilled in working with glass including the removal and cutting of glass, installing window glass, and the use of associated tools.

Group comparison designs A method of research in which two or more groups known to differ on one (independent) variable are investigated with respect to hypothesised differences on other (dependent) variables. This is usually cross-sectional, where data are collected at a single timepoint, but more elaborate designs may involve two or more phases of data collection.

Hate crime Any criminal offence for which there is evidence that it was motivated by hostility towards a group to which the victim(s) belongs; in the majority of cases (though not all) victims are members of minority or marginalised groups.

Heritability (h^2) A statistical estimate for a given population of the relationship between the genotype and the phenotype, that is, the amount of variance in a specified behavioural or psychological characteristic that can be attributed to the influence of genes; usually expressed as a correlation coefficient or as a percentage.

Her Majesty's Pleasure In England and Wales, the mandatory sentence for a person convicted of murder who was aged 10 or over but under 18 at the time of the offence.

Hidden figure of crime In criminology, formerly called the 'dark figure', the gap between officially recorded numbers of crimes and the presumed 'real' number of events that could be defined as crimes but are not reported or recorded.

Hippocratic Oath An oath specific to medical doctors outlining what is considered appropriate behaviour in the care of their patients. The origin is unknown, despite its name, and there is a wide variation in the form that the oath takes, thus some explicitly forbid sexual contact with patients, others do not.

Hospital Order In England and Wales, also known as a Section 37 of the Mental Health Act 1983/2007, a period of hospitalisation without a fixed end date given where a court determines that an individual has a mental disorder that requires assessment or treatment. The hospital can provide treatment without the individual's consent.

Idiographic An approach to knowledge in psychology (and elsewhere) as an attempt to understand experiences or patterns that are found only within a single person, cultural group, language, system of beliefs or other phenomena in a given place at a given time.

Imprisonment for Public Protection (IPP) A type of sentence that existed between 2005 and 2012 in England and Wales that was indeterminate, the offender only being released once a Parole Board considered the person was no longer a risk. This sentence was imposed on people convicted of crimes that did not meet the criteria for a life sentence but who were thought to be dangerous to the public.

Impulsiveness, impulsivity The tendency to act immediately, or quickly, without deliberation or forethought, or consideration of the impact or consequences of one's actions.

Inadmissible evidence Evidence that is not allowed to be presented to whoever is making a decision about the matter of concern. In a criminal case this might be the jury. There are a variety of reasons why evidence might not be admissible. For example, if a judge determines that a piece of evidence is irrelevant or if it not a first-hand account of an event (such second-hand accounts are known as 'hearsay').

Incapacitation In penology, an objective of sentence, designed to control the risk of further offending by removing the offender from crime opportunities, usually through imprisonment but the term may also be used to include curfews, electronic monitoring and other means of restricting individuals' freedom of movement.

Inductive profiling Profiling based on empirical evidence, where research has demonstrated that there is, for example, a link between aspects of a crime and the likely skills and knowledge of the offender, which can then inform the direction of an investigation.

Informed consent Based on the ethical principle of *autonomy*, in order to obtain information from individuals, to provide interventions to them, or to involve them in research, it is essential that they should be able to make voluntary decisions regarding such activities. To do so they should be given clear information about what is being asked of them and why. In psychological as in medical and other research, a formal procedure must be followed for obtaining and recording prospective participants' agreement to proceed.

Interactionism In psychology, an integrative model in which behaviour is understood as a net product of personal and situational factors operating in conjunction.

Investigative psychology The use of psychology to assist criminal investigation by the police, particularly including the study of psychological factors influencing patterns of crime by repeat offenders.

Leading question A question taking a form that suggests a particular answer. For example, if a glass of beer has been stolen a leading question might be, 'did Adrian steal the glass of beer?' whereas a non-leading version would be, 'who stole the glass of beer?'.

Locard's Exchange Principle States that when there is contact between two items, there will be an exchange. Edmond Locard's (1877–1966) idea was that if you touch an object there will be evidence of you having touched the object (perhaps a fingerprint) and evidence that the object was touched by you (perhaps a paint fragment on your finger).

Longitudinal research A type of research design in which a cohort of individuals is followed over an extended period of time and data collected concerning life events, patterns of behaviour or reported experience, and social, psychological, or other variables of interest. See also *birth cohort study*.

Malingering Where an individual is found to be fabricating or exaggerating symptoms of illness or disorder for reasons of personal gain, such as to avoid prosecution, or in the hope of escaping or being made subject to more lenient sanctions.

Mandatory life sentence A life sentence that is given for murder. Strictly speaking it is not a life sentence, there is a minimum sentence imposed (for murder with a knife the starting point is 25 years) and then release is dependent on Parole Board judgments after that minimum has been served. On release the person will be on licence for the rest of his or her life, which means the individual can be recalled if deemed to be a risk.

Manslaughter A partial defence to the charge of murder can reduce the charge to manslaughter. The three partial defences are diminished responsibility, killing as part of a suicide pact, and loss of control. Partial defences are different to complete defences, which include self-defence.

Megan's Law Statutes introduced in the United States from 1994 onwards at both federal and state level, making provision for local communities to be informed of the presence of registered sex offenders living in a neighbourhood, and requiring offenders to keep police informed of changes of address and employment.

Mens rea In law, the mental element of a criminal offence, reflecting an individual's intention to commit a certain act or carelessness as to the consequences of action.

Mental disorder Formally, a term used in psychiatry and related fields to describe an abnormal and dysfunctional mental state, and regarded as such within an individual's culture, that meets specified criteria within a diagnostic system.

Mental health problem A general term for a state of excessive, recurrent continuing distress or dysfunction judged to be outside the range that would typically be expected or attributed to everyday problems in living.

Mental Health Tribunal In England and Wales, a legal body with responsibility for reviewing the detention of individuals in hospital under the Mental Health Act 1983/2007, with powers to discharge them if their case does not meet specified criteria (that he or she suffers from a mental disorder in the meaning of the Act, may be a risk to self or others if discharged, and that there is appropriate medical treatment available in hospital).

Meta-analysis A method of integrating the quantitative findings from a number of basic or primary studies, using statistical analysis to detect trends amongst the results obtained.

Miranda rights In the United States, a set of rights accorded to arrested persons, enabling them to remain silent, to have legal representation, and for steps to be taken to ensure they understand how information they provide may be used. The right to silence exists in many countries but the level of rights information given to arrestees varies considerably.

Miscarriage of justice An instance where an innocent person is convicted of a crime and that conviction is later overturned. In England and Wales it might be possible for the wrongly convicted person to claim compensation. There have been cases where convictions have been overturned after the convicted person has spent a considerable time in prison (27 years in the case of Stephen Downing) or received the death penalty (Derek Bentley).

Misinformation effect A result of using biased or leading questions in interviews, which can influence episodic memory (recall of autobiographical events) by distorting the amount or level of accuracy of the information recalled.

Mock jury In psychological research a mock jury refers to a group of people who are playing the role of a jury in a study concerned with legal processes. This is typically done because research on real juries in real court cases is unlawful. Many studies do not use the same number of people as in a real jury and some do not include jury deliberation. In legal settings a mock jury is used for research by lawyers to examine how their planned arguments and evidence in a case might be understood and perceived by a jury. Here it is acting more like a focus group.

Modelling In Social Learning Theory, a process through which individuals acquire and develop skills or habitual reactions by observing the behaviour of others and wholly or partly imitating or adapting behavioural sequences from it.

Mug shots A slang term for a portrait of a person taken when they have been taken into custody, of the type seen on 'wanted' posters, originating in Europe in the mid-1800s. 'Mug' is slang for 'face'.

Multi-Agency Public Protection Arrangements (MAPPA) A mechanism for assessing and managing the risk of individuals who have been released from prison but are considered to pose a risk of sexual or violent offending. A MAPPA team will include the police, prison and Probation Trust along with other cooperating agencies such as The UK Border Agency, social care and housing.

Multifactorial General term for a causal process where an effect or outcome is the result of different factors acting separately or in combination. In the construction of explanatory models of crime or of mental health problems, this applies to the assumption that in most cases multiple factors are involved in causing them, or are necessary for providing a satisfactory explanation of them.

Multifinality In studies of development, a term which refers to the finding that specific risk factors can be associated with a variety of outcomes.

Multi-modal programme A type of intervention programme with a number of targets of change, each associated with a separate risk factor, including appropriate methods for addressing each.

Necrophilia Also known as a *thanatophilia*, a mental disorder in which person has a sexual attraction to or carries out sexual acts involving corpses.

Neutralisation theory A term used in both criminology and psychology, describing a cognitive event or process in which individuals make statements (to themselves or others) that will counteract or negate unpleasant feelings or other reactions they might have to their own behaviour. *Neutralisation theory* is a model of the maintenance of offending that places emphasis on this process.

Nomothetic An approaching to the accumulation of knowledge in psychology (and elsewhere) as a task centred mainly on discovering patterns that are recurrent across situations, or states of affairs that are replicated across time and place, so allowing the formulation of generalised statements.

Non-maleficence In practical ethics, a principle of acting in ways to ensure no harm is caused to others.

Odds ratio The *odds* of a successful outcome (such as reduction in recidivism) for a given group is defined by the probability that that event will occur, relative to the probability that it will not. The odds ratio is then a statistical expression of the relationship between such odds for experimental and control samples respectively.

Offending behaviour programme A structured sequence of learning opportunities, with the objective of helping to reduce individuals' rates of reoffending, following certain principles and designed to be reproducible on multiple occasions or across multiple sites. Such programmes are usually presented in a printed manual with supporting documentation and requiring training prior to use.

Paedophilia Also known as pedophilic disorder, a type of mental disorder in adults or adolescents aged over 16, characterised by persistent sexual attraction to and sexual interest in prepubescent children.

Paraphilia A term used in psychiatric diagnosis to refer to recurrent and strong sexual arousal to or interest in objects or patterns of activity that are atypical amongst the normative group; sometimes known as sexual *fetishism*.

Parole Release of prisoners from custody on a temporary or long-term basis before the full term of a sentence has expired, in response to good behaviour or evidence of positive change.

PEACE model A model used in investigative interviews, designed to maximise the amount of information gained while observing legal and ethical requirements; the model entails five stages, Preparation and planning, Engagement and explanation, Account, Closure, and Evaluation. The model is authorised and widely used by police forces in England, Wales and Northern Ireland.

Permeable barrier A concept in town planning that considers how easy it is for people to move around their environment. The more permeable a city is the more connected it is. As an example, a river is a barrier to movement, but providing a bridge increases that barrier's permeability, and more bridges increases it further.

Personality disorder In psychiatric diagnosis, a pervasive and enduring configuration of individual experience and behaviour, giving rise to distress, that departs in marked ways from prevailing cultural norms, and is not explicable in terms of other forms of mental disorder. Personality disorder is divided into several types, each defined with reference to specified sets of criteria. There are ongoing disputes concerning the status of definitions in regard to this.

Plea bargaining A discussion and agreement between a defendant (or his/her legal representative) and prosecutor, in which the former agrees to plead guilty, or to do so to a lesser charge than the one initially brought, or to one of several charges: in return for some type of concession, for example that this will be taken into account in sentencing, or that other charges will be dismissed.

Plethysmography A psychophysiological procedure used for assessment of an individual's degree of sexual arousal, by measuring changes in penile circumference or vaginal changes caused by altered blood flow.

Plaintiff The person or group who bring a case to a civil court.

Police and Criminal Evidence Act (PACE) 1984 A framework enacted by an Act of Parliament to provide consistency and balance to the powers of the police whilst also protecting the rights of the individual in England and Wales. It covers such powers as searches, treatment of people in custody, and recording suspect interviews, amongst other issues.

Polygraph A method of measuring arousal thought to result from anxiety under interrogative questioning, considered to be an indicator that the respondent is engaging in deception or dishonesty. Popularly known as a 'lie detector', evidence produced in this way is not acceptable in most court jurisdictions, but is in some American states.

Pre-sentence report A report prepared by a Probation Officer or member of a Youth Offending Team designed to assist the court in making decisions about an offender. The report should include information on the nature and seriousness of the offence and its impact on the victim. Under the Criminal Justice Act 2003 such a report is required before imposition of a custodial sentence.

Primary study, primary analysis Empirical research study that produces data relevant to a scientific investigation; initial analysis of the data collected within it.

Probabilistic A general model of understanding events based on an assumption that they are a complex function of many influences, and also incorporate chance variation. Such a combination makes any specific outcome very difficult to predict. This is sometimes contrasted with a *deterministic* model where outcomes are thought to be predictable and certain. But the general determinist view of the universe (i.e. that events result from a necessary chain of causation) can include the possibility that many specific outcomes are probabilistic in nature.

Profiling A collection of methods of assisting police investigation of serious offences by analysing evidence from the features of an offence or of a crime scene that might indicate possible directions for further investigation, develop hypotheses concerning potential perpetrators (especially across recurrences of events), and enable police to reduce or limit the range of potential suspects.

Programme integrity The extent to which a structured programme adheres to the theoretical model that formed the basis of its design, in terms of the methods of intervention used and the quality and style of delivery of its sessions.

Prosopagnosia Known as 'face blindness' it describes a deficit in the ability to recognise faces. See Bate, S. & Tree, J. (2017). The definition and diagnosis of developmental prosopagnosia. The *Quarterly Journal of Experimental Psychology 70*(2), 193–200.

Protective factor Variables which counter the influence of risk factors and enhance the resilience of those exposed to them; associated with a decreased likelihood of personally or socially undesirable outcomes such as the emergence of criminal offending or a mental health problem.

Psychometric assessment, psychometric test Quantification of variables used in describing and understanding human functioning, resulting in an approach to measurement of a variety of attributes including cognitive abilities, skills, personality, attitudes, or mental states, amongst many others, allowing comparisons to be made between individuals on designated variables.

Public interest In legal terms this is concerned with the best outcome for the public, and may result in an individual being prosecuted in court. Importantly 'public' does not really refer to you and I but society more generally. There are a number of factors that are considered to determine if it is in the public interest one of which is the likely outcome of a prosecution. If it will cost time and money and the likely sentence will be minimal it may be decided that it is not in the public interest (i.e. cost to the taxpayer) to pursue the case.

Punishment In behavioural psychology, an aversive or unpleasant consequence of a behavioural response that reduces the probability of its recurrence. In criminal justice, a set of procedures for conveying society's disapproval of a criminal act and applying sanctions that will induce change in the offender.

Qualitative methods A collection of research methods for in-depth inquiry into individuals' reports of their experiences, their accounts and perceptions of events, or their attribution of meanings in personal interactions, society and culture. Methods include ethnography, grounded theory, thematic analysis, and interpretative phenomenological analysis.

Quarter Sessions Court hearings that were held four times a year in England and Wales. Abolished in 1971 and taken up by the Crown Court.

Quasi-experimental design A type of evaluation research in which two or more groups are compared but they cannot be assumed to be equivalent at outset, as membership of them is assigned on a non-random basis.

Randomised controlled trial (RCT) Research design used in the evaluation of a psychological, medical or other type of intervention in which individuals are allocated to treatment or otherwise on a random basis, so reducing the likelihood that pre-existing differences can account for differences in observed outcomes.

Rape myth A set of stereotypical but widely held erroneous beliefs concerning female and male sexuality, social behaviour and interaction, sexual urges, controllability, and responsibility for action, that serves a facilitating and neutralizing function in relation to male sexual aggression, and influences both interpersonal and legal responses to sexual victimization.

Rape shield laws Legislation to protect victims of rape from being subject to potentially prejudicial questioning, such as their sexual history and previous behaviour.

Rational Choice Theory A highly influential theory of criminal conduct that places emphasis on the process of conscious decision-making by individuals before committing a crime, weighing up the respective advantages and disadvantages from doing so or not doing so. This provides the basis of the view that crime can be controlled by reducing the availability of opportunities, or by increasing the severity of penalties.

Reasonable doubt The standard of proof in the English criminal justice system. If jurors believe, beyond a reasonable doubt, that a defendant committed the offence then s/he should be convicted. Some authors have suggested that beyond a reasonable doubt should be interpreted as a 91 per cent chance that the person did commit the crime.

Reasonable person In law, an artefact, hypothetical or imagined individual who represents the convergence or averaging of a community's views of what would be an appropriate, understandable, and acceptable way to act in a given situation.

Receiver Operating Characteristics (ROC) A statistical concept used to evaluate the accuracy of a prediction or risk assessment method, comparing relative rates of accuracy in predicting alternative outcomes such as the occurrence or non-occurrence of violent acts.

Recidivism Usually taken to refer to repeated involvement in crime or offending behaviour, a person's relapse into criminal activity, typically after they have been previously sanctioned for that activity. This has been defined in specific ways, with reference to self-reported crime, arrests or police contacts, appearances in court, convictions, or in the case of persons with mental disorders, re-admission to hospital.

Reciprocal determinism In Social Learning Theory, the proposal that there is a two-way, bidirectional process of influence between individual and environmental variables.

Rehabilitation In law, one of the objectives of criminal sentencing, focused on promoting an individual's ability to avoid future offending after conviction, through learning to live without resort to crime. In penal and mental health agencies, an approach to providing services that will support that aim, particularly for those who are returning to the community after periods in prison or secure hospital.

Relapse prevention A term derived from research and practice in people with alcohol or other substance abuse problems. It entails a set of self-management and allied methods for enabling individuals who have participated in treatment or training to avoid repetition of the problem behaviour.

Responsivity A design feature that contributes to effectiveness of intervention programmes with offenders. *General responsivity* refers to an overall approach in which activities have clear objectives and structure, and entail active engagement of participants in processes focused on behavioural or attitudinal change. *Specific responsivity* requires taking into account factors that reflect diversity amongst participants in terms of age, gender, ethnicity, language, ability level, or learning style.

Restoration One of the core purposes of sentencing in criminal justice, based on a model in which an individual who has damaged the welfare of another through a criminal offence is invited or authorised to repair the damage, through apology, provision of services or payment of compensation. This is associated with a wider model and set of principles known as *restorative justice*.

Retribution, retributivism In penal philosophy, a conceptual basis for the use of sanctions based on a moral theory in which the advantage gained by an individual who has committed a criminal offence should be rebalanced by depriving him or her of some asset, for example by restriction of liberty. This is the central basis of penology in many jurisdictions throughout the world.

Revictimization Consists of two forms, one in which research has suggested that victims of certain crimes are more likely to be victims of those same crimes again. The second form is where a victim of a crime re-experiences being a victim through, for example, being a witness in court, being interviewed by the police, or through intervention aimed at dealing with trauma.

Risk A measure of the likelihood of an event occurring. In forensic psychology this would typically focus on the likelihood of a person committing crimes or being a victim of a crime. A variety of methods have been used to assess risk including unstructured clinical judgment, structured clinical judgment, and actuarial judgment.

Risk factor An individual or environmental variable which has been shown through empirical research to be associated with greater likelihood of involvement in criminal activity (or other type of problem).

Risk-needs assessment A combined approach to working with offenders, the first stage of which is collecting information concerning the probability of future offending and the factors likely to influence it.

Risk-needs-responsivity principle (RNR) An approach to tertiary prevention, or working with those convicted of criminal offences, used to address offending behaviour and reduce the likelihood of further recidivism. Drawing on basic and evaluation research, the resultant model derives a set of principles for guiding the design and delivery of rehabilitative services in criminal justice settings.

Routine Activity Theory An influential theory in criminology explaining the occurrence of crime in terms of the everyday patterning of behaviour of masses of individuals. This results in combinations of circumstances that produce crime opportunities as a function of there being suitable targets of crime, absence of individuals capable of protecting them, and presence of motivated offenders.

Schema In cognitive and developmental psychology, a hypothesised internal construct, involving a set of relatively enduring relationships between ideas and beliefs, usually outside awareness, through which individuals organise and interpret information about themselves or others; also used as a key concept in some psychological therapies.

Secondary analysis Analysis of an existing dataset, carried out to answer questions not posed in the initial study, or to check for possible errors in previous analyses.

Secure services In the United Kingdom, mental health services for individuals who cannot be managed in other mental health settings due to their risk of harm to self, others, or absconding.

Self-control In criminology, a theory that holds that variations in the likelihood of offending are influenced mainly by individual differences in a psychological construct reflecting the extent to which people can restraint the tendency to act on impulse. In Cognitive Social Learning Theory, the finding that individuals can self-consciously acquire mastery over habitual, automatic modes of thinking or responding that are dysfunctional for themselves or others.

Self-management, Self-regulation An acquired or learned capacity in developing children, usually involving the use of automatic processes and language, in which individual patterns of thoughts, feelings and behaviour become less dependent on the immediate environment.

Self-report survey Any survey where individuals are asked to provide information about themselves. In criminology, the term refers to survey studies in which individuals are asked questions concerning their involvement in criminal acts, whether or not those came to the attention of police or other authorities.

Sentence discount Sentencing guidelines in England and Wales require that courts give consideration to a guilty plea, once the sentence has been decided. For example, if a person pleads guilty as soon as they possibly could it is recommended that their sentence is reduced by one-third. If they do so after the trial has started it is recommended that the reduction be one-tenth.

Sentencing Council In England and Wales, a legal body that formulates guidance for those passing sentence (judges, magistrates) on the appropriate penalties to be imposed for particular types of criminal offence. Originally established as the Sentencing Guidelines Council by the Criminal Justice Act 2003, it was replaced in its present form in 2010.

Sex Offender Register An approach to monitor the behaviour of sexual offenders once released from prison (in some cases, such as the UK, people can be on the register if they are considered to be at risk of offending). Various countries have such a register (UK, USA, Canada, Australia). The application of the register varies by country. In the UK offenders must keep the police informed of data such as address, bank details, foreign travel, amongst other information. Only the US allows the register to be available to the public.

Sexual Offences Prevention Order (SOPO) a list of behaviours and activities that an individual is prohibited from doing on the basis that they are considered a risk of sexual offending, for a fixed period of no less than 5 years or until the order is rescinded. Such behaviours and behaviours may include being in the company of children, using public swimming facilities, being within a certain distance of one's children, for example.

Shame aversion therapy A form of aversion therapy where a positive (but considered deviant) stimulus is paired with an unpleasant sensation. In shame aversion therapy the unpleasant sensation is humiliation. As an example, a person who is aroused by exposing himself (the positive stimulus) does so in a room full of professionals who, in response, laugh, insult his genitalia, and generally demean the person leading to an unpleasant sensation. The idea is that this will reduce the instances of the behaviour as it becomes more strongly associated with a negative outcome.

Situational crime prevention An approach to reducing crime based on an analysis of the places where it occurs and its pattern over time, involving measures to reduce opportunities, strengthen controls, or increase likelihood of being observed.

Social construct, social constructionism In the philosophy of science and in psychology, an approach which asserts that experience of the social world, and thereby understanding of the self, results from a process of interaction and exchange involving the use of language and other symbols. Such a process and its products are viewed as more important than the 'objective' features of the situation.

Social Learning Theory A generalised account of human learning based on behavioural principles, but proposing that a large proportion of learning occurs through indirect experience or observational processes in the interpersonal environment.

Socialisation The totality of experiences of a developing child as he/she interacts with and responds to the behaviour and communications of adult or other caregivers, within a wider familial, social and cultural context, and through which he or she acquires patterns of acting, feeling and thinking that are acceptable in that context.

Standardised mean difference In meta-analysis, a type of statistic that expresses the extent of difference between two groups, commonly used in treatment-outcome research to evaluate relative changes in experimental relative to comparison groups.

Strain Theory In criminology, a theory focusing on the part played by social competition for success and status in contributing to the occurrence of crime.

Structured professional judgment (SPJ) A term denoting a set of risk assessment methods which have in common the use of defined anchors for scoring accompanied by guidelines over professional discretion that can be used at specified points.

Suggestibility Individual differences in the tendency to accept or follow suggestions made by others, found to have a marked influence in some cases where potentially vulnerable individuals are being questioned by police or in other investigative interviews. This entails susceptibility to suggestion or persuasion to the extent that an individual absorbs and believes inaccurate or contrived information.

Summary cases Cases that do not require a jury trial and as such include most offences that are considered 'minor', such as drunk and disorderly and minor criminal damage.

Systematic review A type of research literature review, which involves following a standard set of procedures for locating, synthesising and drawing conclusions from all available studies related to a given research question or testable hypothesis. Systematic review has become a cornerstone of the development of *evidence-based practice*, and sometimes incorporates *meta-analysis*, though whether that is possible or useful depends on the studies found in the review.

Taxometric analysis A set of statistical procedures for examining the distribution pattern of a variable, with particular reference to establishing whether it has a categorical or continuous pattern.

Temperament A collection of patterns or propensities to feel or act in certain ways, evident from shortly after birth onwards, and exhibiting relatively stable differences between individuals. Usually considered to have psychophysiological features, this interacts with socialisation to influence the early development of individuality.

Theory integration Process with criminology, psychology and other social sciences, as an alternative to competitive elimination, in which theoretical concepts from different sources are combined in appropriate ways to construct and test models with greater validity or breadth of reference.

Therapeutic community A specially devised format for delivering therapeutic and social-learning experiences based on the use of everyday group interaction and discussion rather than individual practitioner-led sessions at predetermined intervals. First developed in residential mental health settings, this has since then been extensively used in prisons and community services in criminal justice for individuals with histories of substance misuse, or who have committed serious offences against others.

Therapeutic jurisprudence An approach within law in which legal processes and decisions are studied in terms of their potential therapeutic or anti-therapeutic effects on the individuals involved; representing a combination of ideas from law and behavioural sciences.

Trait A description of how people typically behave that also helps to account for individual differences between them; sometimes used on a purely descriptive level, at other times to denote hypothesised underlying causal patterns that account for relative stability across situations or over time.

Transactional model An integrative theory of human development which emphasises the multi-level interplay of different sets of factors related to parents or other caregivers, the child or adolescent, environmental and situational variables.

Transcript Typically a verbatim, written form of an interview or a conversation, which may be used in research or in evidence.

Transvestism Considered to be a paraphilia this is a desire to wear the clothes of another gender. It is only identified as a disorder if the person who is experiencing it is distressed, impaired, or causes harm to others because of it.

Treatment-outcome evaluation A type of research study designed to test the effectiveness of an intervention in producing its planned outcome effects. In its simplest form this involves a comparison between experimental ('treatment') and comparison ('no treatment') groups in either randomised or quasi-experimental designs.

Underdetermination of theory A principle in the philosophy of science referring to circumstances in which the available data on a given question are compatible with two or more theoretical accounts, with insufficient information to choose between them.

Victim Personal Statements (VPS) Statements that may be presented in court allowing a victim or appropriate relative to describe the wider personal implications for having been a victim of a crime (such as psychological, economic) which they believe should be taken into account before sentencing. In England and Wales the person making the statement can be cross-examined.

Victim survey A method of collecting data on the volume and patterning of crime by interviewing a sample of members of the public and asking about incidents of victimisation. Self-report studies of this kind are conducted in a number of countries and there have also been international surveys. Data are usually compared with police-recorded statistics in order to obtain an estimate of the 'true' level of crime in a society.

Video-links Where there are concerns about the ability of a witness to give their evidence (due to, for example, stress, fear of intimidation, being under the age of 18) that witness may be allowed to provide their evidence over a live video-link rather than appearing in person in the court.

Volume crime A loose term often used to refer to the bulk of less serious criminal activity recorded by the police, consisting of criminal damage, acquisitive offences including theft, burglary and robbery, and assaults, which together typically constitute in the region of two-thirds of recorded offences.

Weapon-focus effect A pattern in victim or witness accounts of offences where a weapon was present, in which attention centred on the weapon is associated with poorer recall of other details of the situation or of the events that occurred.

Bibliography

A

Abbey, A. (2011). Alcohol's role in sexual violence perpetration: Theoretical explanations, existing evidence and future directions. *Drug and Alcohol Review*, 30, 481–489.

Abel, G. G., Becker, J. V. & Cunningham-Rathner, J. (1984). Complications, consent and cognitions in sex between children and adults. *International Journal of Law and Psychiatry*, 7, 89–103.

Abel, G. G., Becker, J. V., Cunningham-Rathner, J., Mittelman, M. & Rouleau, J.-L. (1988). Multiple paraphilic diagnoses among sex offenders. *Bulletin of the American Academy of Psychiatry and Law*, 16, 153–168.

Abel, G. G., Gore, D. K., Holland, C. L., Camp, N., Becker, J. V. & Rathner, J. (1989). The measurement of the cognitive distortions of child molesters. *Annals of Sex Research*, 2, 135–153.

Abel, G. G., Jordan, A., Hand, C. G., Holland, L. A. & Phipps, A. (2001). Classification models of child molesters utilizing the Abel Assessment for Sexual Interest. *Child Abuse and Neglect*, 25, 703–718.

Abramsky, T., Watts, C. H., García-Moreno, C., Devries, K., Kiss, L., Ellsberg, M., Henrica, A. F. M. & Heise, L. (2011). What factors are associated with recent intimate partner violence? Findings from the WHO multi-country study on women's health and domestic violence. *BMC Public Health*, 11, 109. http://www.biomedcentral.com/1471-2458/11/109

Academy for Critical Incident Analysis (2012). *Shooting incidents in educational settings*. New York, NY: John Jay College of Criminal Justice. http://archive.aciajj.org/the-acia-archive/datasets-available-for-analysis/shooting-incidents-in-educational-settings/

Ackerman, M. J. (2006). Forensic report writing. *Journal of Clinical Psychology*, 62, 59–72.

Adams, D. (1982). *Life, the universe and everything*. London: Pan Books.

Adams, D. (2007). *Why Do They Kill? Men Who Murder Their Intimate Partners*. Nashville, TN: Vanderbilt University Press.

Adams, H. E., Wright, L. W. & Lohr, B. A. (1996). Is homophobia associated with homosexual arousal? *Journal of Abnormal Psychology*, 105, 440-445.

Adams, K. (2003). The effectiveness of juvenile curfews at crime prevention. *Annals of the American Academy of Political and Social Science*, 587, 136–159.

Aebi, M. F., Akdeniz, G., Barclay, G., Campistol, C., Caneppele, S., Gruszczyńska, B., Harrendorf, S., Heiskanen, M., Hysi, V., Jehle, J.-M., Jokinen, A., Kensey, A., Killias, M., Lewis, C. G., Savona, E., Smit, P. & Þórisdóttir, R. (2014). *European Sourcebook of Crime and Criminal Justice Statistics*. 5th edition. Helsinki: European Institute for Crime Prevention and Control (HEUNI).

Agnew, R. (1992). Foundation for a General Strain Theory of crime and delinquency. *Criminology*, 30, 47–87.

Agnew, R. (2006a). General Strain Theory: current status and directions for research. In F. T. Cullen, J. P. Wright & K. R. Blevins (eds.), *Taking Stock: The Status of Criminological Theory*. Advances in Criminological Theory, Volume 15. pp. 101–123. New Brunswick, NJ: Transaction Publishers.

Agnew, R. (2006b). Storylines as a neglected cause of crime. *Journal of Research in Crime and Delinquency*, 43, 119–147.

Agnew, R. (2007). *Pressured Into Crime: An Overview of General Strain Theory*. New York, NY: Oxford University Press.

Agnew, R. & White, H. R. (1992). An empirical test of General Strain Theory. *Criminology*, 30, 475–500.

Akers, R. J. & Jensen, G. F. (eds.) (2006). The empirical status of social learning theory of crime and deviance: the past, present, and future. In F. T. Cullen, J. P. Wright & K. R. Blevins (eds.), *Taking Stock: The Status of Criminological Theory*. Advances in Criminological Theory, Volume 15. pp. 37–76. New Brunswick, NJ: Transaction Publishers.

Akers, R. L., Krohn, M. D., Lanza-Kaduce, L. & Radosevich, M. (1979). A social learning theory of deviant behavior. *American Sociological Review*, 44, 635–655.

Alalehto, T. (2003). Economic crime: Does personality matter? *International Journal of Offender*

Therapy and Comparative Criminology, 47, 335–355.

Albright, J. M. (2008). Sex in America online: An exploration of sex, marital status, and sexual identity in internet sex seeking and its impacts. *Journal of Sex Research*, 45, 175–186.

Albright, J. M. (2009). Erratum. *Journal of Sex Research*, 46, 381.

Alexander, M. A. (1999). Sexual offender treatment efficacy revisited. *Sexual Abuse: Journal of Research and Treatment*, 11, 101–116.

Alhabib, S., Nur, U. & Jones, R. (2010). Domestic violence against women: Systematic review of prevalence studies. *Journal of Family Violence*, 25, 369–382.

Ali, A., Hall, I. Blickwedel, J. & Hassiotis, A. (2015). Behavioural and cognitive-behavioural interventions for outwardly-directed aggressive behaviour in people with intellectual disabilities. *Cochrane Database of Systematic Reviews*, Issue 4, Art. No.: CD003406.

Ali, P. A. & Naylor, P. B. (2013a). Intimate partner violence: A narrative review of the biological and psychological explanations for its causation. *Aggression and Violent Behavior*, 18, 373–382.

Ali, P. A. & Naylor, P. B. (2013b). Intimate partner violence: A narrative review of the feminist, social and ecological explanations for its causation. *Aggression and Violent Behavior*, 18, 611–619.

Alison, L., Bennell, C., Mokros, A., and Ormerod, D. (2002). The personality paradox in offender profiling: a theoretical review of the processes involved in deriving background characteristics from crime scene actions. *Psychology, Public Policy, and Law*, 8, 115–135.

Allen, G. & Dempsey, N. (2016). *Prison Population Statistics*. Briefing Paper. London: House of Commons Library.

Allen, G. & Watson, C. (2017). *UK Prison Population Statistics*. Briefing Paper Number SN/SG/04334. London: House of Commons Library.

Allen, L. C., MacKenzie, D. L. & Hickman, L. J. (2001). The effectiveness of cognitive-behavioral treatment for adult offenders: A methodological, quality-based review. *International Journal of Offender Therapy and Comparative Criminology*, 45, 498–514.

Alleyne, E., Gannon, T. A., Ó Ciardha, C. & Wood, J. L. (2014). Community males show multiple-perpetrator rape proclivity: Development and preliminary validation of an interest scale. *Sexual Abuse: A Journal of Research and Treatment*, 26, 82–104.

Alschuler, A. W. (2003). The changing purposes of criminal punishment: A retrospective on the past century and some thoughts about the next. *The University of Chicago Law Review*, 70, 1–22.

Altheimer, I. (2013a). Cultural processes and homicide across nations. *International Journal of Offender Therapy and Comparative Criminology*, 57, 842–863.

Altheimer, I. (2013b). Herding and homicide across nations. *Homicide Studies*, 17, 27–58.

Ambos, K. (2009). What does 'intent to destroy' in genocide mean? *International Review of the Red Cross*, 91, 833–858.

American Educational Research Association, American Psychological Association, & National Council of Measurement in Education (1999). *Standards for educational and psychological testing*. Washington, DC: AERA.

American Psychiatric Association (2013). *Diagnostic and Statistical Manual of Mental and Behavioral Disorders* DSM-5. Washington, DC: American Psychiatric Association.

American Psychological Association (2012). Ethical principles of psychologists and code of conduct. http://www.apa.org/ethics/code/index.aspx

American Psychological Association Ethics Committee. (2002). Report of the Ethics Committee. *American Psychologist, 57*, 646–653.

Anastasi, J. S. & Rhodes, M. G. (2006). Evidence for an Own-Age Bias in Face Recognition. *North American Journal of Psychology*, 8, 237–252.

Anckärsater, H., Radovic, S., Svennerlind, C., Höglund, P. & Radovic, F. (2009). Mental disorder is a cause of crime: The cornerstone of forensic psychiatry. *International Journal of Law and Psychiatry*, 32, 342–347.

Anderson, C. A. (1989). Temperature and aggression: Ubiquitous effects of heat on occurrence of human violence. *Psychological Bulletin*, 106, 74–96.

Anderson, C. A. (2001). Heat and violence. *Current Directions in Psychological Science*, 10, 33–38.

Anderson, C. A. & Bushman, B. J. (2002). Human aggression. *Annual Review of Psychology*, 53, 27–51.

Anderson, C. A. & Carnagey, N. L. (2004). Violent evil and the General Aggression Model. In A. Miller (ed.), *The Social Psychology of Good and Evil*. pp. 168–192. New York, NY: Guilford.

Anderson, N., Schlueter, J. E., Carlson, J. F. & Geisinger, K. F. (2016). *Tests in Print IX: An Index to Tests, Test Reviews, and the Literature on Specific Tests*. Lincoln, NE: University of Nebraska Press.

Anderson, R. C. & Pichert, J. W. (1978). Recall of previously unrecallable information following a shift in perspective. *Journal of Verbal Learning and Verbal Behaviour*, 17, 1–12.

Andrews, D. A. (2001). Principles of effective correctional programs. In L. L. Motiuk & R. C. Serin (Eds.), *Compendium 2000 on Effective Correctional Programming*. Ottawa: Correctional Service Canada.

Andrews, D. A. (2011). The impact of nonprogrammatic factors on criminal-justice interventions. *Legal and Criminological Psychology*, 16, 1–23.

Andrews, D. A., & Bonta, J. (2010). *The psychology of criminal conduct*. 5th edition. Cincinnati, OH: Anderson Publishing.

Andrews, D.A., Bonta, J. & Hoge, R.D. (1990). Classification for effective rehabilitation: rediscovering psychology. *Criminal Justice and Behavior, 17*, 19–52.

Andrews, D. A., Bonta, J. & Wormith, J. S. (2006). The recent past and near future of risk and/ or need assessment. *Crime & Delinquency*, 52, 7–27.

Andrews, D. A., & Dowden, C. (2005). Managing correctional treatment for reduced recidivism: A meta-analytic review of programme integrity. *Legal and Criminological Psychology*, 10, 173–187.

Andrews, D. A. & Dowden, C. (2006). Risk principles of case classification in correctional treatment: a meta-analytic investigation. *International Journal of Offender Therapy and Comparative Criminology*, 50, 88–100.

Andrews, D. A., Zinger, I., Hoge, R. D., Bonta, J., Gendreau, P. & Cullen, F. T. (1990). Does correctional treatment work? A clinically relevant and psychologically informed meta-analysis. *Criminology*, 28, 369–404.

Andrews, G., Slade, T. & Peters, L. (1999). Classification in psychiatry: ICD-10 versus DSM-IV. *British Journal of Psychiatry*, 174, 3–5.

Anglemeyer, A., Horvath, T. & Rutherford, G. (2014). The accessibility of firearms and risk for suicide and homicide victimization among household members: A systematic review and meta-analysis. *Annals of Internal Medicine*, 160, 101–110.

Appleton, C. & Grøver, B. (2007). The pros and cons of life without parole. *British Journal of Criminology*, 47, 597–615.

Ardley, J. (2005). Preparation for the Release of Life Sentenced Prisoners at HM Prison Sudbury. *The Internet Journal of Criminology*. http://www.internetjournalofcriminology.com/Jenny%20Ardley%20-%20HM%20Prison%20Sudbury.pdf

Arnold, L., Gozna, L. & Brown, J. (2007). *Observed strategy use during police-suspect interviews*. Paper presented at the British Psychological Society Forensic Psychology Conference, York 23–25 July.

Arrigo, B. A. & Shipley, S. (2001). The confusion over psychopathy (I): Historical considerations. *International Journal of Offender Therapy and Comparative Criminology*, 45, 325–344.

Arson Prevention Forum (2014). *Arson: a call to action. A 'State of the Nation' report*. Arson Prevention Forum.

Asch, S. E. (1956). Studies of independence and conformity: I. A minority of one against a unanimous majority. *Psychological Monographs: General and Applied*, 70, 1–70.

Ashby, J. S. & Webley, P. (2008). 'But everyone else is doing it': a closer look at the occupational taxpaying culture of one business sector. *Journal of Community & Applied Social Psychology*, 18, 194–210.

Ashworth, A. (2015) *Sentencing and Criminal Justice*. 6th edition. Cambridge: Cambridge University Press.

Ashworth, A. & Redmayne, M. (2010). *The Criminal Process*. 4th edition. Oxford: Oxford University Press.

Ashworth, A. & Roberts, J. (2012). Sentencing: theory, principle, and practice. In M. Maguire, R. M. Morgan & R. Reiner (eds.), *The Oxford Handbook of Criminology*. 5th edition. pp. 866-894. Oxford: Oxford University Press.

Assadi, S. M., Noroozian, M., Pakravannejad, M., Yahyazadeh, O., Aghayan, S., Shariat, S. V. & Fazel, S. (2006). Psychiatric morbidity among sentenced prisoners: prevalence study in Iran. *British Journal of Psychiatry*, 188, 159–164.

Association for the Treatment of Sexual Abusers (ATSA) (2012). *Pharmacological Interventions with Adult Male Sexual Offenders*. Beaverton, OR: ATSA. http://www.atsa.com/pdfs/PharmacologicalInterventionsAdultMaleSexualOffenders.pdf

Association of Chief Police Officers of England, Wales and Northern Ireland (2001). *ACPO Investigation of Volume Crime Manual*. ACPO Crime Committee. http://www.nga.org/files/live/sites/NGA/files/pdf/0903DNAAPCOMANUAL.PDF

Athens, L. (1997). *Violent Criminal Acts and Actors Revisited*. Urbana and Chicago, IL: University of Illinois Press.

Avalon Project (2008). *The Code of Hammurabi*. Lillian Goldman Law Library, Yale University. http://avalon.law.yale.edu/subject_menus/hammenu.asp

Avidan, G., Tanzer, M., Hadj-Bouziane, F., Liu, N., Ungerleider, L. G. & Behrmann, M. (2013). Selective dissociation between core and extended regions of the face processing network in congenital prosopagnosia. *Cerebral Cortex*, first published online January 31, 2013. Doi:10.1093/cercor/bht007.

Axelrod, S. & Apsche, J. (eds.) (1983). *The Effects of Punishment on Human Behavior*. New York, NY: Academic Press.

Aylwin, A. S., Clelland, S. R., Kirkby, L. Reddon, J. R., Studer, L. H. & Johnston, J. (2000). Sexual offense severity and victim gender preference: A comparison of adolescent and adult sex offenders. *International Journal of Law and Psychiatry*, 23, 113–124.

B

Baars, B. J. & Gage, N. M. (2010). *Cognition, Brain and Consciousness: Introduction to Cognitive Neuroscience*. 2nd edition. Bulrington, MA: Academic Press.

Babchishin, K. M., Hanson, R. K. & Hermann, C. A. (2011). The characteristics of online sex offenders: A meta-analysis. *Sexual Abuse: A Journal of Research and Treatment*, 23, 92–123.

Babchishin, K. M., Hanson, R. K. & VanZuylen, H. (2015). Online child pornography offenders are different: A meta-analysis of the characteristics of online and offline sex offenders against children. *Archives of Sexual Behavior*, 44, 45–66.

Babcock, J. C., Green, C. E. & Robie, C. (2004). Does batterers' treatment work? A meta-analytic review of domestic violence treatment. *Clinical Psychology Review*, 23, 1023–1053.

Babiak, P., Neumann, C. S. Hare, R. D. (2010). Corporate psychopathy: Talking the walk. *Behavioral Sciences and the Law*, 28, 174–193.

Bachman, R. & Meloy, M. L. (2008). Epidemiology of violence against the elderly: Implications for primary and secondary prevention. *Journal of Contemporary Criminal Justice*, 24, 186–197.

Bäckman, O. & Nilsson, A. (2011). Pathways to social exclusion – a life-course study. *European Sociological Review*, 27, 107–123.

Badenes-Ribera, L., Frias-Navarro, D., Bonilla-Campos, A., Pons-Salvador, G. & Monterde-i-Bort, H. (2015). Intimate partner violence in self-identified lesbians: a meta-analysis of its prevalence. *Sexuality Research and Social Policy*, 12, 47–59.

Bailey, J. & MacCulloch, M. (1992a). Characteristics of 112 cases discharged directly to the community from a new special hospital and some comparisons of performance. *Journal of Forensic Psychiatry*, 3, 91–112.

Bailey, J. & MacCulloch, M. (1992b). Patterns of reconviction in patients discharged directly to the community from a special hospital: Implications for aftercare. *Journal of Forensic Psychiatry*, 3, 445–461.

Bain, S. A. & Baxter, J. S. (2000). Interrogative suggestibility: the role of interviewer behaviour. *Legal and Criminological Psychology*, 5, 123–133.

Baker, L. A., Jacobson, K. C., Raine, A., Lozano, D. I. & Bezdjian, S. (2007). Genetic and environmental bases of childhood antisocial behaviour: a multi-informant twin study. *Journal of Abnormal Psychology*, 116, 219–235.

Baker, L. A., Raine, A., Liu, J. & Jacobson, K. C. (2008). Differential genetic and environmental influences on reactive and proactive aggression in children. *Journal of Abnormal Child Psychology*, 36, 1265–1278.

Baldwin, J. (1993). Police interview techniques: Establishing truth of proof. *British Journal of Criminology*, 33, 325–352.

Baldwin, J., Bottoms, A. E. & Walker, M. A. (1976). *The Urban Criminal: A Study in Sheffield*. London: Tavistock.

Baller, R. D., Zevenbergen, M. P. & Messner, S. F. (2009). The heritage of herding and Southern homicide: examining the ecological foundations of the code of honor thesis. *Journal of Research in Crime and Delinquency*, 46, 275–300.

Bandura, A. (1977). *Social Learning Theory*. New York, NY: General Learning Press.

Bandura, A. (1990). Selective activation and disengagement of moral control. *Journal of Social Issues*, 46, 27–46.

Bandura, A. (1997). *Self-efficacy: The Exercise of Control*. New York, NY: W.H. Freeman.

Bandura, A. (2001). Social cognitive theory: an agentic perspective. *Annual Review of Psychology*, 52, 1–26.

Bangalore, S. & Messerli, F. H. (2013). Gun ownership and firearm-related deaths. *American Journal of Medicine*, 126, 873–876.

Banks, L., Crandall, C., Sklar, D. & Bauer, M. (2008). A comparison of intimate partner homicide to intimate partner homicide-suicide: One hundred and twenty-four New Mexico cases. *Violence Against Women*, 14, 1065–1078.

Barak, G. (ed.) (1998). *Integrative Criminology*. Aldershot: Ashgate.

Barak, G. (2012). *Theft of a Nation: Wall Street Looting and Federal Regulatory Colluding*. Lanham, MD: Rowman & Littlefield.

Barak, G. (ed.) (2015). *The Routledge International Handbook of the Crimes of the Powerful*. (London and New York: Routledge).

Barbaree, H. E., Blanchard, R. & Langton, C. M. (2003). The development of sexual aggression through the lifespan: The effect of age on sexual arousal and recidivism among sex offenders. *Annals of the New York Academy of Sciences*, 989, 59–71.

Barbaree, H. E., Marshall, W. L. & Lanthier, R. D. (1979). Deviant sexual arousal in rapists. *Behaviour Research and Therapy*, 17, 215–222.

Barbaree, H. E., Seto, M. C., Serin, R. C., Amos, N. L. & Preston, D. L. (1994). Comparisons between sexual and nonsexual rapist subtypes: Sexual arousal to rape, offense precursors, and offense characteristics. *Criminal Justice and Behavior*, 21, 95–114,

Barber, C. W., Azrael, D., Hemenway, D., Olson, L. M., Nie, C., Schaechter, J. & Walsh, S. (2008). Suicides and suicide attempts following homicide: Victim-suspect relationship, weapon type, and presence of antidepressants. *Homicide Studies*, 12, 285–279.

Barelds, D. P. H. & Dijkstra, P. (2005). Reactive, anxious and possessive forms of jealousy and their relation to relationship quality among heterosexuals and homosexuals. *Journal of Homosexuality*, 51, 183–198.

Barker, E. T. & McLaughlin, A. J. (1977). The total encounter capsule. *Canadian Psychiatric Association Journal*, 22, 355–360.

Barlow, J. & Kirby, N. (1991). Residential satisfaction of persons with intellectual disability living in an institution or in the community. *Australia and New Zealand Journal of Developmental Disabilities*, 17, 7–23.

Barner, J. R. & Carney, M. M. (2011). Interventions for intimate partner violence: A historical review. *Journal of Family Violence*, 26, 235–244.

Barnett, J. E., Lazarus, A. A., Vasquez, M. J. T., Moorehead-Slaughter, O. & Johnson, W. B. (2007). Boundary issues and multiple relationships: Fantasy and reality. *Professional Psychology: Research and Practice*, 38, 401–410.

Barnett, O. W., Miller-Perrin, C. L. & Perrin, R. D. (2011). *Family Violence Across the Lifespan: An Introduction*. 3rd edition. Thousand Oaks, CA: Sage.

Barnoux, M. & Gannon, T. A. (2014). A new conceptual framework for revenge firesetting. *Psychology, Crime & Law*, 20, 497–513.

Barnoux, M., Gannon, T. A. & Ó Ciardha, C. (2015). A descriptive model of the offence chain for imprisoned adult male firesetters (descriptive model of adult male firesetting). *Legal and Criminological Psychology*, 20, 48–67.

Barnwell, S. S., Borders, A. & Earleywine, M. (2006). Alcohol-aggression expectancies and dispositional aggression moderate the relationship between alcohol consumption and alcohol-related violence. *Aggressive Behavior*, 32, 517–527.

Baron, L., Straus, M. A. & Jaffee, D. (1988). Legitimate violence, violent attitudes, and rape: a test of the Cultural Spillover Theory. In R. A. Prentky & V. L. Quinsey (eds.) *Human Sexual Aggression: Current Perspectives. Annals of the New York Academy of Sciences*, 528, 79–110.

Barratt, E. S. & Slaughter, L. (1998). Defining, measuring and predicting impulsive aggression: A heuristic model. *Behavioral Sciences and the Law*, 16, 285–302.

Barratt, E. S., Stanford, M. S., Dodwy, L., Liebman, M. J. & Kent, T. A. (1999). Impulsive and premeditated aggression: a factor analysis of self-reported acts. *Psychiatry Research*, 86, 163–173.

Barriga, A. Q., Hawkins, M. A. & Camelia, C. R. T. (2008). Specificity of cognitive distortions to antisocial behaviours. *Criminal Behaviour and Mental Health*, 18, 104–116.

Barsky, A. E. (2012). *Clinicians in Court: A Guide to Subpoenas, Depositions, Testifying, & Everything Else You May Need to Know*. New York, NY: Guilford Press.

Bartholomew, K., Regan, K. V., Oram, D. & White, M. A. (2008). Correlates of partner abuse in male same-sex relationships. *Violence and Victims*, 23, 344–360.

Bartholow, B. D., Anderson, C. A., Carnagey, N. L. & Benjamin, A. J. (2005). Interactive effects of life experience and situational cues on aggression: The weapons priming effect in hunters and nonhunters. *Journal of Experimental Social Psychology*, 41, 48–60.

Bartlett, A. & McGauley, G. (eds.) (2009). *Forensic Mental Health: Concepts, Systems and Practice*. Oxford: Oxford University Press.

Bartlett, F. C. (1932). *Remembering: A study in experimental and social psychology*. London: Cambridge University Press.

Bartol, C. R. & Bartol, A. M. (2006). History of forensic psychology. In I. B. Weiner & A. K. Hess (eds.), *Handbook of Forensic Psychology*. 3rd edition. pp. 3–27. Hoboken, NJ: Wiley.

Bartol, C. R. & Bartol, A. M. (2014). *Introduction to Forensic Psychology: Research and Application*. 4th edition. Thousand Oaks, CA: Sage.

Bartol, C. R. & Freeman, N. J. (2005). History of the American Association for Correctional Psychology. *Criminal Justice and Behavior*, 32, 123–142.

Baskin-Sommers, A. R. & Newman, J. P. (2012). Cognition-emotion interactions in psychopathy: implications for theory and practice. In H. Häkkänen-Nyholm & J.-O. Nyholm (eds.), *Psychopathy and Law: A Practitioner's Guide*. pp. 79–97. Chichester: Wiley-Blackwell.

Bates, E. A., Graham-Kevan, N. & Archer, J. (2014). Testing predictions from the male control theory of men's partner violence. *Aggressive Behavior*, 40, 42–55.

Baumeister, R. F. (2008). Free will in scientific psychology. *Perspectives on Psychological Science,* 3, 14–19.

Bäuml, K-H. & Kuhbandner, C. (2007). Remembering can cause forgetting – but not in negative moods. *Psychological Science*, 18, 111–115.

Baura, G. D. (2006). *Engineering Ethics: An Industrial Perspective*. Burlington, MA: Elsevier Science.

Baxter, D. J., Barbaree, H. E. & Marshall, W. L. (1986). Sexual responses to consenting and forced sex in a large sample of rapists and nonrapists. *Behaviour Research and Therapy*, 24, 513–520.

Bazzett, T. J. (2008). *An Introduction to Behavior Genetics*. Sunderland, MA: Sinauer Associates.

Beardsley, N. L. & Beech, A. R. (2013). Applying the violent extremist risk assessment (VERA) to a sample of terrorist case studies. *Journal of Aggression, Conflict and Peace Research*, 5, 4–15.

Beauregard E. & Lieb, R. (2011). Sex offenders and sex offender policy. In J. Q. Wilson & J. Petersilia (eds.), *Crime and Public Policy*. pp. 345–367. New York, NY: Oxford University Press.

Beaver, K. M., Wright, J. P., DeLisi, M. & Vaughn, M. G. (2008). Genetic influences on the stability of low self-control: results from a longitudinal sample of twins. *Journal of Criminal Justice*, 36, 478–485.

Becker, G. S. (1968). Crime and punishment: An economic approach. *Journal of Political Economy*, 76, 169–217.

Beeble, M. L., Bybee, D. & Sullivan C. M. (2007). Abusive men's use of children to control their partners and ex-partners. *European Psychologist*, 12, 54–61.

Beech, A. R., Craig, L. A. & Browne, K. D. (eds.) (2009). *Assessment and Treatment of Sex Offenders: A Handbook*. Chichester: Wiley-Blackwell.

Beech, A. R., Elliott, I. A., Birgden, A. & Findlater, D. (2008). The Internet and child sexual offending: A criminological review. *Aggression and Violent Behavior*, 13, 216–228.

Beech, A. R., Fisher, D. D. & Thornton, D. (2003). Risk assessment of sex offenders. *Professional Psychology: Research and Practice,* 34, 339–352.

Beech, A. R., Friendship, C., Erikson, M. & Hanson, R. K. (2002). The relationship between static and dynamic risk factors and reconviction in a sample of UK child abusers. *Sexual Abuse: A Journal of Research and Treatment,* 14, 155–167.

Beech, A. R. & Ward, T. (2004). The integration of etiology and risk in sexual offenders: a theoretical framework. *Aggression and Violent Behavior,* 10, 31–63.

Beeghley, L. (2003). *Homicide: A Sociological Explanation*. Lanham, MD: Rowman & Littlefield.

Beesley, F. & McGuire, J. (2009). Gender-role identity and hypermasculinity in violent offending. *Psychology, Crime & Law*, 15, 251–268.

Begany, J. J. & Milburn, M. A. (2002). Psychological predictors of sexual harassment: Authoritarianism, hostile sexism and rape myths. *Psychology of Men & Masculinity*, 3, 119–126.

Bègue, L., Subra, B., Arvers, P., Muller, D., Bricout, V. & Zorman, M. (2009). A message in a bottle: Extrapharmacological effects of alcohol on aggression. *Journal of Experimental Social Psychology*, 45, 137–142.

Behrmann, M., Avidan, G., Thomas, C. & Humphreys, K. (2009). Congenital and acquired prosopagnosia: Flip sides of the same coin? *Perceptual Expertise*, 31, 167–197.

Belknap, J., Larson, D.-L., Abrams, M. L., Garcia, C. & Anderson-Block, K. (2012). Types of intimate partner homicides committed by women: Self-defence, proxy/retaliation and sexual proprietariness. *Homicide Studies*, 16, 359–379.

Bell, B.G. & Grubin, D. (2010). Functional magnetic resonance imaging may promote theoretical understanding of the polygraph test. *Journal of Forensic Psychiatry and Psychology*, 21, 52–65.

Bell, K. M. & Naugle, A. E. (2008). Intimate partner violence theoretical considerations: Moving towards a contextual framework. *Clinical Psychology Review*, 28, 1096–1107.

Bender, D. & Lösel, F. (2011). Bullying at school as a predictor of delinquency, violence and other anti-social behaviour in adulthood. *Criminal Behaviour and Mental Health*, 21, 99–106.

Benis, A. (2004). *Toward Self and Sanity: On the Genetics of the Human Character*. New York, NY: Psychological Dimensions.

Benjamin, L. T. (2007). *A Brief History of Modern Psychology*. Malden, MA: Blackwell.

Bennett, P. (2011). *Abnormal and Clinical Psychology: An Introductory Textbook*. 3rd edition. Maidenhead: Open University Press/McGraw-Hill Education.

Bennett, T. & Brookman, F. (2010). Street robbery. In F. Brookman, M. Maguire, H. Pierpoint & T. Bennett (eds.), *Handbook on Crime*. pp. 270–289. Cullompton: Willan.

Bennett, T. H. & Wright, R. (1984). *Burglars on Burglary: Prevention and the Offender*. Aldershot: Gower.

Bennett, T. & Holloway, K. (2007). *Drug-Crime Connections*. Cambridge: Cambridge University Press.

Bennett, T. & Holloway, K. (2009). The causal connection between drug misuse and crime. *British Journal of Criminology*, 49, 513–531.

Bennett, T. H., Holloway, K. R. & Farrington, D. P. (2008a). *Effectiveness of Neighbourhood Watch in Reducing Crime*. Stockholm: Swedish National Council for Crime Prevention.

Bennett, T. H., Holloway, K. R. & Farrington, D. P. (2008b). The statistical association between drug misuse and crime: A meta-analysis. *Aggression and Violent Behavior*, 13, 107–118.

Bennice, J. A. & Resick, P. A. (2003). Marital rape: History, research, and practice. *Trauma, Violence, & Abuse*, 4, 228–246.

Ben-Shakhar, G. (2002). A critical review of the control question test. In M. Kleiner (ed.), *Handbook of polygraph testing*. pp. 103–126. San Diego, CA: Academic Press.

Bentall, R. (1992). A proposal to classify happiness as a psychiatric disorder. *Journal of Medical Ethics*, 18, 94–98.

Bentall, R. P. (2009). *Doctoring the Mind: Why Psychiatric Treatments Fail*. London: Penguin Books.

Bentall, R. P. & Taylor, J. L. (2006). Psychological processes and paranoia: Implications for forensic behavioural science. *Behavioral Sciences and the Law*, 24, 277–294.

Berkowitz, L. (1993). *Aggression: Its Causes, Consequences, and Control*. New York, NY: McGraw-Hill.

Berkun, M. M., Bialek, H. M., Kern, R. P. & Yagi, K. (1962). Experimental studies of psychological stress in man [Special issue]. *Psychological Monographs: General and Applied*, 76 (15 Whole No. 534).

Bernard, T. J. (1990). Angry aggression among the "truly disadvantaged". *Criminology*, 28, 73–96.

Bernard, T. J. & Snipes, J. B. (1996). Theoretical integration in criminology. *Crime and Justice: A Review of Research*, 20, 301–348.

Bernard, T. J., Snipes, J. B. & Gerould, A. L. (2015). *Vold's Theoretical Criminology*. 7th edition. New York, NY: Oxford University Press.

Bernfeld, G. A. (2001). The struggle for treatment integrity in a "dis-integrated" service delivery system. In G. A. Bernfeld, D. P. Farrington & A. W. Leschied (eds.), *Offender Rehabilitation in Practice: Implementing and Evaluating Effective Programs*. pp. 167–188. Chichester: Wiley.

Bernstein, D. E. & Jackson, J. D. (2004). The *Daubert* Trilogy in the States. *Jurimetrics*, 44. https://ssrn.com/abstract=498786

Bertolote, J. M. & Fleischmann, A. (2002). Suicide and psychiatric diagnosis: A worldwide perspective. *World Psychiatry*, 1, 181–185.

Beyer, K., Mack, S. M. & Shelton, J. L. (2008). Investigative analysis of neonaticide: An exploratory study. *Criminal Justice and Behavior*, 35, 522–535.

Beyer, K., Wallis, A. B. & Hamberger, L. K. (2015). Neighborhood environment and intimate partner violence: A systematic review. *Trauma, Violence, & Abuse*, 16, 16–47.

Bickart, K. C., Wright, C. I., Dautoff, R. J., Dickerson, B. C. & Barrett, L. F. (2010). Amygdala volume and social network size in humans. *Nature Neuroscience*, 14, 163–164.

Bierie, D. M. (2012). Is tougher better? The impact of physical prison conditions on inmate violence. *International Journal of Offender Therapy and Comparative Criminology*, 56, 338–355.

Bijttebier, P. & Roeyers, H. (2009). Temperament and vulnerability to psychopathology: Introduction to the Special Section. *Journal of Abnormal Child Psychology*, 37, 305–308.

Biklen, S. K. & Moseley, C. R. (1988). "Are you retarded?" "No, I'm Catholic": Qualitative methods in the study of people with severe handicaps. *Journal for the Association of People with Severe Handicaps*, 13, 155–162.

Bilby, C., Brooks-Gordon, B. & Wells, H. (2006). A systematic review of psychological interventions for sexual offenders II: Quasi-experimental and qualitative data. *Journal of Forensic Psychiatry & Psychology*, 17, 467–484.

Birkley, E. L. & Eckhardt, C. I. (2015). Anger, hostility, internalizing negative emotions, and intimate partner violence perpetration: A meta-analytic review. *Clinical Psychology Review*, 37, 40–56.

Bjørkly, S. (2013). A systematic review of the relationship between impulsivity and violence in persons with psychosis: Evidence or spin cycle? *Aggression and Violent Behavior*, 18, 753–760.

Bjørkly, S. & Waage, L. (2005). Killing again: a review of research on recidivistic single-victim homicide. *International Journal of Forensic Mental Health*, 4, 99–106.

Black, D. (2004). Violent structures. In M. A. Zahn, H. H. Brownstein & S. L. Jackson (eds.), *Violence: From Theory to Research*. pp. 145–158. Matthew Bender/ LexisNexis.

Blackburn, R. (1993). *The Psychology of Criminal Conduct*. Chichester: Wiley.

Blackburn, R. (1996). What is forensic psychology? *Legal and Criminological Psychology*, 1, 3–16.

Blackburn, R. (2009). Subtypes of psychopath. In M. McMurran & R. Howard (eds.), *Personality, Personality Disorder and Violence*. pp. 113–132. Chichester: Wiley.

Blackman, D. E. (1996). Punishment: an experimental and theoretical analysis. In J. McGuire & B. Rowson (eds.) *Does Punishment Work?* London: Institute for the Study and Treatment of Delinquency.

Blair, R. J. R. (2005). Applying a cognitive neuroscience perspective to the disorder of psychopathy. *Development and Psychopathology*, 17, 865–891.

Blair, R. J. R. (2007). The amygdala and ventromedial prefrontal cortex in morality and psychopathy. *Trends in Cognitive Sciences*, 11, 387–392.

Blair, R. J. R., Mitchell, D. & Blair, K. (2005). *The Psychopath: Emotion and the Brain*. Malden, MA: Blackwell Publishing.

Blair, R. J. R., Monson, J. & Frederickson, N. (2001). Moral reasoning and conduct problems in children with emotional and behavioural difficulties. *Personality and Individual Differences*, 31, 799–811.

Blakemore, C. B., Thorpe, J. G., Barker, J. C., Conway, C. G., & Lavin, N. I. (1963). The application of Faradic Aversion Conditioning in a case of transvestism. *Behavioural Research Therapy, 1,* 29–34.

Blashfield, R. K. & Fuller, A. K. (1996). Predicting the DSM-V. *Journal of Nervous & Mental Disease*, 184, 4–7.

Blickle, G., Schlegel, A., Fassbender, P. & Klein, U. (2006). Some personality correlates of business white-collar crime. *Applied Psychology: An International Review*, 55, 220–233.

Bo, S., Abu-Akel, A., Komgerslev, M., Haahr, U. H. & Simonsen, E. (2011). Risk factors for violence among patients with schizophrenia. *Clinical Psychology Review*, 31, 711–726.

Bobadilla, L., Wampler, M. & Taylor, J. (2012). Proactive and reactive aggression are associated with different physiological and personality profiles. *Journal of Social and Clinical Psychology*, 31, 458–487.

Boccaccini, M. T. & Brodsky, S. L. (2002). Believability of expert and lay witnesses: Implications for trial consultation. *Professional Psychology: Research and Practice,* 33, 384–388.

Böckler, N., Seeger, T., Sitzer, P. & Heitmeyer, W. (eds.) (2013). *School Shootings: International Research, Case Studies and Concepts for Prevention*. New York, NY: Springer.

Boden, J. M., Fergusson, D. M. & Horwood, L. J. (2012). Alcohol misuse and violent behavior: Findings from a 30-year longitudinal study. *Drug and Alcohol Dependence*, 122, 135–141.

Boer, D. P. (ed.) (2016). *The Wiley Handbook on the Theories, Assessment and Treatment of Sexual Offending*. Malden, MA: Wiley-Blackwell.

Boer, D. P., Eher, R., Craig, L. A., Miner, M. H. & Pfäfflin, F. (eds.) (2011). *International Perspectives on the Assessment and Treatment of Sexual Offenders: Theory, Practice and Research*. Chichester: Wiley-Blackwell.

Boland, A., Cherry, G. & Dickson, R. (2017). *Doing a Systematic Review: A Student's Guide*. 2nd edition. London: Sage.

Boles, S. M. & Miotto, K. (2003). Substance abuse and violence: A review of the literature. *Aggression and Violent Behavior*, 8, 155–174.

Bolles, R. C. (1963). Psychological determinism and the problem of morality. *Journal for the Scientific Study of Religion,* 2, 182–189.

Bolton, F. E. (1896). The accuracy of recollection and observation. *Psychological Review,* 3, 286–295.

Boniface, D. (2005). The common sense of jurors vs the wisdom of the law: Judicial directions and warnings in sexual assault trials. *University of New South Wales Law Journal,* 28, 261–271.

Bonnema, M. C. (1992–1993). Trance on trial: An exegesis of hypnotism and criminal responsibility. *The Wayne Law Review,* 39, 1299–1334.

Bonta, J. (1996). Risk-needs assessment and treatment. In A. T. Harland (ed.) *Chooosing Correctional Options That Work: Defining the*

Demand and Evaluating the Supply. pp.18–32. Thousand Oaks, CA: Sage Publications.

Bonta, J. & Andrews, D. A. (2017). *The Psychology of Criminal Conduct*. 6th edition. London & New York, NY: Routledge.

Bonta, J., Blais, J. & Wilson, H. A. (2014). A theoretically informed meta-analysis of the risk for general and violent recidivism for mentally disordered offenders. *Aggression and Violent Behavior*, 19, 278–287.

Bonta, J., Law, M. & Hanson, K. (1998). The prediction of criminal and violent recidivism among mentally disordered offenders: A meta-analysis. *Psychological Bulletin*, 123, 123–142.

Boomsma, D., Busjahn, A. & Peltonen, L. (2002). Classical twin studies and beyond. *Nature Reviews Genetics,* 3, 872–882.

Boose, L. E. (2002). Crossing the River Drina: Bosnian rape camps, Turkish impalement, and Serb cultural memory. *Signs: Journal of Women in Culture and Society,* 28, 71–96.

Borenstein, M., Hedges, L. V., Higgins, J. P. T. and Rothstein, H. R. (2009). *Introduction to Meta-analysis*. New York, NY: Wiley.

Bornstein, B. H. & Greene, E. (2011). Jury decision making: Implications for and from psychology. *Current Directions in Psychological Science,* 20, 63–67.

Bornstein, B. H. & Penrod, S. D. (2008). Hugo who? G. F. Arnold's alternative early approach to psychology and law. *Applied Cognitive Psychology*, 22, 759–768.

Borsboom, D. (2005). *Measuring the Mind: Conceptual Issues in Contemporary Psychometrics*. Cambridge: Cambridge University Oress.

Bourget, D., Grace, J. & Whitehurst, L. (2007). A review of maternal and paternal filicide. *Journal of the American Academy of Psychiatry and the Law*, 35, 74–82.

Bowen, E. (2011). *The Rehabilitation of Partner-Violent Men*. Chichester: Wiley-Backwell.

Boyd, N. (2006). *Investment fraud: The victims of ERON mortgage*. Paper presented at the annual conference of the American Society of Criminology, Los Angeles, November.

Boyer, P. (2002). *Religion Explained: The Evolutionary Origins of Religious Thought*. New York, NY: Vintage.

Boyle, J. (1977). *A Sense of Freedom*. London: Pan Books.

Bracha, H. S., Livingston, R. L., Clothier, J., Linington, B. B., & Karson, C. N. (1993). Correlation of severity of psychiatric patients' delusions with right hemispatial inattention (left-turning behavior). *American Journal of Psychiatry*, 150, 330–332.

Brady, P. Q. & Nobles, M. R. (2015). The dark figure of stalking: Examining the law enforcement response. *Journal of Interpersonal Violence*. Doi: 10.1177/0886260515596979

Braga, A. A., Kennedy, D. M., Waring, E. J. & Piehl. A. M. (2001). Problem-oriented policing, deterrence, and youth violence: an evaluation of Boston's Operation Ceasefire. *Journal of Research in Crime and Delinquency*, 38, 195–225.

Braga, A. A. & Weisburd, D. L. (2015). Focused deterrence and the prevention of violent gun injuries: practice, theoretical principles, and scientific evidence. *Annual Review of Public Health*, 36, 55–68.

Braidwood, R. J., Sauer, J. D., Helbaek, H., Mangelsdorf, P. C., Cutler, H. C., Coon, C. S., Linton, R., Steward, J., & Oppenheim, A. L. (1953). Symposium: Did man once live by beer alone? *American Anthropologist*, 55, 515–526.

Branas, C. C., Richmond, T. S., Culhane, D. P., Ten Have, T. R. & Wiebe, D. J. (2009). Investigating the link between gun possession and gun assault. *American Journal of Public Health*, 99, 2034–2040.

Brandon, S., Boakes, J. Glaser, D. & Green, R. (1998). Recovered memories of childhood sexual abuse. *British Journal of Psychiatry*, 172, 296–307.

Brannon, Y. N, Levenson, J. S., Fortney, T. & Baker, J. N. (2007). Attitudes about community notification: A comparison of sexual offenders and the non-offending public. *Sexual Abuse: A journal of research and treatment,* 19, 369–379.

Brantingham, P. J. & Brantingham, P. L. (1975). The spatial patterning of burglary. *Howard Journal of Penology and Crime Prevention,* 14, 11–24.

Brantigham, P. L. & Brantingham, P. J. (1999). A theoretical model of crime hot spot generation. *Studies on Crime and Crime Prevention,* 8, 7–26.

Brass, M. & Haggard, P. (2010). The hidden side of intentional action: the role of the anterior insular cortex. *Brain Structure and Function,* 214, 603–610.

Braude, L., Heaps, M. M., Rodriguez, P. & Whitney, T. (2007). *Improving Public Safety through Cost-Effective Alternatives to Incarceration in Illinois*. Chicago, IL: Center for Health and Justice.

Bray, S. (2005). Not proven: Introducing a third verdict. *University of Chicago Law Review,* 72, 1299–1329.

Breau, D. L., & Brook, B. (2007). "Mock" Mock Juries. A Field Experiment on the ecological validity of jury simulations. *Law and Psychology Review,* 31, 77–92.

Breiding, M. J., Smith, S. G., Basile, K. C., Walters, M. L., Chen, J. & Merrick, M. T. (2014). *Prevalence and characteristics of sexual violence, stalking, and intimate partner violence victimisation – National Intimate Partner and Sexual Violence Survey, United States, 2011.* Washington, DC: US Department of Health and Human Services, Centers for Disease Control and Prevention.

Brennan, I. R. & Moore, S. C. (2009). Weapons and violence: A review of theory and research. *Aggression and Violent Behavior*, 14, 215–225.

Brennan, I. R., Moore, S. C. & Shepherd, J. P. (2006). Non-firearm weapon use and injury severity: priorities for prevention. *Injury Prevention*, 12, 395–399.

Brennan, M. & Brennan, R. E. (1988). *Strange language – child victims under cross-examination.* Wagga Wagga, NSW: Riverina Murray Institute of Higher Education.

Brewer, N. & Palmer, M. A. (2010). Eyewitness identification tests. *Legal and Criminological Psychology*, 15, 77–96.

Briant, E., Watson, N. & Philo, G. (2013). Reporting disability in the age of austerity: the changing face of media representation of disability and disabled people in the United Kingdom and the creation of new 'folk devils'. *Disability and Society*, 28, 874–889.

Briere, J. & Runtz, M. (1989). University males' sexual interest in children: Predicting potential indices of "pedophilia" in a nonforensic sample. *Child Abuse and Neglect,* 13, 65–75.

Briggs, P., Simon, W. T. & Simonsen, S. (2011). An exploratory study of internet-initiated sexual offenses and the chat room sex offender: Has the internet enabled a new typology of sex offender? *Sexual Abuse: A Journal of Research and Treatment*, 23, 72–91.

Brigham, J. C. (1999). What is forensic psychology, anyway? *Law and Human Behaviour*, 23, 273–298.

Brigham, J. C. & Malpass, R. S. (1985). The role of experience and contact in the recognition of faces of own- and other-race persons. *Journal of Social Issues*, 41, 139–155.

British Psychological Society (n.d.). *Becoming a Forensic Psychologist.* http://www.bps.org.uk/careers-education-training/how-become-psychologist/types-psychologists/becoming-forensic-psychologist accessed on 26/04/2012

British Psychological Society (2008). *Generic Professional Practice Guidelines.* 2nd edition. Leicester: British Psychological Society.

Brodt, S. E. & Tuchinsky, M. (2000). Working together but in opposition: An examination of the "good-cop/bad-cop" negotiating team tactic. *Organizational Behavior and Human Decision Processes*, 81, 155–177.

Brookman, F. (2005). *Understanding Homicide.* London: Sage.

Brookman, F. (2010). Homicide. In F. Brookman, M. Maguire, H. Pierpoint & T. Bennett (eds.), *Handbook on Crime*. pp. 217–244. Cullompton: Willan.

Brookman, F., Maguire, M., Pierpoint, H. & Bennett, T. (eds.) (2010). *Handbook on Crime*. Cullompton: Willan.

Brookman, F. & Nolan, J. (2006). The dark figure of infanticide in England and Wales: Complexities of diagnosis. *Journal of Interpersonal Violence*, 21, 869–889.

Brookman, F. & Robinson, A. (2012). Violent crime. In M. Maguire, R. M. Morgan & R. Reiner (eds.), *The Oxford Handbook of Criminology*. 5th edition. pp. 563–594. Oxford: Oxford University Press.

Brooks-Gordon, B., Bilby, C. & Wells, H. (2006). A systematic review of psychological interventions for sexual offenders I: Randomised control trials. *Journal of Forensic Psychiatry & Psychology*, 17, 442–466.

Brown C. L. & Geiselman, R. E. (1990). Eyewitness testimony of the mentally retarded: effect of the cognitive interview. *Journal of Police and Criminal Psychology*, 6, 14–22.

Brown, J. & Campbell, E. A. (eds.) (2010). *Cambridge Handbook of Forensic Psychology*. Cambridge: Cambridge University Press.

Brown, J. & Sutton, J. (2007). Protection or attack? Young people carrying knives and dangerous implements. *Australian Journal of Guidance and Counselling*, 17, 49–59.

Browne, K. D., Beech, A. R., Craig, L. A. & Chou, S. (eds.) (2017). *Assessments in Forensic Practice: A Handbook*. Chichester: Wiley-Blackwell.

Brownmiller, S. (1975). *Against Our Will: Men, Women, and Rape*. New York, NY: Simon and Schuster.

Brownstein, H. & Crossland, C. (2003). *Toward a Drugs and Crime Research Agenda for the 21st Century*. Washington, DC: National Institute of Justice, US Department of Justice.

Bruce, V., Henderson, Z., Greenwood, K., Hancock, P., Burton, A. M. & Miller, P. (1999). Verification of face identities from images captured on video. *Journal of Experimental Psychology: Applied*, 5, 339–360.

Bruck, M. & Ceci, S. J. (1995). Amicus brief for the case of State of New Jersey v. Michaels presented by Committee of Concerned Social Scientists. *Psychology, Public Policy, and Law*, 1, 272–322.

Brüne, M. (2003). Erotomanic stalking in evolutionary perspective. *Behavioral Sciences and the Law*, 21, 83–88.

Brussel, J. (1968). *Casebook of a Crime Psychiatrist.* New York, NY: Bernard Geis Associates.

Bucci, S., Birchwood, M., Twist, L., Tarrier, N., Emsley, R. & Haddock, G. (2013). Predicting compliance with command hallucinations: anger, impulsivity and appraisals of voices' power and intent. *Schizophrenia Research*, 147, 163–168.

Buchanan, A. (1998). Criminal conviction after discharge from special (high security) hospital: Incidence in the first I0 years. *British Journal of Psychiatry*, 172, 472–476.

Buchanan, N. T. & Harrell, Z. A. (2011). Surviving sexual harassment: coping with, recognizing, and preventing unwanted sexual behaviors in the workplace. In T. Bryant-Davis (ed.), *Surviving Sexual Violence: A Guide to Recovery and Empowerment*. pp. 7–21. Lanham, MD: Rowman and Littlefield.

Buckle, A. & Farrington, D. P. (1994). Measuring shoplifting by systematic observation: a replication study. *Psychology, Crime & Law*, 1, 133–141.

Bucks, R. S., Gidron, Y., Harris, P., Teeling, J., Wesnes, K. A., & Perry, V. H. (2008). Selective effects of upper respiratory tract infection on cognition, mood and emotion processing: A prospective study. *Brain, Behavior, and Immunity,* 22, 399–407.

Bufacchi, V. & Arrigo, J. M. (2006). Torture, terrorism and the state: a refutation of the ticking-bomb argument. *Journal of Applied Philosophy*, 23, 355–373.

Bull, R. & Carson, D. (eds.) (2003). *Handbook of Psychology in Legal Contexts*. 2nd edition. Chichester: Wiley-Blackwell.

Bull, R. & Milne, R. (2004). Attempts to improve the police interviewing of suspects. In G. D. Lassiter (ed.), *Interrogations, Confessions, and Entrapment*. pp. 181–196. New York, NY: Kluwer.

Bureau of Diplomatic Security (2002). *Carjacking: Don't be a victim*. Publication No. 10863. United States Department of State.

Bureau of Justice Statistics (2002). *Recidivism of Prisoners Released in 1994*. Washington, DC: Bureau of Justice Statistics, US Department of Justice.

Bureau of Justice Statistics (2004). *Carjacking, 1993–2002*. Bureau of Justice Statistics, US Department of Justice.

Burgess, A. W., Hartmann, C. R., Ressler, R. K., Douglas, J. E. & McCormack, A. (1986). Sexual homicide: A motivational model. *Journal of Interpersonal Violence*, 1, 251–272.

Burgess, A. W. & Hazelwood, R. R. (2009). Classifying rape and sexual assault. In R. R. Hazelwood & A. W. Burgess (Eds.), *Practical Aspects of Rape Investigation: A Multidisciplinary Approach*. 4th edition. pp. 343–362. Boca Raton, FL: CRC Press/Taylor & Francis Group.

Burgess, C. (2009). Prejudicial publicity: When will it ever result in a permanent stay of proceedings? *University of Tasmania Law Review,* 28, 63–80.

Burnett, A. & Omar, H. A. (2014). Firesetting and maltreatment: A review. *International Journal of Child and Adolescent Health*, 7, 99–101.

Burnett, R. & Maruna, S. (2004). So 'prison works', does it? The criminal careers of 130 men released from prison under Home Secretary Michael Howard. *Howard Journal, 43*(4), 390–404.

Burns, G. (1984). *Somebody's husband, somebody's son: The story of Peter Sutcliffe.* London: William Heinemann.

Burt, M. R. (1980). Cultural myths and supports for rape. *Journal of Personality and Social Psychology*, 38, 217–230.

Bush, J. (1995). Teaching self-risk-management to violent offenders. In J. McGuire (Ed.), *What Works: Reducing Reoffending: Guidelines from Research and Practice*. pp. 139–154. Chichester: Wiley.

Bushman, B. J. (2016). Violent media and hostile appraisals: A meta-analytic review. *Aggressive Behavior*, 42, 605–613.

Bushman, B. J. & Anderson, C. A. (2001). Is it time to pull the plug on the hostile versus instrumental aggression dichotomy? *Psychological Review*, 108, 273–279.

Bushman, B. J., Baumeister, R. F., Thomaes, S., Ryu, E., Begeer, S. & West, S. G. (2009). Looking again, and harder, for a link between low self-esteem and aggression. *Journal of Personality*, 77, 427–446.

Butchart, A., Harvey, A. P., Mian, M. & Fürniss, T. (2006). *Preventing Child Maltreatment: A guide to taking action and generating evidence*. Geneva: World Health Organization and the International

Society for the Prevention of Child Abuse and Neglect.

Byrd, A. L. & Manuck, S. B. (2014). MAOA, childhood maltreatment, and antisocial behavior: meta-analysis of a gene-environment interaction. *Biological Psychiatry*, 75, 9–17.

Byrne, J. M., Pattavina, A. & Taxman, F. S. (2015). International trends in prison upsizing and downsizing: In search of evidence of a global rehabilitation revolution. *Victims and Offenders*, 10, 420–451.

C

Cahalane, H., Duff, S. & Parker, G. (2013). Treatment implications arising from a qualitative analysis of letters written by the nonoffending partners of men who have perpetrated child *sexual abuse. Journal of Child Sexual Abuse*, 22, 720–741.

Caldwell, M. F., Vitacco, M. & Van Rybroek, G. J. (2006). Are violent delinquents worth treating? A cost–benefit analysis. *Journal of Research in Crime and* Delinquency, 43, 148–168.

Cameron, S. (2013). Killing for money and the economic theory of crime. *Review of Social Economy*, 72, 28–41.

Campbell, J. C., Webster, D., Koziol-McLain, J., Block, C., Campbell, D., Curry, M. A., Gary, F., Glass, N., McFarlane, J., Sachs, C., Sharps, F., Ulrich, Y., Wilt, S. A., Manganello, J., Xu, X., Schollenberger, J., Frye, V. & Laughton, K. (2003). Risk factors for femicide in abusive relationships: results from a multisite case control study. *American Journal of Public Health*, 93, 1089–1097.

Campbell, M. A., French, S. & Gendreau, P. (2009). The prediction of violence in adult offenders: a meta-analytic comparison of instruments and methods of assessment. *Criminal Justice and Behavior*, 36, 567–590.

Campbell, R. (2006). Rape survivors' experiences with the legal and medical systems: Do rape victim advocates make a difference? *Violence Against Women*, 12, 30–45.

Campbell, R., Self, T., Barnes, H. E., Ahrens, C. E., Wasco, S. M. & Zaragoza-Diesfeld, Y. (1999). Community services for rape survivors: Enhancing psychological well-being or increasing trauma? *Journal of Consulting and Clinical Psychology*, 67, 847–858.

Camperio Ciani, A. S. & Fontanesi, L. (2012). Mothers who kill their offspring: Testing evolutionary hypothesis in a 110-case Italian sample. *Child Abuse & Neglect*, 36, 519–527.

Cann, J., Falshaw, L., & Friendship, C. (2004). Sexual offenders discharged from prison in England and Wales: A 21-year reconviction study. *Legal and Criminological Psychology*, 9, 1–10.

Cann, J., Falshaw, L., Nugent, F. & Friendship, C. (2003). *Understanding What Works: accredited cognitive skills programmes for adult men and young offenders*. Findings 226. London: Home Office Research, Development and Statistics Directorate.

Cann, J., Friendship, C. & Gozna, L. (2007). Assessing crossover in a sample of sexual offenders with multiple victims. *Legal and Criminological Psychology*, 12, 149–163.

Canter, D. & Fritzon, K. (1998). Differentiating arsonists: a model of firesetting actions and characteristics. *Legal and Criminological Psychology*, 3, 73–96.

Canter, D. V. (1995). *Criminal Shadows*. London: HarperCollins.

Canter, D. V. (2004a). Geographical profiling of criminals. *Medico-Legal Journal*, 72, 53–66.

Canter, D. V. (2004b). Offender profiling and investigative psychology. *Journal of investigative Psychology and Offender Profiling*, 1, 1–15.

Canter, D. V. (2007). *Mapping murder: The secrets of geographic profiling*. London: Virgin Books.

Canter, D. V. & Alison, L. (2000). *Profiling property crime*. Burington, VT: Ashgate Publishing Company.

Canter, D. V. & Heritage, R. (1990). A multivariate model of sexual offence behaviour: Developments in offender profiling. *Journal of Forensic Psychiatry*, 1, 185–212.

Canter, D. V. & Larkin P. (1993). The environmental range of serial rapists. *Journal of Environmental Psychology*, 13, 63–69.

Canter, D. V. & Youngs, D. (2003). Beyond 'offender profiling': The need for an investigative psychology. In D. Carson & R. Bull (eds.), *Handbook of Psychology in Legal Contexts*. 2nd edition. pp. 171–206. Chichester: Wiley.

Canter, D. V., Alison, L. J., Alison, E., & Wentink, N. (2004). The organized/disorganized typology of serial murder: Myth or model? *Psychology, Public Policy, and Law*, 10, 293–320.

Canter, D. V., Coffey, T. Huntley, M. & Missen, C. (2000). Predicting serial killers' home base using a decision support system. *Journal of Quantitative Criminology*, 16, 457–478.

Cantlon, J., Payne, G., & Erbaugh, C. (1996). Outcome-based practice: Disclosure rates of child sexual abuse comparing allegation blind and allegation informed structured interviews. *Child Abuse and Neglect*, 20, 1113–1120.

Cantor, J. M., Kuban, M. E., Blak, T., Klassen, P. E., Dickey, R. & Blanchard, R. (2007). Physical height in pedophilic and hebephilic sexual offenders. *Sex Abuse,* 19, 395–407.

Carlson, J. F., Geisinger, K. F. & Jonson, J. L. (2017). *The Twentieth Mental Measurements Yearbook*. Lincoln, NE: University of Nebraska Press.

Carlson, K., & Russo, J. (2001). Biased interpretation of evidence by mock jurors. *Journal of Experimental Psychology: Applied,* 7, 91–103.

Carrabine, E., Cox, P., Lee, M. & South, N. (2002.) *Crime in Modern Britain*. Oxford: Oxford University Press.

Carré, J. M. & McCormick, C. M. (2008). In your face: Facial metrics predict aggressive behaviour in the laboratory and in varsity and professional hockey players. *Proceedings of the Royal Society B: Biological Sciences,* 275, 2651–2656.

Carré, J. M., McCormick, C. M. & Mondloch, C. J. (2009). Facial structure is a reliable cue of aggressive behaviour. *Psychological Science,* 20, 1194–1198.

Carroll, J. & Weaver, F. (1986). Shoplifters' perceptions of crime opportunities: a process-tracing study. In D. B. Cornish & R. V. Clarke (eds.), *The Reasoning Criminal: Rational Choice Perspectives on Offending*. pp. 19–38. New York, NY: Springer-Verlag.

Carson, D. (2000). The legal context: obstacle or opportunity? In J. McGuire, T. Mason & A. O'Kane (eds.) *Behaviour, Crime and Legal Processes: A Guide for Forensic Practitioners*. pp. 19–37. Chichester: Wiley.

Carson, D. & Bull, R. (eds.) (2003). *Handbook of Psychology in Legal Contexts*. 2nd edition. Chichester: Wiley-Blackwell.

Carswell, K., Maughan, B., Davis, H., Davenport, F. & Goddard, N. (2004). The psychosocial needs of young offenders and adolescents from an inner city area. *Journal of Adolescence*, 27, 415–428.

Carter, A. & Hollin, C. R. (2010). Characteristics of non-serial sexual homicide offenders: a review. *Psychology, Crime & Law*, 16, 25–45.

Carter, P. & Harrison, R. (1991). *Carter and Harrison on Offences of Violence*. London: Waterlow.

Casey, P. & Rottman, D. B. (2000). Therapeutic jurisprudence in the courts. *Behavioral Sciences and the Law,* 18, 445–457.

Caspi, A., Henry, B., McGee, R. O., Moffitt, T. E. & Silva, P. A. (1995). Temperamental origins of child and adolescent behavior problems: from age three to age fifteen. *Child Development*, 66, 55–68.

Caspi, A., McClay, J., Moffitt, T. E., Mill, J., Martin, J., Craig, I. W., Taylor, A. & Poulton, R. (2002). Role of genotype in the cycle of violence in maltreated children. *Science*, 297, 851–854.

Caspi, A., Moffitt, T. E., Silva, P. A., Stouthamer-Loeber, M., Krueger, R. F. & Schmutte, P. A. (1994). Are some people crime-prone? Replications of the personality-crime relationship across countries, genders, races and methods. *Criminology*, 32, 163–196.

Casswell, M., French, P. & Rogers, A. (2012). Distress, defiance or adaptation? A review paper of at-risk mental health states in young offenders. *Early Intervention in Psychiatry*, 6, 219–228.

Cattell, J. M. (1895). Measurements of the accuracy of recollection. *Science,* 2, 761–766.

Caulkins, J. P., Reuter, P. & Coulson, C. (2011). Basing drug scheduling decisions on scientific ranking of harmfulness: false promise from false premises. *Addiction*, 106, 1886–1890.

Cavadino, P., Dignan, J. & and Mair, G. (2013). *The Penal System: An Introduction*. 5th edition. London: Sage.

Ceci, S. J. & Bruck, M. (1993). Suggestibility of the child witness: A historical review and synthesis. *Psychological Bulletin*, 113, 403–439.

Centre for Economic Performance (2012). *How Mental Illness Loses Out in the NHS*. London: Centre for Economic Performance, London School of Economics and Political Science.

Cervone, D. & Pervin, L. A. (2013). *Personality Psychology*. New York, NY: Wiley.

Chamberlain, J. & Miller, M.K. (2008). Stress in the Courtroom: Call for research. *Psychiatry, Psychology and Law,* 15, 237–250.

Chambers, J. C., Horvath, M. A. H. & Kelly, L. (2010). A typology of multiple-perpetrator rape. *Criminal Justice and Behavior*, 37, 1114–1139.

Chan, H.-C. & Heide, K. M. (2009). Sexual homicide: A synthesis of the literature. *Trauma Violence Abuse*, 10, 31–54.

Chappell, A. T. & Piquero, A. R. (2004). Applying social learning theory to police misconduct. *Deviant Behavior*, 25, 89–108.

Chen, M. K. & Shapiro, J. M. (2007). Do harsher prison conditions reduce recidivism? A discontinuity-based approach. *American Law and Economics Review*, 9, 1–29.

Chen, Y.-H., Arria, A. M. & Anthony, J. C. (2003). Firesetting in adolescence and being aggressive, shy, and rejected by peers: New epidemiologic evidence from a national sample survey. *Journal of the American Academy of Psychiatry and the Law*, 31, 44–52.

Chesney-Lind, M. & Pasko, L. (2004). *The Female Offender: Girls, Women and Crime*. 2nd edition. Thousand Oaks, CA: Sage.

Chess, S. & Thomas, A. (1990). Continuities and discontinuities in temperament. In L. N. Robbins and M. Rutter (eds.), *Straight and Devious Pathways from Childhood to Adulthood*. pp. 205–220. Cambridge: Cambridge University Press.

Chiari, G., & Nuzzo, M. L. (1996). Psychological constructivisms: A metatheoretical differentiation. *Journal of Constructivist Psychology, 9*, 163–184.

Child, I. L. (1968). Personality in culture. In E. F. Borgatta and W. W. Lambert (eds.), *Handbook of Personality Theory and Research*. Chicago, IL: Rand McNally.

Chisholm, R. (1967). He could have done otherwise. *Journal of Philosophy*, 64, 409–417.

Chisum, W. J. & Turvey, B. (2000). Evidence dynamics: Locard's exchange principle & crime reconstruction. *Journal of Behavioral Profiling*, 1, January.

Chitsabesan, P. & Bailey, S. (2006). Mental health educational and social needs of young offenders in custody and in the community. *Current Opinion in Psychiatry*, 19, 355–360.

Chitsabesan, P., Kroll, I., Bailey, S., Kenning, C., Sneider, S., MacDonald, W. & Theodosiou, L. (2006). Mental health needs of young offenders in custody and in the community. *British Journal of Psychiatry*, 188, 534–540.

Choice, P., Lamke, L. K., & Pittman, J. F. (1995). Conflicting resolution strategies and marital distress as mediating factors in the link between witnessing interparental violence and wife battering. *Violence and Victims,* 10, 107–119.

Cialdini, R. (2001). *Influence: Science and Practice*. Boston: Alleyn and Bacon.

Cid, J. (2009). Is imprisonment criminogenic? A comparative study of recidivism rates between prison and suspended prison sanctions. *European Journal of Criminology*, 6, 459–480.

Clare, I. (1993). Issues in the assessment and treatment of male sex offenders with mild learning disabilities. *Sexual and Marital Therapy,* 8, 167–179.

Clark, L. A., Watson, D. & Reynolds, S. (1995). Diagnosis and classification of psychopathology: Challenges to the current system and future directions. *Annual Review of Psychology,* 46, 121–153.

Clarke, M., Duggan, C., Hollin, C. R., Huband, N., McCarthy, L. & Davies, S. (2013). Readmission after discharge from a medium secure unit. *Psychiatric Bulletin*, 37, 124–129.

Clarke, R. V. G. (1980). "Situational" crime prevention: Theory and practice. *British Journal of Criminology,* 20, 136–147.

Clarke, R. V. G. (1997). Introduction. In R. G. V. Clarke (ed.), *Situational Crime Prevention: Successful Case Studies*. 2nd edition. pp. 2–43. Guilderland, NY: Harrow and Heston.

Clarke, R. V. G. & Brown, R. (2003). International trafficking in stolen vehicles. *Crime and Justice*, 30, 197–227.

Clarke, R. V. G. & Felson, M. (1993). Introduction: criminology, routine activity, and rational choice. In R. V. Clarke & M. Felson (eds.) *Routine Activity and Rational Choice. Advances in Criminological Theory*, Vol.5. pp. 1–14. New Brunswick, NJ and London: Transaction Publishers.

Clarke, R. V. G. & Mayhew, P. (1988). The British gas suicide story and its criminological implications. *Crime and Justice: A Review of Research*, 10, 79–116.

Clavelle, P. R. & Turner, A. D. (1980). Clinical decision-making among professionals and paraprofessionals. *Journal of Clinical Psychology,* 36, 833–838.

Cleckley, H. R. (1976). *The Mask of Sanity: An attempt to clarify some issues about the so-called psychopathic personality*. 5th edition. St.Louis, MO: C. V. Mosby Company.

Clegg, C. & Fremouw, W. (2009). Phallometric assessment of rapists: A critical review of the research. *Aggression and Violent Behavior*, 14, 115–125.

Cohen, A. (2008). IAPT: A brief history. *Healthcare Counselling and Psychotherapy Journal,* April, 8–11.

Cohen, L. E. & Felson, M. (1979). Social change and crime rate trends: A routine activity approach. *American Sociological Review*, 44, 588–608.

Cohen, M. A. (1988). Some new evidence on the seriousness of crime. *Criminology*, 26, 343–353.

Coid, J. & Ullrich, S. (2009). Antisocial personality disorder is on a continuum with psychopathy. *Comprehensive Psychiatry*, 51, 426–433.

Coid, J., Hickey, N., Kahtan, N. & Zhang, T. (2007). Patients discharged from medium secure forensic psychiatry services: reconvictions and risk factors. *The British Journal of Psychiatry,* 190, 223–229.

Coid, J., Kahtan, N., Gault, S., Cook, A. & Jarman, B. (2001). Medium secure forensic psychiatry services: Comparsion of seven English health regions. *British Journal of Psychiatry*, 178, 55–61.

Coid, J., Yang, M., Ullrich, S., Roberts, A., & Hare, R. (2009a). Prevalence and correlates of psychopathic traits in the household population of Great Britain. *International Journal of Law and Psychiatry*, 32, 65–73.

Coid, J., Yang, M., Ullrich, S., Roberts, A., Moran, P., Bebbington, P., Brugha, T., Jenkins, R., Farrell, M., Lewis, G., Singleton, N. & Hare, R. (2009b). Psychopathy among prisoners in England and Wales. *International Journal of Law and Psychiatry*, 32, 134–141.

Cole, C. B. & Loftus, E. F. (1987). The memory of children. In S. J. Ceci, M. P. Toglia & D. F. Ross (eds.), *Children's Memory*. pp. 178–208. New York, NY: Springer-Verlag.

Coleman, C. & Moynihan, J. (1996). *Understanding Crime Data: Haunted by the dark figure*. Buckingham: Open University Press.

Collie, R. M., Vess, J. & Murdoch, S. (2007). Violence-related cognition: Current research. In T. A. Gannon, T. Ward, A. R. Beech & D. Fisher (eds.), *Aggressive Offenders' Cognition: Theory, Research and Practice*. pp. 179–197. Chichester: Wiley.

Collins, J. M. & Schmidt, F. L. (1993). Personality, integrity, and white collar crime: a construct validity study. *Personnel Psychology*, 46, 295–311.

Collins, R. (2008). *Violence: A Micro-Sociological Theory*. Princeton, NJ: Princeton University Press.

Collins, R. (2009). The micro-sociology of violence. *British Journal of Sociology*, 60, 566–576.

Collins, R. (2013). Entering and leaving the tunnel of violence: Micro-sociological dynamics of self-entrainment in severe violence. *Current Sociology*, 61, 132–151.

Colman, A. M., & Mackay, R. D. (1995). Psychological evidence in court: Legal developments in England and the United States. *Psychology, Crime & Law*, 1, 261–268.

Concannon, D. M. (2013). *Kidnapping: An Investigator's Guide*, 2nd edition. London and Waltham, MA: Elsevier.

Conger, R. D., Ge, X., Elder, G. H. Lorenz, F. O. & Simons, R. L. (1994). Economic stress, coercive family process, and developmental problems of adolescents. *Child Development*, 65, 541-561.

Conroy, M. A. & Murrie, D. C. (2007). *Forensic Assessment of Violence Risk: A Guide for Risk Assessment and Risk Management*. Hoboken, NJ: Wiley.

Conway, K. P. & McCord, J. (2002). A longitudinal examination of the relation between co-offending with violent accomplices and violent crime. *Aggressive Behavior*, 28, 97–108.

Cook, P. J. & Ludwig, J. (2002). *The effects of gun prevalence on burglary: deterrence vs inducement*. National Bureau of Economic Research (NBER), Working Paper 8926. Cambridge, MA: NBER. http://www.nber.org/papers/w8926.pdf

Cooke, D. J. & Michie, C. (2001). Refining the construct of psychopathy: Towards a hierarchical model. *Psychological Assessment*, 13, 171–188.

Cooke, D. J., Michie, C., Hart, S. D. & Clark, D. A. (2004). Reconstructing psychopathy: clarifying the significance of antisocial and socially deviant behavior in the diagnosis of psychopathic personality disorder. *Journal of Personality Disorders*, 18, 337–357.

Cooney, M. (2009). The scientific significance of Collins's *Violence*. *British Journal of Sociology*, 60, 586–594.

Cooper, A. & Smith, E. L. (2011). *Homicide Trends in the United States, 1980–2008*. Washington, DC: Bureau of Justice Statistics, US Department of Justice.

Cooper, C. S. (2003). Drug courts: Current issues and future perspective. *Substance Use & Misuse, 38,* 11–13.

Cooper, H. M., Hedges, L. V. & Valentine, J. C. (Eds.) (2009). *The Handbook of Research Synthesis and Meta-analysis*. 2nd edition. New York, NY: Russell Sage Foundation.

Cooper, J. & Neuhaus, I. M. (2000). The "hired gun" effect: Assessing the effect of pay, frequency of testifying, and credentials on the perception of expert testimony. *Law and Human Behavior, 24,* 149–171.

Cooper, J. O., Heron, T. E. & Heward, W. L. (2007). *Applied Behavior Analysis*. 2nd edition. Upper Saddle River, NJ: Pearson Education.

Cooper, R. M. & Zubek, J. P. (1958). Effects of enriched and restricted early environments on the learning ability of bright and dull rats. *Canadian Journal of Psychology*, 12, 159–164.

Copas, J., & Marshall, P. (1998). The offender group reconviction scale: a statistical reconviction score for use by probation officers. *Applied Statistics*, 47, 159–171.

Copestake, S., Gray, N. S. & Snowden, R. J. (2011). A comparison of a self-report measure of psychopathy with the psychopathy checklist-revised in a UK sample of offenders. *Journal of Forensic Psychiatry & Psychology*, 22, 169–182.

Copson, G. (1995). *Coals to Newcastle? Part 1: A study of offender profiling (Paper 7).* London: Police Research Group Special Interest Series, Home Office.

Corbett, C. & Simon, F. (1992). Decisions to break or adhere to the rules of the road, viewed from the rational choice perspective. *British Journal of Criminology*, 32, 537–549.

Cordella, P. & Siegel, L. (eds.) (1996). *Readings in Contemporary Criminological Theory*. Boston: MA: Northeastern University Press.

Cornell, D. G., Warren, J., Hawk, G., Stafford, E., Oram, G. & Pine, D. (1996). Psychopathy in instrumental and reactive violent offenders. *Journal of Consulting and Clinical Psychology*, 64, 783–790.

Corradi, C. & Stöckl, H. (2014). Intimate partner homicide in 10 European countries: Statistical data and policy development in a cross-national perspective. *European Journal of Criminology*, 11, 601–618.

Correctional Services Accreditation Panel (2010). *Report 2009-2010*. London: Ministry of Justice, Correctional Services Accreditation Panel Secretariat.

Correctional Services Accreditation Panel (2016). *Criteria for Programme Accreditation*. London: Ministry of Justice.

Costanzo, M., Gerrity, E. & Lykes, M. B. (2007). Psychologists and the use of torture in interrogations. *Analyses of Social Issues and Public Policy*, 7, 7–20.

Courtney, K. E. & Polich, J. (2009). Binge drinking in young adults: Data, definitions, and determinants. *Psychological Bulletin*, 135, 124–156.

Cownie, F., Bradney, A. & Burton, M. (2007). *English Legal System in Context*. 4th edition. Oxford: Oxford University Press.

CPS (2010). http://www.cps.gov.uk/victims_witnesses/resources/prosecution.html#a03

CPS (2013). *Charging perverting the course of justice and wasting police time in cases involving allegedly false rape and domestic violence allegations*. Joint report to the Director of Public Prosecutions by Alison Levitt QC, Principal Legal Adviser, and the Crown Prosecution Service Equality and Diversity Unit. http://www.cps.gov.uk/publications/research/perverting_course_of_justice_march_2013.pdf

Crabbé, A., Decoene, S. & Vertommen, H. (2008). Profiling homicide offenders: A review of assumptions and theories. *Aggression and Violent Behavior*, 13, 88–106.

Craig, K. M. (2002). Examining hate-motivated aggression: A review of the social psychological literature on hate crimes as a distinct form of aggression. *Aggression and Violent Behavior*, 7, 85–101.

Craig, L. A. (2008). How should we understand the effect of age on sexual recidivism? *Journal of Sexual Aggression*, 14, 185–198.

Craig, L. A., Browne, K. D. & Beech, A. R. (2008). *Assessing Risk in Sex Offenders: A Practitioner's Guide*. Chichester: Wiley-Blackwell.

Craig, L. A., Dixon, L. & Gannon, T. A. (eds.) (2013). *What Works in Offender Rehabilitation: An Evidence Based Approach to Assessment and Treatment*. Chichester: Wiley-Blackwell

Craig, M. C., Catani, M., Deeley, Q., Latham, R., Daly, E., Kanaan, R., Picchioni. M., McGuire, P. K., Fahy, T. & Murphy, D. G. M. (2009). Altered connections on the road to psychopathy. *Molecular Psychiatry*, 14, 946–953.

Craissati, J., McClurg, G. & Browne, K. D. (2002). Characteristics of perpetrators of child sexual abuse who have been sexually victimised as children. *Sexual Abuse: A Journal of Research and Treatment*, 14, 225–240.

Creighton, S. J. (2004). *Prevalence and incidence of child abuse: international comparisons*. London: National Society for the Prevention of Cruelty to Children.

Crépault, C. & Couture, M. (1980). Men's erotic fantasies. *Archives of Sexual Behaviour*, 9, 565–581.

Cretacci, M. A. (2008). A general test of self-control theory: has its importance been exaggerated? *International Journal of Offender Therapy and Comparative Criminology*, 52, 538-553.

Criminal Injuries Compensation Authority (2012). *A guide to the Criminal Injuries Compensation Scheme 2012*. London: Criminal Injuries Compensation Authority.

Crits-Cristoph, P., Gibbons, M. B. C. & Mukherjee, D. (2013). Psychotherapy process-outcome research. In M. J. Lambert (ed.), *Bergin and Garfield's Handbook of Psychotherapy and Behavior Change*. 6th edition. pp. 298–340. Hoboken, NJ: Wiley.

Cronbach, L. J. (1975). Beyond the two disciplines of scientific psychology. *American Psychologist*, 30, 116–127.

Cross-Disorder Group of the Psychiatric Genomics Consortium (2013). Identification of risk loci with shared effects on five major psychiatric disorders: a genome-wide analysis. *Lancet*, 381, 1371–1379.

Cruceanu, C., Matosin, N. & Binder, E. B. (2017). Interactions of early-life stress with the genome and epigenome: from prenatal stress to psychiatric disorders. *Current Opinion in Behavioral Sciences*, 14, 167–171.

Cullen, F. T., Myer, A. J. & Latessa, E. J. (2009). Eight lessons from *Moneyball*: The high cost of ignoring evidence-based corrections. *Victims & Offenders*, 4, 197–213.

Cullen. F. T., Wright, J. P. & Blevins, K. R. (eds.) (2008). *Taking Stock: The Status of Criminological Theory*. New Brunswick, NJ: Transaction Publishers.

Cummings, K. M., Morley, C. P. & Hyland, A. (2002). Failed promises of the cigarette industry and its effect on consumer misperceptions about the health risks of smoking. *Tobacco Control*, 11, i110–i117.

Curtis, M. (2003). *Web of Deceit: Britain's Real Role in the World*. London: Vintage Books.

Cutler, B. L., Berman, G. L., Penrod, S., & Fisher, R. P. (1994). Conceptual, practical, and empirical issues associated with eyewitness identification test media. In D. F. Ross, J. D. Read, & M. P. Toglia (eds.), *Adult Eyewitness Testimony: Current Trends and Developments*. pp. 163–181. New York, NY: Cambridge University Press.

Cutright, P. & Briggs, C. M. (1995). Structural and cultural determinants of adult homicide in developed countries: age and gender-specific rates, 1955–1989. *Sociological Focus*, 28, 221-243.

Cyr, M. & Lamb, M. E. (2009). Assessing the effectiveness of the NICHD investigative interviewing protocol when interviewing French-speaking alleged victims of child sexual abuse in Quebec. *Child Abuse and Neglect*, 33, 257–268.

D

Dabney, D. A., Dugan, L., Topalli, V., & Hoolinger, R. C. (2006). The impact of implicit stereotyping on offender profiling: Unexpected results from an observational study of shoplifting. *Criminal Justice and Behavior,* 33, 646–674.

Daffern, M., Jones, L., Howells, K., Shine, J., Mikton, C. & Tunbridge, V. (2007). Refining the definition of offence paralleling behaviour. *Criminal Behaviour and Mental Health,* 17(5), 265–273.

Daftary-Kapur, T., Dumas, R. & Penrod, S.D. (2010). Jury decision-making biases and methods to counter them. *Legal and Criminological Psychology,* 15, 133–154.

Dalgaard-Nielsen, A. (2010). Violent radicalization in Europe: What we know and what we do not know. *Studies in Conflict and Terrorism*, 33, 7970814.

Daly, K. & Chesney-Lind, M. (1988). Feminism and criminology. *Justice Quarterly*, 5, 497–538.

Daly, M. & Wilson, M. (1988). *Homicide*. Hawthorne, NY: Aldine.

Dando, C., Wilcock, R., Milne, R. & Henry, L. (2009). A modified cognitive interview procedure for frontline police investigators. *Applied Cognitive Psychology*, 23, 698–716.

Das, E., Bushman, B. J., Bezemer, M. D., Kerkhof, P., Vermeulen, I. E. (2009). How terrorism news reports increase prejudice against outgroups: A terror management account. *Journal of Experimental Social Psychology*, 45, 453–459.

Daubert (1993). *Daubert v Merrell Dow Pharmaceuticals Inc.* 509 U.S., 113 S.Ct. 2786.

David, A. S., Fleminger, S., Kopelman, M. D., Lovestone, S. & Mellers, J. D. C. (2012). *Lishman's Organic Psychiatry: A Textbook of Neuropsychiatry*. 4th revised edition. Chichester: Wiley-Blackwell.

Davies, A. (1997). Specific profile analysis: A data-based approach to offender profiling. In J. L. Jackson (ed.), *Offender Profiling: Theory, Research and Practice*. pp. 191–207. Chichester: Wiley.

Davies, G. (2008). Introduction. In G. Davies, C. Hollin & R Bull (eds.), *Forensic Psychology*. pp. XIII–XXIII. Chichester: Wiley.

Davies, M., Croall, H. & Tyrer, J. (2010). *Criminal Justice*. 4th edition. Harlow: Pearson Education.

Davies, M. & Mouzos, J. (2007). Fatal fires: fire-associated homicide in Australia, 1990–2005. *Trends & Issues in crime and criminal justice*. No. 340. Canberra: Australian Institute of Criminology.

Davies, S., Clarke, M., Hollin, C. & Duggan, C. (2007). Long-term outcomes after discharge from medium secure care: a cause for concern. *British Journal of Psychiatry*, 191, 70–74.

Davis, K. E., Swan, S. C. & Gambone, L. J. (2012). Why doesn't he just leave me alone? Persistent pursuit: A critical review of theories and evidence. *Sex Roles*, 66, 328–339.

Davis, M. R., McMahon, M., & Greenwood, K.M. (2005). The efficacy of mnemonic components of the Cognitive Interview: Towards a shortened variant for time-critical investigations. *Applied Cognitive Psychology*, 19, 75–93.

Davis, R. C. (1961). Physiological responses as a means of evaluating information. In A. D. Biderman & H. Zimmer (eds.), *The manipulation of human behaviour*. pp. 142–168. New York, NY: Wiley.

Dawes, R. M., Faust, D. & Meehl, P. E. (1989). Clinical versus actuarial judgment. *Science,* 243 1668–1674.

Dawes, W., Harvey, P., McIntosh, B., Nunney, F. & Phillips, A. (2011). *Attitudes to guilty plea sentence reductions*. Sentencing Council Research Series 02/11. London: Sentencing Council.

Deakin, J., Smithson, H., Spencer, J. & Medina-Ariza, J. (2007). Taxing on the streets: Understanding the methods and process of street robbery. *Crime Prevention and Community Safety*, 9, 52–67.

De Castro, B. O., Veerman, J. W., Koops, W., Bosch, J. D. & Monshouwer, H. (2002). Hostile attribution of intent and aggressive behaviour: a meta-analysis. *Child Development*, 73, 916–934.

Decker, S. H. & Chapman, M. T. (2008). *Drug Smugglers on Drug Smuggling: Lessons from the Inside*. Philadelphia, PA: Temple University Press.

DeCuyper, M., de Pauw, S., de Fruyt, F., de Bolle, M. & de Clercq, B. J. (2009). A meta-analysis of psychopathy, antisocial PD, and FFM associations. *European Journal of Personality*, 23, 531–565.

DeGue, S. & DiLillo, D. (2009). Is animal cruelty a "red flag" for family violence? Investigating co-occurring violence toward children, partners, and pets. *Journal of Interpersonal Violence*, 24, 1935–1956.

Del Bove, G. & Mackay, S. (2011). An empirically derived classification system for juvenile firesetters. *Criminal Justice and Behavior*, 38, 796–817.

DeLisi, M. & Vaughan, M. G. (2014). Foundations for a temperament-based theory of antisocial behavior and criminal justice system involvement. *Journal of Criminal Justice*, 42, 10–25.

Dempster, F. N. & Corkill, A. J. (1999). Interference and inhibition in cognition and behavior: Unifying themes for educational psychology. *Educational Psychology Review*, 11, 1–88.

Demuth, S. & Brown, S. L. (2004). Family structure, family process, and adolescent delinquency: the significance of parental absence versus parental gender. *Journal of Research in Crime and Delinquency*, 41, 58–81.

Dennis, J. A., Khan, O., Ferriter, M., Huband, N., Powney, M. J. & Duggan, C. (2012). Psychological interventions for adults who have sexually offended or at risk of offending. *Cochrane Database of Systematic Reviews*, Issue 12. Art. No.: CD007507.

Denno, D. W. (1988). Biology and criminal responsibility: Free will or free ride? *University of Pennsylvania Law Review*, 137, 615–671.

Denno, D. W. (2006). Revisiting the legal link between genetics and crime. *Law and Contemporary Problems*, 69, 209–257.

Department of Health (2008). *Refocusing the Care Programme Approach: Policy and Positive Practice Guidance*. London: Department of Health.

Dernevik, M., Beck, A., Grann, M., Hogue, T. & McGuire, J. (2009). The use of psychiatric and psychological evidence in the assessment of terrorist offenders. *Journal of Forensic Psychiatry & Psychology*, 20, 508–515.

De Ruiter, C. & Kaser-Boyd, N. (2015). *Forensic Psychological Assessment in Practice: Case Studies*. New York & London: Routledge.

Desjarlais, D. C., Lyles, C., Crepaz, N., & the TREND Group (2004). Improving the Reporting Quality of Nonrandomized Evaluations of Behavioral and Public Health Interventions: The TREND Statement. *American Journal of Public Health*, 94, 361–366.

Desjarlais, R., Eisenberg, L., Good, B. & Kleinman, A. (1996). *World Mental Health: Problems and Priorities in Low Income Countries*. New York, NY: Oxford University Press.

Deslauriers-Varin, N., Lussier, P. & St-Yves, M. (2011). Confessing their crime: Factors influencing the offender's decision to confess to the police. *Justice Quarterly*, 28, 113–145.

De Visser, R. O. & Smith, J. A. (2007). Alcohol consumption and masculine identity among young men. *Psychology and Health*, 22, 595–614.

Devlin, C., Bolt, O., Patel, D., Harding, D. & Hussain, I. (2014). *Impacts of immigration on UK native employment: An analytical review of the evidence*. London: Home Office and Department for Business, Innovation and Skills.

Devries, K., Watts, C., Yoshihama, M. Kiss, L., Schraiber, L. B., Deyessa, N., Heise, L., Durand, J., Mbwambo, J., Jansen, H., Berhane, Y., Ellsberg, M. & García-Moreno, C., WHO Multi-Country Study Team (2011). Violence against women is strongly associated with suicide attempts: evidence from the WHO multi-country study on women's health and domestic violence against women. *Social Science & Medicine*, 73, 79–86.

DeWall, C. N., Anderson, C. A. & Bushman, B. J. (2011). The General Aggression Model: Theoretical extensions to violence. *Psychology of Violence*, 1, 245–258.

Dezhbakhsh, H., Rubin, P.H. & Shepherd, J.M. (2003). Does capital punishment have a deterrent effect? New evidence from post-moratorium panel data. *American Law and Economics Review*, 5, 344–376.

Dhami, M. K. (2007). White-collar prisoners' perceptions of audience reaction. *Deviant Behavior*, 28, 57–77.

Dickie, I. (2008). Ethical dilemmas, forensic psychology, and therapeutic jurisprudence. *Thomas Jefferson Law Review*, 30, 455–461.

Dietz, P. E. (1986). Mass, serial and sensational homicides. *Bulletin of the New York Academy of Medicine*, 62, 477–491.

Dillehay, T. D., Rossen, J., Ugent, D., Karathanasis, A., Vásquez, V. & Netherly, P. J. (2011). Early Holocene coca chewing in northern Peru. *Antiquity*, 84, 939–953.

Dinos, S., Burrowes, N., Hammond, K. & Cunliffe, C. (2015). A systematic review of juries' assessment of rape victims: Do rape myths impact on juror decision-making? *International Journal of Law, Crime and Justice*, 43, 36–49.

Dishion, T. J., Patterson, G. R. & Kavanagh, K. A. (1992). An experimental test of the Coercion Model: Linking theory, measurement, and intervention. In J. McCord & R. E. Tremblay (eds.), *Preventing Antisocial Behaviour: Interventions from Birth through Adolescence*. pp. 253–282. New York, NY: Guilford Press.

Dixon, L. & Browne, K. (2003). The heterogeneity of spouse abuse: A review. *Aggression and Violent Behavior*, 8, 107–130.

Dixon, L. & Graham-Kevan, N. (2011). Understanding the nature and etiology of intimate partner violence and implications for practice and policy. *Clinical Psychology Review*, 31, 1145–1155.

Dixon, L., Hamilton-Giachristis, C. & Browne. K. (2008). Classifying partner femicide. *Journal of Interpersonal Violence*, 23, 74–93.

Doak, J. (2005). Victims' rights in criminal trials: Prospects for participation. *Journal of Law and Society*, 32, 294–316.

Doan, B. & Snook, B. (2008). A failure to find empirical support for the homology assumption in criminal profiling. *Journal of Police and Criminology Psychology*, 23, 61–70.

Dobash, R. E. & Dobash, R. P. (2000). Evaluating criminal justice interventions for domestic violence. *Crime and Delinquency*, 46, 252–270.

Dobash, R. E. & Dobash, R. P. (2011). What were they thinking? Men who murder an intimate partner. *Violence Against Women*, 17, 111–134.

Dobash, R. P., Dobash, R. E., Cavanagh, K., Smith, D. & Medina-Ariza, J. (2007). Onset of offending and life course among men convicted of murder. *Homicide Studies*, 11, 243–271.

Dodge, K. A. & Pettit, G. S. (2003). A biopsychosocial model of the development of chronic conduct problems in adolescence. *Developmental Psychology*, 39, 349–371.

Dodge, K. A., Pettit, G. S. & Bates, J. E. (1994). Socialisation mediators of the relation between socioeconomic status and child conduct problems. *Child Development*, 65, 649–665.

Doherty, J. L., O'Donovan, M. C. & Owen, M. J. (2011). Recent genomic advances in schizophrenia. *Clinical Genetics*, October. Doi: 10.1111/j.1399-0004.2011.01773.x

Doherty-Sneddon, G. & McAuley, S. (2000). Influence of video-mediation on adult-child interviews: Implications for the use of the live link with child witnesses. *Applied Cognitive Psychology*, 14, 379–392.

Doley, R. (2003). Making sense of arson through classification. *Psychiatry, Psycholgy and Law*, 10, 346–352.

Doley, R. M., Dickens, G. L. & Gannon, T. A. (2016). Introduction: Deliberate firesetting – an overview. In R. M. Doley, G. L. Dickens & T. A. Gannon (eds.), *The Psychology of Arson: A Practical Guide to Understanding and Managing Deliberate Firesetters*. pp. 1–11. Abingdon: Routledge.

Donald, J. (1970). Psychologists in the prison service. *Occupational Psychology*, 44, 237–243.

Donohue, J. & Wolfers, J. (2005). Uses and abuses of statistical evidence in the death penalty debate. *Stanford Law Review*, 58, 791–846.

Doren, D. M. & Yates, P. M. (2008). Effectiveness of sex offender treatment for psychopathic sexual offenders. *International Journal of Offender Therapy and Comparative Criminology*, 52, 234–245.

Dorn, N., Murji, K. & South, N. (1992). *Traffickers: Drug Markets and Law Enforcement*. London: Routledge.

Douglas, J. E., Burgess, A. W., Burgess, A. G. & Ressler, R. K. (2013). *Crime Classification Manual: A Standard System for Investigating and Classifying Violent Crime*. 3rd edition. Hoboken, NJ: Wiley.

Douglas, J. E., Ressler, R. K., Burgess, A. W. & Hatman, C. R. (1986). Criminal profiling from crime scene analysis. *Behavioral Sciences and the Law*, 4, 401–421.

Douglas, K. S., Guy, L. S. & Hart, S. D. (2009). Psychosis as a risk factor for violence to others: A meta-analysis. *Psychological Bulletin*, 135, 679–706.

Douglas, K. S., Hart, S. D., Webster, C. D. & Belfrage, H. (2013). *HCR-20 version 3 – Assessing Risk For Violence v 3*. Ann Arbor, MI: Ann Arbor Publishers.

Douglas, K. S., Lyon, D. R. & Ogloff, J. R. P. (1997). The impact of graphic photographic evidence on mock jurors' decisions in a murder trial: Probative or prejudicial? *Law and Human Behavior*, 21, 485–500.

Dowden, C. & Andrews, D. A. (1999). What works for female offenders: a meta-analytic review. *Crime and Delinquency*, 45, 438–452.

Dowden, C. & Andrews, D. A. (2000). Effective correctional treatment and violent reoffending: A meta-analysis. *Canadian Journal of Criminology and Criminal Justice*, 42, 449–467.

Dowden, C. & Andrews, D. A. (2004). The importance of staff practice in delivering effective correctional treatment: A meta-analytic review of core correctional practice. *International Journal of Offender Therapy and Comparative Criminology*, 48, 203–214.

Dowden, C., Antonowicz, D. & Andrews, D. A. (2003). The effectiveness of relapse prevention with offenders: A meta-analysis. *International Journal of Offender Therapy and Comparative Criminology*, 47, 516–528.

Dowden, C., Blanchette, K. & Serin, R. C. (1999). Anger management programming for federal male inmates: An effective intervention. *Research Report R-82*. Ottawa: Correctional Service of Canada.

Dowden, C. & Brown, S. L. (2002). The role of substance abuse factors in predicting recidivism: A meta-analysis. *Psychology, Crime & Law*, 8, 243–264.

Dowie, M. (1977). Pinto madness. *Mother Jones*, September/October issue. http://www.motherjones.com/politics/1977/09/pinto-madness/

Drago, F., Galbiati, R. & Vertova, P. (2011). Prison conditions and recidivism. *American Law and Economics Review*, 13, 103–130.

Drake, K. & Bull, R. (2011). Individual differences in interrogative suggestibility: life adversity and field dependence. *Psychology, Crime & Law*, 17, 677–687.

Drogin, E. Y., Dattilio, F. M., Sadoff, R. L. & Gutheil, T. G. (eds.) (2011). *Handbook of Forensic Assessment: Psychological and Psychiatric Perspectives*. New York, NY: Wiley.

D'Silva, K., Duggan, C., & McCarthy, L. (2004). Does treatment really make psychopaths worse? A review of the evidence. *Journal of Personality Disorders*, 18, 163–177.

Dubber, M. D. (2006). Comparative criminal law. In M. Reimann & R. Zimmermann (eds.), *The Oxford Handbook of Comparative Law*. pp. 1287–1325. Oxford: Oxford University Press.

Duff, A. (2003). Punishment, communication and community. In D. Matravers & J. Pike (eds.). *Debates in Contemporary Political Philosophy: An anthology*. pp. 387–407. London: Routledge.

Duff, S. C. & Kinderman, P. (2008). Predicting the behaviour of offenders with Personality Disorder: Issues for Investigative Psychology. *Journal of Investigative Psychology and Offender Profiling, 5*, 45–57.

Dugan, L., LaFree, G. & Piquero, A. R. (2005). Testing a rational choice model of airline hijackings. *Criminology*, 43, 1031–1065.

Duggan, L. M., Aubrey, M., Doherty, E., Isquith, P., Levine, M., & Scheiner, J. (1989). The credibility of children as witnesses in a simulated child sex abuse trial. In S. J. Ceci, D. F. Ross, & M. P. Toglia (eds.), *Perspectives on children's testimory*. pp. 23–37. New York: Springer-Verlag.

Dukes, R. L., & Mattley, C. L. (1977). Predicting rape victim reportage. *Sociology and Social Research, 62*, 63–84.

Dunaway, R. G., Cullen, F. T., Burton, V. S. & Evans, T. D. (2000). The myth of social class and crime revisited: An examination of class and adult criminality. *Criminology*, 38, 589–632.

Dunlap, E. E., Hodell, E. C., Golding, J. M. & Wasarhaley, N. E. (2012). Mock jurors' perceptions of stalking: The impact of gender and expressed fear. *Sex Roles, 66*, 405–417.

Duntley, J. D. & Buss, D. M. (2012). The evolution of stalking. *Sex Roles*, 66, 311–327.

Durlauf, S. N. & Nagin, D. S. (2011). Imprisonment and crime: can both be reduced? *Criminology & Public Policy*, 10, 13–54.

Durston, G. (2011). *Evidence: Text and Materials*. 2nd edition. Oxford: Oxford University Press.

Dutton, D. G. (2007). *The Psychology of Genocide, Massacres, and Extreme Violence: Why "Normal" People Come to Commit Atrocities*. Westport, CT: Praeger Security International.

Dutton, D. G., Boyanowsky, E. O. & Bond, M. H. (2005). Extreme mass homicide: From military massacre to genocide. *Aggression and Violent Behavior*, 10, 437–473.

Dutton, D. G., White, K. R. & Fogarty, D. (2013). Paranoid thinking in mass shooters. *Aggression and Violent Behavior*, 18, 548–553.

Dutton, M. A. & Goodman, L. A. (2005). Coercion in intimate partner violence: Toward a new conceptualization. *Sex Roles*, 52, 743–756.

Dvoskin, J. A., Skeem, J. L., Novaco, R. W. & Douglas, K. S. (eds.) (2012). *Using Social Science to Reduce Violent Offending*. New York, NY: Oxford University Press.

Dwyer, C. A. (1996). Cut scores and testing: statistics, judgment, truth and error. *Psychological Assessment*, 8, 360–362.

Dyer, C. (2011). UK Supreme Court abolishes immunity for expert witnesses. *British Medical Journal*. Doi: 10.1136/bmj.d2096.

E

Eades, D. (1995). *Language in Evidence.* Sydney: University of New South Wales Press.

Eastman, N. (2000). Psycho-legal studies as an interface discipline. In J. McGuire, T. Mason & A. O'Kane (eds.) *Behaviour, Crime and Legal Processes: A Guide for Forensic Practitioners.* pp. 83–110. Chichester: Wiley.

Eaton, T. E., Ball, P. J., & O'Callaghan, M. G. (2001). Child-witness and defendant credibility: Child evidence presentation mode and judicial instructions. *Journal of Applied Social Psychology*, 31, 1845–1858.

Eckhardt, C. I., Samper, R. E. & Murphy, C. M. (2008). Anger disturbances among perpetrators of intimate partner violence: Clinical characteristics and outcomes of court-mandated treatment. *Journal of Interpersonal Violence*, 23, 1600–1617.

Eddy, J. M., Leve, L. D. & Fagot, B. I. (2001). Coercive family processes: A replication and extension of Patterson's coercion model. *Aggressive Behavior*, 27, 14–25.

Edelstein, L. (1943). *The Hippocratic Oath: Text, Translation, and Interpretation*. Baltimore: Johns Hopkins Press.

Edens, J. F., Marcus, D. K., Lilienfeld, S. O. & Poythress, N. G. (2006). Psychopathic, not psychopath: taxometric evidence for the dimensional structure of psychopathy. *Journal of Abnormal Psychology*, 115, 131–144.

Egg, R., Pearson, F. S., Cleland, C. M. & Lipton, D. S. (2000). Evaluations of correctional treatment programs in Germany: A review and meta-analysis. *Substance Use and Misuse*, 35, 1967–2009.

Egger, S. (1984). A working definition of serial murder and the reduction of linkage blindness. *Journal of Police Science and Administration*, 12, 348-357.

Eher, R. & Pfäfflin, F. (2011). Adult sexual offender treatment – is it effective? In D. P. Boer, R. Eher, L. A. Craig, M. H. Miner & F. Pfäfflin (eds.), *International Perspectives on the Assessment and Treatment of Sexual Offenders: Theory, Practice and Research*. pp. 3–12. Chichester: Wiley-Blackwell.

Ehrlich, I. (1975). The deterrent effect of capital punishment: A question of life and death. *American Economic Review*, 65, 397–417.

Eisenberg, T., Hannaford-Agor, P. L., Hans, V. P., Waters, N. L., Munsterman, G. T., Schwab, S. J. & Wells, M. T. (2005). Judge-jury agreement in criminal cases: A partial replication of Kalven and Zeisel's The American Jury. *Journal of Empirical Legal Studies*, 2, 171–206.

Eisner, M. (2003). Long-term historical trends in violent crime. *Crime and Justice*, 30, 83–142.

Eklund, J. M. & Klinteberg, B. A. (2003). Childhood behaviour as related to subsequent drinking offences and violent offending: a prospective study of 11- to 14-year-old youths into their fourth decade. *Criminal Behaviour and Mental Health*, 13, 294–309.

Ekman, P. (2003). *Emotions Revealed: Understanding Faces and Feelings*. London: Weidenfeld and Nicholson.

Elbogen, E. B. & Johnson, S. C. (2009). The intricate link between violence and mental disorder: Results from the national epidemiologic survey on alcohol and related conditions. *Archives of General Psychiatry*, 66, 152–161.

Elias, N. (2000). *The Civilizing Process: Sociogenetic and Psychogenetic Investigations.* Revised edition edited by E. Dunning, J. Goudsblom & S. Mennell. Oxford: Blackwell.

Elisha, E., Idisis, Y., Timor, U. & Addad, M. (2010). Typology of intimate partner homicide: Personal, interpersonal and environmental characteristics of men who murdered their female intimate partner. *International Journal of Offender Therapy and Comparatve Criminology*, 54, 494–516.

Ellingson, L. (2003). Interdisciplinary health care teamwork in the clinic backstage. *Applied Communication Research,* 31, 93–117.

Elliott, D. S., Huizinga, D. & Morse, B. J. (1986). Self-reported violent offending: a descriptive analysis of juvenile offenders and their offending careers. *Journal of Interpersonal Violence*, 1, 472–514.

Elliott, I. A. & Beech, A. R. (2009). Understanding online child pornography use: Applying sexual offender theory to internet offenders. *Aggression and Violent Behavior*, 14, 180–193.

Ellis, L. (1988). The victimful-victimless crime distinction, and seven universal demographic correlates of victimful criminal behavior. *Personality and Individual Differences*, 9, 525–548.

Ellis, L. (1991). Monoamine oxidase and criminality: identifying an apparent biological marker for antisocial behaviour. *Journal of Research in Crime and Delinquency*, 28, 227–251.

Ellis, L., Beaver, K. & Wright, J. (2009). *Handbook of Crime Correlates*. Amsterdam: Academic Press.

Ellis, L. & McDonald, J. N. (2001). Crime, delinquency, and social status: a reconsideration. *Journal of Offender Rehabilitation*, 32, 23–52.

Ellis, L. & Walsh, A. (1997). Gene-based evolutionary theories in criminology. *Criminology*, 35, 229–276.

Ellis, P. D. (2010). *The Essential Guide to Effect Sizes: Statistical Power, Meta-Analysis, and the Interpretation of Research Results*. Cambridge: Cambridge University Press.

Ellison, L. (2001). The mosaic art? Cross-examination and the vulnerable witness. *Legal Studies,* 21, 353–375.

Ellison, L. & Munro, V. E. (2010). Getting to (not) guilty: examining jurors' deliberative processes in, and beyond, the context of mock rape trial. *Legal Studies,* 30, 74–97.

Ellsworth, P. C., Carlsmith, J. M. & Henson, A. (1972). The stare as a stimulus to flight in human subjects: a series of field experiments. *Journal of Personality and Social Psychology*, 21, 302–311.

Elsegood, K. J. & Duff, S. C. (2010). Theory of mind in men who have sexually offended against children: a U.K. comparison study between child sex offenders and non-offender controls. *Sexual Abuse: A Journal of Research and Treatment,* 22, 112–131.

Emerick, R. L., & Dutton, W. A. (1993). The effect of polygraphy on the self-report of adolescent sex offenders: Implications for risk assessment. *Annals of Sex Research,* 6, 83–103.

Endrass, J., Urbaniok, F., Hammermeister, L.C., Benz, C., Elbert, T., Laubacher, A., & Rosseger, A. (2009). The consumption of internet child pornography and violent and sex offending. *BMC Psychiatry, 9*(43). Available from: http://www.biomedcentral.com/1471-244X/9/43

Engdahl, O. (2008). The role of money in economic crime. *British Journal of Criminology*, 48, 154–170.

Erez, E., & Hartley, C. C. (2003). Battered immigrant women and the legal system: A therapeutic jurisprudence perspective. *Western Criminology Review,* 4, 155–169.

Erikson, K. (1966). *Wayward Puritans: A Study in the Sociology of Deviance*. New York, NY: Macmillan.

Eron, L. D. & Huesmann, L. R. (1983). *Stability of aggressive behaviour*. Paper presented at the Biennial Meeting of the Society for Research in Child Development, Detroit.

Eronen, M., Hakola, P. & Tiihonen, J. (1996). Factors associated with homicide recidivism in a 13-year sample of homicide offenders in Finland. *Psychiatric Services*, 47, 403–406.

Esquivel-Santoveña, E. E. & Dixon, L. (2012). Investigating the true rate of physical intimate partner violence: A review of nationally representative surveys. *Aggression and Violent Behavior*, 17, 208–219.

Esquivel-Santoveña, E. E., Lambert, T. L. & Hamel, J. (2013). Partner abuse worldwide. *Partner Abuse*, 4, 6–75.

Estrich, S. (1987). *Real Rape*. Cambridge, MA: Harvard University Press.

European Commission (1998). *Sexual harassment in the workplace in the European Union*. Strasbourg: Directorate-General for Employment, Industrial Relations and Social Affairs.

Evensen, J., Røssberg, J. I., Barder, H., Haahr, U., Hegelstad, W. t. V., Hoa, I., Johannessen, J. O., Larsen, T. K., Melle, I., Opjordsmoen, S., Rund, B. R., Simonse, E., Vaglum, P., McGlashan, T. & Friis, S. (2012). Flat affect and social functioning: A 10 year follow-up study of first episode psychosis patents. *Schizophrenia Research*, 139, 99–104.

EWCA Crim 1, [2004] 1 WLR 2607.

EWCA Crim 1020, [2003] 2 FCR 447 (second appeal).

Exum, M. L. (2006). Alcohol and aggression: An integration of findings from experimental studies. *Journal of Criminal Justice*, 34, 131–145.

Eysenck, H. J. (1977). *Crime and Personality*. 3rd edition. London: Routledge and Kegan Paul.

Ezekiel, R. S. (2002). An ethnographer looks at neo-Nazi and Klan groups: The racist mind revisited. *American Behavioral Scientist*, 46, 51–71.

Ezzati, M. & Lopez, A. D. (2003). Estimates of global mortality attributable to smoking in 2000. *Lancet*, 362, 847–852.

F

Faigman, D. L. & Monahan, J. (2005). Psychological evidence at the dawn of the law's scientific age. *Annual Review of Psychology*, 56, 631–659.

Falshaw, L., Friendship, C. & Bates, A. (2003). *Sexual offenders – measuring reconviction, reoffending and recidivism*. Findings 183. London: Home Office Research, Development and Statistics Directorate.

Fals-Stewart, W. (2003). The occurrence of partner physical aggression on days of alcohol consumption: A longitudinal diary study. *Journal of Consulting and Clinical Psychology*, 71, 41–52.

Fajnzylber, P., Lederman, D. & Loayza, N. (2002). Inequality and violent crime. *Journal of Law and Economics*, XLV, 1–40.

Falk, A., Kuhn, A. & Zweimüller, J. (2011). Unemployment and right-wing extremist crime. *Scandinavian Journal of Economics*, 113, 260–285.

Farber, I. (1963). The things people say to themselves. *American Psychologist*, 18, 185–197.

Farrington, D. P. (1996). The explanation and prevention of youthful offending. In J. D. Hawkins (ed.) *Delinquency and Crime: Current Theories*. Cambridge: Cambridge University Press.

Farrington, D. P. (2006). Key longitudinal-experimental studies in criminology. *Journal of Experimental Criminology*, 2, 121–141.

Farrington, D. P. (2007). Childhood risk factors and risk-focused prevention. In M. Maguire, R. Morgan, & R. Reiner (eds.), *The Oxford Handbook of Criminology*. pp. 602–640. 4th edition. Oxford: Oxford University Press.

Farrington, D. P. & Loeber, R. (2011a). Early risk factors for convicted homicide offenders and homicide arrestees. In R. Loeber & D. P. Farrington (eds.), *Young Homicide Offenders and Victims: Risk Factors, Prediction, and Prevention from Childhood*. pp. 57–77. New York, NY: Springer.

Farrington, D. P. & Loeber, R. (2011b). Prediction of homicide offenders out of violent boys. In R. Loeber & D. P. Farrington (eds.), *Young Homicide Offenders and Victims: Risk Factors, Prediction, and Prevention from Childhood*. pp. 79–94. New York, NY: Springer.

Farrington, D. P. & Ttofi, M. M. (2011). Bullying as a predictor of offending, violence and later life outcomes. *Criminal Behaviour and Mental Health*, 21, 90–98.

Farrington, D. P., Jolliffe, D. & Johnstone, L. (2008). *Assessing Violence Risk: A Framework for Practice*. Paisley: Risk Management Authority.

Farrington, D. P., Langan, P. A. & Tonry, M. (eds.) (2004). *Cross-National Studies in Crime and Justice*. NCJ200988. Washington, DC: Bureau of Justice Statistics, US Department of Justice. http://www.ojp.usdoj.gov/bjs

Farrington, D. P., Loeber, R. & Berg, M. T. (2012). Young men who kill: A prospective longitudinal examination from childhood. *Homicide Studies*, 16, 99–128.

Farrington, D. P., Coid, J. W., Harnett, L.M., Jolliffe, D., Soteriou, N., Turner, R. E. & West, D. J. (2006). *Criminal careers up to age 50 and life success up to age 48: new findings from the Cambridge Study in Delinquent Development*. Home Office Research Study 299. 2nd edition. London: Home Office Research, Development and Statistics Directorate.

Farrington, D. P., Jolliffe, D., Loeber, R., Stouthamer-Loeber, M. & Kalb, L. M. (2001). The concentration of offenders in families, and family criminality in the prediction of boys' delinquency. *Journal of Adolescence*, 24, 579–596.

Faust, D. & Ziskin, J. (1988). The expert witness in psychology and psychiatry. *Science*, 241, 31–35.

Fazel, S. & Danesh, J. (2002). Serious mental disorder in 23000 prisoners: a systematic review of 62 surveys. *Lancet*, 359, 545–550.

Fazel, S. & Seewald, K. (2012). Severe mental illness in 33 588 prisoners worldwide: systematic review and meta-regression analysis. *British Journal of Psychiatry*, 200, 364–73.

Fazel, S., Doll, H. & Långström, N. (2008). Mental disorder among adolescents in juvenile detention and correctional facilities: a systematic review and metaregresssion analysis of 25 surveys. *Journal of the American Academy of Child and Adolescent Psychiatry*, 47, 1010–1019.

Fazel, S., Xenitidis, K. & Powell, J. (2008). The prevalence of intellectual disabilities among 12000 prisoners - A systematic review. *International Journal of Law and Psychiatry*, 31, 369–373.

Fazel, S., Singh, J. P., Doll, H. & Grann, M. (2012). Use of risk assessment instruments to predict violence and antisocial behaviour in 73 samples involving 24827 people: systematic review and meta-analysis. *British Medical Journal*, 345, e4692.

Fazel, S., Grann, M., Carlström, E., Lichtenstein, P. & Långström, N. (2009a). Risk factors for violent crime in schizophrenia: A national cohort study of 13,806 patients. *Journal of Clinical Psychiatry*, 70, 362–369.

Fazel, S., Gulati, G., Linsell, L., Geddes, J. R. & Grann. M. (2009b). Schizophrenia and violence: Systematic review and meta-analysis. *PLoS Medicine*, 6: e1000120.

Fazel, S., Långström, N., Hjern, A. Grann, M., & Lichtenstein, P. (2009c). Schizophrenia, substance abuse, and violent crime. *Journal of the American Medical Association*, 301, 2016–2023.

Febres, J., Brasfield, H., Shorey, R. C., Elmquist, J., Ninnemann, A., Schonbrun, Y. C., Temple, J. R., Recupero, P. R. & Stuart, G. L. (2014). Adulthood animal abuse among men arrested for domestic violence. *Violence Against Women*, 20, 1059–1077.

Feder, L. & Wilson, D. B. (2005). A meta-analytic review of court-mandated batterer intervention programs: Can courts affect abusers' behaviour? *Journal of Experimental Criminology*, 1, 239–262.

Feeley, D. (2006). Personality, environment, and the causes of white-collar crime. *Law and Psychology Review*, 30, 201–213,

Feigenson, N. (2010). Emotional influences on judgments of legal blame: How they happen, whether they should, and what to do about it. In B. H. Bornstein & R. L. Wiener (eds.), *Emotion and the law: Psychological perspectives*. pp. 45–96. New York, NY: Springer.

Feiring, C., Taska, L., & Lewis, M. (1999). Age and gender differences in children's and adolescents' adaption to sexual abuse. *Child Abuse & Neglect*, 23, 115–128.

Feldmeyer, B. & Steffensmeier, D. (2012). Patterns and trends in elder homicide across race and ethnicity, 1985-2009. *Homicide Studies*, 17, 204–223.

Felson, M. & Boba, R. L. (2010). *Crime and Everyday Life*. 4th edition. Thousand Oaks, CA: Sage.

Felson, M., & Cohen, L. E. (1980). Human ecology and crime: A routine activity approach. *Human Ecology*, 8, 389–405.

Felson, R. B. & Lane, K. J. (2010). Does violence involving women and intimate partners have a special etiology? *Criminology*, 48, 321–338.

Felson, R. B. & Messner, S. F. (1998). Disentangling the effects of gender and intimacy on victim precipitation in homicide. *Criminology*, 36, 405–423.

Felson, R. B. & Staff, J. (2010). The effects of alcohol intoxication on violent versus other offending. *Criminal Justice and Behavior*, 37, 1343–1360.

Felson, R. B. & Steadman, H. J. (1983). Situational factors in disputes leading to criminal violence. *Criminology*, 21, 59–74.

Fennell, P. (2010). Mental health law: history, policy, and regulation. In L. Gostin, P. Bartlett, P. Fennell, J. McHale & R. Mackay (eds.) *Principles of Mental Health Law and Policy*. pp. 3–70. Oxford: Oxford University Press.

Feresin, E. (2009). Lighter sentence for murderer with 'bad genes'. *Nature*, 30 October. Doi: 10.1038/news.2009.1050

Fergusson, D. M., Horwood, L. J. & Nagin, D. S. (2000). Offending trajectories in a New Zealand birth cohort. *Criminology*, 38, 525–552.

Fessler, D. M. T. (2006). A burning desire: Steps toward an evolutionary psychology of fire learning. *Journal of Cognition and Culture*, 6, 429–451.

Field, H. E. (1932). The psychology of crime: II: the place of psychology in the treatment of delinquents. *British Journal of Medical Psychology*, 12, 241–256.

Field, M., Wiers, R. W., Christiansen, P., Fillmore, M. T. & Verster, J. C. (2010). Acute alcohol effects on inhibitory control and implicit cognition: Implications for loss of control over drinking. *Alcoholism: Clinical and Experimental Research*, 34, 1346–1352.

Finch, E. & Munro, V.E. (2006). Breaking boundaries? Sexual consent in the jury room. *Legal Studies,* 26, 303–320.

Fineman, K. R. (1995). A model for the qualitative analysis of child and adult fire deviant behavior. *American Journal of Forensic Psychology*, 13, 31–60.

Finkelhor, D. (1984). *Child Sexual Abuse: New Theory and Research*. New York, NY: Free Press.

Finkelhor, D. & Araji, S. (1986). Explanations of pedophilia: A four factor model. *Journal of Sex Research*, 22, 145–161.

Finkelhor, D. & Browne, A. (1985). The traumatic impact of child sexual abuse: A conceptualization. *American Journal of Orthopsychiatry*, 55, 530–541.

Finkelhor, D., Ormrod, R. K. & Turner. H. A. (2007). Polyvictimization and trauma in a national longitudinal cohort. *Development and Psychopathology*, 19, 149–166.

Finkelhor, D., Ormrod, R. K. & Turner. H. A. (2009). Lifetime assessment of poly-victimization in a national sample of children and youth. *Child Abuse & Neglect*, 33, 403–411.

Finlay, W. M. L. & Lyons, E. (2001). Methodological issues in interviewing and using self-report questionnaires with people with mental retardation. *Psychological Assessment*, 13, 319–335.

Finney, A. (2003). *Alcohol and sexual violence: key findings from the research*. Home Office Findings No. 215. London: Home Office Research Development and Statistics Directorate.

Finney, A. (2004a). *Violence in the night-time economy: key findings from the research*. Findings 214. London: Home Office Research Development and Statistics Directorate.

Finney, A. (2004b). *Alcohol and intimate partner violence: Key findings from the research*. Findings 216. London: Home Office Research Development and Statistics Directorate.

Fischer, J. M. & Ravizza, M. (1988). *Responsbility and Control: A Theory of Moral Responsibility*. Cambridge: Cambridge University Press.

Fisher, B. S., Daigle, L. E., Cullen, F. T., & Turner, M. G. (2003). Reporting sexual victimization to the police and others: Results from a national-level study of college women. *Criminal Justice and Behavior,* 30, 6–38.

Fisher, C. B. (2003). *Decoding the Ethics Code: A Practical Guide for Psychologists.* Thousand Oaks, CA: Sage.

Fisher, R. & Geiselman, R. (1992). *Memory-enhancing techniques for investigative interviewing: The Cognitive Interview*. Springfield, IL: Charles C. Thomas.

Fisher, R., Geiselman, R. & Amador, M. (1989). Field test of the cognitive interview: Enhancing the recollection of actual victims and witnesses of crime. *Journal of Applied Psychology*, 74, 722–727.

Fitzmaurice, C. & Pease, K. (1986). *The Psychology of Judicial Sentencing*. Manchester: Manchester University Press.

Flannery, D. J., Williams, L. L. & Vazsonyi, A. T. (1999). Who are they with and what are they doing? Delinquent behavior, substance use, and early adolescents' after-school time. *American Journal of Orthopsychiatry*, 69, 247–253.

Flood-Page, C., Campbell, S., Harrington, V. & Miller, J. (2000). *Youth crime: Findings from the 1998/99 Youth Lifestyles Survey*. Home Office Research Study 209. London: Home Office Research, Development and Statistics Directorate.

Flynn, S., Swinson, N., While, D., Hunt, I. M., Roscoe, A., Rodway, C., Windfuhr, K., Kapur, N., Appleby, L. & Shaw, J. (2009). Homicide followed by suicide; a cross-sectional study. *Journal of Forensic Psychiatry & Psychology*, 20, 306–321.

Folkes v Chadd (1782) 3 Doug KB 157.

Follette, W. C. & Bonow, J. T. (2009). The challenge of understanding process in clinical behaviour analysis: The case of functional analytic psychotherapy. *The Behavior Analyst, 32,* 135–148.

Fontaine, R. G. (2007). Disentangling the psychology and law of instrumental and reactive subtypes of aggression. *Psychology, Public Policy, and Law*, 13, 143–165.

Foran, H. M. & O'Leary, K. D. (2008). Alcohol and intimate partner violence: A meta-analytic review. *Clinical Psychology Review*, 28, 1222–1234.

Forbes, G. B., Adams-Curtis, L. E., Pakalka, A. H. & White, K. B. (2006). Dating aggression, sexual coercion, and aggression-supporting attitudes among college men as a function of participation in aggressive high school sports. *Violence Against Women*, 12, 441–455.

Forde, D. R. & Kennedy, L. W. (1997). Risky lifestyles, routine activities, and the general theory of crime. *Justice Quarterly*, 14, 265–294.

Forsyth, A. J. M. (2001). Distorted? A quantitative exploration of drug fatality reports in the popular press. *International Journal of Drug Policy*, 12, 435–453.

Foster, J. H. & Ferguson, C. (2012). Alcohol 'pre-loading': A review of the literature. *Alcohol and Alcoholism*, 49, 213–226.

Foucault, M. (1979). *Discipline and Punish: The Birth of the Prison*. Harmondsworth: Peregrine Books.

Fox, J. A. & DeLateur, M. J. (2014). Mass shootings in America: Moving beyond Newtown. *Homicide Studies*, 18, 125–145.

Fox, J. A. & Levin, J. (2012). *Extreme Killing: Understanding Serial and Mass Murder*. 2nd edition. Thousand Oaks, CA: Sage.

Fox, J. A. & Piquero, A. R. (2003). Deadly demographics: Population characteristics and forecasting homicide trends. *Crime and Delinquency*, 49, 339–359.

Fox, K. A. & Allen, T. (2014). Examining the instrumental-expressive continuum of homicides: incorporating the effects of gender, victim-offender relationships, and weapon choice. *Homicide Studies*, 18, 298–317.

Fox, K. A., Nobles, M. R. & Akers, R. L. (2010). Is stalking a learned phenomenon? An empirical test of social learning theory. *Journal of Criminal Justice*, 39, 39–47.

FRA (European Union Agency for Fundamental Rights) (2014a). *Hate Crime in the European Union*. Vienna: FRA.

FRA (European Union Agency for Fundamental Rights) (2014b). *Violence against women: an EU-wide survey: Main results*. Luxembourg: Publications Office of the European Union.

Frances, A. (2013). *Saving Normal: An Insider's Revolt Against Out-of-Control Psychiatric Diagnosis, DSM-5, Big Pharma, and the Medicalization of Ordinary Life.* New York, NY: HarperCollins.

Frances, A. J. & Widiger, T. (2012). Psychiatric diagnosis: lessons from the DSM-IV past and cautions for the DSM-5 future. *Annual Review of Clinical Psychology*, 8, 109–130.

Francis, B., Soothill, K. & Dittrich, R. (2001). A new approach for ranking 'serious' offences: The use of paired-comparisons methodology. *British Journal of Criminology*, 41, 726–737.

Frazier, S. N. & Vela, J. (2014). Dialectical behaviour therapy for the treatment of anger and aggressive behaviour: A review. *Aggression and Violent Behavior*, 19, 156–163.

Freckelton, I. (2003). Mental health review tribunal decision-making: A therapeutic jurisprudence lens. *Psychiatry, Psychology and Law,* 10, 44–62.

Freckelton, I. & Selby, H. (2002). *Expert Evidence: Law, Practice, Procedure and Advocacy*. Sydney: Lawbook Co.

Freeman, D., Garety, P. A., Kuipers, E., Fowler, D., Bebbington, P. E. & Dunn, G. (2007). Acting on persecutory delusions: the importance of safety seeking, *Behaviour Research and Therapy*, 45, 89–99.

Freeman, N. J. (2006). Socioeconomic status and belief in a just world: Sentencing of criminal defendants. *Journal of Applied Social Psychology*. 36, 2379–2394.

Freeman-Longo, R. (1996). Prevention or problem? *Sexual Abuse: A Journal of Research and Treatment,* 8, 91–100.

Frenda, S. J., Nichols, R. M., & Loftus, E. F. (2011). Current issues and advances in misinformation research. *Current Directions in Psychological Science*, 20, 20–23.

Freshwater, K. & Aldridge, J. (1994). The knowledge and fears about court of child witnesses, schoolchildren and adults. *Child Abuse Review,* 3, 183–195.

Freund, K. (1976). Diagnosis and treatment of forensically significant anomalous erotic preferences. *Canadian Journal of Criminology and Corrections,* 18, 181–189.

Frick, P. J. Hare, R. D. (2001) *Antisocial Process Screening Device*. Toronto: Multi-Health Systems.

Friedman, S. H., Horwitz, S. M. & Resnick, P. J. (2005). Child murder by mothers: A critical analysis of the current state of knowledge and a research agenda. *American Journal of Psychiatry*, 162, 1578–1587.

Friedman, S. H., Hrouda, D. R., Holden, C. E., Noffsinger, S. G. & Resnick, P. J. (2005). Filicide-suicide: Common factors in parents who kill their children and themselves. *Journal of the American Academy of Psychiatry and the Law*, 33, 496–504.

Friendship, C., Mann, R. E. & Beech, A. R. (2003). Evaluation of a national prison-based treatment programme for sexual offenders in England and Wales. *Journal of Interpersonal Violence*, 18, 744–759.

Friendship, C. Blud, L., Erikson, M. & Travers, R. (2002). *An evaluation of cognitive-behavioural treatment for prisoners*. Findings 161. London: Home Office Research, Development and Statistics Directorate.

Friendship, C., McClintock, S., Rutter, S. & Maden. T. (1999). Re-offending: patients discharged from a Regional Secure Unit. *Criminal Behaviour and Mental Health*, 9, 226–236.

Frisher, M., Croime, I., Macleod, J., Bloor, R. & Hickman, M. (2007). *Predictive factors for illicit drug use among young people: a literature review*. Home Office Online Report 05/07. London: Home Office.

Fritzon, K. (2001). An examination of the relationship between distance travelled and motivational aspects of firesetting behaviour. *Journal of Environmental Psychology,* 21, 45–60.

Fry, D. P. (2011). Human nature: The nomadic forager model. In R. W. Sussman & C. R. Cloninger (eds.), *Origins of Altruism and Cooperation*. pp. 227–247. New York, NY: Springer.

Furnham, A., Richards, S. C. & Paulhus, D. L. (2013). The dark triad of personality: A 10 year review. *Social and Personality Psychology Compass*, 7, 199–216.

G

Gaes, G. G. (1998). Correctional treatment. In M. Tonry (ed.), *The Handbook of Crime and Punishment*. Oxford: Oxford University Press.

Gaes, G. G. & Camp, S. D. (2009). Unintended consequences: experimental evidence for the criminogenic effect of prison security level placement on post-release recidivism. *Journal of Experimental Criminology*, 5, 139–162.

Gage, E. A. (2008). Gender attitudes and sexual behaviors: Comparing center and marginal athletes and nonathletes in a collegiate setting. *Violence Against Women*, 14, 1014–1032.

Gallagher, C. A., Wilson, D. B., Hirschfield, P., Coggeshall, M. B. & MacKenzie, D. L. (1999). A quantitative review of the effects of sexual offender treatment on sexual reoffending. *Corrections Management Quarterly*, 3, 19–29.

Galton, F. (1870, republished 1965). Hereditary genius: An inquiry into its laws and consequences. In A. Anastasi (ed.), *Individual Differences*. pp. 239–248. New York, NY: Wiley.

Galton, F. (1877). Address. *Nature, 16,* 344–347.

Galton, F. (1883). *Inquiries into Human Faculty and its Development.* London: Dent & Dutton.

Gannon, T. A. (2009). Social cognition in violent and sexual offending: An overview. *Psychology, Crime & Law*, 15, 97–118.

Gannon, T. A. (2016). Explanations of firesetting: typologies and theories. In R. M. Doley, G. L. Dickens & T. A. Gannon (eds.), *The Psychology of Arson: A Practical Guide to Understanding and Managing Deliberate Firesetters*. pp. 13–27. Abingdon: Routledge.

Gannon, T. A. & Polaschek, D. L. L. (2006). Cognitive disstorions in child molesters: A re-examination of key theories and research. *Clinical Psychology Review*, 26, 1000–1019.

Gannon, T. A., Beech, A. R. & Ward, T. (2008). Does the polygraph lead to a better risk prediction for sexual offenders? *Aggression and Violent Behavior*, 13, 29–44.

Gannon, T. A., Ó Ciardha, C., Doley, R. M. & Alleyne, E. (2012). The multi-trajectory theory of adult firsesetting (M-TTAF). *Aggression and Violent Behavior*, 17, 107–121.

Gannon, T. A., Rose, M. R. & Ward, T. (2008). A descriptive model of the offense process for female sexual offenders. *Sexual Abuse: A Journal of Research and Treatment*, 20, 352–374.

Gannon, T. A., Ward, T., Beech, A. R. & Fisher, D. (eds.) (2007). *Aggressive Offenders' Cognition: Theory, Research and Practice*. Chichester: Wiley.

Gannon, T. A., Wood, J. L., Pina, A., Tyler, N., Barnoux, M. F. L. & Vasquez, E. A. (2013). An evaluation of mandatory polygraph testing for sexual offenders in the United Kingdom. *Sexual Abuse: A Journal of Research and Treatment*, 26, 178–203

Garcia-Bajos, E. & Migueles, M. (2003). False memories for script actions in a mugging account. *European Journal of Cognitive Psychology*, 15, 195–208.

García-Moreno, C., Pallitto, C., Devries, K., Stöcki, H., Watts, C. & Abrahams, N. (2013). *Global and regional estimates of violence against women: prevalence and health effects of intimate partner violence and non-partner sexual violence*. Geneva: World Health Organization.

García-Moreno, C., Zimmerman, C., Morris-Gehring, Heise, L., Amin, A., Abrahams, N., Montoya, O., Bhate-Doesthali, P., Kilonzo, N. & Watts, C. (2015). Addressing violence against women: a call to action. *Lancet*, 385, 1685–1695.

Gardner, W., Lidz, C. W., Mulvey, E. P., & Shaw, E. C. (1996). Clinical versus actuarial predictions of violence in patients with mental illness. *Journal of Consulting and Clinical Psychology*, 64, 602–609.

Garland, D. (1990). *Punishment and Modern Society*. Oxford: Clarendon Press.

Garrett, C. G. (1985). Effects of residential treatment on adjudicated delinquents: A meta-analysis. *Journal of Research in Crime and Delinquency*, 22, 287–308.

Garside, R. (2006). Right for the wrong reasons: making sense of criminal justice failure. In R. Garside and W. McMahon (eds.), *Does Criminal Justice Work? The 'Right for the wrong reasons' debate*. pp. 9–39. London: Crime and Society Foundation.

Gavin, H. (2005). The social construction of the child sex offender explored by narrative. *The Qualitative Report*, 10, 395–413.

Geis, G. (2000). On the absence of self-control as the basis for a general theory of crime: a critique. *Theoretical Criminology*, 4, 35–53.

Geis, G. & Goff, C. (1983). Introduction. E. H. Sutherland: *White Collar Crime: The Uncut Version*. New Haven, CT: Yale University Press.

Gendreau, P. (1996). The principles of effective intervention with offenders. In A. T. Harland (ed.), *Choosing Correctional Options That Work: Defining the Demand and Evaluating the Supply*. pp. 117–230. Thousand Oaks, CA: Sage.

Gendreau, P., Goggin, C. & Cullen, F. T. (1999). *The Effects of Prison Sentences on Recidivism*. Report to the Corrections Research and Development and Aboriginal Policy Branch. Ottawa: Solicitor General of Canada.

Gendreau, P., Goggin, C. & Smith, P. (1999). The forgotten issue in effective correctional treatment: program implementation. *International Journal of Offender Therapy and Comparative Criminology*, 43, 180–187.

Gendreau, P., Little, T. & Goggin, C. (1996). A meta-analysis of the predictors of adult offender recidivism: What works! *Criminology*, 34, 575–607.

Gendreau, P., Goggin, C., Cullen, F. T. & Andrews, D. A. (2001). The effects of community sanctions and incarceration on recidivism. In L. L. Motiuk & R. C. Serin (Eds.), *Compendium 2000 on Effective Correctional Programming*. pp. 18–26. Ottawa: Correctional Services Canada.

Gerstenfeld, P. B. (2013). *Hate Crimes: Causes, Controls, and Controversies*. Thousand Oaks, CA: Sage.

Giancola, P. R. (2006). Influence of subjective intoxication, breath alcohol concentration, and expectancies on the alcohol-aggression relationship. *Alcoholism, Clinical and Experimental Research*, 30, 844–850.

Giancola, P. R., Josephs, R. A., Parrott, D. J. & Duke, A. A. (2010). Alcohol myopia revisited: clarifying aggression and other acts of disinhibition through a distorted lens. *Perspectives on Psychological Science*, 5, 265–278.

Gibbs, J. P. (1986). Deterrence theory and research. In G. B. Melton (ed.) *The Law as a Behavioral Instrument: Nebraska Symposium on Motivation 1985*. pp. 87–130. Lincoln and London: University of Nebraska Press.

Gibbs, W. W. (2003). The unseen genome: gems among the junk. *Scientific American*, 289, 47–53.

Gibson, C. L. & Krohn. M. D. (eds.) (2013). *Handbook of Life-Course Criminology: Emerging Trends and Directions for Future Research*. New York, NY: Springer.

Gibson, J. J. (1977). The theory of affordances. In R. E. Shaw & J. Bransford (eds.), *Perceiving, Acting, and Knowing: Toward an Ecological Psychology*. pp. 67–82. Hillsdale, NJ: Lawrence Erlbaum Associates.

Gilbert, R., Fluke, J., O'Donnell, M., Gonzalez-Izquierdo, A., Brownell, M., Gulliver, P., Janson, S. & Sidebotham, P. (2012). Child maltreatment: variation in trends and policies in six developed countries. *Lancet*, 379, 758–772.

Gilbert, R., Widom, C. S., Browne, K., Fergusson, D., Webb, E. & Janson, S. (2008). Burden and consequences of child maltreatment in high-income countries. *Lancet*, 373, 68–81.

Gilinskiy, Y. (2006). Crime in contemporary Russia. *European Journal of Criminology*, 3, 259–292.

Gill, C. (2016). Community interventions. In D. Weisburd, D. P. Farrington & C. Gill (eds.), *What Works in Crime Prevention and Rehabilitation: Lessons from Systematic Reviews*. pp. 77–109. New York, NY: Springer.

Gilmore, I. & Daube, M (2014). How a minimum unit price for alcohol was scuppered. *British Medical Journal*, 348:g23. Doi: 10.1136/bmj.g23

Gini, G., Pozzoli, T. & Hymel, S. (2014). Moral disengagement among children and youth: A meta-analytic review of links to aggressive behaviour. *Aggressive Behavior*, 40, 56–58.

Glaser, B. (2003). Therapeutic jurisprudence: An ethical paradigm for therapists in sex offender treatment programs. *Western Criminology Review*, 4, 143–154.

Glass, G. V., McGaw, B. & Smith, M. L. (1981). *Meta-analysis in Social Research*. Newbury Park, CA: Sage.

Glenn, A. L. & Raine, A. (2009). Psychopathy and instrumental aggression: Evolutionary, neurobiological, and legal perspectives. *International Journal of Law and Psychiatry*, 32, 253–258.

Glenn, H. P. (2006). Comparative legal families and comparative legal traditions. In M. Reimann & R. Zimmermann (eds.), *The Oxford Handbook of Comparative Law*. pp. 421–440. Oxford: Oxford University Press.

Global Terrorism Index (2016). *Measuring and Understanding the Impact of Terrorism*. Institute for Economics and Peace, National Consortium for the Study of Terrorism and Responses to Terrorism, US Department of Homeland Security.

Godwin, G. M. (2008). *Hunting Serial Predators*. 2nd edition. Boston, MA: Jones and Bartlett.

Godwin, G. M. & Rosen, F. (2005). *Tracker: Hunting Down Serial Killers*. New York, NY: Thunder's Mountain Press.

Godwin, M. & Canter, D. (1997). Encounter and death: The spatial behaviour of US serial killers. *Policing: An International Journal of Police Strategies & Management*, 20, 24–38.

Golan, T. (2007). *Laws of men and laws of nature: The history of scientific expert testimony in England and America*. Cambridge, MA: Harvard University Press.

Golding, J. M., Dunlap, E. E. & Hodell, E. C. (2009). Jurors' perceptions of children's eyewitness testimony. In B. L. Bottoms (ed.), *Children as Victims, Witnesses and Offenders: Psychological Science and the Law*. pp188–208. New York, NY: Guilford Press.

Goldstein, A. P. (2002). Low-level aggression: definition, escalation, intervention. In J. McGuire (ed.) *Offender Rehabilitation and Treatment: Effective Programmes and Policies to Reduce Re-Offending*. pp. 169–192. Chichester: Wiley.

Goldstein, A. P., Nensén, R., Daleflod, B. & Kalt, M. (eds.) (2004). *New Perspectives on Aggression Replacement Training*. Chichester: Wiley.

Goldstein, P. J. (1985). The drugs/violence nexus: A tripartite conceptual framework. *Journal of Drugs Isssues*, 39, 143–174.

Goldstein, P. J., Brownstein, H. H., Ryan, P. J. & Bellucci, P. A. (1989). Crack and homicide in New York City, 1988: a conceptually based event analysis. *Contemporary Drug Problems*, 16, 651–687.

Goode, E. (1997). *Deviant Behavior*. 5th edition. Upper Saddle River, NJ: Prentice-Hall.

Goode, E. (ed.) (2008). *Out of Control: Assessing the General Theory of Crime*. Stanford, CA: Stanford University Press.

Goodman, G. S., Golding, J. M. & Haith, M. M. (1984). Jurors' reactions to child witnesses. *Journal of Social Issues*, 40, 139–156.

Goodman, G. S. & Reed, R. S. (1986). Age differences in eyewitness testimony. *Law and Human Behavior*, 10, 317.

Goodman-Delahunty, J. (1997). Forensic psychological expertise in the wake of Daubert. *Law and Human Behavior, 61*, 121–140.

Gornall, J. (2014). Under the influence. *British Medical Journal*, 348:f7646. Doi: 10.1136/bmj.f7646

Gosling, S. D. (2001). From mice to men: what can we learn about personality from animal research? *Psychological Bulletin*, 127, 45–86.

Gossop, M., Trakada, K., Stewart, D. & Witton, J. (2005). Reduction in criminal convictions after addiction treatment: 5-year follow-up. *Drug and Alcohol Dependence*, 79, 295–302.

Gottfredson, M. R. (2008). The empirical status of control theory in criminology. In F. T. Cullen, J. P. Wright & K. R. Blevins (eds.), *Taking Stock: The Status of Criminological Theory*. Advances in Criminological Theory, Volume 15. New Brunswick, NJ: Transaction Publishers.

Gottfredson, S. D. & Moriarty, L. J. (2006). Statistical risk assessment. Old problems and new applications. *Crime and Delinquency*, 52, 178–200.

Gottlieb, G. (1998). Normally occurring environmental and behavioral influences on gene activity from central dogma to probabilistic epigenesist. *Psychological Review*, 105, 792–802.

Gottlieb, G. (2000). Environmental and behavioral influences on gene activity. *Current Directions in Psychological Sciences*, 8, 93–97.

Graduate Institute of International and Development Studies (2007). *Small Arms Survey 2007: Guns and the City*. Geneva: Graduate Institute. http://www.smallarmssurvey.org/publications/by-type/yearbook/small-arms-survey-2007.html

Graham, J. & Bowling, B. (1995). *Young people and crime*. Home Office Research Study 145. London: Home Office Research and Statistics Department.

Graham, K. & West, P. (2001). Alcohol and crime: examining the link. In N. Heather, T. J. Peters & T. Stockwell (eds.), *International Handbook of Alcohol Dependence and Problems*. pp. 439–470. Chichester: Wiley.

Graham, K., Bernards, S., Osgood, D. W. & Wells, S. (2006). Bad nights or bad bars? Multi-level analysis of environmental predictors of aggression in late-night large-capacity bars and clubs. *Addiction*, 101, 1569–1580.

Graham, L. Parkes, T., McAuley, A. & Doi, L. (2012). *Alcohol problems in the criminal justice system: an opportunity for intervention*. Copenhagen: World Health Organization, Regional Office for Europe.

Granhag, P. A., Vrij, A. & Vershuere, B. (2015). *Detecting Deception: Current Challenges and Cognitive Approaches*. Chichester: Wiley.

Granic, I. & Dishion, T. J. (2003). Deviant talk in adolescent friendships: A step toward measuring a pathogenic attractor process. *Social Development*, 12, 314–334.

Granic, I. & Patterson, G. R. (2006). Toward a comprehensive model of antisocial development: A dynamic systems approach. *Psychological Review*, 113, 101–131.

Grasmick, H. G., Tittle, C. R., Bursik, R. J. & Arneklev, B. J. (1993). Testing the core empirical implications of Gottfredson and Hirschi's general theory of crime. *Journal of Research in Crime and Delinquency*, 30, 5–29.

Gray, N. S., MacCulloch, S., Smith, J., Morris, M. & Snowden, R. J. (2003). Violence viewed by psychopathic murderers. *Nature*, 423, 497–498.

Gray, N. S., Snowden, R. J., MacCulloch, S., Phillips, H., Taylor, J. & MacCulloch, M. J. (2004). Relative efficacy of criminological, clinical and personality measures of future risk of offending in mentally disordered offenders: A comparative study of HCR-20, PCL:SV and OGRS. *Journal of Consulting and Clinical Psychology*, 72, 523–530.

Gray, N. S, Taylor, J. & Snowden, R. J. (2008). Predicting violent reconvictions using the HCR–20. *British Journal of Psychiatry*, 192, 384–387.

Grayling, A. C. (2007). *Towards the Light: The Story of the Struggles for Liberty & Rights That Made the Modern West*. London: Bloomsbury Publishing.

Grechenig, K., Nicklisch, A. & Thöni, C. (2010). Punishment despite reasonable doubt – A public goods experiment with sanctions under uncertainty. *Journal of Empirical Legal Studies*, 7, 847–867.

Greenberg, S. A. & Shuman, D. W. (1997). Irreconcilable conflict between therapeutic and forensic roles. *Professional Psychology: Research and Practice, 28*, 50–157.

Greenberg, S. A. & Shuman, D. W. (2007). When worlds collide: Therapeutic and forensic roles. *Professional Psychology: Research and Practice*, 38, 129–132.

Greenberg, S. W., Rohe, W. M. & Williams, J. R. (1982). Safety in urban neighbourhoods: A comparison of physical characteristics and informal territorial control in high and low crime neighbourhoods. *Population and Environment*, 5, 141–165.

Greene, E. & Bornstein, B. (2000). Precious little guidance: Jury instructions on damage awards. *Psychology, Public Policy, and Law*, 6, 743–768.

Greenfield, V. A. & Paoli, L. (2013). A framework to assess the harms of crimes. *British Journal of Criminology*, 53, 864–885.

Gregory, M. (2012). Masculinity and homicide-suicide. *International Journal of Law, Crime and Justice*, 40, 133–151.

Gregory, R. J. (2011). *Psychological Testing: History, Principles, and Applications*. 6th edition. Boston, MA: Allyn and Bacon.

Greve, K. W. & Bianchini, K. J. (2004). Setting empirical cut-offs on psychometric indicators of negative response bias: a methodological commentary with recommendations. *Archives of Clinical Neuropsychology*, 19, 533–541.

Griffin, D. & O'Donnell, I. (2012). The life sentence and parole. *British Journal of Criminology*, 52, 611–629.

Grisso, T. (1986). *Evaluating Competencies: Forensic Assessments and Instruments*. New York, NY: Plenum.

Grisso, T. (1998). *Assessing understanding and appreciation of Miranda Rights: Manual and materials*. Sarasota, FL: Professional Resources.

Groombridge, N. (2006). Pathology. In E. McLaughlin and J. Muncie (eds.), *The Sage Dictionary of Criminology*. 2nd edition. pp. 285-286. London: Sage.

Gross, S. R., Jacoby, K., Matheson, D. J., Montgomery, N., & Patil, S. (2005). Exonerations in the United States 1989 through 2003. *The Journal of Criminal Law and Criminology*, 95, 523–560.

Groth, A. N. & Birnbaum, H. J. (1979). *Men Who Rape: The Psychology of the Offender*. London and New York, NY: Plenum Press.

Groth, A. N., Burgess, A. W. & Holstrom, L. L. (1977). Rape: power, anger and sexuality. *American Journal of Psychiatry*, 134, 1239–1243.

Groth, A. N., Longo, R. E. & McFadin, J. B. (1982). Undetected recidivism among rapists and child molesters. *Crime and Delinquency*, 28, 450–58.

Grove, W. M. & Meehl, P. E. (1996). Comparative efficiency of informal (subjective, impressionistic) and formal (mechanical, algorithmic) prediction procedures. *Psychology, Public Policy and Law*, 2, 293–323.

Groves, N. & Thomas, T. (2014). *Domestic Violence and Criminal Justice*. Abingdon: Routledge.

Grubin, D. (1998). *Sex offending against children: Understanding the risk*. Police Research Series Paper 99. London: Home Office Policing and Reducing Crime Unit.

Grubin, D. (2004). The risk assessment of sex offenders. In H. Kemshall & G. McIvor (Eds.) *Managing Sex Offender Risk*. pp. 91–110. London: Jessica Kingsley.

Grubin, D. (2008). The case for polygraph testing of sex offenders. *Legal and Criminological Psychology*, 13, 177–189.

Grubin, D. (2010). The polygraph and forensic psychiatry. *Journal of the American Academy of Psychiatry and the Law*, 38, 446–451.

Grusec, J. E. & Hastings, P. D. (eds.) (2015). *Handbook of Socialization: Theory and Research*. 2nd edition. New York, NY: Guilford Press.

Guay, J.-P., Ruscio, J., Knight, R. A. & Hare, R. D. (2007). A taxometric analysis of the latent structure of psychopathy: evidence for dimensionality. *Journal of Abnormal Psychology*, 116, 701–716.

Gudjonsson, G. H. (1984). A new scale of interrogative suggestibility. *Personality and Individual Differences*, 5, 303–314.

Gudjonsson, G. H. (2003a). *The Psychology of Interrogations and Confessions: A Handbook*. Chichester: Wiley-Blackwell.

Gudjonsson, G. H. (2003b). Psychology brings justice: the science of forensic psychology. *Criminal Behaviour and Mental Health*, 13, 159–167.

Gudjonsson, G. H. (2006). Disputed confessions and miscarriages of justice in Britain: Expert psychological and psychiatric evidence in court. *The Manitoba Law Journal*, 31, 489–521.

Gudjonsson, G. H. & Haward, L. R. C. (1998). *Forensic Psychology: A Guide to Practice*. London: Routledge.

Gudjonsson, G. H., Sigurdsson, J. F., Young, S., Newton, A. K. & Peersen, M. (2009). Attention Deficit Hyperactivity Disorder (ADHD). How do ADHD symptoms relate to personality among prisoners? *Personality and Individual Differences*, 47, 64–68.

Guerette, R. T. & Bowers, K. J. (2009). Assessing the extent of crime displacement and diffusion of benefits: a review of situational crime prevention evaluations. *Criminology*, 47, 1331–1368.

Guerra, N. G., Tolan, P. H. & Hammond, W. R. (1994). Prevention and treatment of adolescent violence. In L. D. Eron, J. H. Gentry & P. Schlegel (Eds.), *Reason to Hope: A Psychosocial Perspective on Violence and Youth*. pp. 383-403. Washington, DC: American Psychological Association.

Guerrini, I., Quadri, G. & Thomson, A. D. (2014). Genetic and environmental interplay in risky drinking in adolescents: a literature review. *Alcohol and Alcoholism*, 49, 138–142.

Guilaine, J. & Zammit, J. (2005). *The Origins of War: Violence in Prehistory*. Malden, MA: Blackwell Publishing.

Gurian, E. A. (2013). Explanations of mixed-sex partnered homicide: A review of sociological and psychological theory. *Aggression and Violent Behavior*, 18, 520–526.

Guttridge, P., Gabrielli, W. F., Mednick, S. A. & Van Dusen, K. T. (1983). Criminal violence in a birth cohort. In K. T. Van Dusen & S. A. Mednick (eds.) *Prospective Studies of Crime and Delinquency*. pp. 211–224. Hingham, MA: Kluwer Nijhoff.

Guy, L. S., Packer, I. K. & Warnken, W. (2012). Assessing risk of violence using structured professional judgment guidelines. *Journal of Forensic Psychology Practice*, 12, 270–283.

H

Haas, L. J. & Malouf, J. L. (1995). *Keeping Up the Good Work: A Practitioner's Guide to Mental Health Ethics*. Sarasota, FL: Professional Resource Exchange.

Hackett, S., Masson, H., Balfe, M. & Phillips, J. (2013). Individual, family and abuse characteristics of 700 British child and adolescent sexual abusers. *Child Abuse Review*, 22, 232–245.

Haddock, G., Eisner, E., Davies, G., Coupe, N. & Barrowclough, C. (2013). Psychotic symptoms, self-harm and violence in individuals with schizophrenia and substance misuse problems. *Schizophrenia Research*, 151, 215–220.

Haggard-Grann, U., Hallqvist, J., Langström, N. & Möller, J. (2006). The role of alcohol and drugs in triggering criminal violence: a case cross-over study. *Addiction*, 101, 100–108.

Haines, J., Williams, C. L. & Lester, D. (2010). Murder-suicide: A reaction to interpersonal crises, *Forensic Science International*, 202, 93–96.

Hald, G. M., Malamuth, N. M., & Yuen, C. (2010). Pornography and attitudes supporting violence against women: Revisiting the relationship in nonexperimental studies. *Aggressive Behavior,* 36, 14–20.

Hale, V. E. & Strassberg, D. S. (1990). The role of anxiety on sexual arousal. *Archives of Sexual Behavior*, 19, 569–581.

Hall, C., Hogue, T., & Guo, K. (2011). Differential gaze pattern towards sexually preferred and non-preferred human figures. *Journal of Sex Research,* 48, 461–469.

Hall, G. C. N. (1995). Sexual offender recidivism revisited: A meta-analysis of recent treatment studies. *Journal of Consulting and Clinical Psychology*, 63, 802–809.

Hall, N. (2013). *Hate Crime*. 2nd edition. London and New York, NY: Routledge.

Hall, W., Carter, A. & Forline, C. (2015). The brain disease model of addiction: is it supported by the evidence and has it delivered on its promises? *Lancet Psychiatry*, 2, 105–110.

Hämäläinen, M. & Pulkkinen, L. (1995). Aggressive and non-prosocial behaviour as precursors of criminality. *Studies on Crime and Crime Prevention*, 4, 6–20.

Hanawalt, B. A. & Wallace, D. (1998). *Medieval Crime and Social Control*. Minneapolis, MN: University of Minnesota Press.

Handelsman, M. M. (1986). Problems with ethics training by 'osmosis'. *Professional Psychology: Research and Practice,* 17, 371–372.

Haney, C., Banks, W. C. & Zimbardo, P. G. (1973). Interpersonal dynamics in a simulated prison. *International Journal of Criminology and Penology*, 1, 69–97.

Hannah-Moffat, K. (1999). Moral agent or actuarial subject: Risk and Canadian women's imprisonment. *Theoretical Criminology,* 3, 71–94.

Hannawa, A. F., Spitzberg, B. H., Wiering, L. & Teranishi, C. (2006). "If I can't have you, no-one can": Development of a Relational Entitlement and Proprietariness Scale (REPS). *Violence and Victims*, 21, 539–560.

Hanoch, Y., Gummerum, M. & Rolison, J. (2012). Second-to-fourth digit ratio and impulsivity: A comparison between offenders and nonoffenders. *PLoS ONE,* 7, e47140.

Hanson, R. K. (2000). Will they do it again? Predicting sex-offense recidivism. *Current Directions in Psychological Science*, 9, 106–109.

Hanson, R. K. & Bussière, M. (1998). Predicting relapse: a meta-analysis of sexual offender recidivism studies. *Journal of Consulting and Clinical Psychology,* 66, 348–362.

Hanson, R. K & Morton-Bourgon, K. E. (2005). The characteristics of persistent sexual offenders: A meta-analysis of recidivism studies. *Journal of Consulting and Clinical Psychology,* 73, 1154–1163.

Hanson, R. K & Morton-Bourgon, K. E. (2009). The accuracy of recidivism risk assessments for sexual offenders: A meta-analysis of 118 prediction studies. *Psychological Assessment*, 21, 1–21.

Hanson, R. K., Bourgon, G., Helmus, L. & Hodgson, S. (2009). The principles of effective correctional treatment also apply to sexual offenders: A meta-analysis. *Criminal Justice and Behavior*, 36, 865–891.

Hanson, R. K., Harris, A. J. R., Helmus, L. & Thornton, D. (2014). High-risk sex offenders may not be high risk forever. *Journal of Interpersonal Violence*, 29, 2792–2813.

Hanson, R. K., Gordon, A., Harris, A. J. R., Marques, J. K., Murphy, W., Quinsey, V. L. & Seto, M. C. (2002). First report of the Collaborative Outcome Data Project on the effectiveness of psychological treatment for sex offenders. *Sexual Abuse: A Journal of Research and Treatment*, 14, 169–194.

Hare, R. D. (1996). Psychopathy: A clinical construct whose time has come. *Criminal Justice and Behavior*, 23, 25–54.

Hare, R. D. (1999). *Without Conscience: The Disturbing World of the Psychopaths Among Us*. New York, NY: Guilford Press.

Hare, R. D. (2003). *Hare Psychopathy Check List-Revised: Technical Manual*. 2nd edition. North Tonawanda, NY: Multi-Health Systems, Inc.

Hare, R. D. & Neumann, C. S. (2008). Psychopathy as a clinical and empirical construct. *Annual Review of Clinical Psychology*, 4, 217–246.

Harenski, C. L., Harenski, K. A., Shane, M. S. & Kiehl, K. A. (2010). Aberrant neural processing of moral violations in criminal psychopaths. *Journal of Abnormal Psychology*, 119, 863–874.

Hargreaves, C. & Francis, B. (2014). The long term recidivism risk of young sexual offenders in England and Wales – enduring risk or redemption? *Journal of Criminal Justice*, 42, 164–172.

Harkins, L. & Beech, A. R. (2007). A review of the factors that can influence the effectiveness of sexual offender treatment: Risk, need, responsivity, and process issues. *Aggression and Violent Behavior*, 12, 615–627.

Harmon, L. D. & Julesz, B. (1973). Masking in visual recognition: Effects of two-dimensional noise. *Science*, 180, 1194–1197.

Harper, C. A. & Hogue, T. E. (2015). The emotional representation of sexual crime in the national British press. *Journal of Language and Social Psychology*, 34, 3–24.

Harper, D. W. & Voigt, L. (2007). Homicide followed by suicide: An integrated theoretical perspective. *Homicide Studies*, 11, 295–318.

Harrendorf, S., Heiskanen, M. & Malby, S. (eds.) (2010). *International Statistics on Crime and Justice*. HEUNI Publication Series No.64. Helsinki and Vienna: European Institute for Crime Prevention and Control & United Nations Office on Drugs and Crime.

Harris, A. J. R. & Hanson, R. K. (2004). *Sex offender recidivism: A simple question*. Ottawa: Public Safety and Emergency Preparedness Canada.

Harris, D. A., Mazerolle, P. & Knight, R. A. (2009). Understanding male sexual offending: A comparison of general and specialist theories. *Criminal Justice and Behavior*, 36, 1051–1069.

Harris, G. T., Rice, M. E. & Cormier, C. A. (1994). Psychopaths: is a therapeutic community therapeutic? *Therapeutic Communities. Special Issue: Therapeutic Communities for offenders*, 15, 283–299.

Harris, G. T., Rice, M. E. & Quinsey, V. L. (1994). Psychopathy as a taxon: Evidence that psychopaths are a discrete class. *Journal of Consulting and Clinical Psychology*, 62, 387–397.

Harris, G. T., Skilling, T. A. & Rice, M. E. (2001).The construct of psychopathy. *Crime and Justice*, 28, 197–264.

Harris, G. T., Rice, M. E., Quinsey, V. L. & Cormier, C. A. (2015). *Violent Offenders: Appraising and Managing Risk*. 3rd edition. Washington, DC: American Psychological Association.

Harrison, M. A. & Bowers, T. G. (2010). Autogenic massacre as a maladaptive response to status threat. *Journal of Forensic Psychiatry & Psychology*, 21, 916–932.

Harrow, M. & Jobe, T. H. (2007). Factors involved in outcome and recovery in schizophrenia patients not on antipsychotic medications: A 15-year multifollow-up study. *Journal of Nervous and Mental Disease*, 195, 406–414.

Hart, D. & Marmorstein, N. R. (2009). Neighborhoods and genes and everything in between: Understanding adolescent aggression in social and biological contexts. *Development and Psychopathology*, 21, 961–973.

Hart, S. D., Michie, C. & Cooke, D. J. (2007). Precision of actuarial risk assessment instruments: Evaluating the 'margins of error' of group v. individual predictions of violence. *British Journal of Psychiatry*, 190, 60–65.

Hart, S., Sturmey, P., Logan, C. & McMurran, M. (2011). Forensic case formulation. *International Journal of Forensic Mental Health*, 10, 118–126.

Hartley, R. D. (2008). *Corporate Crime: A Reference Handbook*. Santa Barbara, CA: ABC-CLIO.

Haskett, M. E., Wayland, K., Hutcheson, J. S., & Tavana, T. (1995). Substantiation of sexual abuse allegations: Factors involved in the decision-making process. *Journal of Child Sexual Abuse*, 4, 19–44.

Haslam, N. (2011). The latent structure of personality and psychopathology: A review of trends in taxometric research. *The Scientific Review of Mental Health Practice*, 8, 17–29.

Haslam, N., Holland, E. & Kuppens, P. (2012). Categories versus dimensions in personality and psychopathology: a quantitative review of taxometric research. *Psychological Medicine*, 42, 903–920.

Haverkamp, B. E. (2005). Ethical perspectives on qualitative research in applied psychology. *Journal of Counseling Psychology*, 52, 146–155.

Haward, L. R. C. (1981). *Forensic Psychology: A Guide to Practice*. London: Routledge.

Hawkins, J. D., Smith, B. H., Kill, K. J., Kosterman, R., Catalano, R. F. & Abbott, R. D. (2003) Understanding and preventing crime and violence: findings from the Seattle Social Development Project. In T. P. Thornberry & M. D. Krohn (eds.) *Taking Stock of Delinquency: An Overview of Findings from Contemporary Longitudinal Studies*. pp. 255–312. New York, NY: Kluwer Academic / Plenum.

Haydock, R. & Sonsteng, J. (1994). *Advocacy*. Eagan, MN: West Publishing Company.

Hayhurst, K. P., Pierce, M., Hickman, M., Seddon, T., Dunn, G., Keane, J. & Millar, T. (2017). Pathways through opiate use and offending: A systematic review. *International Journal of Drug Policy*, 39, 1–13.

Haynes, S. N., O'Brien, W. H. & Kaholokula, J. K. (2011). *Behavioral Assessment and Case Formulation*. New York, NY: Wiley.

Haynie, D. L., Giordano, P. C., Manning, W. D. & Longmore, M. A. (2005). Adolescent romantic relationships and delinquency involvement. *Criminology*, 43, 177–210.

Hazelwood, R. R. (2009). Analyzing the rape and profiling the offender. In R. R. Hazelwood & A. W. Burgess (Eds.), *Practical Aspects of Rape Investigation: A Multidisciplinary Approach*. 4th edition. pp. 97–122. Boca Raton, FL: CRC Press/ Taylor & Francis Group.

Health and Care Professions Council (2008). *Standards of conduct, performance and ethics.* http://www.hpc-uk.org/assets/documents/10002367FINALcopyofSCPEJuly2008.pdf

Health and Care Professions Council (2010). *Guidance on conduct and ethics for students.* http://www.hpc-uk.org/assets/documents/10002C16Guidanceonconductandethicsforstudents.pdf

Heerde, J. A., Hemphill, S. A. & Scholes-Balog, K. E. (2014). 'Fighting' for survival: A systematic review of physically violent behavior perpetrated and experienced by homeless young people *Aggression and Violent Behavior*, 19, 50–66.

Heide, K. M. (2003). Youth homicide: A review of the literature and a blueprint for action. *International Journal of Offender Therapy and Comparative Criminology*, 47, 6–36.

Heide, K. M. (2013). *Understanding Parricide: When Sons and Daughters Kill Parents*. New York, NY: Oxford University Press.

Heide, K. M. & Frei, A. (2010). Matricide: A critique of the literature. *Trauma, Violence, & Abuse*, 11, 3–17.

Heide, K. M. & Petee, T. A. (2007). Parricide: An empirical analysis of 24 years of US data. *Journal of Interpersonal Violence*, 22, 1382–1399.

Heil, P., Ahlmeyer, S. & Simons, D. (2003). Crossover sexual offences. *Sexual Abuse: A Journal of Research and Treatment*, 15, 221–236.

Heise, L. L. (1998). Violence against women: An integrated, ecological framework. *Violence Against Women*, 4, 262–290.

Helfgott, J. B. (2008). *Criminal Behavior: Theories, Typologies, and Criminal Justice*. Thousand Oaks, CA: Sage.

Helmus, L., Hanson, R.K., Babchishin, K. M. & Mann, R. E. (2013). Attitudes supportive of sexual offending predict recidivism: A meta-analysis. *Trauma, Violence, & Abuse*, 14, 34–53.

Henderson, Z., Bruce, V. & Burton, A. M. (2001). Matching the faces of robbers captured on video. *Applied Cognitive Psychology*, 15, 445–464.

Henham, R. (1997). Protective sentences: Ethics, rights and sentencing policy. *International Journal of the Sociology of Law*, 25, 45–63.

Henning, K. R. & Frueh, B. C. (1996). Cognitive-behavioral treatment of incarcerated offenders: An evaluation of the Vermont Department of Corrections' Cognitive Self-Change Program. *Criminal Justice and Behavior*, 23, 523–542.

Henry, S. & Einstadter, W. (eds.) (1998). *The Criminological Theory Reader*. New York, NY: New York University Press.

Henshaw, M., Ogloff, J. R. P. & Clough, J. A. (2015). Looking beyond the screen: A critical review of the literature on the online child pornography offender. *Sexual Abuse: A Journal of Research and Treatment*, 1–30. Doi: 10.1177/1079063215603690

Henwood, K. S., Chou, S. & Browne, K. D. (2015). A systematic review and meta-analysis on the effectiveness of CBT informed anger management. *Aggression and Violent Behavior*, 25, 280–292.

Hepburn, L. M. & Hemenway, D. (2004). Firearm availability and homicide: A review of the literature. *Aggression and Violent Behavior*, 9, 417–440.

Herek, G. M., Gillis, J. R., Cogan, J. C. & Glunt, E. K. (1997). Hate crime victimisation among lesbian, gay, and bisexual adults: Prevalence, psychological correlates, and methodological issues. *Journal of Interpersonal Violence*, 12, 195–215.

Heres, S., Davis, J., Maino, K., Jetzinger, E., Kissling, W. & Leucht, S. (2006). Why Olanzapine beats Risperidone, Risperidone beats Quetiapine, and Quetiapine beats Olanzapine: An exploratory analysis of head-to-head comparison studies of second generation antipsychotics. *American Journal of Psychiatry*, 163, 185–194.

Hernández, P., Engstrom, D. & Gangsei, D. (2010). Exploring the impact of trauma on therapists: Vicarious resilience and related concepts in training. *Journal of Systemic Therapies*, 29, 67–83.

Herrero, J., Torres, A., Fernández-Suárez, A. & Rodríguez-Díaz, F. J. (2016). Generalists versus specialists: Toward a typology of batterers in prison. *The European Journal of Psychology Applied to Legal Context*, 8, 19–26.

Herring, J. (2016). *Criminal Law: Text, Cases and Materials*. 7th edition. Oxford: Oxford University Press.

Hess, A. K. (2006). Defining forensic psychology. In I. B. Weiner & A. K. Hess (eds.), *Handbook of Forensic Psychology*. 3rd edition. pp. 28–58. Hoboken, NJ: Wiley.

Heuer, L. & Penrod, S. (1994). Trial complexity: A field investigation of its meaning and effects. *Law and Human Behavior*, 18, 29–51.

Hewitt, S. K. (1998). *Assessing Allegations of Sexual Abuse in Preschool Children: Understanding Small Voices*. Thousand Oaks, CA: Sage.

Hickey, E. W. (2013). *Serial Murderers and Their Victims*. 6th edition. Belmont, CA: Wadsworth/Cengage Learning.

Hicks, D. C. (2010). Money laundering. In F. Brookman, M. Maguire, H. Pierpoint & T. Bennett (eds.), *Handbook on Crime*. pp. 712–725. Cullompton: Willan.

Hicks, M. M., Rogers, R., & Cashel, M. (2000). Predictions of violent and total infractions among institutionalized male juvenile offenders. *Journal of the American Academy of Psychiatry and the Law*, 28, 183–190.

Hicks, S. J. & Sales, B. D. (2006). *Criminal profiling: Developing an effective science and practice*. Washington, DC: American Psychological Association.

Hillbrand, M. & Cipriano, T. (2007). Commentary: Parricides – unanswered questions, methodological obstacles, and legal considerations. *Journal of the American Academy of Psychiatry and the Law*, 35, 13–16.

Hillbrand, M., Alexandre, J. W., Young, J. L. & Spitz, R. T. (1999). Parricides: Characteristics of offenders and victims, legal factors, and treatment issues. *Aggression and Violent Behavior*, 4, 179–190.

Hillier, B., Burdett, R., Peponis, J. & Penn, A. (1987). Creating life: Or, does architecture determine anything? *Architecture & Behaviour*, 3, 233–250.

Hillyard, P. & Tombs, P. (2008). Beyond criminology? In W. McMahon (ed.), *Criminal Obsessions? Why Harm matters more than Crime*. 2nd edition. pp. 9–23. London: Centre for Crime and Justice Studies, King's College.

Hirsch, J. B., Galinksy, A. D. & Zhong, C.-B. (2011). Drunk, powerful, and in the dark: How general processes of disinhibition produce both prosocial and antisocial behavior. *Perspectives on Psychological Science*, 6, 415–427.

Hirschi, T. (1979). Separate and unequal is better. *Journal of Research in Crime and Delinquency*, 16, 34–38.

Hirschi, T., & Gottfredson, M. R. (1995). Control theory and the life-course perspective. *Studies on Crime and Crime Prevention*, 4, 131–142.

HM Inspectorate of Constabulary (2014). *Everyone's business: Improving the police response to domestic abuse*. London: HMIC. https://www.justiceinspectorates.gov.uk/hmicfrs/wp-content/uploads/2014/04/improving-the-police-response-to-domestic-abuse.pdf

HM Inspectorate of Constabulary (2015). *Increasingly everyone's business: A progress report on the police response to domestic abuse*. London: HMIC.

HM Prison Service (2005). *Offender assessment and sentence management – OASys*. http://www.justice.gov.uk%2Fdownloads%2Foffenders%2Fpsipso%2Fpso%2FPSO_2205_offender_assessment_and_sentence_management.doc&ei=MDf0UJiZHoLJ0AWu44DQBA&usg=AFQjCNH3sK8rvunLtQOhkh-BjlneVAhkcQ&bvm=bv.1357700187,d.d2k

HMSO (1981). *Contempt of Court Act 1981*. Retrieved from http://www.opsi.gov.uk/acts/acts1981/1981o4o.htm

HM Treasury and Home Office (2015). *UK national risk assessment of money laundering and terrorist financing*. Crown copyright.

Ho, D. K. & Ross, C. C. (2012). Editorial: Cognitive behaviour therapy for sex offenders. Too good to be true? *Criminal Behaviour and Mental Health*, 22, 1–6.

Ho, H., Thomson, L. & Darjee, R. (2009). Violence risk assessment: the use of the PCL-SV, HCR-20, and VRAG to predict violence in mentally disordered offenders discharged from a medium secure unit in Scotland. *Journal of Forensic Psychiatry and Psychology*, 20, 523–541.

Hobbs, T. (2010a). Extortion. In F. Brookman, M. Maguire, H. Pierpoint & T. Bennett (eds.), *Handbook on Crime*. pp. 726–737. Cullompton: Willan.

Hobbs, T. (2010b). Stealing commercial cash: from safe-cracking to armed robbery. In F. Brookman, M. Maguire, H. Pierpoint & T. Bennett (eds.), *Handbook on Crime*. pp. 290–307. Cullompton: Willan.

Hoberman, H. M. (2016). Forensic psychotherapy for sexual offenders: has its effectiveness yet been demonstrated? In A. Phenix & H. M. Hoberman (eds.), *Sexual Offending: Predisposing Antecedents, Assessments and Management*. pp. 605–666. New York, NY: Springer.

Hochschild, A. (1998). *King Leopold's Ghost: A Story of Greed, Terror and Heroism in Colonial Africa*. Boston: Mariner Books/Houghton Mifflin Harcourt.

Hochstetler, A., Copes, H. & DeLisi, M. (2002). Differential association in group and solo offending. *Journal of Criminal Justice*, 30, 559–566.

Hockenhull, J. C., Whittington, R., Leitner, M., Barr, W., McGuire, J., Cherry, M. G., et al. (2012). A systematic review of prevention and intervention strategies for populations at high risk of engaging in violent behaviour: update 2002–8. *Health Technology Assessment*, 16 (3).

Hodson, G., Hooper, H., Dovidio, J.F., & Gaertner, S.L. (2005). Aversive racism in Britain: The use of inadmissible evidence in legal decisions. *European Journal of Social Psychology*, 35, 437–448.

Hoeve, M., Dubas, J. S., Eichelsheim, V. I., van der Laan, P. H., Smeenk, W. & Gerris, J. R. M. (2009). The relationship between parenting and delinquency: A meta-analysis. *Journal of Abnormal Child Psychology*, 37, 749–775.

Hoeyer, K. (2009). Informed consent: The making of a ubiquitous rule in medical practice. *Organization*, 16, 267–288.

Holden, R. T. (1986). The contagiousness of aircraft hijacking. *American Journal of Sociology*, 91, 874–904.

Hollin, C. R. (1995). The meaning and implications of program integrity. In J. McGuire (Ed.), *What Works: Reducing Reoffending: Guidelines from Research and Practice*. pp. 195-208. Chichester: Wiley.

Hollin, C. R. (ed.) (2001). *Handbook of Offender Assessment and Treatment*. Chichester: Wiley.

Hollin, C. R. (2006). Offending behaviour programmes and contention: evidence-based practice, manuals, and programme evaluation. In C. R. Hollin & E. J. Palmer (eds.), *Offending Behaviour Programmes: Development, Application, and Controversies*. pp. 33–67. Chichester: Wiley.

Hollin, C. R. (2008). Evaluating offending behaviour programmes: Does only randomization glitter? *Criminology and Criminal Justice*, 8, 89–106.

Hollin, C. R. (2012). Criminological psychology. In M. Maguire, R. Morgan, & R. Reiner (eds.), *The Oxford Handbook of Criminology*. 5th edition. pp. 43–77. Oxford: Oxford University Press.

Hollin, C. R. (2013). *Psychology and Crime*. 2nd edition. Abingdon: Routledge.

Hollin, C. R. & Palmer, E. J. (eds.) (2006). *Offending Behaviour Programmes: Development, Application, and Controversies*. Chichester: Wiley.

Hollin, C. R., McGuire, J., Hatcher, R. M., Bilby, C. A. L., Hounsome, J. & Palmer, E. J. (2008) Cognitive skills offending behavior programs in the community: A reconviction analysis. *Criminal Justice and Behavior*, 34, 269–283.

Hollis, V. (2007). *Reconviction Analysis of Interim Accredited Programmes Software (IAPS) data*. London: Research Development Statistics, National Offender Management Service.

Holloway, K. R. & Bennett, T. H. (2016). Drug interventions. In D. Weisburd, D. P. Farrington and C. Gill (eds.), *What Works in Crime Prevention and Rehabilitation: Lessons from Systematic Reviews*. pp. 219–236. New York, NY: Springer.

Holloway, K., Bennett, T. & Farrington, D. (2005). *The effectiveness of criminal justice and treatment programmes in reducing drug related crime: A systematic review*. Home Office Online report 26/05. London: Home Office.

Holmberg, U. & Christianson, S-Å. (2002). Murderers' and sexual offenders' experiences of police interviews and their inclination to admit or deny crimes. *Behavioral Sciences and the Law*, 20, 31–45.

Holmes, G. (2002). DCP update: Some thoughts on why clinical psychologists should not have formal powers under the new Mental Health Act. *Clinical Psychology*, 12, 40–43.

Holmes, R. M. & Holmes, S. T. (2009). *Profiling Violent Crimes: An investigative tool*. 4th edition. Thousand Oaks, CA: Sage.

Holmes, R. M. & Holmes, S. T. (2010). *Serial Murder*. 3rd edition. Thousand Oaks, CA: Sage.

Homel, R., Carvolth, R., Hauritz, M., McIlwain, G. & Teague, R. (2004). Making licensed venues safer for patrons: what environmental factors should be the focus of interventions? *Drug and Alcohol Review*, 23, 19–29.

Home Office (1993a). *Royal Commission on Criminal Justice Report* (para. 182). London: Her Majesty's Stationery Office.

Home Office (1993b). *Digest 2: Information on the Criminal Justice System in England and Wales*. London: Home Office Research and Statistics Department.

Home Office (1999). *The Stephen Lawrence Inquiry: Report of an Inquiry by Sir William Macpherson of Cluny*. Cm 4262. London: The Stationery Office.

Home Office (2012). *Statistical News Release: Hate Crimes, England and Wales 2011/12*. London: Home Office.

Home Office (2016a). *List of most commonly encountered drugs currently controlled under the misuse of drugs legislation*. London: Home Office.

Home Office (2016b). *Drug Misuse: Findings from the 2015/16 Crime Survey for England and Wales*. 2nd edition. London: Home Office.

Home Office (2016c). *Fire Statistics Monitor: April 2015 to March 2016*. Statistical Bulletin 09/19. London: Home Office.

Home Office/Scottish Executive (2001). *Consultation Paper on the Review of Part 1 of the Sex Offenders Act 1997*. London: HMSO.

Honderich, T. (2006). *Punishment: The Supposed Justifications Revisited*. Revised edition. London: Pluto Press.

Hood, R. & Hoyle, C. (2015). *The Death Penalty: A Worldwide Perspective*. 5th edition. Oxford: Oxford University Press.

Hope, L. & Wright, D. (2007). Beyond unusual? Examining the role of attention in the weapon focus effect. *Applied Cognitive Psychology*, 21, 951–961.

Horney, J. (2001). Criminal events and criminal careers: An integrative approach to the study of violence. In R. F. Meier, L. W. Kennedy & V. F. Sacco (eds.), *The Process and Structure of Crime: Criminal Events and Crime Analysis. Advances in Criminological Theory*, Vol. 9. pp. 141–167. New Brunswick, NJ and London: Transaction Publishers.

Horney, J., Osgood, D. W. & Marshall, I. H. (1995). Criminal careers in the short-term: Intra-individual variability in crime and its relation to local life circumstances. *American Sociological Review*, 60, 655–673.

Horowitz, I. A., Bordens, K. S., Victor, E., Bourgeois, M. J. & ForsterLee, L. (2001). The effects of complexity on jurors' verdicts and construction of evidence. *Journal of Applied Psychology*, 86, 641–652.

Horsley, T. A., de Castro, B. O. & Van der Schoot, M. (2010). In the eye of the beholder: eye-tracking assessment of social information processing in aggressive behavior. *Journal of Abnormal Child Psychology*, 38, 587–599.

Horwitz, A. & Wakefield, J. (2007). *The Loss of Sadness: How Psychiatry Transformed Normal Sorrow into Depressive Disorder*. New York, NY: Oxford University Press.

Hough, M. (2004). Crimes against statistics. *The Guardian*, 14 October.

House, J. C. (1997). Towards a practical application of offender profiling: The RNC's Criminal Suspect Prioritization System. In J. L. Jackson (ed.), *Offender Profiling: Theory, Research and Practice*. pp. 177–190. Chichester: Wiley.

House of Commons (2011). *Committee on Arms Export Controls: First Report*. London: The Stationery Office.

Houtepen, J. A. B. M., Sijtsema, J. J. & Bogaerts, S. (2014). From child pornography offending to child sexual abuse: A review of child pornography offender characteristics and risks for cross-over. *Aggression and Violent Behavior*, 19, 466–473.

Howard, P. D., Barnett, G. D. & Mann, R. E. (2014). Specialization in and within sexual offending in England and Wales. *Sexual Abuse: A Journal of Research and Treatment*, 26, 225–251.

Howard, P., Francis, B., Soothill, K. & Humphreys, I. (2009). *OGRS 3: the revised Offender Group Reconviction Scale*. London: Ministry of Justice. http://www.justice.gov.uk/publications/docs/oasys-research-summary-07-09-ii.pdf

Howells, K. & Day, A. (2003). Readiness for anger management. *Clinical Psychology Review*, 23, 319-337.

Howitt, D. (2015). *Introduction to Forensic and Criminal Psychology*. 5th edition. Harlow: Pearson Education.

Huang, Y., Kotov, R., de Girolamo, G., Preti, A., Angermeyer, M., Benjet, C., Demyttenaere, D., de Graaf, R., Gureje, O., Karam, A. N., Lee, S., Lépine, J. P., Matschinger, H., Posada-Villa, J., Suliman, S., Vilagut, G. & Kessler, R. C. (2009). DSM-IV personality disorders in the WHO World Mental Health Surveys. *British Journal of Psychiatry*, 195, 46–53.

Huesman, L. R., Eron, L. D. & Dubow, E. F. (2002). Childhood predictors of adult criminality: are all risk factors reflected in childhood aggressiveness? *Criminal Behaviour and Mental Health*, 12, 185–208.

Huffman, M. L., Warren, A. R., & Larson, S. M. (1999). Discussing truth and lies in interviews with children: Whether, why, and how? *Applied Developmental Science*, 3, 6–15.

Hughes, B., Parker, H. & Gallagher, B. (1996). *Policing and Sexual Abuse: The View from Police Practitioners*. Police Research Group. London: Home Office.

Hughes, J. R. (2007). Review of medical reports on pedophilia. *Clinical Pediatrics*, 46, 667–682.

Hughes, K., Anderson, Z., Morleo, M. & Bellis, M. A. (2008). Alcohol, nightlife and violence: the relative contributions of drinking before and during nights out to negative health and criminal justice outcomes. *Addiction*, 103, 60–5.

Huizinga, D., Weiher, A. W., Espiritu, E. & Esbensen, F. (2003). Delinquency and crime: some highlights from the Denver Youth Survey. In T. P. Thornberry and M. D. Krohn (eds.) *Taking Stock of Delinquency: An Overview of Findings from Contemporary Longitudinal Studies*. pp. 47–91. New York, NY: Kluwer Academic / Plenum.

Huizinga, D., Haberstsick, B. C., Smolen, A., Menard, S., Young, S. E., Corley, R. P., Stallings, M. C., Grotpeter, J. & Hewitt, J. K. (2006). Childhood maltreatment, subsequent antisocial behavior, and the role of Monoamine Oxidase A genotype. *Biological Psychiatry*, 60, 677–683.

Humphreys, D. K., Gasparrini, A. & Wiebe, D. J. (2017). Evaluating the impact of Florida's "Stand your ground" self-defense law on homicide and suicide by firearm: An interrupted time series study. *JAMA Internal Medicine*, 177, 44–50.

Humphreys, L. (1970). *Tea room trade. Impersonal sex in public places.* Chicago: Aldine Publishing Company.

Hungerford, A., Wait, S. K., Fritz, A. M. & Clements, C. M. (2012). Exposure to intimate partner violence and children's psychological adjustment, cognitive functioning, and social competence: A review. *Aggression and Violent Behavior*, 17, 373–382.

Huss, M. T. (2009). *Forensic Psychology: Research, Clinical Practice, and Applications*. Chichester: Wiley-Blackwell.

Huss, M. T. & Ralston, A. (2008). Do batterer subtypes actually matter? Treatment completion, treatment response, and recidivism across a batterer typology. *Criminal Justice and Behavior*, 35, 710–724.

Hyman, S. (2010). The diagnosis of mental disorders: The problem of reification. *Annual Review of Clinical Psychology*, 6, 155–179.

I

Iganski, P. (2001). Hate crimes hurt more. *American Behavioral Scientist*, 45, 626–638.

Iganski, P. (2010). Hate crime. In F. Brookman, M. Maguire, H. Pierpoint & T. Bennett (eds.), *Handbook on Crime*. pp. 351–365. Cullompton: Willan.

Ilyas, S. & Moncrieff, J. (2012). Trends in prescriptions and costs of drugs for mental disorders in England, 1998–2010. *British Journal of Psychiatry*, 200, 393–398.

International Crime Victims Survey (2010). *ICVS 2010 – preliminary results on safety feelings and victimisation*. http://62.50.10.34/icvs/About_ICVS_2010/News_and_updates/Latest_news/Conference_report_ICVS_Final_Conference_Freiburg_October_13th_2010

International Labour Organization (2011). *World Statistic: The enormous burden of poor working conditions*. Moscow: International Labour Organisation. http://www.ilo.org/public/english/region/eurpro/moscow/areas/safety/statistic.htm

International Schizophrenia Consortium (2009). Common polygenic variation contributes to the risk of schizophrenia and bipolar disorder. *Nature*, 460, 748–452.

Interpol (2014). *Analytic Report: Motor Vehicle Crime in Global Perspective*. Lyon: Interpol.

Ioannidis, J. P. A. (2011). Excess significance bias in the literature on brain volume abnormalities. *Archives of General Psychiatry*, 68, 773–780.

Iodice, A. J., Dunn, A. G., Rosenquist, P., Hughes, D .L. & McCall, W. V. (2003). Stability over time of patients' attitudes towards ECT. *Psychiatry Research*, 117, 89–91.

Ireland, C. & Craig, L. A. (2011). Adult sexual offender assessment. In D. P. Boer, R. Eher, L. A. Craig, M. H. Miner & F. Pfäfflin (eds.), *International Perspectives on the Assessment and Treatment of Sexual Offenders: Theory, Practice and Research*. pp. 13–33. Chichester: Wiley-Blackwell.

Ireland, J. L. (2010). Legal consulting: providing expertise in written and oral testimony. In. C. A. Ireland & M. J. Fisher (eds.), *Consultancy and Advising in Forensic Practice: Empirical and Practical Guidelines*. pp. 108–122. Chichester: BPS-Blackwell.

Itsukushima, Y., Nishi, M., Maruyama, M. & Takahashi, M. (2006). The effect of presentation medium of post-event information: impact of co-witness information. *Applied Cognitive Psychology, 20,* 575–581.

Iverson, G. (2008). Assessing for exaggeration, poor effort, and malingering in neuropsychological assessment. In A. M. Horton & D. Wedding (eds.) *The Neuropsychology Handbook*. 3rd edition. pp. 125–182. New York, NY: Springer.

Ivey, A. E., Ivey, M. B. & Zalaquett, C. P. (2014). *Intentional Interviewing and Counseling: Facilitating Client Development in a Multicultural Society*. 8th edition. Belmont, CA: Brooks-Cole.

J

Jackson, H. F., Glass, C. & Hope, S. (1987). A functional analysis of recidivistic arson. *British Journal of Clinical Psychology*, 26, 175–185.

Jacobs, B. A. & Wright, R. (1999). Stick-up, street culture, and offender motivation. *Criminology*, 37, 149–173.

Jakob, R. (1992). On the development of psychologically oriented legal thinking in German speaking countries. In F. Lösel, D. Bender & T. Bliesener (eds.) *Psychology and Law: International Perspectives*. pp. 519–525. Berlin: Walter De Gruyter.

James, D. C. & Farnham, F. R. (2003). Stalking and serious violence. *Journal of the American Academy of Psychiatry and the Law*, 31, 432–439.

James, J. W. & Haley, W. E. (1995). Age and health bias in practicing clinical psychologists. *Psychology and Ageing*, 10, 610–616.

James, M. & Seager, J. A. (2006). Impulsivity and schemas for a hostile world: Postdictors of violent behaviour. *International Journal of Offender Therapy and Comparative Criminology*, 50, 47–56.

Jamieson, L. & Taylor, P. J. (2004). A re-conviction study of special (high security) hospital patients. *British Journal of Criminology*, 44, 783–802.

Janson, C.-G. (1983). Delinquency among metropolitan boys: a progress report. In K. T. Van Dusen & S. A. Mednick (eds.) *Prospective Studies of Crime and Delinquency*. pp. 147–180. Hingham, MA: Kluwer Nijhoff.

Janus, E. S. & Meehl, P. E. (1997). Assessing the legal standard for predictions of dangerousness in sex offender commitment proceedings. *Psychology, Public Policy, and Law, 3,* 33–64.

Jarvis, G. & Parker, H. (1989). Young heroin users and crime: How do the 'new users' finance their habits? *British Journal of Criminology*, 28, 175–89.

Jenkins, A., Millar, S. & Robins, J. (2011). Denial of pregnancy – a literature review and discussion of ethical and legal issues. *Journal of the Royal Society of Medicine*, 104, 286–291.

Jensen, G. F. & Akers, R. L. (2003). "Taking social learning global": Micro-macro transitions in criminological theory. In R. J. Akers & G. F. Jensen (eds.), *Social Learning Theory and the Explanation of Crime*. Advances in Criminological Theory, Volume 11. pp. 9–37. New Brunswick, NJ: Transaction Publishers.

Jesperson, A. F., Lalumière, M. L. & Seto, M. C. (2009). Sexual abuse history among adult sex offenders and non-sex offenders: A meta-analysis. *Child Abuse & Neglect*, 33, 179–192.

Jewkes, R., Levin, J. & Penn-Kekana, L. (2002). Risk factors for domestic violence: findings from a South African cross-sectional study. *Social Science & Medicine*, 55, 1603–1617.

Jewkes, R., Fulu, E., Roselli, T., García-Moreno, C. on behalf of the UN Multi-country Cross-sectional Study on Men and Violence research team (2013). Prevalence of and factors associated with non-partner rape perpetration: findings from the UN Multi-country Crosssectional Study on Men and Violence in Asia and the Pacific. *Lancet Global Health*, 1, e208–18.

Jewkes, Y., Crewe, B. & Bennett, J. (eds.) (2016). *Handbook on Prisons*. 2nd edition. Abingdon: Routledge.

Jha, P., Kester, M. A., Kumar, R., Ram, F., Ram, U., Aleksandrowicz, L., Bassani, D. G., Chandra, S. & Banthia, J. K. (2011). Trends in selective abortion of female foetuses in India: analysis of nationally representative birth histories from 1990 to 2005 and census data from 1991 to 2011. *Lancet*, 377, 1921–1928.

Johansen, M., Karterud, S., Pedersen, G., Gude, T. & Falkum, E. (2004). An investigation of the prototype validity of the borderline DSM-IV construct. *Acta Psychiatrica Scandanavica*, 109, 289–298.

Johnson, B. R. & Becker, J. V. (1997). Natural born killers? The development of the sexually sadistic serial killer. *Journal of the American Academy of Psychiatry and the Law*, 25, 335–348.

Johnson, M. K. & Foley, M. A. (1984). Differentiating fact from fantasy: The reliability of children's memory. *Journal of Social Issues*, 40, 33–55.

Johnson, M. K. & Rye, C. L. (1981). Reality monitoring. *Psychological Review, 88,* 67–85.

Johnson, M. P. (2008). *A Typology of Domestic Violence: Intimate Terrorism, Violent Resistance, and Situational Couple Violence*. Lebanon, NH: Northeastern University Press.

Johnson, S. (2006). *The Ghost Map*. New York: Riverhead.

Johnson, S. D., Guerette, R. T. & Bowers, K. J. (2014). Crime displacement: what we know, what we don't know, and what it means for crime reduction. *Journal of Experimental Criminology*, 10, 549–571.

Jolliffe, D. & Farrington, D. P. (2007). *A systematic review of the national and international evidence on the effectiveness of interventions with violent offenders*. Ministry of Justice Research Series 16/07. London: Ministry of Justice, Research Development Statistics.

Jolliffe, D. & Farrington, D. P. (2009). A systematic review of the relationship between childhood impulsiveness and later violence. In M. McMurran & R. Howard (eds.), *Personality,*

Personality Disorder and Violence. pp. 41–61. Chichester: Wiley-Blackwell.

Jonason, P. K. & Webster, G. D. (2010). The Dirty Dozen: A concise measure of the dark triad, *Psychological Assessment*, 22, 420–432.

Jones v Kaney (2011) UKSC 13; [2011] WLR (D) 109.

Jones, A. (2017). *Genocide: A Comprehensive Introduction*. 3rd edition. Abingdon: Routledge.

Jones, D. P. H. & Krugman, R. D. (1986). Can a three year-old child bear witness to her sexual assault and attempted murder? *Child Abuse and Neglect*, 10, 253–8.

Jones, L., Bates, G., Bellis, M., Beynon, C., Duffy, P., Evans-Brown, M., Mackridge, A., McCoy, E., Sumnall, H. & McVeigh, J. (2011). *A summary of the health harms of drugs*. London: Department of Health.

Jones, S. E., Miller, J. D. & Lynam, D. R. (2011). Personality, antisocial behavior, and aggression: A meta-analytic review. *Journal of Criminal Justice*, 39, 329–337.

Joyal, C. C., Beaulieu-Plante, J. & de Chantérac, A. (2014). The neuropsychology of sex offenders: A meta-analysis. *Sexual Abuse: A Journal of Research and Treatment*, 26, 149–177.

Joyce, P. (2009). *Criminology and Criminal Justice: A study guide*. Cullompton: Willan Publishing.

Jütte, S., Bentley, H., Miller, P. & Jetha, N. (2014). *How safe are our children?* London: National Society for the Prevention of Cruelty to Children. http://www.nspcc.org.uk/Inform/research/findings/howsafe/indicator01_wdf95539.pdf

K

Kacou, A. (2013). Five arguments on the rationality of suicide terrorists. *Aggression and Violent Behavior*, 18, 539–547.

Kafka, M. P. (2010). The DSM diagnostic criteria for paraphilia not otherwise specified. *Archives of Sexual Behavior*, 39, 373–376.

Kagan, J. & Snidman, N. (2004). *The Long Shadow of Temperament*. Cambridge, MA: The Belknap Press of Harvard University Press.

Kagan, J., Snidman, N., Khan, V. & Towsley, S. (2007). The preservation of two infant temperaments into adolescence. *Monographs of the Society for Research in Child Development*, 72, 1–95.

Kalmus, E., & Beech, A. R. (2005). Forensic assessment of sexual interest: A review. *Aggression and Violent Behavior*, 10, 193–217.

Kamisar, Y. (1980). *Police Interrogation and Confession: Essays in Law and Policy*. Ann Arbor: University of Michigan.

Kamphuis, J., Meerlo, P., Koolhaas, J. M. & Lancel, M. (2012). Poor sleep as a potential causal factor in aggression and violence. *Sleep Medicine*, 13, 327–334.

Kamphuis, J. H., & Emmelkamp, P. M. G. (2000). Stalking – a contemporary challenge for forensic and clinical psychiatry. *British Journal of Psychiatry*, 176, 206–209.

Kandel, D. & Kandel, E. (2015). The Gateway Hypothesis of substance abuse: developmental, biological and societal perspectives. *Acta Pædiatrica*, 104, 130–137.

Kane, R. (2005). *A Contemporary Introduction to Free Will*. Oxford: Oxford University Press.

Kant, I. (1797, republished 1967). *Kritik der praktischen Vernunft* [Critique of practical reason]. Hamburg, Germany: Felix Meiner Verlag.

Kao, A. B. & Couzin, I. D. (2014). Decision accuracy in complex environments is often maximized by small group sizes. *Proceedings of the Royal Society*, B281, 1–8.

Kapardis, A. (2014). *Psychology and Law: A Critical Introduction*. 4th edition. Cambridge: Cambridge University Press.

Kaplan, J. (1967–1968). Decision theory and the factfinding process. *Stanford Law Review*, 20, 1065–1092.

Karson, M. & Nadkarni, L. (2013). *Principles of Forensic Report Writing*. Washington, DC: American Psychological Association.

Kassin, S. M. (2008). False confessions: Causes, consequences, and implications for reform. *Current Directions in Psychological Science*, 17, 249–253.

Kassin, S. M. & Fong, C. T. (1999). "I'm innocent!" Effects of training on judgments of truth and deception in the interrogation room. *Law and Human Behavior*, 23, 499–516.

Kassin, S. M. & Sukel, H. (1997). Coerced confessions and the jury: An experimental test of the 'harmless error' rule. *Law and Human Behavior*, 21, 27–46.

Kassin, S. M. & Wrightsman, L. S. (1988). *The American Jury on Trial: Psychological Perspectives*. Philadelphia, PA: Hemisphere.

Kassinove, H. & Tafrate, R. C. (2002). *Anger Management: The Complete Treatment Guidebook for Practitioners*. Atascadero, CA: Impact.

Katz, J. (1972). *Experimentation with Human Beings*. New York, NY: Russel Sage Foundation.

Kavanagh, K. (1995). Don't ask, don't tell: Deception required, disclosure denied. *Psychology, Public Policy, and Law*, 1, 142–160.

Kazdin, A. E. (1986). Comparative outcome studies of psychotherapy: methodological issues and strategies. *Journal of Consulting and Clinical Psychology*, 54, 95–105.

Kazdin, A. E. & Blase, S. L. (2011). Rebooting psychotherapy research and practice to reduce the burden of mental illness. *Perspectives on Psychological Science*, 6, 21–37.

Kebbell, M. R., Milne, R., & Wagstaff, G. F. (1999). The cognitive interview: a survey of its forensic effectiveness. *Psychology, Crime & Law*, 5, 101–115.

Kemp, R., Towell, N. & Pike, G. (1997). When seeing should not be believing: Photographs, credit cards and fraud. *Applied Cognitive Psychology*, 11, 211–222.

Kemshall, H., Mackenzie, G., Wood, J., Bailey, R. & Yates, J. (2005). Strengthening Multi-Agency Public Protection Arrangements (MAPPAs). *Home Office Development and Practice Report,* 45, 1–28.

Kemshall, H. & Wood, J. (2007). High-risk offenders and public protection. In L. Gelsthorpe and R. Morgan (eds.) *Handbook of Probation*. pp. 381–397. Cullompton, Devon: Willan Publishing.

Kendell, R. & Jablensky, A. (2003). Distinguishing between the validity and utility of psychiatric diagnoses. *American Journal of Psychiatry*, 160, 4–12.

Kennedy, L. W. & Baron, S. W. (1993). Routine activities and a subculture of violence: A study of violence on the street. *Journal of Research in Crime and Delinquency*, 30, 88–112.

Kennedy, L. W. & Forde, D. R. (1996). Pathways to aggression: A factorial study of "routine conflict". *Journal of Quantitative Criminology*, 12, 417–438.

Kenny, D. T., Lennings, C. J. & Nelson, P. K. (2007). The mental health of young offenders serving orders in the community: Implications for rehabilitation. *Mental Health issues in the Criminal Justice System*, 123–148.

Keogh, A. (2010). *Blackstone's Magistrates' Court Handbook 2010*. Oxford: Oxford University Press.

Kerig, P. K., Ludlow, A. & Wenar, C. (2012). *Developmental Psychopathology*. 6th edition. New York, NY: McGraw-Hill.

Kerr, N. J., Nerenz, D. R. & Herrick, D. (1979). Role playing and the study of jury behavior. *Sociological Methods and Research,* 7, 337–355.

Kershaw, C. (1999). *Reconviction of offenders sentenced or released from prison in 1994*. Research Findings No.90. London: Home Office Research, Development and Statistics Directorate.

Kershaw, C., Goodman, J. & White, S. (1999). *Reconviction of offenders sentenced or released from prison in 1995*. Research Findings No.101. London: Home Office Research, Development and Statistics Directorate

Kessler, R. (1993). *The FBI*. New York, NY: Pocket Books.

Kessler, R. C., Berglund, P., Demler, O., Jin, R., Merikangas, K. R. & Walters, E. E. (2005). Lifetime prevalence and age-of-onset distributions of *DSM-IV* disorders in the National Comorbidity Survey replication. *Archives of General Psychiatry*, 62, 593–602.

Khiroya, R., Weaver, T. & Maden, T. (2009). Use and perceived utility of structured violence risk assessments in English medium secure forensic units. *Psychiatric Bulletin*, 33, 129–132.

Kiehl, K. A. (2006). A cognitive neuroscience perspective on psychopathy: Evidence for paralimbic system dysfunction. *Psychiatry Research*, 142, 107–128.

Killias, M. & Markwalder, N. (2012). Firearms and homicide in Europe. In M. C. A. Liem & W. A. Pridemore (eds.), *Handbook of European Homicide Research: Patterns, Explanations and Country Studies*. Springer Science+Business Media. Doi: 10.1007/978-1-4614-0466-8_16

Kim, B., Benekos, P. J. & Merlo, A. V. (2016). Sex offender recidivism revisited: Review of recent meta-analyses on the effects of sex offender treatment. *Trauma, Violence, & Abuse*, 17, 105–117.

Kim-Cohen, J., Caspi, A., Taylor, A., Williams, B., Newcombe, R., Craig, I. W. & Moffitt, T. E. (2006). MAOA, maltreatment, and gene-environment interaction predicting children's mental health: new evidence and a meta-analysis. *Molecular Psychiatry*, 11, 903–913.

King, L. W. (1915). *The Code of Hammurabi* (trans: L. W. King). Yale University. http://avalon.law.yale.edu/subject_menus/hammenu.asp

King, M. & Taylor, D. M. (2011). The radicalization of homegrown jihadists: A review of theoretical models and social psychological evidence. *Terrorism and Political Violence*, 23, 602–622.

Kiss, L., Schraiber, L. B., Heise, L., Zimmerman, C., Gouveia, N. & Watts, C. (2012). Gender-based violence and socioeconomic inequalities: Does living in deprived neighbourhoods increase women's risk of intimate partner violence? *Social Science and Medicine*, 74, 1172–1179.

Kitchener, K. S. & Anderson, S. K. (2011). *Foundations of Ethical Practice, Research, and*

Teaching in Psychology and Counseling. 2nd edition. New York, NY: Taylor & Francis.

Kleck, G. & Barnes, J. C. (2010). Do more police lead to more crime deterrence? *Crime and Delinquency*, online first.

Klement, C. (2015). Comparing the effects of community service and imprisonment on reconviction: results from a quasi-experimental Danish study. *Journal of Experimental Criminology*, 11, 237–261

Klemfuss, J. Z., Quas, J. A. & Lyon, T. D. (2014). Attorneys' questions and children's productivity in child sexual abuse criminal trials. *Applied Cognitive Psychology,* 28, 780–788.

Klinteberg, B. A., Andersson, T., Magnusson, D. & Stattin, H. (1993). Hyperactive behaviour in childhood as related to subsequent alcohol problems and violent offending: A longitudinal study of male subjects. *Personality and Individual Differences*, 15, 381–388.

Kloess, J. A., Beech, A. R. & Harkins, L. (2014). Online child sexual exploitation: Prevalence, process, and offender characteristics. *Trauma, Violence, & Abuse*, 15, 126–139.

Klusemann, S. (2010). Micro-situational antecedents of violent atrocity. *Sociological Forum*, 25, 272–295.

Klusemann, S. (2012). Massacres as process: A micro-sociological theory of internal patterns of mass atrocities. *European Journal of Criminology*, 9, 468–480.

Knapp, S. & Slattery, J. M. (2004). Professional boundaries in non-traditional settings. *Professional Psychology: Research and Practice,* 35, 553–558.

Knight, R. A. & Prentky, R. A. (1990). Classifying sexual offenders: The development and corroboration of taxonomic models. In W. L. Marshall, D. R. Laws & H. E. Barbaree (eds.), *Handbook of Sexual Assault: Issues, Theories, and Treatment of the Offender*, pp. 23–52. New York and London: Plenum Press.

Knight, R. A. & Thornton, D. (2007). *Evaluating and improving risk assessment schemes for sexual recidivism: A long-term follow-up of convicted sexual offenders*. Washington, DC: US Department of Justice.

Knoll IV, J. L. (2010a). The "pseudocommando" mass murderer: Part I, the psychology of revenge and obliteration. *Journal of the American Academy of Psychiatry and the Law*, 38, 87–94.

Knoll IV, J. L. (2010b). The "pseudocommando" mass murderer: Part II, the language of revenge. *Journal of the American Academy of Psychiatry and the Law*, 38, 363–372.

Kocsis, R. N. (ed.) (2008). *Serial Murder and the Psychology of Violent Crimes*. Totowa, NJ: Humana Press.

Köhnken, G., Milne, R., Memon, A. & Bull, R. (1999). The cognitive interview: A meta-analysis. *Psychology, Crime & Law*, 5, 3–27.

Kokko, K. & Pulkkinen, L. (2005). Stability of aggressive behaviour from childhood to middle age in women and men. *Aggressive Behavior*, 31, 485–497.

Kon, Y. (1994). Amok. *British Journal of Psychiatry*, 165, 685–689.

Konopasek, J. E. (2015). Expeditious disclosure of sexual history via polygraph testing: Treatment outcome and sex offense recidivism. *Journal of Offender Rehabilitation*, 54, 194–211.

Kovandzic, T. V., Sloan, J. J. & Vieraitis, L. M. (2004). "Striking out" as crime reduction policy: The impact of "three strikes" laws on crime rates in U.S. cities. *Justice Quarterly*, 21, 207–239.

Kovandzic, T. V., Vieraitis, L. M. & Boots, D. P. (2009). Does the death penalty save lives? New evidence from state panel data, 1977 to 2006. *Criminology & Public Policy*, 8, 803–843.

Kraanen, F. L. & Emmelkamp, P. M. G. (2011). Substance misuse and substance use disorders in sex offenders: A review. *Clinical Psychology Review*, 31, 478–489.

Kraanen, F. L., Scholing, A. & Emmelkamp, P. M. G. (2012). Substance use disorders in forensic psychiatry: Differences among different types of offenders. *International Journal of Offender Therapy and Comparative Criminology*, 56, 1201–1219.

Kraemer, G. W., Lord, W. D. & Heilbrun, K. (2004). Comparing single and serial homicide offenses. *Behavioral Sciences and the Law*, 22, 325–343.

Krahé, B. (2013). *The Social Psychology of Aggression*. 2nd edition. Hove: Psychology Press.

Krahé, B., Tomaszewska, P., Kuyper, L. & Vanwesenbeeck, I. (2014). Prevalence of sexual aggression among young people in Europe: A review of the evidence from 27 EU countries. *Aggression and Violent Behavior*, 19, 545–558.

Kratzer, L. & Hodgins, S. (1997). Adult outcomes of child conduct problems: A cohort study. *Journal of Abnormal Child Psychology*, 25, 65–81.

Krauss, D. A. & Goldstein, A. M. (2007). The role of forensic mental health experts in Federal sentencing proceedings. In A. M. Goldstein (ed.) *Forensic Psychology: Emerging topics and expanding roles*. pp. 359–384. Hoboken, NJ: Wiley.

Krienert, J. L. & Walsh, J. A. (2010). Eldercide: A gendered examination of elderly homicide in the United States, 2000-2005. *Homicide Studies*, 14, 52–71.

Kring, A. M., Johnson, S. L., Davison, G. C. & Neale, J. M. (2017). *Abnormal Psychology: The Science and Treatment of Psychological Disorders*. 13th edition. Hoboken, NJ: Wiley.

Krischer, M. K., Stone, M. H., Sevecke, K. & Steinmeyer, E. M. (2007). Motives or maternal filicide: Results from a study with female forensic patients. *International Journal of Law and Psychiatry*, 30 191–200.

Kristof, N. D. (2009). Priority test: health care or prisons? *The New York Times*, August 20.

Kroll, B. & Taylor, A. (2003). *Parental Substance Misuse and Child Welfare*. London: Jessica Kingsley.

Kross, E., Mischel, W. & Shoda, Y. (2010). Enabling self-control: a Cognitive-Affective Processing System approach to problematic behaviour. In J. E. Maddux & J. P. Tangney (eds.), *Social Psychological Foundations of Clinical Psychology*. pp. 375–394. New York, NY: Guilford Press.

Krueger, A. B. & Malečková, J. (2003). Education, poverty and terrorism: Is there a causal connection? *Journal of Economic Perspectives*, 17, 119–144.

Krug, E. G., Dahlberg, L. L., Mercy, J. A., Zwi, A. B. & Lozano, R. (eds.) (2002). *World report on violence and health*. Geneva: World Health Organization.

Kuhns, J. B., Exum, M. L., Clodfelter, T. A. & Bottia, M. C. (2014). The prevalence of alcohol-involved homicide offending: A meta-analytic review. *Homicide Studies*, 18, 251–270.

Kuhns, J. B., Wilson, D. B., Clodfelter, T. A., Maguire, E. R. & Ainsworth, S. A. (2011). A meta-analysis of alcohol toxicology study findings among homicide victims. *Addiction*, 106, 62–72.

Kutchins, H. A. & Kirk, S. A. (1997). *Making Us Crazy: DSM: The Psychiatric Bible and the Creation of Mental Disorders*. Glencoe, IL: The Free Press.

Kyle, D. (2004). Correcting miscarriages of justice: the role of the Criminal Cases Review Commission. *Drake Law Review*, 52, 657–676.

L

Lacey, N. & Zedner, L. (2012). Legal constructions of crime. In M. Maguire, R. Morgan & R. Reiner (eds.), *The Oxford Handbook of Criminology*. 5th edition. pp. 159–181. Oxford: Oxford University Press.

Lacourse, E., Dupéré, V. & Loeber, R. (2008). Developmental trajectories of violence and theft. In R. Loeber, D. P. Farrington, M. Stouthamer-Loeber & H. R. White (eds.). *Violence and Serious Theft: Development and Prediction from Childhood to Adulthood*. pp. 231–268. New York, NY: Routledge.

Lader, D., Singleton, N. & Meltzer, H. (2000). *Psychiatric Morbidity among Young Offenders in England and Wales*. London: Office for National Statistics.

LaFree, G. & Birkbeck, C. (1991). The neglected situation: A cross-national study of the situational characteristics of crime. *Criminology*, 29, 73–98.

Lahey, B. B. & Waldman, I. D. (2003). A developmental propensity model of the origins of conduct problems during childhood and adolescence. In B. B. Lahey, E. Moffitt & A. Caspi (eds.), *Causes of Conduct Disorder and Juvenile Delinquency*. pp. 76–117. New York, NY: Guilford Press.

Lahey, B. B. & Waldman, I. D. (2005). A developmental model of the propensity to offend during childhood and adolescence. In D. P. Farrington (ed.), *Integrated Developmental & Life-Course Theories of Offending*. pp. 15–50. New Brunswick and London: Transaction Publishers.

Lamb, M. E. & Garretson, M. E. (2003). The effects of interviewer gender and child gender on the informativeness of alleged child sexual abuse victims in forensic interviews. *Law and Human Behavior*, 27, 157–171.

Lamb, M. E., Orbach, Y., Sternberg, K. J., Esplin, P. W., & Hershkowitz, I. (2002). The effects of forensic interview practices on the quality of information provided by alleged victims of child abuse. In H. L. Westcott, G. M. Davies, & R. H. C. Bull (eds.) *Children's Testimony: A Handbook of Psychological Research and Forensic Practice*. pp. 131–145. Chichester: Wiley.

Lambie, I. & Randell, I. (2011). Creating a firestorm: A review of children who deliberately light fires. *Clinical Psychology Review*, 31, 307–327.

Land, K. C., McCall, P. L. & Cohen, L. E. (1990). Structural covariates of homicide rates: are there any invariances across time and social space? *American Journal of Sociology*, 95, 922–963.

Langan, P. A., Schmitt, E. L. & Durose, M. R. (2003). *Recidivism of sex offenders released from prison in 1994*. Washington, DC: Office of Justice Programs, US Department of Justice.

Langenderfer, L. (2013). Alcohol use among partner violent adults: Reviewing recent literature to inform intervention. *Aggression and Violent Behavior*, 18, 152–158.

Langer, W. (1972). *The Mind of Adolf Hitler*. New York, NY: New American Library.

Langhinrichsen-Rohling, J., Misra, T. A., Selwyn, C. & Rohling, M. L. (2012). Rates of bidirectional versus unidirectional intimate partner violence across samples, sexual orientations, and race/ethnicities: A comprehensive review. *Partner Abuse*, 3, 199–230.

Langman, P. (2009a). Rampage school shooters: A typology. *Aggression and Violent Behavior*, 14, 79–86.

Langman, P. (2009b). *Why Kids Kill: Inside the Minds of School Shooters*. New York, NY: Palgrave Macmillan.

Langman, P. (2013). Thirty-five rampage school shooters: Trends, patterns, and typology. In N. Böckler, T. Seeger, P. Sitzer & W. Heitmeyer (eds.), *School Shootings: International Research, Case Studies and Concepts for Prevention*. pp. 131–156. New York, NY: Springer.

Långström, N., Sjöstedt, G. & Grann, M. (2004). Psychiatric disorders and recidivism in sexual offenders. *Sexual Abuse: A Journal of Research and Treatment*, 16, 139–150.

Långström, N., Enebrink, P., Laurén E.-M., Lindblom, J., Werkö, S. & Hanson, R. K. (2013). Preventing sexual abusers of children from reoffending: systematic review of medical and psychological interventions. *British Medical Journal*, 347:f4630. Doi: 10.1136/bmj.f4630

Lankford, A. (2010). Do suicide terrorists exhibit clinically suicidal risk factors? A review of initial evidence and call for future research. *Aggression and Violent Behavior*, 15, 334–340.

Lankford, A. & Hakim, N. (2011). From Columbine to Palestine: A comparative analysis of rampage shooters in the United States and volunteer suicide bombers in the Middle East. *Aggression and Violent Behavior*, 16, 98–107.

Lansford, J. E., Miller-Johnson, S., Berlin, L. J., Dodge, K. A., Bates, J. E. & Pettit, G. S. (2007). Early physical abuse and later violent delinquency: A prospective longitudinal study. *Child Maltreatment*, 12, 233–245.

Larcombe, W. (2011). Falling rape conviction rates: (Some) feminist aims and measures for rape law. *Feminist Legal Studies*, 19, 27–45.

Large, M., Smith, G., & Neilssen, O. (2009). The epidemiology of homicide followed by suicide. A systematic and quantitative review. *Suicide and Life-Threatening Behavior*, 39, 294–306.

Larson, R. & Ham, M. (1993). Stress and "Storm and Stress" in early adolescence: The relationship of negative events with dysphoric affect. *Developmental Psychology*, 29, 130–140.

Larsson, H., Andershed, H. & Lichtenstein, P. (2006). A genetic factor explains most of the variation in the psychopathic personality. *Journal of Abnormal Psychology*, 115, 221–230.

Lasher, M. P. & McGrath, R. J. (2012). The impact of community notification on sex offender reintegration: A quantitative review of the research literature. *International Journal of Offender Therapy and Comparative Criminology*, 56, 6–28.

Lassiter, G. D. & Irvine, A. A. (1986). Videotaped confessions: The impact of camera point of view on judgments of coercion. *Journal of Applied Social Psychology*, 16, 268–276.

Lassiter, G. D., Geers, A. L., Handley, I. M., Weiland, P. E., & Munhall, P. J. (2002). Videotaped interrogations and confessions: A simple change in camera perspective alters verdicts in simulated trials. *Journal of Applied Psychology*, 87, 867–874.

Latimer, J., Dowden, C. & Muise, D. (2005). The effectiveness of restorative justice practices: A meta-analysis. *The Prison Journal*, 85, 127–144.

Law Commission (2011). *Expert Evidence in Criminal Proceedings in England and Wales*. London: The Stationery Office.

Law Commission (2014). *Simplification of Criminal Law: Kidnapping and Related Offences*. Law Com No 355. www.gov.uk/government/publications

Laws, D. R. & O'Donohue, W. T. (eds.) (2008). *Sexual Deviance: Theory, Assessment, and Treatment*. New York, NY: Guilford Press.

Layard, R., Clark, D., Knapp, M. & Mayraz, G. (2007). Cost-benefit analysis of psychological therapy. *National Institute Economic Review*, 202, 90–98.

Leahy, T. H. (2003). *A History of Psychology: Main Currents in Psychological Thought*. 6th edition. Upper Saddle River, NJ: Prentice Hall.

Learned Hand (1901). Historical and practical considerations regarding expert testimony. *Harvard Law Review*, 15, 40–58.

Lee, L. K., Fleegler, E. W., Farrell, C., Avakame, E., Srinivasan, S., Hemenway, D. & Monuteaux, M. C. (2017). Firearm laws and firearm homicides: A systematic review. *JAMA Internal Medicine*, 177, 106–119.

Lee, S., Aos, S. & Pennucci, A. (2015). *What works and what does not? Benefit-cost findings from WSIPP*. (Doc. No. 15-02-4101). Olympia: Washington State Institute for Public Policy. http://www.wsipp.wa.gov/ReportFile/1602/Wsipp_What-Works-and-What-Does-Not-

Benefit-Cost-Findings-from-WSIPP_Report.pdf

LeGresley, E. M., Muggli, M. E. & Hurt, R. D. (2005). Playing hide-and-seek with the tobacco industry. *Nicotine and Tobacco Research*, 7, 27–40.

Leschied, A., Chiodo, D., Nowicki, E. & Rodger, S. (2008). Childhood predictors of adult criminality: A meta-analysis drawn from the prospective longitudinal literature. *Canadian Journal of Criminology and Criminal Justice*, 435–467.

Leslie, O., Young, S., Valentine, T. & Gudjonsson, G. (2007). Criminal barristers' opinions and perceptions of mental health expert witnesses. *The Journal of Forensic Psychiatry & Psychology,* 18, 394–410.

Lester, D. (1990). The effects of detoxification of domestic gas on suicide in the United States. *American Journal of Public Health*, 80, 80–81.

Leukefeld, C., Gullotta, T. P & Gregrich, J. (eds.) (2011). *Handbook of Evidence-Based Substance Abuse Treatment in Criminal Justice Settings*. New York, NY: Springer.

Levenson, J. S. & Cotter, L. P. (2005). The effect of Megan's Law on sex offender reintegration. *Journal of Contemporary Criminal Justice,* 21, 49–66.

Levenson, J. S., Brannon, Y. N., Fortney, T. & Baker, J. (2007). Public perceptions about sex offenders and community protection policies. *Analysis of Social Issues and Public Policy,* 7, 137–161.

Levi, K. (1981). Becoming a hit man: Neutralization in a very deviant career. *Journal of Contemporary Ethnography*, 10, 47–63.

Levi, M. (2009). Suite revenge? The shaping of folk devils and moral panics about white-collar crimes. *British Journal of Criminology*, 49, 48–67.

Levi, M. (2012). The organization of serious crimes for gain. In M. Maguire, R. Morgan, & R. Reiner (eds.), *The Oxford Handbook of Criminology.* 5th edition. pp. 595-622. Oxford: Oxford University Press.

Levinson, C. A., Giancola, P. R. & Parrott, D. J. (2011). Beliefs about aggression moderate alcohol's effects on aggression. *Experimental and Clinical Psychopharmacology*, 19, 64–74.

Levitt, S. D. & Venkatesh, S. A. (2000). An economic analysis of a drug-selling gang's finances. *The Quarterly Journal of Economics*, 115, 755–789.

Levy, D. M. (1968). Beginnings of the Child Guidance Movement. *American Journal of Orthopsychiatry*, 38, 799–804.

Lewin, K. (1951). *Field theory in social science: Selected theoretical papers.* New York, NY: Harper & Row.

Lewis, M. (2015). *The Biology of Desire: Why Addiction is Not a Disease*. New York, NY: PublicAffairs.

Lewis, M. (2017). Addiction and the brain: Development, not disease. *Neuroethics*. Doi: 0.1007/s12152-016-9293-4

Lewis, R. (2011). *Human Genetics: The Basics*. London and New York, NY: Routledge.

Lewis, T., Leeb, R., Kotch, J., Smith, J., Thompson, R., Black, M. M., Pelaez-Merrick, M., Briggs, E. & Coyne-Beasley, T. (2007). Maltreatment history and weapon carrying among early adolescents. *Child Maltreatment*, 12, 259–268.

Lewis, V., Oates, J., Martin, S., & Duffy. H (2007) Teaching of research methods in undergraduate psychology courses: a survey of provision in HE institutions and colleges in the UK. *Psychology Learning and Teaching,* 6, 6–11.

Lewontin, R. C. (2006). The analysis of variance and the analysis of causes. *International Journal of Epidemiology*, 35, 520-525. Doi:10.1093/ije/dyl062

Lexchin, J., Bero, L. A., Djulbegovic, B. & Clark, O. (2003). Pharmaceutical industry sponsorship and research outcome and quality: systematic review. *British Medical Journal*, 326, 1–10.

Liem, M. (2010). Homicide followed by suicide: A review. *Aggression and Violent Behavior*, 15, 153–163.

Liem, M. & Reichelmann, A. (2014). Patterns of multiple family homicide. *Homicide Studies*, 18, 44–58.

Liem, M. & Roberts, D. W. (2009). Intimate partner homicide by the presence or absence of a self-destructive act. *Homicide Studies*, 13, 339–354.

Liem, M., Levin, J., Holland, C. & Fox, J. A. (2013). The nature and prevalence of familicide in the United States, 2000-2009. *Journal of Family Violence*, 28, 351–358.

Liem, M., Barber, C., Markwalder, N., Killias, M. & Nieuwbierta, P. (2011). Homicide-suicide and other violent deaths: An international comparison. *Forensic Science International*, 207, 70–76.

Lilienfeld, S. C. & Widows, M. R. (2005). *Psychopathic Personality Inventory: Revised*. Odessa, FL: Psychological Assessment Resources.

Lilly, J. R., Cullen, F. T. & Ball, R. A. (2014). *Criminological Theory: Context and Consequences*. 6th edition. Thousand Oaks, CA: Sage.

Lindegaard, M. R., Bernasco, W., Jacques, S. & Zevenbergen, B. (2014). Posterior gains and immediate pains: Offender emotions before, during and after robberies. In J. L. van Gelder, H. Elffers, D. Nagin, & D. Reynald (eds.), *Affect and*

Cognition in Criminal Decision Making. pp. 58-76. New York, NY: Routledge.

Lindsay, R. C. L., Nosworthy, G. J., Martin, R. & Martynuck, C. (1994). Using mug shots to find suspects. *Journal of Applied Psychology*, 79, 121–130.

Lininger, T. (2005). Bearing the cross. *Fordham Law Review*, 74, 1353–1423.

Link, B. G., Stueve, A. & Phelan, J. (1998). Psychotic symptoms and violent behaviors: Probing the components of "threat/control-override" symptoms. *Social Psychiatry and Psychiatric Epidemiology*, 22, S55–S60.

Lipsey, M. W. (1995). What do we learn from 400 studies on the effectiveness of treatment with juvenile delinquents? In J. McGuire (Ed.), *What Works: Reducing Re-offending: Guidelines from Research and Practice*. pp. 63–78. Chichester: Wiley.

Lipsey, M. W. (1999). Can rehabilitative programs reduce the recidivism of juvenile offenders? An inquiry into the effectiveness of practical programs. *Virginia Journal of Social Policy and the Law*, 6, 611–641.

Lipsey, M. W. & Cullen, F. T. (2007). The effectiveness of correctional rehabilitation: A review of systematic reviews. *Annual Review of Law and Social Science*, 3, 297–320.

Lipsey, M. W. & Derzon, J. H. (1998). Predictors of violent or serious delinquency in adolescence and early adulthood: A synthesis of longitudinal research. In R. Loeber & D. P. Farrington (eds.), *Serious and violent juvenile offenders: Risk factors and successful interventions*. pp. 86–105. London: Sage.

Lipsey, M. W. & Wilson, D. B. (1993). The efficacy of psychological, educational, and behavioral treatment: confirmation from meta-analysis. *American Psychologist*, 48, 1181–1209.

Lipsey, M. W. & Wilson, D. B. (1998). Effective intervention for serious juvenile offenders: a synthesis of research. In R. Loeber & D. P. Farrington (eds.), *Serious and Violent Juvenile Offenders: Risk Factors and Successful Interventions*. pp. 313–345. Thousand Oaks, CA: Sage.

Lipsey, M. W. & Wilson, D. B. (2001). *Practical Meta-Analysis*. Thousand Oaks, CA: Sage.

Lipsey, M. W., Landenberger N. A. & Wilson S. J. (2007). Effects of cognitive-behavioral programs for criminal offenders. *Campbell Systematic Reviews*. Doi: 10.4073/csr.2007.6

Lipsitt, P. D. (2007). Ethics and forensic psychological practice. In A. M. Goldstein (Ed.). *Forensic Psychology: Emerging topics and expanding roles*. pp. 171–189. Hoboken, NJ: Wiley, Inc.

Lipton, D. S., Pearson, F. S., Cleland, C. M. & Yee, D. (2002a). The effects of therapeutic communities and milieu therapy on recidivism. In J. McGuire (ed.), *Offender Rehabilitation and Treatment: Effective Programmes and Policies to Reduce Re-Offending*. pp. 39–77. Chichester: Wiley.

Lipton, D. S., Pearson, F. S., Cleland, C. M. & Yee, D. (2002b). The effectiveness of cognitive-behavioural treatment methods on recidivism. In J. McGuire (Ed.), *Offender Rehabilitation and Treatment: Effective Programmes and Policies to Reduce Re-Offending*. pp. 79–112. Chichester: Wiley.

Listwan, S. J., Sullivan, C. J., Agnew, R., Cullen, F. T. & Colvin, M. (2013). The pains of imprisonment revisited: Impact of strain on inmate recidivism. *Justice Quarterly*, 30, 144–168.

Livesley, J. (2012). Editorial: Tradition versus empiricism in the current DSM-5 proposal for revising the classification of personality disorders. *Criminal Behaviour and Mental Health*, 22, 81–90.

Livesley, W. J. & Larstone, R. (eds.) (2018). *Handbook of Personality Disorders: Theory, Research and Treatment*. New York, NY: Guilford.

Lloyd, M. & Dean, C. (2015). The development of structured guidelines for assessing risk in extremist offenders. *Journal of Threat Assessment and Management*, 2, 40–52.

Lloyd, C., Mair, G., & Hough, M. (1994). *Explaining reconviction rates: A critical* analysis. Home Office Research Study No. 136. London: Her Majesty's Stationery Office.

Locard, E. (1934). *La police et les méthodes scientifiques*. Paris: Les Editions Rieder.

Loeber, R. & Farrington, D. P. (eds.) (1998). *Serious and Violent Juvenile Offenders: Risk Factors and Successful Interventions*. Thousand Oaks, CA: Sage.

Loeber, R., Farrington, D. P. & Jolliffe, D. (2008). Comparing arrests and convictions with reported offending. In R. Loeber, D. P. Farrington, M. Stouthamer-Loeber. & H. R. White (eds.). *Violence and Serious Theft: Development and Prediction from Childhood to Adulthood*. pp. 105–136. New York, NY: Routledge.

Loeber, R., Farrington, D. P., Stouthamer-Loeber, M. & White, H. R. (2008a). *Violence and Serious Theft: Development and Prediction from Childhood to Adulthood*. New York, NY: Routledge.

Loeber, R., Farrington, D. P., Stouthamer-Loeber, M. & White, H. R. (2008b). Introduction and key questions. In Loeber, R., Farrington, D. P.,

Stouthamer-Loeber, M. & White, H. R. (eds.), *Violence and Serious Theft: Development and Prediction from Childhood to Adulthood*. pp. 3–23. New York, NY: Routledge.

Loeber, R. Pardini, D., Homish, D. L., Wes, E. H., Crawford, A. M., Farrington, D. P., Stouthamer-Loeber, M., Creemers, J., Koehler, S. A. & Rosenfeld, R. (2005). The prediction of violence and homicide in young men. *Journal of Consulting and Clinical Psychology*, 73, 1074-1088.

Loftus, E. F. (1993). The reality of repressed memories. *American Psychologist*, 48, 518–537.

Loftus, E. F. (1996). *Eyewitness Testimony*. Cambridge, MA: Harvard University Press.

Loftus, E. F. (1997). Creating childhood memories. *Applied Cognitive Psychology*, 11, S75–S86.

Loftus, E. F. (2011). Intelligence gathering post-9/11. *American Psychologist*, 66, 532–541.

Loftus, E. F., Loftus, G. R. & Messo, J. (1987). Some facts about 'weapon focus'. *Law and Human Behavior*, 11, 55–62.

Logan, C. & Johnstone, L. (2010). Personality disorders and violence: making the link through risk formulation. *Journal of Personality Disorders*, 24, 610–633.

Logan, C., Nathan, R. & Brown, A. (2011). Formulation in clinical risk assessment and management. In R. Whittington & C. Logan (eds.), *Self-Harm and Violence: Towards Best Practice in Managing Risk in Mental Health Services*. pp. 187–204. Chichester: Wiley-Blackwell.

Logar, R. and the WAVE team (2016). *WAVE Report 2015: On the role of specialist women's support services in Europe*. Vienna: Women against Violence Europe. http://fileserver.wave-network.org/researchreports/WAVE_Report_2015.pdf

Lohr, B. A., Adams, H. E. & Davis, J. M. (1997). Sexual arousal to erotic and aggressive stimuli in sexually coercive and noncoercive men. *Journal of Abnormal Psychology*, 106, 230–242.

Lombroso, C. (1876/2006). *Criminal Man*. Translated by M. Gibson & N. H. Rafter. Durham, NC: Duke University Press.

Lopez, V. A. & Emmer, E. T. (2000). Adolescent male offenders: A grounded theory study of cognition, emotion, and delinquent crime contexts. *Criminal Justice and Behavior*, 27, 292–311.

Lopez, V. A. & Emmer, E. T. (2002). Influences of beliefs and values on male adolescents' decision to commit violent offenses. *Psychology of Men and Masculinity*, 3, 28–40.

Loranger, A. W. (1999). *International Personality Disorder Examination: DSM-IV and ICD-10 Interviews*. Lutz, FL: Psychological Assessment Resources.

Loranger, A. W., Janca, A. & Sartorius, N. (1997). *Assessment and diagnosis of personality disorders: The ICD-10 international personality disorder examination (IPDE)*. Cambridge: Cambridge University Press.

Lorenz, K. & Ullman, S. E. (2016). Alcohol and sexual assault victimization: Research findings and future direction. *Aggression and Violent Behavior*, 31, 82–94.

Lösel, F. (2001). Evaluating the effectiveness of correctional programs: Bridging the gap between research and practice. In G. A. Bernfeld, D. P. Farrington & A. W. Leschied (eds.), *Offender Rehabilitation in Practice: Implementing and Evaluating Effective Programs*. pp. 67–92. Chichester: Wiley.

Lösel, F. (2012). Offender treatment and rehabilitation: what works? In M. Maguire, R. Morgan & R. Reiner (eds.), *The Oxford Handbook of Criminology*. 5th edition. pp. 986–1016. Oxford: Oxford University Press.

Lösel, F. (2017). Evidence comes by replication, but needs differentiation: the reproducibility issue in science and its relevance for criminology. *Journal of Experimental Criminology*, 13. Doi: 10.1007/s11292-017-9297-z

Lösel, F. & Koferl, P. (1989). Evaluation research on correctional treatment in West Germany: A meta-analysis. In H. Wegener, F. Lösel & J. Haisch (eds.), *Criminal Behavior and the Justice System: Psychological Perspectives*. pp. 334–355. New York, NY: Springer-Verlag.

Lösel, F. & Schmucker, M. (2005). The effectiveness of treatment for sexual offenders: A comprehensive meta-analysis. *Journal of Experimental Criminology*, 1, 117–146.

Lovbakke, J. (2007). Public perceptions. In S. Nicholas, C. Kershaw & A. Walker (eds.) *Crime in England and Wales 2006/07*. London: Home Office Research, Development and Statistics Directorate. http://www.homeoffice.gov.uk/rds/pdfs07/hosb1107.pdf

Lovén, J., Herlitz, A., & Rehnman, J. (2011). Women's own-gender bias in face recognition memory: the role of attention at encoding. *Experimental Psychology*, 58, 333–340.

Lowenkamp, C. T., Flores, A. W., Holsinger, A. M., Makarios, M. D. & Latessa, E. J. (2010). Intensive supervision programs: Does program philosophy and the principles of effective intervention matter? *Journal of Criminal Justice*, 38, 368–375.

Lowenkamp, C. T., Latessa, E. J. & Holsinger, A. M. (2006). The risk principle in action: What have we learned from 13,676 offenders and 97 correctional programs? *Crime and Delinquency*, 52, 77–93.

Lowenkamp, C. T., Latessa, E. J., & Smith, P. (2006). Does correctional program quality really matter: The impact of adhering to the principles of effective intervention. *Criminology & Public Policy*, 5, 201–220.

Loza, W. (2003). Predicting violent and nonviolent recidivism of incarcerated male offenders. *Aggression and Violent Behaviour*, 8, 175–203.

Lucia, S. & Killias, M. (2011). Is animal cruelty a marker of interpersonal violence and delinquency? Results of a Swiss national self-report study. *Psychology of Violence*, 1, 93–105.

Luckenbill, D. F. (1977). Criminal homicide as a situated transaction. *Social Problems*, 25, 176–186.

Luckenbill, D. F. (1981). Generating compliance: The case of robbery. *Urban Life (Journal of Contemporary Ethnography)*, 10, 25–46.

Luckenbill, D. F. & Doyle, D. P. (1989). Structural position and violence: Developing a cultural explanation. *Criminology*, 27, 419–436.

Lum, C. & Yang, S.-M. (2005). Why do evaluation researchers in crime and justice use non-experimental methods? *Journal of Experimental Criminology*, 1, 191–213.

Lundholm, L., Haggård, U., Möller, J., Hallqvist, J. & Thiblin, I. (2013). The triggering effect of alcohol and illicit drugs on violent crime in a remand prison population: A case crossover study. *Drug and Alcohol Dependence*, 129, 110–115.

Lundström, R. (2013). Framing fraud: Discourse on benefit cheating in Sweden and the UK. *European Journal of Communication*, 28, 630–645.

Lussier, P. & Cale, J. (2013). Beyond sexual recidivism: A review of the sexual criminal career parameters of adult sex offenders. *Aggression and Violent Behavior*, 18, 445–457.

Lussier, P., LeClerc, B., Cale, J. & Proulx, J. (2007). Developmental pathways of deviance in sexual aggressors. *Criminal Justice and Behavior*, 34, 1441–1462.

Lussier, P., Proulx, J. & LeBlanc, M. (2005). Criminal propensity, deviant sexual interests and criminal activity of sexual aggressors against women: A comparison of explanatory models. *Criminology*, 43, 249–281.

Lykken, D. T. (1957). A study of anxiety in the sociopathic personality. *Journal of Abnormal and Social Psychology*, 55, 6–10.

Lynam, D. R., Caspi, A., Moffitt, T. E., Loeber, R., & Stouthamer-Loeber, M. (2007). Longitudinal evidence that psychopathy scores in early adolescence predict adult psychopathy. *Journal of Abnormal Psychology*, 116, 155–165.

M

Maas, C., Herrenkohl, T. I. & Sousa, C. (2008). Review of research on child maltreatment and violence in youth. *Trauma Violence Abuse*, 9, 56–67.

Maccoby, E. E. (2015). Historical overview of socialization theory and research. In J. E. Grusec & P. D. Hastings (eds.), *Handbook of Socialization: Theory and Research*. 2nd edition. pp. 3–32. New York, NY: Guilford Press.

MacCulloch, M., Snowden, P. R., Wood, P. J. & Mills, H. E. (1983). Sadistic fantasy, sadistic behaviour and offending. *British Journal of Psychiatry*, 143, 20–29.

Mackay, R. D. (2010). Mental disability at the time of the offence. In L. Gostin, P. Bartlett, P. Fennell, J. McHale & R. Mackay (eds.), *Principles of Mental Health Law and Policy*. pp. 721–755. Oxford: Oxford University Press.

Mackay, R. D. & Colman, A. M. (1996). Equivocal rulings on expert psychological and psychiatric evidence: Turning a muddle into a nonsense. *Criminal Law Review*, 88–95.

MacKenzie, D. L. (2006). *What Works in Corrections: Reducing the Criminal Activities of Offenders and Delinquents*. Cambridge: Cambridge University Press.

MacKenzie, D. L. & Farrington, D. P. (2015). Preventing future offending of delinquents and offenders: what have we learned from experiments and meta-analyses? *Journal of Experimental Criminology*, 11, 565–595.

MacKenzie, D. L., Wilson, D. B. & Kider, S. B. (2001). Effects of correctional boot camps on offending. *Annals of the American Academy of Political and Social Science*, 578, 126–143.

MacLeod, M. D. (2002). Retrieval-induced forgetting in eyewitness memory: forgetting as a consequence of remembering. *Applied Cognitive Psychology*, 16, 135–149.

McAdams, D. P. (2009). *The person: An introduction to the science of personality psychology*. 5th edition. New York, NY: Wiley.

McCabe, M. P. & Wauchope, M. (2005). Behavioral characteristics of men accused of rape: Evidence for different types of rapists. *Archives of Sexual Behavior*, 34, 241–253.

McCall, G. S. & Shields, N. (2008). Examining the evidence from small-scale societies and early prehistory and implications for modern theories and aggression and violence. *Aggression and Violent Behavior*, 13, 1–9.

McCall, P. S., Land, K. C. & Parker, K. F. (2011). Heterogeneity in the rise and decline of city-level homicide rates, 1976-2005: A latent trajectory analysis. *Social Science Research*, 40, 363–378.

McCall, P. S., Parker, K. F. & McDonald, J. M. (2008). The dynamic relationship between homicide rates and social, economic, and political factors from 1970 to 2000. *Social Science Research*, 37, 721–735.

McCarthy, D. (2012). How can the Sandy Hook atrocity happen? *The Media Transformation*. http://www.themediatransformation.com/2012/12/16/how-can-the-sandy-hook-atrocity-happen-a-statistical-look-at-the-perpetrators-of-school-violence/

McConkey, K. M. & Roche, S.M. (1989). Knowledge of eyewitness memory. *Australian Psychologist,* 24, 377–84.

McCord, J. (1979). Some child-rearing antecedents of criminal behavior in adult men. *Journal of Personality and Social Psychology*, 37, 1477–1486.

McCord, J. (1992). The Cambridge-Somerville Youth Study: A pioneering longitudinal experimental study of delinquency prevention. In J. McCord & R. E. Tremblay (eds.), *Preventing Antisocial Behavior*. pp. 196–206. New York, NY: Guilford Press.

McCoy, A. (2006). *A question of torture: CIA interrogation, from the cold war to the war on terror*. New York: Metropolitan Books/Henry Holt.

McDevitt, J., Levin, J. & Bennett, S. (2002). Hate crime offenders: An expanded typology. *Journal of Social Issues*, 58, 303–317.

McDougall, C., Cohen, M. A., Swaray, R. & Perry, A. (2003). The costs and benefits of sentencing: A systematic review. *Annals of the American Academy of Political and Social Science*, 587, 160–177.

McDowall, D., Wiersema, B. & Loftin, C. (1989). Did mandatory firearm ownership in Kennesaw really prevent burglaries? *Sociology and Sociological Research*, 74, 48–51.

McEwan, J. (2000). Decision making in legal settings. In J. McGuire, T. Mason, & A. O'Kane (eds.) *Behaviour, Crime and Legal Processes: A Guide for Forensic Practitioners*. pp. 111–131. Chichester: Wiley.

McEwan, T. E. & Ducat, L. (2016). The role of mental disorder in firesetting behaviour. In R. M. Doley, G. L. Dickens & T. A. Gannon (eds.), *The Psychology of Arson: A Practical Guide to Understanding and Managing Deliberate Firesetters*. pp. 211–227. Abingdon: Routledge.

McEwan, T., Pathé, M. & Ogloff, J. R. P. (2011). Advances in stalking risk assessment. *Behavioral Sciences and the Law*, 29, 180–201.

McEwan, T., Shea, D. E., Daffern, M., MacKenzie, R. D., Ogloff, J. R. P. & Mullen, P. E. (2016). The reliability and predictive validity of the Stalking Risk Profile. *Assessment.* Doi: 10.1177/1073191116653470

McGuire, J. (ed.) (1995). *What Works: Reducing Reoffending: Guidelines from Research and Practice*. Chichester: Wiley.

McGuire, J. (1997). Ethical dilemmas in forensic clinical psychology. *Legal and Criminological Psychology*, 2, 177–192.

McGuire, J. (2000). Can the criminal law ever be therapeutic? *Behavioral Sciences and the Law,* 18, 413–426.

McGuire, J. (2001). Defining correctional programs. In L. L. Motiuk & R. C. Serin (eds.), *Compendium 2000 on Effective Correctional Programming*. pp. 1-8. Ottawa: Correctional Service Canada.

McGuire, J. (2002). Criminal sanctions versus psychologically-based interventions with offenders: a comparative empirical analysis. *Psychology, Crime & Law*, 8, 183–208.

McGuire, J. (2003). Property offenders. In C. R. Hollin (ed.), *The Essential Handbook of Offender Assessment and Treatment*. pp. 264–288. Chichester: Wiley.

McGuire, J. (2004a). *Understanding Psychology and Crime: Perspectives on Theory and Action*. Maidenhead; Open University Press/McGraw-Hill Education.

McGuire, J. (2004b). Minimising harm in violence risk assessment: practical solutions to ethical problems? *Health, Risk, & Society,* 6, 327–345.

McGuire, J. (2008). A review of effective interventions for reducing aggression and violence. *Philosophical Transactions of the Royal Society B*, 363, 2577–2597.

McGuire, J. (2013). "What Works" to reduce reoffending: 18 years on. In L. Craig, J. Dixon & T. A. Gannon (eds.), *What Works in Offender Rehabilitation: An Evidence Based Approach to Assessment and Treatment*. pp. 20–49. Chichester: Wiley-Blackwell.

McGuire, J. (2017a). Crime and punishment: what works? In G. Davies & A. R. Beech (eds.), *Forensic Psychology*. 3rd edition. pp. 481–511. Chichester: Wiley.

McGuire, J. (2017b). Assessing risk of violence in offenders with mental disorders. In K. D. Browne, A. R. Beech, L. A. Craig & S. Chou (eds.), *Assessments in Forensic Practice: A Handbook*. pp. 139–171. Chichester: Wiley-Blackwell.

McGuire, J. (2017c). Evidence-based practice and adults: What works? What works best? In P. Sturmey (ed.), *The Wiley Handbook of Violence and Aggression*. New York, NY: Wiley.

McGuire, J., Mason, T. & O'Kane, A. (2000). Effective interventions, service and policy implications. In J. McGuire, T. Mason, & A. O'Kane (eds.) *Behaviour, Crime and Legal Processes: A Guide for Forensic Practitioners*. pp. 289–314. Chichester: Wiley.

McGuire, J., Bilby, C. A. L., Hatcher, R. M., Hollin, C. R., Hounsome, J. C. & Palmer, E. J. (2008). Evaluation of structured cognitive-behavioural programs in reducing criminal recidivism. *Journal of Experimental Criminology*, 4, 21–40.

McGuire, R. J., Carlisle, J. M. & Young, B. G. (1964). Sexual deviations as conditioned behaviour: a hypothesis. *Behaviour Research and Therapy*, 2, 185–190.

McLaughlin, E. & Newburn, T. (eds.) (2010). *The Sage Handbook of Criminological Theory*. London: Sage.

McLaughlin, J., O'Carroll, R. E. & O'Connor, R. C. (2012). Intimate partner abuse a suicidality: a systematic review. *Clinical Psychology Review*, 32, 677–689.

McLean, I. & Urken, A. B. (1995). *Classics of Social Choice*. Ann Arbor, MI: University of Michigan Press.

McLean, J., Maxwell, M., Platt, S., Harris, F. & Jepson, R. (2008). *Risk and protective factors for suicide and suicidal behaviour: A literature review*. Edinburgh: Scottish Government Social Research. www.scotland.gov.uk/socialresearch

McManus, S., Meltzer, H., Brugha, T., Bebbington, P. & Jenkins, R. (2009). *Adult Psychiatric Morbidity in England, 2007: Results of a Household Survey*. London: NHS Information Centre for Health and Social Care.

McMurran, M. (ed.) (2002). *Motivating Offenders to Change: A Guide to Enhancing Engagement in Therapy*. Chichester: Wiley.

McMurran, M. (2007). The relationships between alcohol-aggression proneness, general alcohol expectancies, hazardous drinking, and alcohol-related violence in adult male prisoners. *Psychology, Crime & Law*, 13, 275–284.

McMurran, M. (2009). Personality, personality disorder, and violence: An introduction. In M. McMurran & R. Howard (eds.), *Personality, Personality Disorder, and Violence*. pp. 3–18. Chichester: Wiley-Blackwell.

McMurran, M. (2011). Anxiety, alcohol intoxication, and aggression. *Legal and Criminological Psychology*, 16, 357–371.

McMurran, M. & Duggan, C. (2005). The manualisation of a treatment programme for personality disorder. *Criminal Behaviour and Mental Health*, 15, 17–27.

McMurran, M. & McGuire, J. (eds.) (2005). *Social Problem-Solving and Offending: Evidence, Evaluation and Evolution*. Chichester: Wiley.

McMurran, M., Hoyte, H. & Jinks, M. (2012). Triggers for alcohol-related violence in young male offenders. *Legal and Criminological Psychology*, 17, 307–321.

McMurran, M., Khalifa, N. & Gibbon, S. (2009). *Forensic Mental Health*. Cullompton: Willan Publishing.

McNally, M. R. & Fremouw, W. J. (2014). Examining risk of escalation: A critical review of the exhibitionistic behavior literature. *Aggression and Violent Behavior*, 19, 474–485.

McNiel, D. E., Eisner, J. P. & Binder, R. L. (2000). The relationship between command hallucinations and violence. *Psychiatric Services*, 51, 1288–1292.

McVay, D., Schiraldi, V. & Ziedenberg, J. (2004). *Treatment or Incarceration? National and State Findings on the Efficacy and Cost Savings of Drug Treatment Versus Imprisonment*. Washington, DC: Justice Policy Institute.

McVicar, J. (2004). *McVicar by Himself*. 3rd edition. Artnik.

McVilly, K. R. (1995). Interviewing people with a learning disability about their residential service. *British Journal of Learning Disabilities*, 23, 138–142.

Maddux, J. E., Gosselin, J. T. & Winstead, B. A. (2015). Conceptions of psychopathology: A social constructionist perspective. In J. E. Maddux & B. A. Winstead (eds.), *Psychopathology: Foundations for a Contemporary Understanding*. 4th edition. pp. 3–17. New York, NY: Routledge.

Maddux, J. E. & Winstead, B. E. (eds.) (2015). *Psychopathology: Foundations for a Contemporary Understanding. 4th edition*. New York, NY: Routledge.

Maden, A., Scott, F., Burnett, R., Lewis, G. H. & Skapinakis, P. (2004). Offending in psychiatric patients after discharge from medium secure units: prospective national cohort study. *British Medical Journal*, 328, 1534.

Magaletta, P. R., Faust, E., Bickart, W. & McLearen, A. M. (2014). Exploring clinical and personality characteristics of adult male internet-only child pornography offenders. *International Journal of Offender Therapy and Comparative Criminology*, 58, 137–53.

Maguire, M. (2012). Crime statistics and the construction of crime. In M. Maguire, R. Morgan, & R. Reiner (eds.) *The Oxford Handbook of Criminology*. 5th edition. pp. 206–244. Oxford: Oxford University Press.

Maguire, M., Grubin, D., Lösel, F. & Raynor, P. (2010). 'What Works' and the Correctional Services Accreditation Panel: Taking stock from an insider perspective. *Criminology and Criminal Justice*, 10, 37–58.

Maguire, M., Morgan, R. & Reiner, R. (eds.) (2012). *The Oxford Handbook of Criminology*. Oxford: Oxford University Press.

Maher, G. (2005). Age and criminal responsibility. *Ohio State Journal of Criminal Law*, 2, 493–512.

Mahoney, M. J. (1974). *Cognition and Behavior Modification.* Cambridge, MA: Ballinger.

Malamuth, N. M. (1981). Rape proclivity among males. *Journal of Social Issues,* 37, 138–157.

Malby, S. (2010). Homicide. In S. Harrendorf, M. Heiskanen & S. Malby (eds.), *International Statistics on Crime and Justice*. HEUNI Publication Series No.64. pp. 7–20. Helsinki and Vienna: European Institute for Crime Prevention and Control & United Nations Office on Drugs and Crime.

Males, M. (2011). *Striking out: California's "three strikes and you're out" law has not reduced violent crime: A 2011 update*. Research Brief, Center on Juvenile and Criminal Justice. http://www.cjcj.org/uploads/cjcj/documents/Striking_Out_Californias_Three_Strikes_And_Youre_Out_Law_Has_Not_Reduced_Violent_Crime.pdf

Maletzky, B. M. & George, F. S. (1973). The treatment of homosexuality by 'assisted' covert sensitization. *Behavior Research & Therapy,* 11, 655–657.

Mallender, J. & Tierney, R. (2016). Economic analyses. In D. Weisburd, D. P. Farrington and C. Gill (eds.), *What Works in Crime Prevention and Rehabilitation: Lessons from Systematic Reviews*. pp. 291–309. New York, NY: Springer.

Malmquist, C. P. (2010). Adolescent parricide and a clinical and legal problem. *Journal of the American Academy of Psychiatry and the Law*, 38, 73–79.

Malmquist, C. P. (2013). Infanticide/neonaticide: the outlier situation in the United States. *Aggression and Violent Behavior*, 18, 399–408.

Malpass, R. S., Tredoux, C. G. & McQuiston-Surrett, D. (2009). Public policy and sequential lineups. *Legal and Criminological Psychology*, 14, 1–12.

Maniglio, R. (2009). The impact of child sexual abuse on health: A systematic review of reviews. *Clinical Psychology Review*, 29, 647–657.

Mann, R. E., Hanson, R. K. & Thornton, D. (2010). Assessing risk for sexual recidivism: some proposals on the nature of psychologically meaningful risk factors. *Sexual Abuse: A Journal of Research and Treatment*, 22, 191–217.

Mann, S., Vrij, A., Shaw, D. J., Leal, S., Ewens, S., Hillman, J., Granhag, P. A., & Fisher, R. P. (2013). Two heads are better than one? How to effectively use two interviewers to elicit cues to deception. *Legal and Criminological Psychology*, 18, 324–340.

Mannarino, A. P. & Cohen, J. A. (2001). Treating sexually abused children and their families: Identifying and avoiding professional role conflicts. *Trauma, Violence, & Abuse,* 2, 331–342.

Marbe, K. (1913). *Grundzüge Der Forensischen Psychologie.* [Foundations of Forensic Psychology]. München: C. H. Beck.

Marcus, D. K., John, S. L. & Edens, J. F. (2004). A taxometric analysis of psychopathic personality. *Journal of Abnormal Psychology*, 113, 626–635.

Mark, T. L., Levit, K. R., Buck, J. A., Coffey, R. M. & Vandivort-Warren, R. (2007). Mental health treatment expenditure trends, 1986–2003. *Psychiatric Services*, 48, 1041–1048.

Marquart, J.W. & Sorensen, J.R. (1989). A national study of the Furman-commuted inmates: assessing the threat to society from capital offenders. *Loyola of Los Angeles Law Review,* 23, 101–20.

Marsh, A. A., Finger, E. C., Mitchell, D. G. V., Reid, M. E., Sims, C., Kosson, D. S., Towbin, K. E., Leibenluft, E., Pine, D. S. & Blair, R. J. R. (2008). Reduced amygdala response to fearful expressions in children and adolescents with callous-unemotional traits and disruptive behavior disorders. *American Journal of Psychiatry*, 165, 712–720.

Marsh, K., Fox, C. & Sarmah, R. (2009). Is custody an effective sentencing option for the UK? Evidence from a meta-analysis of existing studies. *Probation Journal: The Journal of Community and Criminal Justice,* 56, 129–151.

Marshall, W. L. & Fernandez, Y. (2003). Sexual preferences: Are they useful in the assessment and treatment of sexual offenders? *Aggression and Violent Behavior*, 8, 131–143.

Marshall, W. L. & Kennedy, P. (2003). Sexual sadism in sexual offenders: An elusive diagnosis. *Aggression and Violent Behavior*, 8, 1–22.

Marshall, W. L., Fernandez, Y., Marshall, L. E. & Serran, G. A. (Eds.) (2006). *Sexual Offender Treatment: Controversial Issues*. Chichester: Wiley.

Marston, W. M. (1917). Systolic blood pressure symptoms of deception. *Journal of Experimental Psychology*, 2, 117–163.

Marston, W. M. (1920). Reaction-time symptoms of deception. *Journal of Experimental Psychology*, 3, 72–87.

Marston, W. M. (1921). Psychological possibilities in deception tests. *Journal of the American Institute of Criminal Law and Criminology*, 11, 551–570.

Mart, E. G. (2004). Factitious disorder by proxy: a call for the abandonment of an outmoded diagnosis. *Journal of Psychiatry and Law*, 32, 297–314.

Martens, W. H. J. & Palermo, G. B. (2005). Loneliness and associated violent antisocial behavior: Analysis of the case reports of Jeffrey Dahmer and Dennis Nilsen. *International Journal of Offender Therapy and Comparative Criminology*, 49, 298–307.

Martin, G. (2016). *Understanding Terrorism: Challenges, Perspectives, and Issues*. 5th edition. Thousand Oaks: Sage.

Martin, J. (2014). *The English Legal System*. Abingdon: Routledge.

Martin, M. S., Dorken, S. K., Wamboldt, A. D. & Wootten, S. E. (2012). Stopping the revolving door: A meta-analysis on the effectiveness of interventions for criminally involved individuals with major mental disorders. *Law and Human Behavior*, 36, 1–12.

Martinson, R. (1974). What works? – Questions and answers about prison reform. *The Public Interest*, 10, 22–54.

Martire, K. (2010). An examination of the implications of financial strain for forensic psychology. *Journal of Forensic Psychology Practice*, 10, 159–176.

Maruna, S. (2001). *Making Good: How Ex-convicts Reform and Rebuild Their Lives*. Washington, DC: American Psychological Association.

Maruna, S. & Copes, H. (2005). What have we learned from five decades of neutralization research? *Crime and Justice*, 32, 221–320.

Maruna, S. & LeBel, T.P. (2003). Welcome home? Examining the "re-entry court" concept from a strength-based perspective. *Western Criminology Review*, 42, 91–107.

Maruna, S. & Mann, R. E. (2006). A fundamental attribution error? Rethinking cognitive distortions. *Legal and Criminological Psychology*, 11, 155–177.

Masip, J., Alonso, H., Garrido, E. & Anton, C. (2005). Generalized Communicative Suspicion (GCS) among police officers: Accounting for the investigator bias effect. *Journal of Applied Social Psychology*, 35, 1046–1066.

Mason, D. A. & Frick, P. J. (1994). The heritability of antisocial behaviour: a meta-analysis of twin and adoption studies. *Journal of Psychopathology and Behavioral Assessment*, 16, 301–323.

Masters, B. (1985). *Killing for Company: The Case of Dennis Nilsen*. London: Jonathan Cape.

Masuda, T. & Nisbett, R. E. (2006). Culture and change blindness. *Cognitive Science*, 30, 381–399.

Matsueda, R. L. & Anderson, K. (1998). The dynamics of delinquent peers and delinquent behavior. *Criminology*, 36, 269–308.

Mattei, U. (1997). Three patterns of law: Taxonomy and change in the world's legal systems. *American Journal of Comparative Law*, 45, 5–44.

Matthews, K., Shepherd, J. & Sivarajasingham, V. (2006). Violence-related injury and the price of beer in England and Wales. *Applied Economics*, 38, 661–670.

Mattson, M. & Rengert, G. (1995). Danger, distance, and desirability: Perceptions of inner city neighborhoods. *European Journal of Criminal Policy and Research*, 3, 70–78.

Mayhew, P. (1979). Defensible Space: the current status of a crime prevention theory. *Howard Journal of Penology and Crime Prevention*, 18, 150–159.

Mayhew, P., Clarke, R. V. G. & Elliot, D. (1989). Motorcycle theft, helmet legislation and displacement. *Howard Journal of Criminal Justice*, 28, 1–8.

Mazur, A. (2009). A hormonal interpretation of Collins's micro-sociological theory of violence. *Journal for the Theory of Social Behaviour*, 39, 434–447.

Meehl, P. E. (1992). Factors and taxa, traits and types, differences of degree and differences in kind. *Journal of Personality*, 60, 117–174.

Meichenbaum, D. H. (1977). *Cognitive-Behavior Modification: An Integrative Approach*. New York, NY: Plenum Press.

Meier, R. F., Kennedy, L. W. & Sacco, V. F. (2001). Crime and the criminal event perspective. In R. F. Meier, L. W. Kennedy & V. F. Sacco (eds.), *The Process and Structure of Crime: Criminal Events and Crime Analysis. Advances in Criminological Theory*, Vol. 9. pp. 1–27. New Brunswick, NJ and London: Transaction Publishers.

Meijer, E. H., Verschuere, B., Merckelbach, H. L. G. J. Crombez, G. (2008). Sex offender management using the polygraph: a critical review. *International Journal of Law and Psychiatry*, 31, 423–429.

Melnyk, T., Bloomfield, S. & Benell, C. (2007). *Classifying serial sexual homicide: Validating Keppel and Walter's (1999) Model.* Poster presented at the annual meeting of the Society for Police and Criminal Psychology, Springfield, MA.

Meloy, J. R. & Felthous, A. R. (2004). Introduction to this issue: Serial and mass homicide. *Behavioral Sciences and the Law*, 22, 289–290.

Meloy, J. R., Hempel, A. G., Mohandie, K., Shiva, A. A. & Gray, B. T. (2001). Offender and offense characteristics of a nonrandom sample of adolescent mass murderers. *Journal of the American Academy of Child and Adolescent Psychiatry*, 40, 719–728.

Meloy, J. R., Hempel, A. G., Gray, B. T., Mohandie, K., Shiva, A. A. & Richards, T. C. (2004). A comparative analysis of North American adolescent and adult mass murderers. *Behavioral Sciences and the Law*, 22, 291–309.

Melton, G.B., Petrila, J. Pothress, N.G., Slobogin, C., Otto, R. K., Mossman, D. & Condie, L. O. (2018). *Psychological evaluations for the courts: A handbook for mental health professionals and lawyers.* 4th edition. New York, NY: Guilford Press.

Memon, A., Vrij, A. & Bull, R. (2003). *Psychology & Law: Truthfulness, Accuracy and Credibility of Victims, Witnesses and Suspects*. 2nd edition. Chichester: Wiley-Interscience.

Memon, A., Wark, L., Bull, R. & Koehnken, G. (1997). Isolating the effects of the cognitive interview techniques. *British Journal of Psychology*, 88, 179–197.

Merdian, H. L. & Jones, D. T. (2011). Phallometric assessment of sexual arousal. In D. P. Boer, R. Eher, L. A. Craig, M. H. Miner & F. Pfäfflin (eds.), *International Perspectives on the Assessment and Treatment of Sexual Offenders: Theory, Practice and Research*. pp. 142–169. Chichester: Wiley-Blackwell.

Mews, A., Di Bella, L. & Purver, M. (2017). *Impact evaluation of the prison-based Core Sex Offender Treatment Programme*. Ministry of Justice Analytical Series. London: Ministry of Justice.

Middleton, D., Elliot, I. A., Mandeville-Norden, R. & Beech, A. R. (2006). An investigation into the applicability of the Ward and Siegert Pathways Model of child sexual abuse with internet offenders. *Psychology, Crime & Law*, 12, 589–603.

Miethe, T. D. & Lu, H. (2005). *Punishment: A Comparative Historical Perspective*. Cambridge: Cambridge University Press.

Miethe, T. D., Olson, J. & Mitchell, O. (2006). Specialization and persistence in the arrest histories of sex offenders: A comparative analysis of alternative measures and offence types. *Journal of Reseach in Crime and Delinquency*, 43, 204–229.

Miethe, T. D. & Regoeczi, W. C. (2004). *Rethinking Homicide: Exploring the Structure and Process Underlying Deadly Situations.* Cambridge: Cambridge University Press.

Miles, D. R. and Carey, G. (1997). Genetic and environmental architecture of human aggression. *Journal of Personality and Social Psychology*, 72, 207–217.

Milgram, S. (1963). Behavioral study of obedience. *Journal of Abnormal and Social Psychology*, 67, 371–378.

Miller, A. D. & Perry, R. (2012). The reasonable person. *New York University Law Review,* 87, 323–392.

Miller, J. (1997). *Search and Destroy: African-American Males in the Criminal Justice System*. Cambridge: Cambridge University Press.

Miller, J. M. (2007). Conceptualizing the hijacking threat to civil aviation. *Criminal Justice Review*, 32, 209–232.

Miller, L. (2012). Stalking: Patterns, motives, and intervention strategies. *Aggression and Violent Behavior*, 17, 495–506.

Miller, L. (2014a). Serial killers: I. Subtypes, patterns, and motives. *Aggression and Violent Behavior*, 19, 1–11.

Miller, L. (2014b). Serial killers: II. Development, dynamics, and forensics. *Aggression and Violent Behavior*, 19, 12–22.

Miller, L. (2014c). Rape: I. Sex crime, act of violence, or naturalistic adaptation? *Aggression and Violent Behavior*, 18, 67–81.

Miller, M., Drake, E. & Nafziger, M. (2013). *What works to reduce recidivism by domestic violence offenders?* (Document No. 13-01-1201). Olympia, WA: Washington State Institute for Public Policy.

Miller, M., Hemenway, D. & Azrael, D. (2007). State-level homicide victimization rates in the US in relation to survey measures of household firearm ownership. 2001–2003. *Social Science & Medicine*, 64, 656–664.

Miller, M. K. & Bornstein, B. H. (2004). Juror stress: Causes and interventions. *Thurgood Marshall Law Review*, 30, 237–269.

Miller, M. K., & Flores, D. M. (2007). Addressing the problem of Courtroom stress. *Judicature*, 91, 60–69.

Miller, P. G., Curtis, A., Sønderlund, A., Day, A., & Droste, N. (2015). Effectiveness of interventions for convicted DUI offenders in reducing recidivism: a systematic review of the peer-reviewed scientific literature. *American Journal of Drug and Alcohol Abuse*, 41, 16–29.

Mills, J. E., Kroner, D. G. & Morgan, R. D. (2011). *Clinician's Guide to Violence Risk Assessment*. New York, NY: Guilford Press.

Milne, R. & Bull, R. (1999). *Investigative Interviewing: Psychology and Practice*. Chichester: Wiley.

Milne, R. & Bull, R. (2001). Interviewing witnesses with learning disabilities for legal purposes. *British Journal of Learning Disabilities*, 29, 93–97.

Milne, R. & Bull, R. (2002). Back to basics: A componential analysis of the original cognitive interview mnemonics with three age groups. *Applied Cognitive Psychology*, 16, 743–753.

Milne, R. & Bull, R. (2003). Does the cognitive interview help children to resist the effects of suggestive questioning? *Legal and Criminological Psychology*, 8, 21–38.

Milne, R., Clare, I. C. H., & Bull, R. (1999). Using the cognitive interview with adults with mild learning disabilities. *Psychology, Crime, and Law*, 5, 81–99.

Min, M., Farkas, K., Minnes, S. & Singer, L. T. (2007). Impact of childhood abuse and neglect on substance abuse and psychological distress in adulthood. *Journal of Traumatic Stress*, 20, 833–844.

Ministry of Justice (2012). *The Criminal Injuries Compensation Scheme 2012*. London: Ministry of Justice.

Ministry of Justice (2013a). *Attitudes to Sentencing and Trust in Justice: Exploring Trends from the Crime Survey for England and Wales*. London: Ministry of Justice.

Ministry of Justice (2013b). *Communicating Sentencing: exploring new ways to explain adult sentences*. London: Ministry of Justice.

Ministry of Justice (2013c). *Proven Re-offending Statistics Quarterly Bulletin, April 2010 to March 2011, England and Wales*. London: Ministry of Justice.

Ministry of Justice (2016). *A guide to criminal court statistics*. London: Office for National Statistics and Ministry of Justice.

Ministry of Justice (2017a). *Proven Reoffending Statistics Quarterly Bulletin, April 2014 to March 2015*. London: Ministry of Justice.

Ministry of Justice (2017b). *Guide to Offender Management Statistics: England and Wales*. Ministry of Justice Guidance Documentation.

Ministry of Justice & Office for National Statistics (2017a). *Criminal Justice Statistics Quarterly, England and Wales, July 2016 to June 2017 (provisional)*. London: Ministry of Justice and Office for National Statistics.

Ministry of Justice & Office for National Statistics (2017b). *Offender Management Statistics Quarterly*: Prison receptions: April to June 2017. (Excel spreadsheet). https://www.gov.uk/government/collections/offender-management-statistics-quarterly

Ministry of Justice & Office for National Statistics (2017c). *Offender Management Statistics Quarterly: Probation: April to June 2017*. (Excel spreadsheet). https://www.gov.uk/government/collections/offender-management-statistics-quarterly

Ministry of Justice, Home Office & Office for National Statistics (2013). *An Overview of Sexual Offending in England and Wales. Statistical Bulletin*. London: Office for National Statistics.

Minkes, J. (2010). Corporate financial crimes. In F. Brookman, M. Maguire, H. Pierpoint & T. Bennett (eds.), *Handbook on Crime*. pp. 653–677. Cullompton: Willan.

Minkes, J. & Minkes, L. (2010). Income tax evasion and benefit fraud. In F. Brookman, M. Maguire, H. Pierpoint & T. Bennett (eds.), *Handbook on Crime*. pp. 87–99. Cullompton: Willan Publishing.

Mischel, W. (1973). Toward a cognitive social learning reconceptualization of personality. *Psychological Review*, 80, 252–283.

Mischel, W. (2004). Toward an integrative science of the person. *Annual Review of Psychology*, 55, 1–22.

Mischel, W. & Shoda, Y. (1995). A cognitive-affective system theory of personality: reconceptualising situations, dispositions, dynamics and invariance in personality structure. *Psychological Review*, 102, 246–268.

Mitchell, O., Wilson, D. B., Eggers, A. & MacKenzie, D. L. (2012). Drug courts' effects on criminal offending for juveniles and adults. *Campbell Systematic Reviews*. Doi:10.4073.

Mitchell, O., Wilson, D. B. & MacKenzie, D. L. (2006). The effectiveness of incarceration-based drug treatment on criminal behaviour. *Campbell Systematic Reviews*. Doi: 10.4073/csr.2006.11

Mize, K. D. & Shackelford, T. K. (2008). Intimate partner homicide methods in heterosexual, gay, and lesbian relationships. *Violence and Victims*, 23, 98–114.

Moffitt, T. E. (1993) Adolescence-limited and life-course-persistent antisocial behavior: a developmental taxonomy. *Psychological Review*, 100, 674–701.

Moffitt, T. E. (2003). Life-course-persistent and adolescence-limited antisocial behaviour: A 10-year research review and a research agenda. In B. B. Lahey, T. E. Moffitt & A. Caspi (eds.), *Causes of Conduct Disorder and Delinquency*. pp. 49–75. New York, NY: Guilford Press.

Moffitt, T. E. (2005) Genetic and environmental influences on antisocial behaviours: evidence from behaviour-genetic research. *Advances in Genetics*, 55, 41–104.

Moffitt, T. E. & Caspi, A. (2007). Evidence from behavioural genetics for environmental contributions to antisocial conduct. In. J. E. Grusex & P. D. Hastings (eds.), *Handbook of Socialisation: Theory and Research*. pp. 96–123. New York, NY: Guilford Press.

Moffitt, T. E., Caspi, A., Rutter, M. & Silva, P. A. (2001). *Sex Differences in Antisocial Behaviour: Conduct Disorder, Delinquency and Violence in the Dunedin Longitudinal Study*. Cambridge: Cambridge University Press.

Moffitt, T. E., Caspi, A., Taylor, A., Kokaua, J., Milne, B. J., Polanczyk, G. & Poulton, R. (2010). How common are common mental disorders? Evidence that lifetime prevalence rates are doubled by prospective versus retrospective ascertainment. *Psychological Medicine*, 40, 899–909.

Mokros, A. & Alison, L. J. (2002). Is profiling possible? Testing the predicted homology of crime scene actions and background characteristics in a sample of rapists. *Legal & Criminological Psychology*, 7, 25–43.

Mokros, A., Gebhard, M., Heinz, V., Marschall, R. W., Nitschke, J., Glasgow, D. V., Gress, C. L. Z. & Laws, D. R. (2012). Computerized assessment of pedophilic sexual interest through self-report and viewing time: reliability, validity and classification accuracy of the Affinity Program. *Sexual Abuse: A Journal of Research and Treatment*, 25, 230–258.

Monahan, J. (1981). *The Clinical Prediction of Violent Behavior*. Washington, DC: Government Printing Office.

Monahan, J. (2012). The individual risk assessment of terrorism. *Psychology, Public Policy, and Law*, 18, 167–205.

Monahan, J. & Walker, L. (2009). *Social Science in Law: Cases and Materials*. 7th edition. New York, NY: Foundation Press.

Moncrieff, J. (2009). *The Myth of the Chemical Cure: A Critique of Psychiatric Drug Treatments*. Basingstoke: Palgrave Macmillan.

Moncrieff, J. & Cohen, D. (2005). Rethinking models of psychotropic drug action. *Psychotherapy and Psychosomatics*, 74, 145–153.

Montana, J. A. (1995). An ineffective weapon in the fight against child sexual abuse: New Jersey's Megan's Law. *Journal of Law and Policy*, 3, 569–604.

Montgomery, C., Fisk, J. E., Murphy, P. N., Ryland, I. & Hilton, J. (2012). The effects of heavy social drinking on executive function: a systematic review and meta-analytic study of existing literature and new empirical findings. *Human Psychopharmacology: Clinical and Experimental*, 27, 187–199.

Moore, C. (2008). Moral disengagement in processes of organizational corruption. *Journal of Business Ethics*, 80, 129–139.

Moore, D. (2001). The anthropology of drinking. In N. Heather, T. J. Peters & T. Stockwell (eds.), *International Handbook of Alcohol Dependence and Problems*. pp. 471–487. Chichester: Wiley.

Moore, K., Mason, P. & Lewis, J. (2008). *Images of Islam in the UK: The Representation of British Muslims in the National Print News Media 2000-2008*. Cardiff University: Cardiff School of Journalism, Media and Cultural Studies.

Moore, T. J., Glenmullen, J. & Furberg, C. D. (2010). Prescription drugs associated with reports of violence towards others. *PLOS ONE*, 5(12): e15337. Doi: 10.1371/journal.pone.0015337

Moore, T. M., Stuart, G. L., Meehan, J. C., Rhatigan, D. L., Hellmuth, J. C. & Keen, S. M. (2008). Drug abuse and aggression between intimate partners: A meta-analytic review. *Clinical Psychology Review*, 28, 247–274.

Morgan, R. D., Flora, D. B., Kroner, D. G., Mills, J. F., Varghese, F. & Steffan, J. S. (2012). Treating offenders with mental illness: A research synthesis. *Law and Human Behavior*, 36, 37–50.

Morgan, S. (1999). Prison lives: critical issues in reading prisoner autobiography. *Howard Journal of Criminal Justice*, 38, 328–340.

Morris, S., Humphreys, D. & Reynolds, D. (2006). Myth, marula, and elephant: an assessment of voluntary alcohol intoxication of the African elephant (*Loxodonta africana*) following feeding on the fruit of the marula tree (*Sclerocarya birrea*). *Physiological and Biochemical Zoology*, 79, 363–369.

Morrison, S. & O'Donnell, I. (1994) *Armed Robbery: A Study in London*. Oxford: Centre for Criminological Research.

Mosher, C. J., Miethe, T. D. & Hart, T. C. (2011). *The Mismeasurement of Crime*. 2nd edition. Thousand Oaks, CA: Sage.

Mossman, D. (1994). Assessing predictions of violence: Being accurate about accuracy. *Journal of Consulting and Clinical Psychology*, 62, 783–792.

Motiuk, L. L. & Serin, R. C. (eds.) (2001). *Compendium 2000 on Effective Correctional Programming*. Ottawa: Correctional Service Canada.

Mouzos, J. & Venditto, J. (2003). *Contract Killings in Australia*. Research and Public Policy Series, No. 53. Canberra: Australian Institute of Criminology.

Müllberger, A. (2009). Teaching psychology to jurists: Initiatives and reactions prior to World War I. *History of Psychology*, 12, 60–86.

Mullen, P. E. (2004). The autogenic (self-generated) massacre. *Behavioral Sciences and the Law*, 22, 311–323.

Mullen, P. E., Pathé, M. & Purcell, R. (2001). The management of stalking. *Advances in Psychiatric Treatment*, 7, 335–342.

Mullen, P. E., Pathé, M., Purcell, R. & Stuart, G. W. (1999). Study of stalkers. American Journal of Psychiatry, 156, 1244–1249.

Mullen, P. E., Mackenzie, R., Ogloff, J. R. P., Pathé, M., McEwan, T. & Purcell, R. (2006). Assessing and managing the risks in the stalking situation. *Journal of the American Academy of Psychiatry and the Law*, 34, 439–450.

Muller, D.A. (2000). Criminal profiling: real science or just wishful thinking? *Homicide Studies*, 4, 234–264

Muncie, J. (2001). The construction and deconstruction of crime. In J. Muncie & E. McLaughlin (eds.), *The Problem of Crime*. 2nd edition. London: Sage in association with the Open University.

Münsterberg, H. (1907). *On the Witness Stand: Essays on Psychology and Crime*. Garden City, NY: Doubleday, Page & Company. Reprinted by the University of Michigan Library.

Murnen, S. K. & Kohlman, M. H. (2007). Athletic participation, fraternity membership, and sexual aggression among college men: A meta-analytic review. *Sex Roles*, 57, 145–157.

Murphy, C. M., Winters, J., O'Farrell, T. J., Fals-Stewart, W. & Murphy, M. (2005). Alcohol consumption and intimate partner violence by alcoholic men: Comparing violent and nonviolent conflicts. *Psychology of Addictive Behaviors*, 19, 35–42.

Murphy, J. M. (1976). Psychiatric labelling in cross-cultural perspective. *Science*, 191, 1019–1028.

Murray, H. A. (1938). *Explorations in Personality*. New York, NY: Oxford University Press.

Murrie, D. C., Boccaccini, M. T., Johnson, J. T. & Janke, C. (2008). Does interrater (dis)agreement on Psychopathy Checklist scores in sexually violent predator trials suggest partisan allegiance in forensic evaluations? *Law and Human Behavior*, 32, 352–362.

Myers, W. C. (2004). Serial murder by children and adolescents. *Behavioral Sciences and the Law*, 22, 357–374.

Myers, W. C., Hustead, D. S., Safarik, M. E. & O'Toole, M. E. (2006). The motivation behind serial sexual homicide: Is it sex, power, and control, or anger? *Journal of Forensic Science*, 51, 900–907.

N

Nagin, D. S., Cullen, F. T. & Jonson, C. L. (2009). Imprisonment and reoffending. In Michael H. Tonry (ed.), *Crime and Justice: A Review of Research*, Vol. 38. pp. 115–200. Chicago, IL: University of Chicago Press.

Nagin, D. S. & Pepper, J. V. (eds.) (2012). *Deterrence and the Death Penalty*. Washington, DC: National Academies Press.

Naimark, N. M. (2017). *Genocide: A World History*. New York, NY: Oxford University Press.

Nair, M. (2016). Pharmacotherapy for sexual offenders. In A. Phenix & H. M. Hoberman (eds.), *Sexual Offending: Predisposing Antecedents, Assessments and Management*. pp. 755–767. New York, NY: Springer.

Napier, M. (2010). *Behavior, truth and deception: Applying profiling and analysis to the interview process*. Boca Raton, FL: CRC Press.

Nathanson, R. & Saywitz, K. J. (2003). The effects of the courtroom context on children's memory and anxiety. *The Journal of Psychiatry and Law*, 31, 67–98.

National Crime Victimization Survey (NCVS) (2003). Weapon use and violent crime. Bureau of Justice Statistics Special Report. http://www.bjs.gov/content/pub/pdf/wuvc01.pdf

National Crime Victimization Survey (NCVS) (2009). Criminal victimization, 2009. Bureau of Justice Statistics Bulletin. http://www.bjs.gov/content/pub/pdf/cv09.pdf

National Fraud Authority (2013). *Annual Fraud Indicator: June 2013*. National Fraud Authority.

National Institute of Health and Clinical Excellence (NICE) (2007). *Drug Misuse: Psychosocial Interventions*. NICE Clinical guideline 51. London: NICE.

National Institute of Health and Clinical Excellence (NICE) (2011a). *Common mental health problems: identification and pathways to care*. NICE Clinical guideline 123. London: NICE.

National Institute of Health and Clinical Excellence (NICE) (2011b). *Alcohol-use disorders: Diagnosis, assessment and management of harmful drinking and alcohol dependence*. NICE Clinical guideline 115. London: NICE.

National Institute on Drug Abuse (2009). *Principles of Drug Addiction Treatment: A Research-based guide*. 2nd edition. Washington, DC: National Institutes of Health, US Department of Health and Human Services.

National Probation Service (2004). *General Offending Behaviour/Cognitive Skills Programmes: Evaluation Manual and Scoring Supplement*. London: Home Office, National Probation Directorate.

National Research Council (2003). *The Polygraph and Lie Detection*. Washington, DC: The National Academies Press. https://doi.org/10.17226/10420.

Naylor, R. T. (2003). Towards a general theory of profit-driven crimes. *British Journal of Criminology*, 43, 81–101.

Nee, C. & Meenaghan, A. (2006). Expert decision making in burglars. *British Journal of Criminology*, 46, 935–949.

Needs, A. (2008). Forensic psychology. In G. J. Towl, D. P. Farrington, D. A. Crighton & G. Hughes (eds.), *Dictionary of Forensic Psychology*. pp. 75–77. Cullompton: Willan Publishing.

Nelken, D. (2012). Comparing criminal justice. In In M. Maguire, R. Morgan & R. Reiner (eds.) *The Oxford Handbook of Criminology*. 5th edition. pp. 138–156. Oxford: Oxford University Press.

Nellis, M. (2002). Community justice, time and the new National Probation Service. *Howard Journal*, 41, 59–86.

Nesca, M. & Dalby, J. T. (2013). *Forensic Interviewing in Criminal Court Matters: A Guide for Clinicians*. Springfield, Il: Charles C. Thomas.

Nettler, G. (1984). *Explaining Crime*. 3rd edition. New York, NY: McGraw-Hill.

Neumann, P. R. (2010). *Prisons and Terrorism: Radicalisation and De-radicalisation in 15 Countries*. International Centre for the Study of Radicalisation and Political Violence, King's College London.

Newburn, T. (ed.) (2009). *Key Readings in Criminology*. Cullompton: Willan Publishing.

Newburn, T. (2017). *Criminology*. 3rd edition. London: Routledge.

Newman, G. (1977). Social institutions and the control of deviance: a cross-national opinion survey. *European Journal of Social Psychology*, 7, 39–59.

Newman, J. P., Curtin, J. J., Bertsch, J. D. & Baskin-Sommers, A. R. (2010). Attention moderates the fearfulness of psychopathic offenders. *Biological Psychiatry*, 67, 66–70.

Newman, K. S. (2013). Adolescent culture and the tragedy of rampage school shootings. In N. Böckler, T. Seeger, P. Sitzer & W. Heitmeyer (eds.), *School Shootings: International Research, Case Studies and Concepts for Prevention*. pp. 55–77. New York, NY: Springer.

Newman, K. S., Fox, C., Harding, D. J., Mehta, J. & Roth, W. (2004). *Rampage: The Social Roots of School Shootings*. New York, NY: Basic Books.

Newman, O. (1996). *Creating Defensible Space*. Washington, DC: US Department of Housing and Urban Development. http://www.huduser.org/publications/pdf/def.pdf

Newman, O. & Franck, K. A. (1982). The effects of building size on personal crime and fear of crime. *Population and Environment*, 5, 203–20.

Nicholls, T. L., Pritchard, M. M., Reeves, K. A. & Hilterman, E. (2013). Risk assessment in intimate partner violence: A systematic review of contemporary approaches. *Partner Abuse*, 4, 76–168.

Nieberding, R. J., Frackowiak, M., Bobholdt, R. H. & Rubel, J. G. (2000). Beware the razorwire: Psychology behind bars. *Journal of Police and Criminal Psychology*, 15, 11–20.

Niebuhr, R. (1963). *Moral man and immoral society*. London: SCM Press.

Nisbett, R. E. & Cohen, D. (1996). *Culture of Honor: The Psychology of Violence in the South*. Oxford: Westview Press.

Nofzinger, E. A. & Wettstein, R. M. (1995). Homicidal behavior and sleep apnea: A case report and medicolegal discussion. *Sleep*, 18, 776–782.

Noor-Mohamed, M. K. (2015). The definitional ambiguities of kidnapping and abduction, and its categorisation: The case for a more inclusive typology. *Howard Journal of Criminal Justice*, 53, 83–100.

Norlander, B. & Eckhardt, C. (2005). Anger, hostility, and male perpetrators of intimate partner violence: A meta-analytic review. *Clinical Psychology Review*, 25, 119–152.

North East Public Health Observatory (2010). *Improving Access to Psychological Therapies: A review of the progress made by the sites in the first roll-out year.* Stockton-on-Tees.

Northfield, J. (2004). BILD factsheet – what is a learning disability? http://www.bild.org.uk/pdfs/05faqs/ld.pdf

Nosworthy, G. J. & Lindsay, R. C. (1990). Does nominal lineup size matter? *Journal of Applied Psychology*, 75, 358–361.

Novaco, R. W. (1975). *Anger Control: The Development and Evaluation of an Experimental Treatment.* Lexington, KT: D. C. Heath.

Novaco, R. W. (1994). Anger as a risk factor for violence among the mentally disordered. In J. Monahan & H. J. Steadman (eds.) *Violence and Mental Disorder: Developments in Risk Assessment.* pp. 21–60. Chicago, IL: University of Chicago Press.

Novaco, R. W. (1997). Remediating anger and aggression with violent offenders. *Legal and Criminological Psychology*, 2, 77–88.

Novaco, R. W. (2007). Anger dysregulation. In T. A. Cavell & K. T. Malcolm (eds.) *Anger, Aggression and Interventions for Interpersonal Violence*, pp. 3–54. Mahwah, NJ: Lawrence Erlbaum Associates.

Nugent, W. R., Williams, M. & Umbreit, M. S. (2004). Participation in victim-offender mediation and the prevalence of subsequent delinquent behaviour: A meta-analysis. *Research on Social Work Practice*, 14, 408–416.

Nunes, K. L. & Jung, S. (2012). Are cognitive distortions associated with denial and minimization among sex offenders? *Sexual Abuse: A Journal of Research and Treatment*, 25, 166–188.

Nuňez, N., Schweitzer, K., Chai, C. A. & Myers, B. (2015). Negative emotions felt during trial: the effect of fear, anger, and sadness on juror decision making. *Applied Cognitive Psychology,* 29, 200–209.

Nutt, D. & Nestor, L. (2013). *Addiction*. Oxford: Oxford University Press.

Nutt, D., King, L. A. & Phillips, L. D. (2010). Drug harms in the UK: a multicriteria decision analysis. *Lancet*, 376, 1558–1565.

Nutt, D., King, L. A., Saulsbury, W. & Blakemore, C. (2007). Development of a rational scale to assess the harm of drugs of potential misuse. *Lancet*, 369, 1047–1053.

O

O'Boyle, G. (2002). Theories of justification and political violence: Examples from four groups. *Terrorism and Political Violence*, 14, 23–46.

O'Kelly, C. M. E., Kebbell, M. R., Hatton, C. & Johnson, S. D. (2003). Judicial intervention in court cases involving witnesses with and without learning disabilities. *Legal and Criminological Psychology,* 8, 229–240.

Odeshoo, J. R. (2004). Of penology and perversity: The use of penile plethysmography on convicted child offenders. *Temple Political & Civil Law Review,* 14, 1–44.

Office for National Statistics (ONS) (2013). *Focus on: Violent Crime and Sexual Offences, 2011/12.* London: ONS Statistical Bulletin.

Office for National Statistics (ONS) (2014). *Chapter 2 - Homicide.* London: ONS Statistical Bulletin.

Office for National Statistics (2015). *Crime in England and Wales, Year Ending March 2015.* London: ONS.

Office for National Statistics (ONS) (2016a). *Crime in England and Wales, Year Ending March 2016.* London: ONS.

Office for National Statistics (ONS) (2016b). *Focus on Violent Crime and Sexual Offences: Year Ending March 2015*. London: ONS.

Office for National Statistics (ONS) (2016c). *Crime in England and Wales: Year Ending June 2016.* London: ONS.

Office for National Statistics (ONS) (2016d). *Intimate personal violence and partner abuse.* Compendium. London: ONS.

Office for National Statistics (2016e). *Research outputs: developing a Crime Severity Score for England and Wales using data on crimes recorded by the police*. London: ONS.

Office for National Statistics (ONS) (2017). *Focus on Violent Crime and Sexual Offences: Year Ending March 2016*. London: ONS.

Ogloff, J. R. P. (2006). Psychopathy/antisocial personality disorder conundrum. *Australian and New Zealand Journal of Psychiatry*, 40, 519–528.

Olafson, E., Corwin, D. L & Summit, R. C. (1993). Modern history of child sexual abuse awareness: Cycles of discovery and suppression. *Child Abuse & Neglect*, 17, 7–24.

Olfson, M. & Marcus, S. C. (2010). National trends in outpatient psychotherapy. *American Journal of Psychiatry*, 167, 1456–1463.

Olsson, N., Juslin, P. & Winman, A. (1998). Realism of confidence in earwitness versus eyewitness identification. *Journal of Experimental Psychology: Applied*, 4, 101–118.

Olver, M. E. & Wong, S. C. P. (2013). A description and research review of the Clearwater Sex Offender Treatment Programme. *Psychology, Crime & Law*, 19, 477–492.

Olweus, D. (1979) Stability of aggressive reaction patterns in males: a review. *Psychological Bulletin*, 86, 852–875.

Olweus, D. (1988). Environmental and biological factors in the development of aggressive behaviour. In W. Buikhuisen & S. A. Mednick (eds.) *Explaining Criminal Behaviour*. Leiden: E. J. Brill.

Olweus, D. (2011). Bullying at school and later criminality: Findings from three Swedish community samples of males. *Criminal Behaviour and Mental Health*, 21, 151–156.

Opinion Matters (2010). *Wake up to Rape Research: Summary Report*. London: Opinion Matters.

Orlinsky, D. E., Rønnestad, M. H. & Willutzki, U. (2004). Fifty years of psychotherapy process-outcome research: Continuity and change. In M. J. Lambert (ed.), *Bergin and Garfield's Handbook of Psychotherapy and Behavior Change*. 5th edition. pp. 307–389. Hoboken, NJ: Wiley.

Ormerod, D. & Laird, K. (2015). *Smith and Hogan's Criminal Law*. 14th edition. Oxford: Oxford University Press.

Otto, R. K. & Douglas, K. S. (eds.) (2010). *Handbook of Violence Risk Assessment*. New York, NY: Routledge.

Otto, R. K. & Ogloff, J. (2014). Defining forensic psychology. In I. B. Weiner & R. K. Otto (eds.), *The Handbook of Forensic Psychology*. 4th edition. pp. 35–55. New York, NY: Wiley.

Ownby, R. L. (1997). *Psychological Reports: A Guide to Report Writing in Professional Psychology*. 3rd edition. New York, NY: Wiley.

P

Paas, L. & Kuijlen, T. (2001). Acquisition pattern analyses for recognising cross-sell opportunities in the financial services sector. *Journal of Targeting, Measurement and Analysis for Marketing*, 9, 230–240.

Pack, R. P., Wallander, J. L., & Browne, D. (1998). Health risk behaviors of African American adolescents with mild mental retardation: Prevalence depends on measurement method. *American Journal on Mental Retardation*, 102, 409–420.

Packer, I. K. (2009). *Evaluation of Criminal Responsibility*. New York: Oxford University Press.

Padfield, N. (1996). The Mandatory Life Sentence in the Balance. *New Law Journal*, 26, 98–99.

Padfield, N. (2000). Detaining the dangerous. *The Journal of Forensic psychiatry*, 11, 497–500.

Padfield, N., Liebling, A. & Arnold, H. (2000). *Discretionary lifer panels: an exploration of decision-making.* London: Home Office. Research and Statistics Dept.

Padfield, N., Morgan, R. & Maguire, M. (2012). Out of court, out of sight? Criminal sanctions and non-judicial decision-making. In M. Maguire, R. M. Morgan & R. Reiner (eds.), *The Oxford Handbook of Criminology*. 5th edition. pp. 955–985. Oxford: Oxford University Press.

Palasinski, M. (2013). Security, respect and culture in British teenagers' discourses of knife-carrying. *Safer Communities*, 12, 71–78.

Palermo, G. B. (1997). The berserk syndrome: A review of mass murder. *Aggression and Violent Behavior*, 2, 1–8.

Palermo, G. B. (2008). Narcissism, sadism, and loneliness: the case of serial killer Jeffrey Dahmer. In R. N. Kocsis (ed.), *Serial Murder and the Psychology of Violent Crimes*. pp. 85–100. Totowa, NJ: Humana Press.

Palermo, G. B. (2010). Parricide: A crime against nature. *International Journal of Offender Therapy and Comparative Criminology*, 54, 3–5.

Palmer, E. J., McGuire, J., Hounsome, J. C., Hatcher, R. M., Bilby, C. A. L. & Hollin, C. R. (2007). Offending behaviour programmes in the community: The effects on reconviction of three programmes with adult male offenders. *Legal and Criminological Psychology*, 12, 251–264.

Palmer, T. (1995). Programmatic and nonprogrammatic aspects of successful intervention: New directions for research. *Crime and Delinquency*, 41, 100–131.

Paluck, E. L. & Green, D. P. (2009). Prejudice reduction: What works? A review and assessment of research and practice. *Annual Review Psychology*, 60, 339–367.

Panczak, R., Geussbühler, M., Zwahlen, M, Killias, M., Tal, K. & Egger, M. (2013). Homicide-suicides compared to homicides and suicides: Systematic review and meta-analysis. *Forensic Science International*, 233, 28–36.

Pantucci, R., Ellis, C. & Chaplais, L. (2015). *Lone-Actor Terrorism: Literature Review*. London: Royal United Services Institute for Defence and Security Studies.

Pardo, M. S. & Patterson, D. (2014). *Minds, Brains, and Law: The Conceptual Foundations of Law and Neuroscience*. Oxford: Oxford University Press.

Pardue, A. D., Robinson, M. B. & Arrigo, B. A. (2013a). Psychopathy and corporate crime: A preliminary examination, Part 1. *Journal of Forensic Psychology Practice*, 13, 116–144.

Pardue, A. D., Robinson, M. B. & Arrigo, B. A. (2013b). Psychopathy and corporate crime: A preliminary examination, Part 2. *Journal of Forensic Psychology Practice*, 13, 145–169.

Parhar, K. K., Wormith, J. S., Derkzen, D. M. & Beauregard, A. M. (2008). Offender coercion in treatment: A meta-analysis of effectiveness. *Criminal Justice and Behavior*, 35, 1109–1135.

Parker, H. & Newcombe, R. (1987). Heroin use and acquisitive crime in an English community. *British Journal of Sociology*, 38, 331–350.

Parole Board (2016). *Statement on IPP prisoners from Parole Board Chairman*. 26 July. https://www.gov.uk/government/news/statement-on-ipp-prisoners-from-parole-board-chairman

Parrot, A. & Cummings, N. (2006). *Forsaken Females: The Global Brutalization of Women*. Lanham, MD: Rowman & Littlefield.

Parrott, D. J. & Giancola, P. R. (2007). Addressing "The criterion problem" in the assessment of aggressive behavior: Development of a new taxonomic system. *Aggression and Violent Behavior*, 12, 280–299.

Parrott, D. J., Gallagher, K. E., Vincent, W. & Bakeman, R. (2010). The link between alcohol use and aggression toward sexual minorities: An event-based analysis. *Psychology of Addictive Behaviors*, 24, 516–521.

Parry, J. (2004). Escalation and necessity: Defining torture at home and abroad. In S. Levenson (ed.). *Torture: A Collection*. pp.145–164. Oxford: Oxford University Press.

Parton, D. A., Hansel, M. & Stratton, J. R. (1991). Measuring crime seriousness: Lessons from the National Survey of Crime Severity. *British Journal of Criminology*, 31, 72–85.

Paternoster, R. & Deise, J. (2011). A heavy thumb on the scale: The effect of victim impact evidence on capital decision making. *Criminology*, 49, 129–161.

Patrick, C. J. (ed.) (2018). *Handbook of Psychopathy*. 2nd edition. New York, NY: Guilford Press.

Patrick, C. J., Venables, N. C. & Skeem, J. (2012). Psychopathy and brain function: empirical findings and legal implications. In H. Häkkänen-Nyholm & J.-O. Nyholm (eds.), *Psychopathy and Law: A Practitioner's Guide*. pp. 39–77. Chichester: Wiley-Blackwell.

Patterson, G. R. (1982). *Coercive Family Process*. Eugene, OR: Castalia.

Patterson, G. R., Dishion, T. J. & Bank, L. (1984). Family interaction: A process model of deviancy training. *Aggressive Behavior*, 10, 253–267.

Patterson-Kane, E. G. & Piper, H. (2009). Animal abuse as a sentinel for human violence: A critique. *Journal of Social Issues*, 65, 589–614.

Patton, C. L., Nobles, M. R. & Fox, K. A. (2010). Look who's stalking: Obsessive pursuit and attachment theory. *Journal of Criminal Justice*, 38, 282–290.

Paulhus, D. L. & Williams, K. M. (2002). The dark triad of personality: Narcissism, Machiavellianism, and psychopathy. *Journal of Research in Personality*, 35, 556–563.

Pearson, F. S. & Lipton, D. S. (1999). A meta-analytic review of the effectiveness of corrections-based treatments for drug abuse. *The Prison Journal*, 79, 384–410.

Peay, J. (2012). Mentally disordered offenders, mental health, and crime. In M. Maguire, R. Morgan & R. Reiner (eds.), *The Oxford Handbook of Criminology*. 5th edition. pp. 426–449. Oxford: Oxford University Press.

Penner, E. K., Roesch, R. & Viljoen, J. L. (2011). Young offenders in custody: An international comparison of mental health services. *International Journal of Forensic Mental Health*, 10, 215–232.

Pereda, N., Guilera, G., Forns, M. Gómez-Benito J. (2009a). The international epidemiology of child sexual abuse: A continuation of Finkelhor (1994). *Child Abuse & Neglect*, 33, 331–342.

Pereda, N., Guilera, G., Forns, M. Gómez-Benito J. (2009b). The prevalence of child sexual abuse in community and student samples: A meta-analysis. *Clinical Psychology Review*, 29, 328–338.

Perry, A. E. (2016). Sentencing and deterrence. In D. Weisburd, D. P. Farrington and C. Gill (eds.), *What Works in Crime Prevention and Rehabilitation: Lessons from Systematic Reviews*. pp. 169–191. New York, NY: Springer.

Perry, A. E., Newman, M., Hallam, G., Johnson, G., Sinclair, J. & Bowles, R. (2009). *A Rapid Evidence Assessment of the effectiveness of interventions with persistent/prolific offenders in reducing re-offending*. Ministry of Justice Research Series 12/09. London: Ministry of Justice, Research Development Statistics.

Petersilia, J. & Turner, S. (1993). Intensive probation and parole. *Crime and Justice: A Review of Research*, 17, 281–335.

Peterson, Z. D., Voller, E. K., Polusny, M. A. & Murdoch, M. (2011). Prevalence and consequences of adult sexual assault of men: Review of empirical findings and state of the literature. *Clinical Psychology Review*, 31, 1–24.

Petrella, R. C. & Poythress, N. G. (1983). The quality of forensic evaluations: An interdisciplinary study. *Journal of Consulting and Clinical Psychology*, 51, 76–85.

Petrosino, A., J., Turpin-Petrosino, C. & Finckenauer, J. O. (2000). Well-meaning programs can have harmful effects! Lessons from experiments of programs such as Scared Straight. *Crime and Delinquency*, 46, 354–379.

Petrunik, M. & Deutschmann, L. (2008). The exclusion-inclusion spectrum in state and community response to sex offenders in Anglo-American and European jurisdictions. *International Journal of Offender Therapy and Comparative Criminology,* 52, 499–519.

Petty, G. M. & Dawson, B. (1989). Sexual aggression in normal men: Incidence, beliefs, and personality characteristics. *Personality and Individual Differences,* 10, 355–362.

Pfuhl, E. H. (1983). Police strikes and conventional crime – a look at the data. *Criminology*, 21, 489–503.

Pfungst, O., Rahn, C. L., Stumpf, C. & Angell, J. R. (1911). *Clever Hans (The horse of Mr. von Osten): A contribution to experimental animal and human psychology* (trans. C. L. Rahn). New York, NY: Henry Holt. (Originally published in German, 1907).

Phenix, A. & Hoberman, H. M. (eds.) (2016). *Sexual Offending: Predisposing Antecedents, Assessments and Management*. New York, NY: Springer.

Phillips, H. K., Gray, N. S., MacCulloch, S. I., Taylor, J., Moore, S. C., Huckle, P. & MacCulloch, M. J. (2005). Risk assessment in offenders with mental disorders: relative efficacy of personal demographic, criminal history, and clinical variables. *Journal of Personal Violence*, 20, 833–847.

Phillipson, M. (1971). *Sociological Aspects of Crime and Delinquency*. London: Routledge & Kegan Paul.

Pickel, K. L. (1999). The influence of context on the 'weapon focus' effect. *Law and Human Behavior*, 23, 299–311.

Pickel, K. L., French, T. A., & Betts, J. M. (2003). A cross-modal weapon focus effect: The influence of a weapon's presence on memory for auditory information. *Memory*, 11, 277–292.

Piechowski, L. D. (2014). Conducting personal injury evaluations. In I. B. Weiner & R. K. Otto (eds.). *The Handbook of Forensic Psychology*. pp. 171–196. New York, NY: Wiley.

Pimentel, D., Cooperstein, S., Randell, H., Filiberto, D., Sorrentino, S., Kaye, B., Nicklin, C., Yagi, J., Brian, J., O'Hern, J., Habas, A. & Weinstein, C. (2007). Ecology of increasing diseases: Population growth and environmental degradation. *Human Ecology*, 35, 653–668.

Pina, A. & Gannon, T. A. (2012). An overview of the literature on antecedents, perceptions and behavioural consequences of sexual harassment. *Journal of Sexual Aggression*, 18, 209–232.

Pina, A., Gannon, T. A. & Saunders, B. (2012). An overview of the literature on sexual harassment: Perpetrator, theory, and treatment issues. *Aggression and Violent Behavior*, 14, 126–138.

Pinderhughes, H. (1993). The anatomy of racially motivated violence in New York City: a case study of youth in Southern Brooklyn. *Social Problems*, 40, 478–492.

Pinker, S. (2002). *The Blank Slate: The modern denial of human nature.* New York, NY: Viking.

Pipe, M., Orbach, Y., Lamb, M., Abbott, C. & Stewart, H. (2008). *Do Best Practice Interviews with Child Sexual Abuse Victims Influence Case Outcomes*? Final report for the National Institute of Justice. Washington, DC: National Institute of Justice, NCJ 224524.

Piquero, A. R., Carriaga, M. L., Diamond, B., Kazemian, L. & Farrington, D. P. (2012). Stability in aggression revisited. *Aggression and Violent Behavior*, 17, 365–372.

Piquero, A. R. & Moffitt, T. (2005). Explaining the factors of crime: how the developmental taxonomy replies to Farrington's invitation. In D. P. Farrington (ed.), *Integrated Developmental and Life-Course Theories of Offending*. Advances in Criminological Theory, Vol. 14. pp. 51–72. New Brunswick, NJ: Transaction Publishers.

Piquero, A. R., Jennings, W. C. & Farrington, D. P. (2010). On the malleability of self-control: Theoretical and policy implications regarding a general theory of crime. *Justice Quarterly*, 27, 803–834.

Piquero, N. L., Exum, M. L. & Simpson, S. S. (2005). Integrating the desire-for-control and rational choice in a corporate crime context. *Justice Quarterly*, 22, 252–280.

Piquero, N. L., Schoepfer, A. & Langton, L. (2010). Completely out of control or the desire to be in complete control? How low self-control and the desire for control relate to corporate offending. *Crime and Delinquency*, 56, 627–647.

Pitt, S. E. & Bale, E. M. (1995). Neonaticide, infanticide, and filicide: A review of the literature. *Bulletin of the American Academy of Psychiatry and the Law*, 23, 375–386.

Planty, M. & Truman, J. L. (2013). *Firearm Violence, 1993-2011*. Washington, DC: Bureau of Justice Statistics, Office of Justice Programs, US Department of Justice.

Plass, P. S. (1998). A typology of family abduction events. *Child Maltreatment*, 3, 244–250.

Plotnikoff, J. & Woolfson, R. (2004). *In Their Own Words: the experiences of 50 young witnesses in criminal proceedings*. NSPCC Policy Practice Research Studies in partnership with Victim Support.

Plutchik, R. (1995). Outward and inward directed aggressiveness: The interaction between violence and suicidality. *Pharmacopsychiatry*, 28 (Supplement), 47–57.

Polaschek, D. & Daly, T. E. (2013). Treatment and psychopathy in forensic settings. *Aggression and Violent Behavior*, 18, 592–603.

Polaschek, D. L. L. & Gannon, T. A. (2004). The implicit theories of rapists: What convicted offenders tell us. *Sexual Abuse: A Journal of Research and Treatment*, 16, 299–314.

Polaschek, D. L. L. & Ward, T. (2002). The implicit theories of potential rapists: what our questionnaires tell us. *Aggression and Violent Behavior*, 7, 385–406.

Polaschek, D. L. L., Wilson, N. J., Townsend, M. R. & Daly, L. R. (2005). Cognitive-behavioral rehabilitation for high-risk violent offenders: An outcome evaluation of the violence prevention unit. *Journal of Interpersonal Violence*, 29, 1611–1627.

Polizzi, D. M., MacKenzie, D. L., & Hickman, L. J. (1999). What works in adult sex offender treatment? A review of prison- and non-prison-based treatment programs. *International Journal of Offender Therapy and Comparative Criminology*, 43, 357–374.

Pollak, J.M. & Kubrin, C.E. (2007). Crime in the news: How crimes, offenders and victims are portrayed in the media. *Journal of Criminal Justice and Popular Culture,* 14, 59–83.

Polman, H., de Castro, B. O., Koops, W., van Boxtel, H. W. & Merk, W. W. (2007). A meta-analysis of the distinction between reactive abd proactive aggression in children and adolescents. *Journal of Abnormal Child Psychology*, 35, 522–535.

Porter, L. E. & Alison, L. J. (2006). Examining group rape: a descriptive analysis of offender and victim behaviour. *European Journal of Criminology*, 3, 357–381.

Porter, S., Birt, A. R., & Boer, D. P. (2001). Investigation of the criminal and conditional release profiles of Canadian federal offenders as a function of psychopathy and age. *Law and Human Behavior,* 25, 647–661.

Porter, T. & Gavin, H. (2010). Infanticide and neonaticide: A review of 40 years of research literature on incidence and causes. *Trauma, Violence, & Abuse*, 11, 99–112.

Powell, M. B., Fisher, R. P. & Wright, R. (2005). Investigative interviewing. In N. Brewer & D. D. Williams (eds.) *Psychology and Law: An Empirical Perspective*. pp. 11–42. New York, NY: Guilford Press.

Power, S. (2013). *"A Problem from Hell": America and the Age of Genocide*. 2nd edition. New York, NY: Basic Books.

Poythress, N. G. & Hall, J. R. (2011). Psychopathy and impulsivity reconsidered. *Aggression and Violent Behavior*, 16, 120–134.

Poythress, N. G. & Petrila, J. P. (2010). PCL-R psychopathy: Threats to sue, peer review, and potential implications for science and law. A Commentary. *International Journal of Forensic Mental Health*, 9, 3–10.

Pratarelli, M. E., & Mize, K. D. (2002). Biological determinism/fatalism: Are they extreme cases of the use of inference in evolutionary psychology? *Theory & Science,* 3. Retrieved from: http://theoryandscience.icaap.org/volume3issue1.php

Pratt, T. C. & Cullen, F. T. (2000). The empirical status of Gottfredson and Hirschi's general theory of crime: A meta-analysis. *Criminology*, 38, 931–964.

Pratt, T. C. & Cullen, F. T. (2005). Assessing macro-level predictors and theories of crime: A meta-analysis. *Crime and Justice*, 32, 373–450.

Pratt, T. C., Cullen, F. T., Sellers, C. S., Winfree, L. T., Madensen, T. D., Daigle, L. E., Fearn, N. E. & Gau, J. M. (2010). The empirical status of social learning theory: A meta-analysis. *Justice Quarterly*, 27, 765–802.

Prendergast, M. L., Podus, D. & Chang, E. (2000). Program factors and treatment outcomes in drug dependence treatment: An examination using meta-analysis. *Substance Use and Misuse*, 35, 1931–1965.

Prendergast, M. L., Podus, D., Chang, E. & Urada, D. (2002). The effectiveness of drug abuse treatment: A meta-analysis of comparison group studies. *Drug and Alcohol Dependence*, 67, 53–72.

Prentky, R. A. & Burgess, A. W. (1990). Rehabilitation of child molesters: A cost-benefit analysis. *American Journal of Orthopsychiatry*, 60, 108–117.

Pressman, D. E. & Flockton, J. (2012). Calibrating risk for violent political extremists and terrorists: the VERA 2 structured assessment. *British Journal of Forensic Practice*, 14, 237–251.

PricewaterhouseCoopers (2007). *Economic crime: people, culture and controls. The 4th Biennial Global Economic Crime Survey*. London: PricewaterhouseCoopers, Investigations and Forensic Services. http://www.pwc.com/en_GX/gx/economic-crime-survey/pdf/pwc_2007gecs.pdf

PricewaterhouseCoopers (2011). *Cybercime: Protecting against the growing threat. Global Economic Crime Survey*. London: PricewaterhouseCoopers LLP. www.pwc.com/crimesurvey

Prins, H. (1995). *Offenders, Deviants, or Patients?* 2nd edition. London: Routledge.

Pulkkinen, L., Kyyra, A.-L. & Kokko, K. (2009). Life success of males on nonoffender, adolescence-limited, persistent, and adult-onset antisocial pathways: follow-up from age 8 to 42. *Aggressive Behavior*, 35, 117–135.

Purcell, C. E. & Arrigo, B. A. (2006). *The Psychology of Lust Murder: Paraphilia, Sexual Killing and Serial Homicide*. Amsterdam: Academic Press/Elsevier.

Putkonen, H., Amon, S., Eronen, M., Klier, C. M., Almiron, M. P., Cederwall, J. Y. & Weizmann-Henelius, G. (2011). Gender differences in filicide offense characteristics – A comprehensive register-based study of child murder in two European countries. *Child Abuse & Neglect*, 35, 319–328.

Q

Quayle, E., Vaughan, M. & Taylor, M. (2006). Sex offenders, Internet child abuse images and emotional avoidance: The importance of values. *Aggression and Violent Behavior*, 11, 1–11.

Quigley, B. M., Leonard, K. E. & Collins, R. E. (2003). Characteristics of violent bars and bar patrons. *Journal of Studies on Alcohol*, 64, 765–772.

Qureshi, A. (2016). *The 'Science' of Pre-Crime: The Secret 'Radicalisation' Study Underpinning Prevent*. London: CAGE Advocacy.

R

R. v. Turner (1975). *Law Reports, Queen's Bench* (Court of Appeal), 834–843.

Rachlinski, J. J., Johnson, S. L., Wistrich, A. J. & Guthrie, C. (2008). Does unconscious racial bias affect trial judges? *Notre Dame Law Review,* 84, 1195–1246.

Radelet, M. L. & Lacock, T. L. (2009). Do executions lower homicide rates? The views of leading criminologists. *The Journal of Criminal Law and Criminology,* 99, 489–508.

Radford, L., Corral, S., Bradley, C., Fisher, H., Bassett, C., Howat, N. & Collishaw, S. (2011). *Child abuse and neglect in the UK today*. London: National Society for the Prevention of Cruelty to Children.

Radovic, S. & Högland, P. (2014). Explanations for violent behaviour – an interview study among forensic in-patients. *International Journal of Law and Psychiatry*, 37, 142–148.

Ragatz, L. & Fremouw, W. (2010). A critical examination of research on the psychological profiles of white-collar criminals. *Journal of Forensic Psychology Practice*, 10, 373–402.

Ragatz, L., Fremouw, W. & Baker, E. (2012). The psychological profile of white-collar offenders: demographics, criminal thinking, psychopathic traits, and psychopathology. *Criminal Justice and Behavior*, 39, 978–997.

Raine, A. (2002). Biosocial studies of antisocial and violent behaviour in children and adults: A review. *Journal of Abnormal Child Psychology,* 30, 311–326.

Raine, A. (2008). From genes to brain to antisocial behaviour. *Current Directions in Psychological Science*, 17, 323–328.

Raine, A. & Yang, Y. (2006). Neural foundations to moral reasoning and antisocial behavior. *Scan,* 1, 203–213.

Raistrick, D., Heather, N. & Godfrey, C. (2006). *Review of the Effectiveness of Treatment for Alcohol Problems*. London: NHS National Treatment Agency for Substance Misuse.

Ramchand, R., MacDonald, J. M., Haviland, A. & Morral, A. R. (2009). A developmental approach for measuring the severity of crimes. *Journal of Quantitative Criminology*, 25, 129–153.

Rapley, M., Moncrieff, J. & Dillon, J. (2011). Carving nature at its joints? DSM and the medicalization of everyday life. In M. Rapley, J. Moncrieff & J. Dillon (eds.), *De-Medicalizing Misery: Psychiatry, Psychology and the Human Condition*. pp. 1–9. Basingstoke: Palgrave MacMillan.

Raspberry, W. (1999). Brain study raises many questions. *The Albany Herald*, 24th July.

Ratchford, M. & Beaver, K. M. (2009). Neuropsychological deficits, low self-control, and delinquent involvement: Toward a biosocial explanation of delinquency. *Criminal Justice and Behavior*, 36, 147–162.

Ray, L. (2013). Violent crime. In C. Hale, K. Hayward, A. Wahidin & E. Wincup (eds.), *Criminology*. 3rd edition. pp. 187–209. Oxford: Oxford University Press.

Raynor, P. (2004). The Probation Service 'Pathfinders': Finding the path and losing the way? *Criminal Justice*, 4, 309–325.

Raynor, P. (2012). Community penalties, probation, and offender management. In M. Maguire, R. M. Morgan & R. Reiner (eds.), *The Oxford Handbook of Criminology*. 5th edition. pp. 928–954. Oxford: Oxford University Press.

Read, J. (2004). A history of madness. In J. Read, L. R. Mosher & R. P. Bentall (eds.), *Models of Madness: Psychological, Social and Biological Approaches to Schizophrenia*. pp. 9-20. Hove: Brunner-Routledge.

Read, J., van Os, J., Morrison, A. P. & Ross, C. A. (2005). Childhood trauma, psychosis, and schizophrenia: a literature review with theoretical and clinical implications. *Acta Psychiatrica Scandinavica*, 112, 330–350.

Rebellon, C. J. (2006). Do adolescents engage in delinquency to attract the social attention of peers? An extension and longitudinal test of the social reinforcement hypothesis. *Journal of Research in Crime and Delinquency*, 43, 387–411.

Rebellon, C. J., Straus, M. A. & Medeiros, R. (2008). Self-control in global perspective: An empirical assessment of Gottfredson and Hirschi's General Theory within and across 32 national settings. *European Journal of Criminology*, 5, 331–362.

Reder, P., Lucey, C. & Fellow-Smith E. (1993). Surviving cross-examination in court. *Journal of Forensic Psychiatry*, 4, 489–496.

Redlich, A. D. (2006). The susceptibility of juveniles to false confessions and false guilty pleas. *Rutgers Law Review*, 62, 943–957.

Redlich, A. D., Summers, A. & Hoover, S. (2010). Self-reported false confessions and false guilty please among offenders with mental illness. *Law and Human Behavior*, 34, 79–90.

Redondo, S., Sánchez-Meca, J. & Garrido, V. (2002).Crime treatment in Europe: A review of outcome studies. In J. McGuire (ed.), *Offender Rehabilitation and Treatment: Effective Programmes and Policies to Reduce Re-Offending*. pp. 113–141. Chichester: Wiley.

Reid, J. B., Patterson, G. R. & Snyder, J. (2002). *Antisocial Behavior in Children and Adolescents: A Developmental Analysis and Model for Intervention*. Washington, DC: American Psychological Association.

Reid, S. (2017). Compulsive criminal homicide: A new nosology for serial murder. *Aggression and Violent Behavior*, 34, 290–301.

Reid, S., Wilson, N. J. & Boer, D. P. (2011). Risk, needs and responsivity principles in action: tailoring rapist's treatment to rapist typologies. In D. P. Boer, R. Eher, L. A. Craig, M. H. Miner & F. Pfäfflin (Eds.), *International Perspectives on the Assessment and Treatment of Sexual Offenders: Theory, Practice, and Research*. pp. 287–297. Chichester: Wiley-Blackwell.

Reidy, D. E., Kearns, M. C. & DeGue, S. (2013). Reducing psychopathic violence: A review of the treatment literature. *Aggression and Violent Behavior*, 18, 527–538.

Reiman, J. & Leighton, P. (2017). *The Rich Get Richer and the Poor Get Prison: Ideology, Class, and Criminal Justice*. 11th edition. New York, NY: Routledge.

Reiner, R. (2000). *The Politics of the Police*. 3rd edition. Oxford: Oxford University Press.

Reiner, R. (2007). Media made criminality: The representation of crime in the mass media. In M. Maguire, R. Morgan & R. Reiner (eds.), *The Oxford Handbook of Criminology*. 4th edition. pp. 302–337. Oxford: Oxford University Press.

Reiss, A. J. & Farrington, D. P. (1991). Advancing knowledge about co-offending: results from a prospective longitudinal study of London males. *Journal of Criminal Law and Criminology*, 82, 360–395.

Reith, M. (1998). *Community Care Tragedies: A Practice Guide to Mental Health Inquiries*. Birmingham: Venture Press.

Reitzel, L. R. & Carbonell, J. L. (2006). The effectiveness of sexual offender treatment for juveniles as measured by recidivism: A meta-analysis. *Sexual Abuse: A Journal of Research and Treatment*, 18, 401–421.

Rengert, G. F. (2004). The journey to crime. In G. Bruinsma, H. Elffers, & J. de Keijser (Eds.). *Punishment, places and perpetrators: Developments in criminology and criminal justice*. pp. 169–181. Cullompton: Willan Publishing.

Resnick, P. J. (1969). Child murder by parents: A psychiatric review of filicide. *American Journal of Psychiatry*, 126, 325-334.

Ressler, R. K. & Burgess, A. W. (1985). Crime scene and profile characteristics of organized and disorganized murders. *FBI Law Enforcement Bulletin*, 54, 18–25.

Ressler, R. K., Burgess, A. W., Douglas, J. E., Hartman, C. R. & D'Agostino, R. B. (1986). Sexual killers and their victims: Identifying patterns through crime scene analysis. *Journal of Interpersonal Violence*, 1, 288–308.

Retz, W. & Rösler, M. (2009). The relation of ADHD and violent aggression: What can we learn from epidemiological and genetic studies? *International Journal of Law and Psychiatry*, 32, 235–243.

Rex, S. (1999). Desistance from offending: Experiences of probation. *Howard Journal*, 38, 366–383.

Rhee, S. H. & Waldman, I. D. (2002). Genetic and environmental influences on antisocial behaviour: a meta-analysis of twin and adoption studies. *Psychological Bulletin*, 128, 490–529.

Rice, M. E., & Harris, G. T. (1995). Violent recidivism: Assessing predictive validity. *Journal of Consulting and Clinical Psychology*, 63, 737–748.

Rice, M. E., Harris, G. T. & Cormier, C. A. (1992). An evaluation of a maximum security therapeutic community for psychopaths and other mentally disordered offenders. *Law and Human Behaviour*, 16, 399–412.

Richards, K. (2011). *Misperceptions about child sex offenders*. Trends & Issues in crime and criminal justice. No. 429. Canberra: Australian Institute of Criminology.

Rind, B., Tromovitch, P. & Bauserman, R. (1998). A meta-analytic examination of assumed properties of child sexual abuse using college samples. *Psychological Bulletin*, 124, 22–53.

Rind, B., Tromovitch, P. & Bauserman, R. (2000). Condemnation of a scientific article: A chronology and refutation of the attacks and discussion of threats to the integrity of science. *Sexuality and Culture*, 4(2), 1–62.

Rittner, C. & Roth, J. K. (Eds.) (2012). *Rape: Weapon of War and Genocide*. St.Paul, MN: Paragon House.

Robertiello, G. & Terry, K. J. (2007). Can we profile sex offenders? A review of sex offender typologies. *Aggression and Violent Behavior*. 12, 508–518.

Roberts, A. & Willits, D. (2011). Lifestyle, routine activities, and felony-related eldercide. *Homicide Studies*, 17, 184–203.

Roberts, A. D. L. & Coid, J. W. (2009). Personality disorder and offending behaviour: findings from the national survey of male prisoners England and Wales. *Journal of Forensic Psychiatry & Psychology*, 21, 221–237.

Roberts, A. R. (1996). Battered women who kill: A comparative study of incarcerated participants with a community sample of battered women. *Journal of Family Violence*, 11, 291-304.

Roberts, A. R., Zgoba, K. M. & Shahidullah, S. M. (2007). Recidivism among four types of homicide offenders: An exploratory analysis of 336 homicide offenders in New Jersey. *Aggression and Violent Behavior*, 12, 493–507.

Robinson, M. B. & Murphy, D. S. (2008). *Greed is Good: Maximization and Elite Deviace in America*. Boston, MA: Rowman and Littlefield.

Robinson, W. & Hassle, J. (2001). *Alcohol Problems and the Family: From Stigma to Solution*. London: Alcohol Recovery Project and National Society for the Prevention of Cruelty to Children.

Rock, P. (1993). *The Social World of an English Crown Court*. Oxford: Clarendon Press.

Rock, P. (2007). Sociological theories of crime. In M. Maguire, R. Morgan & R. Reiner (eds.) *The Oxford Handbook of Criminology*. 4th edition. Oxford: Oxford University Press.

Rodway, C., Norrington-Moore, V., While, D., Hunt. I. M., Flynn, S., Swinson, N., Roscoe, A., Appleby, L. & Shaw, J. (2011). A population-based study of juvenile perpetrators of homicide in England and Wales. *Journal of Adolescence*, 34, 19–28.

Roesch, R., Zapf, P. A. & Eaves, D. (2006). *Fitness Interview Test - Revised: A structured interview for assessing competency to stand trial*. Sarasota, FL: Professional Resource Press.

Rogers, R. (2000). The uncritical acceptance of risk assessment in forensic practice. *Law and Human Behavior*, 24, 595–605.

Rogers, R. & Shuman, D. W. (2000). *Conducting Insanity Evaluations*. 2nd edition. New York, NY: Guilford Press.

Rose, N. (2011). Will the new Corporate Homicide Act save lives? *The Guardian*, 22 February.

Rosenhan, D. (1973). On being sane in insane places. *Science*, 10, 250–258.

Rosenthal, R. (1994). Parametric measures of effect size. In H. Cooper & L. V. Hedges (Eds.), *Handbook of Research Synthesis*. New York, NY: Russell Sage Foundation.

Ross, D. F., Hopkins, S., Hanson, E., Lindsay, R. C. L., Hazen, K., & Eslinger, T. (1994). The impact of protective shields and videotape testimony on conviction rates in a simulated trial of child sexual abuse. *Law and Human Behavior*, 18, 553–566.

Ross, J., Quayle, E., Newman, E. & Tansey, L. (2013). The impact of psychological therapies on violent behaviour in clinical and forensic settings: A systematic review. *Aggression and Violent Behavior*, 18, 761–773.

Ross, L. & Nisbett, R. E. (1991/2011). *The Person and the Situation: Perspectives of Social Psychology*. London: Pinter and Martin.

Rossegger, A., Gerth, J., Seewald, K., Urbaniok, F., Singh, J. P. & Endrass, J. (2013). Current obstacles in replicating risk assessment findings: A systematic review of commonly used actuarial instruments. *Behavioral Sciences and the Law*, 31, 154–164.

Rossmo, D. K. (2000). *Geographic profiling*. Boca Raton, FL: CRC Press.

Roth, A. & Fonagy, P. (2005). *What Works for Whom? A Critical Review of Psychotherapy Research*. 2nd edition. New York, NY: Guilford Press.

Rothbart, M. K. (2011). *Becoming Who We Are: Temperament and Personality in Development*. New York, NY: Guilford Press.

Rothbart, M. K., Derryberry, D. & Posner, M. I. (1994). A psychobiological approach to the development of temperament. In J. E. Bates & T. D. Wachs (eds.), *Temperament: Individual Differences at the Interface of Biology and Behavior*. pp. 83–116. Washington, DC: American Psychological Association.

Rothbart, M. K. & Posner, M. I. (2006). Temperament, attention, and developmental psychopathology. In D. Cicchetti & D. J. Cohen (eds.), *Developmental Psychopathology*. Vol. 2. pp. 465–501. 2nd edition. New York, NY: Wiley.

Royal College of Psychiatrists (2016). *Counter-terrorism and psychiatry*. Position Statement PS04/16. London: Royal College of Psychiatrists.

Ruby, C. L. (2002). Are terrorists mentally deranged? *Analyses of Social Issues and Public Policy*, 2, 15–26.

Runyan, D. K., Curtis, P., Hunter, W., Black, M. M., Kotch, J. B., Bangdiwala, S., et al. (1998). LONGSCAN: A consortium for longitudinal studies of maltreatment and the life course of children. *Aggression and Violent Behavior*, 3, 275–285.

Ruscio, J. (2007). Taxometric analysis: an empirically grounded approach to implementing the method. *Criminal Justice and Behavior*, 34, 1588–1622.

Russell, M. N. (2002). Changing beliefs of spouse abusers. In J. McGuire (ed.), *Offender Rehabilitation and Treatment: Effective Programmes and Policies to Reduce Re-offending*. pp.243–258. Chichester: Wiley.

Ryan, E. B., Kennaley, D. E., Pratt, M. W., & Shumovich, M. A. (2000). Evaluations by staff, residents, and community seniors of patronizing speech in the nursing home: Impact of passive, assertive, or humorous responses. *Psychology of Aging*, 15, 272–285.

S

Sabates, R. & Dex, S. (2012). *Multiple Risk Factors in Young Children's Development*. CLS Cohort Studies, Working paper 2012/1. London: Centre for Longitudinal Studies, Institute of Education, University of London.

Sabin, L. N. (1996). Doe v. Poritz: a constitutional yield to an angry society. *California Western Law Review*, 32, 331–357.

Sachdev, P. S. & Chen, X. (2008). Neurosurgical treatment of mood disorders: traditional psychosurgery and the advent of deep brain stimulation. *Current Opinion in Psychiatry*, 22, 25–31.

Sageman, M. (2004). *Understanding Terror Networks*. Philadelphia, PA: University of Pennsylvania Press.

Saini, M. (2009). A meta-analysis of the psychological treatment of anger: Developing guidelines for evidence-based practice. *Journal of the American Academy of Psychiatry and the Law*, 37, 473–488.

Saks, M. J. & Marti, M. W. (1997). A meta-analysis of the effects of jury size. *Law and Human Behavior*, 21, 451–467.

Sakuta, T. (1995). A study of murder followed by suicide. *Medicine and Law*, 14, 141–153.

Salekin, R. T. (2002). Psychopathy and therapeutic pessimism: Clinical lore or clinical reality? *Clinical Psychology Review*, 22, 79–112.

Salekin, R. T., Rogers, R., & Sewell, K. W. (1996). A review and meta-analysis of the Psychopathy Checklist and the Psychopathy Checklist-Revised: Predictive validity of dangerousness. *Clinical Psychology: Science and Practice*, 3, 203–215.

Salerno, J. & Diamond, S. (2010). The promise of a cognitive perspective on jury deliberation. *Psychonomic Bulletin & Review*, 17, 174–179.

Sales, E., Baum, M., & Shore, B. (1984). Victim readjustment following assault. *Journal of Social Issues*, 40, 117–136.

Sameroff, A. (2009). The transactional model. In A. Sameroff (ed.), *The Transactional Model of Development: How Children and Contexts Shape Each Other*. pp. 3-21. Washington, DC: American Psychological Association.

Sameroff, A. J. & Chandler, M. J. (1975). Reproductive risk and the continuum of caretaking casualty. In F. Horowitz, J. Hetherington, S. Scarr-Salapatek & G. Siegel (eds.), *Review of Child Development Research*. pp. 187–244. Chicago: University of Chicago Press.

Sample, S., Wakai, S., Trestman, R. L. & Keeney, E. M. (2008). Functional analysis of behavior in corrections: empowering inmates in skills training groups. *Journal of Behavior Analysis and Offender and Victim Treatment and Prevention*, 1, 42–51.

Sanday, P. R. (2004). *Women at the Center: Life in a Modern Matriarchy*. Ithaca, NY: Cornell University Press.

Santilla, P., Häkkänen, H., Canter, D. & Elfgren, T. (2003). Classifying homicide offenders and predicting their characteristics from crime scene behaviour. *Scandinavian Journal of Psychology*, 44, 107–118.

Santilla, P., Ritvannen, A. & Mokros, A. (2004). Predicting burglar characteristics from crime scene behaviour. *International Journal of Police Science and Management*, 6, 136–154.

Sapsford, R. J. (1978). Life-sentence prisoners: Psychological changes during sentence. *British Journal of Criminology*, 18, 128–145.

Saradjian, J., Murphy, N. & McVey, D. (2013). Delivering effective therapeutic interventions for men with severe personality disorder within a high secure prison. *Psychology, Crime & Law*, 19, 433–447.

Satel, S. L. & Lilienfeld, S. O. (2014). Addiction and the brain-disease fallacy. *Frontiers in Psychiatry*, 4, 1–11. Doi: 10.3389/fpsyt.2013.00141

Saunders, R. (1998). The legal perspective on stalking. In J. R. Meloy (ed.), *The psychology of stalking: Clinical and forensic perspectives*. pp. 25–49. San Diego, CA: Academic Press.

Savitz, L. D., Kumar, K. S. & Zahn, M. A. (1991). Quantifying Luckenbill. *Deviant Behavior: An Interdisciplinary Journal*, 12, 19–29.

Saywitz, K. J. & Nathanson, R. (1993). Children's testimony and their perceptions of stress in and out of the Courtroom. *Child Abuse and Neglect*, 17, 613–622.

Schaeffer, N. C. & Presser, S. (2003). The science of asking questions. *Annual Review of Sociology*, 29, 65–88.

Schall, C. M. & McDonough, J. T. (2010). Autism spectrum disorders in adolescence and early adulthood: Characteristics and issues. *Journal of Vocational Rehabilitation*, 32, 81–88.

Schank, R. C. & Abelson, R. P. (1977). *Scripts, Plans, Goals and Understanding: An Inquiry into Human Knowledge Structures*. Hillsdale, NJ: Erlbaum.

Schilling, C. M., Walsh, A. & Yun, I. (2011). ADHD and criminality: A primer on the genetic, neurobiological, evolutionary and treatment literature for criminologists. *Journal of Criminal Justice*, 39, 3–11.

Schlesinger, L. B. (2009). Psychological profiling: Investigative implications from crime scene analysis. *The Journal of Psychiatry and Law*, 37, 73–84.

Schmid, J. & Fiedler, K. (1998). The backbone of closing speeches: The impact of prosecution versus defense language on judicial attributions. *Journal of Applied Social Psychology*, 28, 1140–1172.

Schmucker, M. & Lösel, F. (2015). The effects of sexual offender treatment on recidivism: an international meta-analysis of sound quality evaluations. *Journal of Experimental Criminology*, 11, 597–630.

Schmucker, M. & Lösel, F. (2017). Sexual offender treatment for reducing recidivism among convicted sex offenders: a systematic review and meta-analysis. *Campbell Systematic Reviews*, 2017:8. Doi: 10.4073/csr.2017.8

Schoepfer, A., Piquero, N. L. & Langton, L. (2014). Low self-control versus the desire-for-control: An empirical test of white-collar crime and conventional crime. *Deviant Behavior*, 35, 197–214.

Schooler, J. W. and Loftus, E. F. (1986). Individual differences and experimentation: complementary approaches to interrogative suggestibility. *Social Behavior*, 1, 105–112.

Schuller, R. A., Terry, D., & McKimmie, B. (2001). The impact of an expert's gender on jurors' decisions. *Law and Psychology Review*, 25, 59–79.

Schweinhart, L. J. (2013). Long-term follow-up of a preschool experiment. *Journal of Experimental Criminology*, 9, 389–409.

Schweinhart, L. J., Barnes, H. V. & Weikart, D. P. (1993). *Significant Benefits: The High/Scope Perry Preschool Project*. Ypsilanti, MI: High/Scope Press.

Scott, D. (2008). Creating ghosts in the penal machine: prison officer occupational morality and the techniques of denial. In J. Bennett, B. Crewe & A. Wahidin (eds.), *Understanding Prison Staff*. pp. 168–186. Abingdon: Routledge.

Scottish Government (2003). *Homicide in Scotland*. Statistical Bulletin Criminal Justice Series CrJ/2003/9. Edinburgh: Scottish Government.

Scottish Government (2013). *Homicide in Scotland, 2012-2013*. Crime and Justice Series. Edinburgh: Scottish Government.

Seager, J. A. (2005). Violent men: The importance of cognitive schema and impulsivity. *Criminal Justice and Behavior*, 32, 26–49.

Segal, D. L. & Hersen, M. (eds.) (2010). *Diagnostic Interviewing*. 4th edition. New York, NY: Springer.

Sentencing Council (2014). *Sexual Offences: Definitive Guideline.* https://www.sentencingcouncil.org.uk/wp-content/uploads/Final_Sexual_Offences_Definitive_Guideline_content_web1.pdf

Sentencing Council (2017). *Magistrates' Court Sentencing Guidelines: Definitive Guideline.* https://www.sentencingcouncil.org.uk/wp-content/uploads/MCSG-April-2017-FINAL-2.pdf

Serba, L. & Nathan, G. (1984). Further explorations in the scaling of penalties. *The British Journal of Criminology*, 23, 221–249.

Serber, M. (1970). Shame aversion therapy. *Journal of Behavior Therapy and Experimental Psychiatry*, 1, 213–215.

Serran, G. & Firestone, P. (2004). Intimate partner homicide: a review of the male proprietariness and the self-defense theories. *Aggression and Violent Behavior*, 9, 1–15.

Seto, M. C. (2008) Pedophilia. In D. R. Laws & W. T. O'Donohue (eds.), *Sexual Deviance: Theory, Assessment, and Treatment*. pp. 164–182. New York, NY: Guilford Press.

Seto, M. C. (2009). Pedophilia. *Annual Review of Clinical Psychology*, 5, 391–407.

Seto, M. C. & Eke, A. W. (2005). The criminal histories and later offending of child pornography offenders. *Sexual Abuse: A Journal of Research and Treatment*, 17, 201–210.

Seto, M. C. & Lalumière, M. L. (2010). What is so special about male adolescent sexual offending? A review and test of explanations using meta-analysis. *Psychological Bulletin,* 136, 526–575.

Seto, M. C., Murphy, W. D., Page, J., & Ennis, L. (2003). Detecting anomalous sexual interests in juvenile sex offenders. *Annals of the New York Academy of Sciences,* 989, 118–130.

Sharp, S. F. (2005). *The Effects of the Death Penalty on Families of the Accused.* New Brunswick, NJ: Rutgers University Press.

Shaver, P. R. & Mikulincer, M. (eds.) (2011). *Human Aggression and Violence: Causes, Manifestations, and Consequences*. Washington, DC: American Psychological Association.

Shaw, J. A. & Budd, E. C. (1982). Determinants of acquiescence and naysaying of mentally retarded persons. *American Journal of Mental Deficiency*, 87, 108–110.

Shaw, J., Hunt, I. M., Flynn, S., Amos, T., Meehan, J., Robinson, J., Bickley, H., Parsons, R., McCann, K., Burns, J., Kapur, N. & Appleby, L. (2006). The role of alcohol and drugs in homicides in England and Wales. *Addiction*, 101, 1117–1124.

Shaw, J. I. & Skolnick, P. (1994). Sex differences, weapon focus, and eyewitness reliability. *Journal of Social Psychology*, 134, 413–420.

Shawyer, A., Milne, B., & Bull, R. (2009). Investigative interviewing in the UK. In T. Williamson, B. Milne, & S. P. Savage (eds.), *International Developments in Investigative Interviewing*. pp. 24–38. Cullompton: Willan Publishing.

Shawyer, F., Mackinnon, A., Farhall, J., Sims, E., Blaney, S., Yardley, P., Daly, M., Mullen, P. & Copolov, D. (2008). Acting on harmful command hallucinations in psychotic disorders: an integrative approach. *Journal of Nervous and Mental Disease*, 196, 390–398.

Sheehan, I. S. (2014). Are suicide terrorists suicidal? A critical assessment of the evidence. *Innovations in Clinical Neuroscience*, 11, 81–92.

Sheldon, K., Davies, J. & Howells, K. (eds.) (2011). *Research in Practice for Forensic Professionals.* London and New York, NY: Routledge.

Sheldon, K. & Howitt, D. (2007). *Sex Offenders and the Internet*. Chichester: Wiley,

Shelton, S. T. (2006). Jury decision making: Using group theory to improve deliberation. *Politics & Policy,* 34, 706–725.

Shepherd, E. (1986). The conversational core of policing. *Policing*, 2, 294–303.

Shepherd, E. (2007). *Investigative Interviewing: The Conversation Management Approach*. Oxford: Oxford University Press.

Shuker, R. & Sullivan, E. (eds.) (2010). *Grendon and the Emergence of Forensic Therapeutic Communities: Developments in Research and Practice*. Chichester: Wiley-Blackwell.

Shuman, D. W., Hamilton, J. A., Daley, C. E., Behinfar, D. J., Bitner, R. H., Bolton, D., Cordobes, S., Doucet, J. A., Drake, T. E., Goheen, G. P., Jackson, M. S., Landry, C. C., Pugh, C. K., Richardson, K., Soli, K. M., Vaughan, K. A. & Whitmore, J. J. (1994). The health effects of jury service. *Law & Psychology Review,* 18, 267–307.

Sibley, C. G. & Duckitt, J. (2008). Personality and prejudice: A meta-analysis and theoretical review. *Personality and Social Psychology Review*, 12, 248–279.

Sidgwick, H. (1874). *The Methods of Ethics.* London: Macmillan.

Siegel, L. J. (2012). *Criminology*. 11th edition. Belmont, CA: Wadsworth.

Silva, J. A., Ferrari, M. M. & Leong, G. B. (2002). The case of Jeffrey Dahmer: Sexual serial homicide from a neuropsychiatric developmental perspective. *Journal of Forensic Science*, 47, 1–13.

Silver, E. (2006). Understanding the relationship between mental disorder and violence: the need for a criminological perspective. *Law and Human Behavior*. 30, 685–706.

Silver, E., Mulvey, E., & Monahan, J. (1999). Assessing violence risk among discharged psychiatric patients: Toward an ecological approach. *Law and Human Behavior*, 23, 237–255.

Sim, D. J. & Proeve, M. (2010). Crossover and stability of victim type in child molesters. *Legal and Criminological Psychology*, 15, 401–413.

Simons, D. J. & Chabris, C. F. (1999). Gorillas in our midst: Sustained inattentional blindness for dynamic events. *Perception*, 28, 1059–1074.

Simons, D. J. & Levin, D. T. (1998). Failure to detect changes to people in a real-world interaction. *Psychonomic Bulletin and Review*, 5, 644–649.

Sinaceur, M., Adam, H., Van Kleef, G. A. & Galinsky, A. D. (2013). The advantages of being unpredictable: How emotional inconsistency extracts concessions in negotiation. *Journal of Experimental Social Psychology*, 49, 498–508.

Singh, J. P. & Fazel, S. (2010). Forensic risk assessment: A metareview. *Criminal Justice and Behavior*, 37, 965–988.

Singh, J. P., Grann, M. & Fazel, S. (2011). A comparative study of violence risk assessment tools: A systematic review and metaregression analysis of 68 studies involving 25,980 participants. *Clinical Psychology Review*, 31, 499–513.

Singleton, N., Meltzer, H., Gatward, R., Coid, J. & Deasy, D. (1998) *Psychiatric Morbidity among Prisoners: Summary Report*. London: Office for National Statistics.

Sirdifield, C., Gojkovic, D., Brooker, C. & Ferriter, M. (2009). A systematic review of research on the epidemiology of mental health disorders in prison populations: a summary of findings. *Journal of Forensic Psychiatry & Psychology*, 20, S78–S101.

Skeem, J. L. & Cooke, D. (2010). Is criminal behavior a central component of psychopathy? Conceptual directions for resolving the debate. *Psychological Assessment*, 22, 446–454.

Skeem, J. L., Douglas, K. S. & Lilienfeld, S. O. (eds.) (2009). *Psychological Science in the Courtroom: Consensus and Controversy*. New York, NY: Guilford Press.

Slapper, G. & Kelly, D. (2009). *The English Legal System*. 10th edition. London: Routledge-Cavendish.

Slick, D. J., Sherman, E. M. S. & Iverson, G. L. (1999). Diagnostic criteria for malingered neurocognitive dysfunction: proposed standards for clinical practice and research. *Clinical Neuropsychologist*, 13, 545–561.

Sloan, J. H., Kellerman, A. L., Reay, D. T., Ferris, J. A., Koepsell, T., Rivara, F. P., Rice, C., Gray, L. & LoGerfo, J. (1988). Handgun regulations, crime, assaults and suicide: A tale of two cities. *New England Journal of Medicine*, 319, 1256–1262.

Smallbone, S. & Cale, J. (2015). An integrated life-course developmental theory of sexual offending. In A. Blokland & P. Lussier (eds.), *Sex Offenders: A Criminal Career Approach*. pp. 43–69. Chichester: Wiley-Blackwell.

Smid, W. J., Kamphuis, J. H., Wever, E. C. & Van Beek, D. (2013). Treatment referral for sex offenders based on clinical judgement versus actuarial risk assessment: Match and analysis of mismatch. *Journal of Interpersonal Violence*, 28, 2273–2289.

Smid, W. J., Kamphuis, J. H., Wever, E. C. & Van Beek, D. J. (2014). A comparison of the predictive properties of nine sex offender risk assessment instruments. *Psychological Assessment*, 26, 691–703.

Smith, J. (2003). *The nature of personal robbery*. Home Office Research Study 254. London: Home Office Research, Development and Statistics Directorate.

Smith, M. D. & Zahn, M. A. (eds.) (1999). *Homicide: A Sourcebook of Social Research*. Thousand Oaks, CA: Sage.

Smith, M. E. (1984). Will the real alternatives please stand up? *New York University Review of Law and Social Change*, 12, 171–197.

Smith, M. L., Glass, G. V. & Miller, T. I. (1980). *The Benefits of Psychotherapy*. Baltimore, MD: Johns Hopkins University Press.

Smith, R. (2006). Principles in cross-examination in criminal cases. http://www.parkcourtchambers.co.uk/seminar-handouts/27.9.06%20Pr%20of%20X%20Exam%20_R%20Smith%20QC_.pdf

Smith, S. A. (1993). Confusing the terms "guilty" and "not guilty": Implications for alleged offenders with mental retardation. *Psychological Reports*, 73, 675–678.

Snodgrass, J. (1984). William Healy (1869-1963): Pioneer child psychiatrist and criminologist. *Journal of the History of the Behavioral Sciences*, 20, 332–339.

Snook, B., Cullen, R. M., Bennell, C., Taylor, P. & Gendreau, P. (2008). The criminal profiling illusion: What's behind the smoke and mirrors? *Criminal Justice and Behavior*, 35, 1257–1276.

Snowden, P. (1985). A survey of the Regional Secure Unit programme. *British Journal of Psychiatry*, 147, 499–507.

Snyder, J., Reid, J. & Patterson, G. (2003). A social learning model of child and adolescent antisocial behaviour. In B. B. Lahey, T. E. Moffitt & A. Caspi (eds.) *Causes of Conduct Disorder and Delinquency*. pp. 27–48. New York, NY: Guilford Press.

Solomon, E. & Silvestri, A. (2008). *Community Sentences Digest*. London: Centre for Crime and Justice Studies.

Soothill, K., Francis, B. & Ackerley, E. (2007). Kidnapping: A criminal profile of persons convicted 1979-2001. *Behavioral Sciences and the Law*, 25, 69–84.

Soothill, K., Francis, B. & Liu, J. (2008). Does serious offending lead to homicide? *British Journal of Criminology*, 48, 522–537.

Soothill, K., Humphreys, L. & Francis, B. (2012). Middle-class offenders: a 35-year follow-up. *British Journal of Criminology*, 52, 765–785.

Soothill, K., Francis, B., Sanderson, B. & Ackerley, E. (2000). Sex offenders: Specialists, generalists – or both? *British Journal of Criminology*, 40, 56–67.

Soothill, K., Francis, B., Ackerley, E. & Fligelstone, R. (2002). *Murder and serious sexual assault: What criminal histories can reveal about future serious offending*. Police Research Series, paper 144.

London: Home Office, Policing and Reducing Crime Unit.

Sorensen, J., Wrinkle, R., Brewer, V. & Marquart, J. (1999). Capital punishment and deterrence: Examining the effect of executions on rates of murder in Texas. *Crime and Delinquency*, 45, 481-493.

Spitzberg, B. H. & Cupach, W. R. (2007). The state of the art of stalking: Taking stock of the emerging literature. *Aggression and Violent Behavior*, 12, 64–86.

Spitzberg, B. H. & Cupach, W. R. (2014). *The Dark Side of Relationship Pursuit: From Attraction to Obsession and Stalking*. 2nd edition. New York and London: Routledge.

Spitzberg, B. H., Cupach, W. R. & Ciceraro, L. D. L. (2010). Sex differences in stalking and obsessional relational instrusion: Two meta-analyses. *Partner Abuse*, 1, 259–285.

Spitzer, R. J. (2012). *The Politics of Gun Control*. 5th edition. Boulder, CO: Paradigm.

Spitzer, R. L. (2003). Can some gay men and lesbians change their sexual orientation? 200 participants reporting a change from homosexual to heterosexual orientation. *Archives of Sexual Behavior,* 32, 403–17; discussion 419–72.

Springer, D. W., McNeece, C. A. & Arnold, E. M. (2003). *Substance Abuse Treatment for Chronic Offenders: An Evidence-Based Guide for Practitioners*. Washington, DC: American Psychological Association.

Sreenivasan, S. & Weinberger, L. E. (2016). Surgical castration and sexual recidivism risk. In A. Phenix & H. M. Hoberman (eds.), *Sexual Offending: Predisposing Antecedents, Assessments and Management*. Pp.769–777. New York, NY: Springer.

Stack, S. (1984). Income inequality and property crime: A cross-national analysis of relative deprivation theory. *Criminology*, 22, 229–257.

Stalans, L. J. (1993). Citizens' crime stereotypes, biased recall and punishment preferences in abstract cases: The educative role of interpersonal sources. *Law and Human Behavior*, 17, 451–470.

Stallard, P., Thomason, J. & Churchyard, S. (2003). The mental health of young people attending a Youth Offending team: a descriptive study. *Journal of Adolescence*, 26, 33–43.

Stams, G. J., Brugman, D., Deković, M., van Rosmalen, L., van der Laan, P. & Gibbs, J. C. (2006). The moral judgment of juvenile delinquents: A meta-analysis. *Journal of Abnormal Child Psychology*, 34, 697–713.

Stanley, S. (2009). What works in 2009: progress or stagnation? *Probation Journal*, 56, 153–174.

Stanton, J. & Simpson, A. (2002). Filicide: A review. *International Journal of Law and Psychiatry*, 25, 1–14.

Staub, E. (1989). *The Roots of Evil: The Origins of Genocide and other Group Violence*. New York, NY: Plenum Press.

Staub, E. (1999). The roots of evil: Social conditions, culture, personality, and basic human needs. *Personality and Social Psychology Review*, 3, 179–192.

Staub, E. (2000). Genocide and mass killing: Origins, prevention, healing and reconciliation. *Political Psychology*, 21, 367–382.

Staunton, C. & Hammond, S. (2011). An investigation of the Guilty Knowledge Test polygraph examination. *Journal of Criminal Psychology,* 1, 1–14.

Steadman, H. J., Mulvey, E. P., Monahan, J., Robbins, P. C., Appelbaum, P. S., Grisso, T., Roth, L. H. & Silver, E. (1998). Violence by people discharged from acute psychiatric inpatient facilities and by others in the same neighborhoods. *Archives of General Psychiatry*, 55, 393–401.

Steadman, H. J., Osher, F. C., Robbins, P. C., Case, B., & Samuels, S. (2009). Prevalence of serious mental illness among jail inmates. *Psychiatric Services*, 60, 761–765.

Steele, C. M. & Josephs, R. A. (1990). Alcoholic myopia: its prized and dangerous effects. *American Psychologist*, 45, 921–933.

Stelfox, P. (2009). *Criminal Investigation: An introduction to principles and practice*. Cullompton: Willan Publishing.

Stelmaszek, B. & Fisher, H. (2012). *Country Report 2012. Reality check on data collection and European services for women and children survivors of violence: A Right for Protection and Support?* Vienna: WAVE-office/Austrian Women's Shelter Network.

Stephens, S. & Seto, M. C. (2016). Hebephilic sexual offending. In A. Phenix & H. M. Hoberman (eds.), *Sexual Offending: Predisposing Antecedents, Assessments and Manag*ement. pp. 29–43. New York, NY: Springer.

Stern, W. (1910). Abstracts of lectures on the psychology of testimony and on the study of individuality. *American Journal of Psychology,* 21, 270–282.

Stern, W. (1939). The psychology of testimony. *Journal of Abnormal and Social Psychology,* 34, 3–30.

Stevens, M. J. (2005). What is terrorism and can psychology do anything about it? *Behavioral Sciences and the Law*, 23, 507–526.

Stevens, P. & Harper, D. J. (2007). Professional accounts of electroconvulsive therapy: A discourse analysis. *Social Science and Medicine*, 64, 1475–1486.

Steward, M. S., Steward, D. S., Farquar, L., Myers, J. E. B., Reinhart, M., Welker, J., Joy, N., Driskill, J. & Morgan, J. (1996). Interviewing young children about body touch and handling. *Monographs of the Society for Research in Child Development*, 61, (4–5, Serial No. 248).

Stinson, J. D. & Becker, J. V. (2013). *Treating sex offenders: An evidence-based manual.* New York, NY: Guilford Press.

Stith, S. M., Liu, T., Davies, C., Boykin, E. L., Alder, M. C., Harris, J. M., Som, A., McPherson, M. & Dees, J. E. M. (2009). Risk factors in child maltreatment: a meta-analytic review of the literature. *Aggression and Violent Behavior*, 14, 13–29.

Stockdale, M. S., Vaux, A. & Cashin, J. (1995). Acknowledging sexual harassment: A test of alternative models. *Basic and Applied Social Psychology*, 17, 469–496.

Stocking, B. (1992). Bringing about change; the introduction of secure units. *Journal of the Royal Society of Medicine*, 85, 279–281.

Stöckl, H., Devries K., Rotstein, A., Abrahams, N., Campbell, J., Watts, C. & Moreno, C. G. (2013). The global prevalence of intimate partner homicide: a systematic review. *Lancet*, 382, 859–865.

Storbeck, J. & Clore, G.L (2005). With sadness comes accuracy; with happiness false memory. *Psychological Science*, 16, 785–791.

Stotland, E. (1977). White collar criminals. *Journal of Social Issues*, 33, 179–96.

Strand, S. & McEwan, T. (2012). Violence among female stalkers. *Psychological Medicine*, 42, 545–555.

Straus, M. A. (2008). Dominance and symmetry in partner violence by male and female university students in 32 nations. *Children and Youth Services Review*, 30, 252–275.

Straus, M. A. (2010). Thirty years of denying the evidence on gender symmetry in partner violence: Implications for prevention and treatment. *Partner Abuse*, 1, 332–362.

Straus, M. A. (2014). Addressing violence by female partners is vital to prevent or stop violence against women: Evidence from the Multisite Batterer Intervention Programme. *Violence Against Women*, 20, 889–899.

Straus, M. A. and the International Dating Violence Research Consortium (2004). Prevalence of violence against dating partners by male and female university students worldwide. *Violence Against Women*, 10, 790–811.

Strentz, T. (1988). A terrorist psychosocial profile: Past and present. *FBI Law Enforcement Bulletin*, 57, 13–18.

Stroebe, W. (2013). Firearm possession and violent death: A critical review. *Aggression and Violent Behavior*, 18, 709–721.

Strong, M. (2009). *Erased: Missing Women, Murdered Wives*. San Francisco, CA: Jossey-Bass.

Studer, L. H., Aylwin, A. S., Sribney, C. & Reddon, J. R. (2011). Uses, misuses, and abuses of risk assessment with sexual offenders. In D. P. Boer, R. Eher, L. A. Craig, M. H. Miner & F. Pfäfflin (eds.), *International Perspectives on the Assessment and Treatment of Sexual Offenders: Theory, Practice and Research*. pp. 193–212. Chichester: Wiley-Blackwell.

Sturmey, P. (ed.) (2017). *The Wiley Handbook of Violence and Aggression*. New York, NY: Wiley-Blackwell.

Sturmey, P. & Lindsay, W. R. (2017). Case formulation and risk assessment. In K. D. Browne, A. R. Beech, L. A. Craig & S. Chou (eds.), *Assessments in Forensic Practice: A Handbook*. pp. 7–27. Chichester: Wiley-Blackwell.

Sturmey, P. & McMurran, M. (eds.) (2011). *Forensic Case Formulation*. Chichester: Wiley-Blackwell.

St-Yves, M. (2002). Interrogatoire de police et crime sexuel: Profil du suspect collaborateur [Police interrogation of sexual offenders: Profile of the collaborative suspect]. *Revue Internationales de Criminologie et de Police Technique et Scientifique*, 1, 81–96.

Sullivan, E. A. & Kosson, D. S. (2006). Ethnic and cultural variations in psychopathy. In C. J. Patrick (ed.), *Handbook of Psychopathy*. pp. 437–458. New York, NY: Guilford Press.

Sullivan, E. B., Dorcus, R. M., Allen, B. M. & Koontz, L. K. (1950). Grace Maxwell Fernald, 1879–1950. *Psychological Review*, 57, 319–321.

Summers, R. S. (1999). Formal legal truth and substantive truth in judicial fact-finding – their justified divergence in some particular cases. *Cornell Law Faculty Publications*. Paper 1186.

Sutherland, E. H. (1940). White collar criminality. *American Sociological Review*, 5, 2–10.

Sutherland, E. H. (1983). *White Collar Crime: The Uncut Version*. New Haven and London: Yale University Press.

Sutherland, E. H. & Cressey, D. (1970). *Criminology*. 8th edition. Philadelphia, PA: Lippincott.

Suzuki, L. A. & Ponterotto, J. G. (eds.) (2008). *Handbook of Multicultural Assessment: Clinical,*

Psychological, and Educational Applications. 3rd edition. San Francisco, CA: Jossey-Bass/Wiley.

Swart, J. & Mellor, L. (eds.) (2016). *Homicide: A Forensic Psychology Casebook*. Boca Raton, FL: CRC Press / Taylor and Francis.

Swim, J., Borgida, E., & McCoy, K. (1993). Videotaped vs. in-court witness testimony: Is protecting the child witness jeopardizing due process? *Journal of Applied Social Psychology*, 23, 603–631.

Swinburne Romine, R. E., Miner, M. H., Poulin, D., Dwyer, S. M. & Berg, D. (2012). Predicting re-offense for community-based sexual offenders: An analysis of 30 years of data. *Sexual Abuse: A Journal of Research and Treatment,* 24, 501–514.

Sykes, G. & Matza, D. (1957). Techniques of neutralization: a theory of delinquency. *American Sociological Review*, 22, 664–673.

Szmuckler, G. (2003). Risk assessment: 'numbers' and 'values'. *The Psychiatrist,* 27, 205–207.

Szmukler, G. & Rose, N. (2013). Risk assessment in mental health care: values and costs. *Behavioral Sciences and the Law*, 31, 125–140.

T

Tafrate, R. C. & Mitchell, D. (2013). *Forensic CBT: A Handbook for Clinical Practice*. Chichester: Wiley.

Tahamont, S. & Chalfin, A. (2016). The effect of prisons on crime. In J, Wooldredge & P. Smith (eds.), *The Oxford Handbook of Prisons and Imprisonment*. pp. 1-32. New York, NY: Oxford University Press. http://www.oxfordhandbooks.com/view/10.1093/oxfordhb/9780199948154.001.0001/oxfordhb-9780199948154-e-29

Tait, D. (2003). The ritual environment of the Mental Health Tribunal hearing: Inquiries and reflections. *Psychiatry, Psychology & Law,* 10, 91–96.

Tajfel, H. & Turner, J. C. (1986). The social identity theory of intergroup behaviour. In S. Worchel and W. G. Austin (eds.), *Psychology of Intergroup Relations*. 2nd edition. pp. 7–24. Chicago, Il: Nelson-Hall.

Tanaka, J. W. & Pierce, L. J. (2009). The neural plasticity of other-race face recognition. *Cognitive, Affective, & Behavioral Neuroscience*, 9, 122–131.

Tanner, B. A. (1973). Shock intensity and fear of shock in the modification of homosexual behavior in males by avoidance learning. *Behavior Research & Therapy,* 11, 213–218.

Tapp, J. L. (1976). Psychology and the law: an overture. *Annual Review of Psychology*, 27, 359–404.

Taslitz, A. E. (2007). Forgetting Freud: The courts' fear of the subconscious in date rape (and other) cases. *Boston University Public Interest Law Journal*, 16, 145–194.

Tax Justice Network (2011). *The Cost of Tax Abuse*. London: Tax Justice Network. http://www.taxjustice.net/2014/04/01/cost-tax-abuse-2011/

Tax Justice Network (2012). *The Price of Offshore Revisited*. London: Tax Justice Network. http://www.taxjustice.net/cms/upload/pdf/Price_of_Offshore_Revisited_120722.pdf

Taylor, A. & Kim-Cohen, J. (2007). Meta-analysis of gene-environment interactions in developmental psychopathology. *Development and Psychopathology*, 19, 1029–1037.

Taylor, M., Holland, G. & Quayle, E. (2001). Typology of paedophile picture collections. *Police Journal*, 74, 97–107.

Telep, C. W., Weisburd, D., Gill, C. E., Vitter, Z. & Teichman, D. (2014). Displacement of crime and diffusion of crime control benefits in large-scale geographic areas: a systematic review. *Journal of Experimental Criminology*, 10, 515–548.

Temcheff, C. E., Serbin, L. A., Martin-Stoyey, A., Stack, D. M., Hodgins, S., Ledingham, J. & Schwartzman, A. E. (2008). Continuity and pathways from aggression in childhood to family violence in adulthood: A 30-year longitudinal study. *Journal of Family Violence*, 23, 231–242.

Ten Berge, M. A. & De Radd, B. (1999). Taxonomies of situations from a trait psychological perspective: A review. *European Journal of Personality*, 13, 337–360.

Teoh, Y-S., Yang, P-J., Lamb, M. E., & Larsson, A. S. (2010). Do human figure diagrams help alleged victims of sexual abuse provide elaborate and clear accounts of physical contact with alleged perpetrators? *Applied Cognitive Psychology*, 24, 287–300.

Terpstra, D. E., Rozell, E. J. & Robinson, R. K. (1993). The influence of personality and demographic variables on ethical decisions related to insider trading. *Journal of Psychology*, 127, 375–389.

Tharp, A. L. T., Sharp, C., Stanford, M. S., Lake, S. L., Raine, A. & Kent, T. A. (2011). Correspondence of aggressive behavior classifications among young adults using the Impulsive Premeditated Aggression Scale and the Reactive Proactive Questionnaire. *Personality and Individual Differences*, 50, 279–285.

Thienel, T. (2006). The admissibility of evidence obtained by torture under international law. *European Journal of International Law*, 17, 349–367.

Thierry, K., Lamb, M. E., Orbach, Y., & Pipe, M. E. (2005). Developmental differences in the function and use of anatomical dolls during interviews with alleged sexual abuse victims. *Journal of Consulting and Clinical Psychology*, 73, 1125–1134.

Thomas, K. A., Dichter, M. E. & Matejkowski, J. (2011). Intimate versus nonintimate partner murder: A comparison of offender and situational characteristics. *Homicide Studies*, 15, 291–311.

Thompson, C. M. & Dennison, S. (2004). Graphic evidence of violence: The impact on juror decision-making, the influence of judicial instructions and the effect of juror bias. *Psychiatry, Psychology and Law,* 11, 323–337.

Thornberry, T. P & Krohn, M. D. (eds.) (2003). *Taking Stock of Delinquency: An Overview of Findings from Contemporary Longitudinal Studies*. New York, NY: Kluwer Academic / Plenum.

Thornberry, T. P., Lizotte, A. J., Krohn, M. D., Smith, C. A. & Porter, P. K. (2003). Causes and consequences of delinquency: findings from the Rochester Youth Development Study. In T. P. Thornberry & M. D. Krohn (eds.), *Taking Stock of Delinquency: An Overview of Findings from Contemporary Longitudinal Studies*. pp. 11–46. New York, NY: Kluwer Academic / Plenum.

Thornberry, T. P., Smith, C. A., Rivera, C., Huizinga, D. & Stouthamer-Loeber, M. (1999). *Family Disruption and Delinquency*. Washington, DC: Office of Juvenile Justice and Delinquency Prevention, Office of Justice Programs, US Department of Justice.

Thornton, D. (2002). Constructing and testing a framework for dynamic risk assessment. *Sexual Abuse: A Journal of Research and Treatment*, 14, 139–153.

Thornton, D. (2013). Implications of our developing understanding of risk and protective factors in the treatment of adult male sexual offenders. *International Journal of Behavioral Consultation and Therapy*, 8, 62–65.

Thornton, D. M., Curran, L., Grayson, D. & Holloway, V. (1984). *Tougher Regimes in Detention Centres: Report of an Evaluation by the Young Offender Psychology Unit.* London: Her Majesty's Stationery Office.

Thorpe, J. G., Schmidt, E., Castell, D. (1963). A comparison of positive and negative (aversive) conditioning in the treatment of homosexuality. *Behavior Research & Therapy,* 1, 357–362.

Tiihonen, J., Isohanni, M., Räsänen, P., Koiranen, M. & Moring, J. (1997). Specific major mental disorders and criminality: A 26-year prospective study of the 1966 Northern Finland Birth Cohort. *American Journal of Psychiatry*, 154, 840–845.

Tolan, P., Henry, D., Schoeny, M., Bass, A., Lovegrove, P. & Nichols, E. (2013). Mentoring interventions to affect juvenile delinquency and associated problems: a systematic review. *Campbell Systematic Reviews,* 2013:10. Doi: 10.4073/csr.2013.10

Tomlinson, M. F., Brown, M. & Hoaken, P. N. S. (2016). Recreational drug use and human aggressive behavior: A comprehensive review since 2003. *Aggression and Violent Behavior*, 27, 9–29.

Tong, L. S. J. & Farrington, D. P. (2006). How effective is the "Reasoning and Rehabilitation" programme in reducing re-offending? A meta-analysis of evaluations in three countries. *Psychology, Crime & Law*, *12*, 3–24.

Tong, S., Bryant, R. P., & Horvath, M. A. H. (2009). *Understanding Criminal Investigation*. Chichester: Wiley.

Tong, Y. & Phillips, M. R. (2010). Cohort-specific risk of suicide for different mental disorders in China. *British Journal of Psychiatry*, 196, 467–473.

Tonkin, M., Bond, J.W. & Woodhams, J. (2009). Fashion conscious burglars? Testing the principles of offender profiling with footwear impressions recovered at domestic burglaries. *Psychology, Crime & Law,* 15, 327–345.

Topalli, V., Jacques, S. & Wright, R. (2015). "It takes skills to take a car": Perceptual and procedural expertise in carjacking. *Aggression and Violent Behavior*, 20, 19–25.

Topalli, V. & Wright, R. (2014). Emotion and the dynamic foreground of predatory street crime: Desperation, anger, and fear. In J. L. Van Gelder, H. Effers, D. Nagin, & D. Reynald (eds.), *Affect and Cognition in Criminal Decision-Making*. pp. 42–57. New York, NY: Routledge.

Topalli, V., Wright, R. & Fornango, R. (2002). Drug dealers, robbery and retaliation: Vulnerability, deterrence and the contagion of violence. *British Journal of Criminology*, 42, 337–351.

Totten, S. & Parsons, W. S. (eds.) (2009). *Century of Genocide: Critical Essays and Eyewitness Accounts.* 3rd edition. New York, NY: Routledge.

Tourangeau, R. & Smith, T. W. (1996). Asking sensitive questions: The impact of data collection mode, question format, and question context. *Public Opinion Quarterly,* 60, 275–304.

Towl, G. J., Farrington, D. P., Crighton, D. A. & Hughes, G. (eds.) (2008). *Dictionary of Forensic Psychology*. Cullompton, Devon: Willan Publishing.

Tracy, P. E., Wolfgang, M. E. & Figlio, R. M. (1985). *Delinquency in Two Birth Cohorts: Executive*

Summary. Washington, DC: US Department of Justice.

Trades Union Congress (2013). *Support for benefit cuts dependent on ignorance, TUC-commissioned poll finds*. http://www.tuc.org.uk/social-issues/child-poverty/welfare-and-benefits/tax-credits/support-benefit-cuts-dependent

Travers, R., Mann, R. E. & Hollin, C. R. (2014). Who benefits from cognitive skills programs? Differential impact by risk and offense type. *Criminal Justice and Behavior*, 41, 1103–1129.

Traverso, G. B. & Manna, P. (1992). Law and psychology in Italy. In F. Lösel, D. Bender & T. Bliesener (eds.) *Psychology and Law: International Perspectives*. pp. 535–545. Berlin: Walter De Gruyter.

Tremblay, R. E., Vitaro, F., Nagin, D. S., Pagani, L. & Séguin, J. R. (2003). The Montreal Longitudinal and Experimental Study: rediscovering the power of descriptions. In T. P. Thornberry & M. D. Krohn (eds.) *Taking Stock of Delinquency: An Overview of Findings from Contemporary Longitudinal Studies*. pp. 205–254. New York, NY: Kluwer Academic / Plenum.

Trevena, J. & Weatherburn, D. (2015). Does the first prison sentence reduce the risk of further offending? *Contemporary Issues in Crime and Justice*, No.187. New South Wales Bureau of Crime Statistics and Research.

Tryon, R. C. (1930). Studies in individual differences in maze ability. I. The measurement of the reliability of individual differences. *Journal of Comparative Psychology*, 11, 145–170.

Tryon, R. C. (1931). Studies in individual differences in maze ability. IV. The constancy of individual differences: correlation between learning and relearning. *Journal of Comparative Psychology*, 12, 303–345.

Tryon, R. C. (1940). Genetic differences in maze-learning ability in rats. *Yearbook of the National Society for Studies in Education*, 39, 111–119.

Ttofi, M. M., Farrington, D. P., Lösel, F. & Loeber, R. (2011). The predictive efficiency of school bullying versus later offending: A systematic/meta-analytic review of longitudinal studies. *Criminal Behaviour and Mental Health*, 21, 80–89.

Tucker-Drob, E. M. & Bates, T. C. (2016). Large cross-national differences in gene x socio-economic status interaction on intelligence. *Psychological Science*, 27, 138–149.

Tully, R. J., Chou, S. & Browne, K. D. (2013). A systematic review on the effectiveness of sex offender risk assessment tools in predicting sexual recidivism of adult male sex offenders. *Clinical Psychology Review*, 33, 287–316.

Tulving, E. & Thomson, D. M. (1973). Encoding specificity and retrieval processes in episodic memory. *Psychological Review*, 80, 353–370.

Turco, R. N. (1990). Psychological profiling. *International Journal of Offender Therapy and Comparative Criminology*, 34, 147–154.

Turkheimer, E., Haley, A., Waldron, M., D'Onofrio, B. & Gottesman, I. I. (2003). Socioeconomic status modifies the heritability of IQ in young children. *Psychological Science*, 14, 623–628.

Turner, M. (1998). Kidnapping and politics. *International Journal of the Sociology of Law*, 26, 145–160.

Turner, M. G., & Piquero, A. R. (2002). The stability of self-control. *Journal of Criminal Justice*, 30, 457-471.

Turquet, L., Seck, P., Azcona, G., Menon, R., Boyce, C., Pierron, N. & Harbour, E. (2011). *Progress of the World's Women 2011-2012*. New York, NY: UN Women (United Nations Entity for Gender Equality and the Empowerment of Women).

Turvey, B. (1999). *Criminal profiling: An introduction to behavioural evidence analysis*. New York, NY: Academic Press.

Tuvblad, C., Raine, A., Zheng, M., & Baker, L. A. (2009). Genetic and environmental stability differs in reactive and proactive aggression. *Aggressive Behavior*, 35, 437–452.

Tyler, K. A. (2002). Social and emotional outcomes of childhood sexual abuse: A review of recent research. *Aggression and Violent Behavior*, 7, 567–589.

Tyler, N. & Gannon, T. A. (2012). Explanations of firesetting in mentally disordered offenders: A review of the literature. *Psychiatry*, 75, 150–166.

Tyler, N., Gannon, T. A., Lockerbie, L., King, T., Dickens, G. L. & De Burca, C. (2014). A firesetting offence chain for mentally disordered offenders. *Criminal Justice and Behavior*, 41, 512–530.

Tyler, T. R. (2006). *Why People Obey the Law*. Princeton, NJ: Princeton University Press.

U

United Nations Office on Drugs and Crime (2013). *CTS2013_SexualViolence.xls*.

United Nations Office on Drugs and Crime (2016). *World Drug Report 2016*. Vienna: UNODC.

Usher, A. M. & Stewart, L. (2014). Effectiveness of correctional programs with ethnically diverse offenders: A meta-analytic study. *International Journal of Offender Therapy and Comparative Criminology*, 58, 209–230.

V

Van der Bruggen, M. & Grubb, A. (2014). A review of the literature relating to rape victim blaming: An analysis of the impact of observer and victim characteristics on attribution of blame in rape cases. *Aggression and Violent Behavior*, 19, 523–531.

Van Dijk, J., van Kesteren, J. & Smit, P. (2007). *Criminal Victimisation in International Perspective: Key Findings from the 2004–2005 ICVS and EU ICS*. Den Haag: Wetenschappelijk Onderzoeken Documentatiecentrum.

Van Kesteren, J., van Dijk, J. & Mayhew, P. (2014). The International Crime Victim Surveys: A retrospective. *International Review of Victimology*, 20, 49–69.

Van Koppen, M. V., de Poot, C. J., Kleemans, E. R. & Nieuwbeerta, P. (2010). Criminal trajectories in organised crime. *British Journal of Criminology*, 50, 102–123.

Van Os, J., Hanssen, M., Bijl, R. V. & Ravelli, A. (2000). Strauss (1969) revisited: a psychosis continuum in the general population? *Schizophrenia Research*, 45, 11–20.

VanderEnde, K. E., Yount, K. M., Dynes, M. M. & Sibley, L. M. (2012). Community-level correlates of intimate partner violence against women globally: A systematic review. *Social Science and Medicine*, 75, 1143–1155.

Vandevelde, S., Broekaert, E., Yates, R. & Kooyman, M. (2004). The development of the therapeutic community in correctional establishments: A comparative retrospective account of the 'democratic' Maxwell Jones TC and the hierarchical concept-based TC in prison. *International Journal of Social Psychiatry*, 50, 66–79.

Vandiver, J. (1982). Crime profiling shows promise. *Law and Order*, 30, 33–78.

Van Vugt, E., Gibbs, J., Stams. G. J., Bijleveld, C., Hendriks, J. & can der Laan, P. (2011). Moral development and recidivism: A meta-analysis. *International Journal of Offender Therapy and Comparative Criminology*, 55, 1234–1250.

Vaughn, M. G., Fu, Q., DeLisi, M., Wright, J. P., Beaver, K. M., Perron, B. E. & Howard, M. O. (2010). Prevalence and correlates of fire-setting in the United States: results from the National Epidemiological Survey on Alcohol and Related Conditions. *Comprehensive Psychiatry*, 51, 217–223.

Vazsonyi, A. T., Pickering, L. E., Belliston, L. M., Hessing, D. & Junger, M. (2002). Routine activities and deviant behaviors: American, Dutch, Hungarian and Swiss youth. *Journal of Quantitative Criminology*, 18, 397–422.

Vazsonyi, A. T., Pickering, L. E., Junger, M. & Hessing, D. (2001). An empirical test of a general theory of crime: a four-nation comparative study of self-control and the prediction of deviance. *Journal of Research in Crime and Delinquency*, 38, 91–131.

Vazsonyi, A. T., Wittekind, J. E. C., Belliston, L. M. & Van Loh, T. D. (2004). Extending the general theory of crime to 'the East': Low self-control in Japanese late adolescents. *Journal of Quantitative Criminology*, 20, 189–216.

Verheul, R., Bartak, A. & Widiger, T. (2007). Prevalence and construct validity of personality disorder not otherwise specified. *Journal of Personality Disorders*, 21, 359–370.

Verheul, R. & Widiger, T. (2004). A meta-analysis of the prevalence and usage of the personality disorder not otherwise specified (PDNOS) diagnosis. *Journal of Personality Disorders*, 18, 309–319.

Vess, J. (2008). Risk formulation with sex offenders: integrating functional analysis and actuarial measures. *Journal of Behavior Analysis and Offender and Victim Treatment and Prevention*, 1, 29–41.

Vess, J., Murphy, C. & Arkowitz, S. (2004). Clinical and demographic differences between sexually violent predators and other commitment types in a state forensic hospital. *Journal of Forensic Psychiatry & Psychology*, 15, 669–681.

Vess, J. & Skelton, A. (2010). Sexual and violent recidivism by offender type and actuarial risk: reoffending rates for rapists, child molesters and mixed-victim offenders. *Psychology, Crime & Law*, 16, 541–554.

Viding, E., Blair, R. J. R., Moffitt, T. E. & Plomin, R. (2005). Evidence for substantial genetic risk for psychopathy in 7-year-olds. *Journal of Child Psychology and Psychiatry*, 46, 592–597.

Vikman, E. (2005a). Ancient origins: Sexual violence in warfare, Part I. *Anthropology & Medicine*, 12, 21–31.

Vikman, E. (2005b). Modern combat: Sexual violence in warfare, Part II. *Anthropology & Medicine*, 12, 33–46.

Villejoubert, G., Almond, L. & Alison, L. (2009). Interpreting claims in offender profiles: The role of probability phrases, base-rates and perceived dangerousness. *Applied Cognitive Psychology*, 23, 36–54.

Villetaz, P., Killias, M. & Zoder, I. (2006). The effects of custodial vs. non-custodial sentences on re-offending: A systematic review of the state of knowledge. *Campbell Systematic Reviews*, 13. Doi: 10.4073/csr.2006.13

Visher, C. A. (1986). The RAND inmate survey: A re-analysis. In A. Blumstein, J. Cohen, J. A. Roth & C. A. Visher (eds.), *Criminal Careers and Career Criminals*. Volume II. pp. 161–211. Washington, DC: National Academy Press.

Visher, C. A., Winterfield, L. & Coggeshall, M. B. (2005). Ex-offender employment programs and recidivism: A meta-analysis. *Journal of Experimental Criminology*, 1, 295–315.

Vitale, J. A. & Newman, J. P. (2007). Psychopathic violence: a cognitive-attention perspective. In M. McMurran & R. Howard (eds.), *Personality, Personality Disorder and Violence*. pp. 247–263. Chichester: Wiley.

Vohs, K. D., Baumeister, R. F., Schmeichel, B. J., Twenge, J. M., Nelson, N. M. & Tice, D. M. (2008). Making choices impairs subsequent self-control: A limited-resource account of decision making, self-regulation, and active initiative. *Journal of Personality and Social Psychology*, 94, 883–898.

Volkow, N. D., Koob, G. F. & McLellan, A. T. (2016). Neurobiologic advances from the brain disease model of addiction. *New England Journal of Medicine*, 374, 363–371.

Von Hirsch, A., Bottoms, A. E., Burney, E. and Wikström, P. O. (1999). *Criminal Deterrence and Sentencing Severity: An Analysis of Recent Research*. Oxford: Hart Publishing.

Von Hirsch, A. & Jareborg, N. (1991). Gauging criminal harms: A living standard analysis. *Oxford Journal of Legal Studies*, 11, 1–38.

Von Hofer, H. (2000). Crime statistics as constructs: the case of Swedish rape statistics. *European Journal on Criminal Policy and Research*, 8, 77–89.

Von Lampe, K. (2016). *Organized Crime: Analyzing Illegal Activities, Criminal Structures, and Extra-Legal Governance*. Thousand Oaks, CA: Sage.

Voss, M., Moore, J., Hauser, M., Gallinat, J., Heinz, A. & Haggard, P. (2010). Altered awareness of action in schizophrenia: a specific deficit in predicting action consequences. *Brain: A Journal of Neurology*, 133, 3104–3112.

Vul, E., Harris, C., Winkielman, P. & Pashler, H. (2009). Puzzlingly high correlations in fMRI studies of emotion, personality and social cognition. *Perspectives on Psychological Science*, 4, 274–290.

W

Wagenaar, A. C., Salois, M. J. & Komro, K. A. (2009). Effects of beverage alcohol price and tax levels on drinking: a meta-analysis of 1003 estimates from 112 studies. *Addiction*, 104, 179–190.

Waites, M. (2005). *The Age of Consent: Young People, Sexuality and Citizenship*. Basingstoke: Palgrave Macmillan.

Wakeling, H., Beech, A. R. & Freemantle, N. (2013). Investigating treatment change and its relationship to recidivism in a sample of 3773 sex offenders in the UK. *Psychology, Crime & Law*, 19, 233–252.

Walfish, S. (2006). Conducting personal injury evaluations. In I.B. Weiner & A.K. Hess (Eds.), *The Handbook of Forensic Psychology*. 3rd edition. pp. 124–139. Hoboken, NJ: Wiley.

Walker, C. & Starmer, K. (1999). *Miscarriages of Justice: A review of justice in error*. Oxford: Oxford University Press.

Walker, F. O. (2007). Huntington's disease. *Lancet*, 369, 218–228.

Walker, P. L. (2001). A bioarchaeological perspective on the history of violence. *Annual Review of Anthropology*, 30, 573–596.

Walker, S. P. & Louw, D. A. (2005). The court for sexual offences: Perceptions of the victims of sexual offences. *International Journal of Law and Psychiatry*, 28, 231–245.

Walker, S. P. & Louw, D. A. (2007). The court for sexual offences: Perceptions of the professionals involved. *International Journal of Law and Psychiatry*, 30, 136–146.

Waller, J. (2007). *Becoming Evil: How ordinary people commit genocide and mass killing*. 2nd edition. Oxford: Oxford University Press.

Walmsley, R. (2016). *World Prison Population List*. 11th edition. Institute for Criminal Policy Research and Birkbeck University of London.

Walsh, J., Scaife, V., Notley, C., Dodsworth, J. & Schofield, G. (2011). Perception of need and barriers to access: the mental health needs of young people attending a Youth Offending Team in the UK. *Health and Social Care in the Community*, 19, 420–428.

Walters, G. D. (1992). A meta-analysis of the gene-crime relationship. *Criminology*, 30, 595–613.

Walters, G. D. (2003). Predicting institutional adjustment and recidivism with the Psychopathy Checklist factor scores: A meta-analysis. *Law and Human Behaviour*, 27, 541–558.

Walters, G. D. (2004). The trouble with psychopathy as a general theory of crime. *International*

Journal of Offender Therapy and Comparative Criminology, 48, 133–148.

Walters, G. D. (2005). Recidivism in released Lifestyle Change Program participants. *Criminal Justice and Behavior*, 32, 50–68.

Walters, G. D. (2013). Testing the specificity postulate of the violence graduation hypothesis: meta-analyses of the animal cruelty–offending relationship. *Aggression and Violent Behavior*, 18, 797–802.

Walters, G. D. (2014). The latent structure of psychopathy in male adjudicated delinquents: a cross-domain taxometric analysis. *Personality Disorders: Theory, Research and Treatment*, 5, 348–355.

Walters, G. D., Ermer, E., Knight, R. A. & Kiehl, K. A. (2015). Paralimbic biomarkers in taxometric analyses of psychopathy: does changing the indicators change the conclusion? *Personality Disorders: Theory, Research, and Treatment*, 6, 41–52.

Walters, G. D., Knight, R. A., Looman, J. & Abracen, J. (2016). Child molestation and psychopathy: a taxometric analysis. *Journal of Sexual Aggression*, 22, 379–393.

Walton, J. S. & Duff, S. (2017). "I'm not homosexual or heterosexual, I'm paedosexual": Exploring sexual preference for children using interpretive phenomenology. *The Journal of Forensic Practice*, 19, 151–161.

Ward, T. (2000). Sex offenders' cognitive distortions as implicit theories. *Aggression and Violent Behavior*, 5, 491–507.

Ward, T. & Beech, A. (2006). An integrated theory of sexual offending. *Aggression and Violent Behavior*, 11, 44–63.

Ward, T. & Beech, A. (2008). An integrated theory of sexual offending. In D. R. Laws & W. T. O'Donohue (eds.), *Sexual Deviance: Theory, Assessment, and Treatment*. pp. 21–36. New York, NY: Guilford Press.

Ward, T. & Hudson, S. M. (1998). The construction and development of theory in the sexual offending area: A metatheoretical framework. *Sexual Abuse: A Journal of Research and Treatment*, 10, 47–63.

Ward, T. & Hudson, S. M. (2001). Finkelhor's precondition model of child sexual abuse: A critique. *Psychology, Crime & Law*, 7, 291–307.

Ward, T. & Keenan, T. (1999). Child molesters' implicit theories. *Journal of Interpersonal Violence*, 14, 821–838.

Ward, T. & Maruna, S. (2007). *Rehabilitation: Beyond the Risk Paradigm*. London and New York: Routledge.

Ward, T. & Siegert, R. J. (2002). Toward a comprehensive theory of child sexual abuse: A theory knitting perspective. *Psychology, Crime, and Law*, 8, 319–351.

Ward, T. & Stewart, C. (2003). Criminogenic needs and human needs: A theoretical model. *Psychology, Crime & Law*, 9, 125–143.

Ward, T., Fisher, S. & Beech, A. R. (2016). An integrated theory of sexual offending. In A, Phenix & H. M. Hoberman (eds.), *Sexual Offending: Predisposing Antecedents, Assessments and Management*. pp. 1–11. New York, NY: Springer.

Ward, T. & Hudson, S. M. & France, K. G. (1993). Self-reported reasons for offending behavior in child molesters. *Annals of Sex Research*, 6, 139–148.

Ward, T., Hudson, S. M., Johnston, L. & Marshall, W. L. (1997). Cognitive distortions in sex offenders: An integrative review. *Clinical Psychology Review*, 17, 479–507.

Ward, T., Louden, K., Hudson, S. M. & Marshall, W. L. (1995). A descriptive model of the offense chain for child molesters. *Journal of Interpersonal Violence*, 10, 452–472.

Warr, M. & Stafford, M. (1991). The influence of delinquent peers: what they think or what they do? *Criminology*, 29, 851–866.

Washington Post (2011). *Editorial: Arms sales to repressive Bahrain misplaced*. 30 September. http://www.washingtonpost.com/opinions/arms-sales-to-repressive-bahrain-misplaced/2011/09/29/gIQASnhH8K_story.html

Watkins, R. E. (1992). *An Historical Review of the Role and Practice of Psychology in the field of Corrections*. Research Report No. R-28. Ottawa: Correctional Service Canada.

Webb, L., Craissati, J. & Keen, S. (2007). Characteristics of internet child pornography offenders: A comparison with child molesters. *Sex Abuse*, 19, 449–465.

Webster, C. D. (1984). On gaining acceptance: Why the courts accept only reluctantly findings from experimental and social psychology. *International Journal of Law and Psychiatry*, 7, 407–414.

Wecht, C. H. (2005). The history of legal medicine. *Journal of the American Academy of Psychiatry and the Law Online*, 33, 245–251.

Weiner, I. B. & Hess, A. K. (eds.) (2006). *Handbook of Forensic Psychology*. 3rd edition. Hoboken, NJ: Wiley.

Weiner, I. B. & Otto, R. K. (eds.) (2014). *Handbook of Forensic Psychology*. 4th edition. Hoboken, NJ: Wiley.

Weisburd, D., Farrington, D. P. & Gill, C. (eds.) (2016). *What Works in Crime Prevention and Rehabilitation: Lessons from Systematic Reviews*. New York, NY: Springer.

Weisburd, D., Farrington, D. P., Gill, C., Ajzenstadt, M., Bennett, T., Bowers, K., Caudy, M. S., Holloway, K., Johnson, S., Lösel, F., Mallender, J., Perry, A., Tang, L. L., Taxman, F., Telep, C., Tierney, R., Ttofi, M. M., Watson, C., Wilson, D. B. & Wooditch, A. (2017). What works in crime prevention and rehabilitation: An assessment of systematic reviews. *Criminology & Public Policy*, 16, 415–449.

Weisburd, D., Lum, C. M. & Yang, S.-M. (2003). When can we conclude that treatments or programs "don't work"? *Annals of the American Academy of Political and Social Science*, 587, 31–48.

Wells, G. L. (1993). What do we know about eye-witness identification? *American Psychologist*, 48, 553–571.

Wells, G. L. & Olson, E. A. (2003). Eyewitness testimony. *Annual Review of Psychology*, 54, 277–295.

Wells-Parker, E., Bangert-Drowns, R., McMillen, R. & Williams, M. (1995). Final results from a meta-analysis of remedial interventions with drink/drive offenders. *Addiction*, 9, 907–926.

Welner, M. (2013). Classifying crimes by severity from aggravators to depravity. In J. E. Douglas, A. W. Burgess, A. G. Burgess & R. K. Ressler, *Crime Classification Manual: A Standard System for Investigating and Classifying Violent Crime*. 3rd edition. pp. 91-107. Hoboken, NJ: Wiley.

Weist, J. (1981). Treatment of violent offenders. *Clinical Social Work Journal*, 9, 271–281.

Welsh, B. C. & Farrington, D. P. (2000). Correctional intervention programs and cost benefit analysis. *Criminal Justice and Behavior*, 27, 115–133.

Welsh, B. C. & Farrington, D. P. (2003). Effects of closed-circuit television on crime. *Annals of the American Academy of Political and Social Science*, 587, 110–135.

Welsh, B. C. & Farrington, D. P. (2007). *Improved Street Lighting and Crime Prevention*. Stockholm: Swedish National Council for Crime Prevention.

Wermink, H., Blokland, A., Nieuwbeerta, P., Nagin, D. & Tollenaar, N. (2010). Comparing the effects of community service and short-term imprisonment on recidivism: a matched samples approach. *Journal of Experimental Criminology*, 6, 325–349.

Werner, E. E. (1989). High-risk children in young adulthood: A longitudinal study from birth to 32 years. *American Journal of Orthopsychiatry*, 59, 72–81.

West, A. (2000). Clinical assessment of homicide offenders: the significance of crime scene in offense and offender analysis. *Homicide Studies*, 4, 219–233.

West, A. G. & Greenall, P. V. (2011). Incorporating index offence analysis into forensic clinical assessment. *Legal and Criminological Psychology*, 16, 144–159.

West, D. J. (1977). *Homosexuality re-examined.* Minneapolis, MN: University of Minnesota Press.

West, R. & Brown, J. (2013). *Models of Addiction*. 2nd edition. Chichester: Wiley-Blackwell

Westcott, H. L. & Page, M. (2002). Cross-examination, sexual abuse and child witness identity. *Child Abuse Review,* 11, 137–152.

Whitaker, R. (2005). Anatomy of an epidemic: Psychiatric drugs and the astonishing rise of mental illness in America. *Ethical Human Psychology and Psychiatry*, 7, 23–35.

Whitaker, R. (2010). *Anatomy of an Epidemic: Magic Bullets, Psychiatric Drugs and the Astonishing Rise of Mental Illness*. New York, NY: Broadway Paperbacks.

White, M. (2011). *Atrocitology: Humanity's 100 Deadliest Achievements*. Edinburgh and London: Canongate.

Whittington, R., Hockenhull, J. C., McGuire, J., Leitner, M., Barr, W., Cherry, M. G., Flentje, R., Quinn, B., Dundar Y. & Dickson, R. (2013). A systematic review of risk assessment strategies for populations at high risk of engaging in violent behaviour: update 2002–8. *Health Technology Assessment*, 17(50), 1–128.

Widiger, T. A. (2015). Classification and diagnosis: historical development and contemporary issues. In J. E. Maddux & B. A. Winstead (eds.) *Psychopathology: Foundations for a Contemporary Understanding*. 4th edition. pp. 97–110. New York and London: Routledge.

Widiger, T. A. & Trull, T. J. (2007). Plate tectonics in the classification of personality disorder: shifting to a dimensional model. *American Psychologist*, 6, 71–83.

Widom, C. S. (1989). The cycle of violence. *Science*, 244, 160–166.

Widom, C. S. & Morris, S. (1997). Accuracy of adult recollections of childhood victimization: Part 2. Childhood sexual abuse. *Psychological Assessment*, 9, 34-46.

Widom, C. S. & Shepard, R. L. (1996). Accuracy of adult recollections of childhood victimization:

Part 1. Childhood physical abuse. *Psychological Assessment*, 8, 412–421.

Wieczorek, W. F., Welte, J. W. & Abel, E.L. (1990). Alcohol, drugs and murder: a study of convicted homicide offenders. *Journal of Criminal Justice*, 18, 217–227.

Wikström, P. (ed.) (1990). *Crime and Measures against Crime in the City*. Stockholm: National Council for Crime Prevention.

Wikström, P.-O. (2006). Individuals, settings, and acts of crime: situational mechanisms and the explanation of crime. In P.-O. Wikström & R. J. Sampson (eds.), *The Explanation of Crime*. pp. 61–107. Cambridge: Cambridge University Press.

Wikström, P.-O., Ceccato, V., Hardie, B. & Treiber, K. (2010). Activity fields and the dynamics of crime: Advancing knowledge about the role of the environment in crime causation. *Journal of Quantitative Criminology*, 26, 55–87.

Wikström, P.-O. & Treiber, K. (2007). The role of self-control in crime causation: Beyond Gottfredson and Hirschi's General Theory of Crime. *European Journal of Criminology*, 4, 237–264.

Wilcox, D. T. (2009). Overview: Opportunities and responsibilities. In D. T. Wilcox (ed.) *Assessing, Treating and Supervising Sex Offenders: A Practitioner's Guide*. pp. 1–7. Chichester: Wiley.

Wilkinson, D. L. (2001). Violent events and social identity: specifying the relationship between respect and masculinity in inner-city youth violence. *Sociological Studies of Children and Youth*, 8, 235–269.

Wilkinson, D. L. & Hamerschlag, S. J. (2005). Situational determinants in intimate partner violence. *Aggression and Violent Behavior*, 10, 333–361.

Wilkinson, R. (2004). Why is violence more common where inequality is greater? *Annals of the New York Academy of Sciences*, 1036, 1–12.

Wilkinson, R. & Pickett, K. (2009). *The Spirit Level: Why more equal societies almost always do better*. London: Allen Lane.

Willness, C. R., Steel, P. & Lee, K. (2007). A meta-analysis of the antecedents and consequences of workplace sexual harassment. *Personnel Psychology*, 60, 127–162.

Willott, S. & Griffin, C. (1999). Building your own lifeboat: working-class male offenders talk about economic crime. *British Journal of Social Psychology*, 38, 445–460.

Wilson, D. B. (2001). Meta-analytic methods for criminology. *Annals of the American Academy of Political and Social Science*, 578, 71–89.

Wilson, D. B. (2016). Correctional programs. In D. Weisburd, D. P. Farrington & C. Gill (eds.), *What Works in Crime Prevention and Rehabilitation: Lessons from Systematic Reviews*. pp. 193–217. New York, NY: Springer.

Wilson, D. B., Bouffard, L. A. & Mackenzie, D. L. (2005). A quantitative review of structured, group-oriented, cognitive-behavioral programs for offenders. *Criminal Justice and Behavior*, 32, 172–204.

Wilson, D. B., Gallagher, C. A. & MacKenzie, D. L. (2000). A meta-analysis of corrections-based education, vocation and work programs for adult offenders. *Journal of Research in Crime and Delinquency*, 37, 568–581.

Wilson, D. B., Olaghere, A. & Gill, C. (2016). Juvenile curfew effects on criminal behavior and victimization: a Campbell Collaboration systematic review. *Journal of Experimental Criminology*, 12, 167–186.

Wilson, J. Q. & Herrnstein, R. J. (1985). *Crime and Human Nature*. New York, NY: Simon & Schuster.

Wilson, N. J. & Tamatea, A. (2013). Challenging the 'urban myth' of psychopathgy untreatability: the High-Risk Personality Programme. *Psychology, Crime & Law*, 19, 493–510.

Wilson, P. R., Lincoln, R. & Kocsis, R. (1997). Validity, utility and ethics of criminal profiling for serial and violent sexual offenders. *Psychiatry, Psychology and the Law*, 4, 1–12.

Wilson, S. J. & Lipsey, M. W. (2000). Wilderness challenge programs for delinquent youth: A meta-analysis of outcome evaluations. *Evaluation and Program Planning*, 23, 1–12.

Wilson, S. J., Lipsey, M. W. & Soydan, H. (2003). Are mainstream programs for juvenile delinquency less effective with minority youth than majority youth? A meta-analysis of outcomes research. *Research on Social Work Practice*, 13, 3–26.

Wing, J. K., Sartorius, N. & Üstün, T. B. (1998). *Diagnosis and clinical measurement in psychiatry: A reference manual for SCAN*. Cambridge: Cambridge University Press.

Winick, B. J. (1997). *Therapeutic Jurisprudence Applied: Essays on Mental Health Law*. Durham, NC: Carolina Academic Press.

Winick, B. J. (1998). Sex offender law in the 1990s: a therapeutic jurisprudence analysis. *Psychology, Public Policy, and the Law*, 4, 505–570.

Wodahl, E. J., Boman, J. H. & Garland, B. E. (2015). Responding to probation and parole violations: Are jail sanctions more effective than community-based graduated sanctions? *Journal of Criminal Justice*, 43, 242–250.

Wogalter, M. S. (1996). *Describing faces from memory: Accuracy and effects on subsequent recognition performance*. Proceedings of the Human Factors and Ergonomics Society 40th Annual Meeting, 536–540.

Wolak, J., Finkelhor, D., Mitchell, K. J. & Ybarra, M. L. (2008). Online "predators" and their victims: Myths, realities, and implications for prevention and treatment. *American Psychologist*, 63, 111–128.

Wolfgang, M. E. (1958). *Patterns in Criminal Homicide*. Philadelphia, PA: University of Pennsylvania Press.

Wolfgang, M. E., Figlio, R. M., Tracy, P. E. & Singer, S. I. (1985). The *National Survey of Crime Severity*. NCJ-96017. Washington, DC: Bureau of Justice Statistics, US Department of Justice.

Wong, S., Gordon, A., Gu, D., Lewis, K. & Olver, M. E. (2012). The effectiveness of violence reduction treatment for psychopathic offenders: Empirical evidence and a treatment model. *International Journal of Forensic Mental Health*, 11, 336–349.

Wood, R. (2010). UK: the reality behind 'kinfe crime' debate. *Race & Class*, 52, 97–103.

Woodhouse, J. (2017). *Alcohol: minimum pricing*. Briefing Paper Number 5021. London: House of Commons Library.

Woody, W. D. & Greene, E. (2012). Jurors' use of standards of proof in decisions about punitive damages. *Behavioral Sciences and the Law,* 30, 856–872.

World Health Organization (1992). *International Classification of Diseases* (ICD-10). Geneva: WHO.

World Health Organization (1994). *Lexicon of Alcohol and Drug Terms*. Geneva: WHO.

World Health Organization (2001). *The World Health Report 2001: Mental Health: New Understanding, New Hope*. Geneva: WHO.

World Health Organization (2011a). *Global status report on alcohol and health*. Geneva: WHO.

World Health Organization (2011b). *Mental Health Atlas 2011*. Geneva: WHO.

World Health Organization (2013). *Global Health Estimates Summary Tables: Deaths by Cause, Age and Sex*. Available from: http://www.who.int/healthinfo/global_burden_disease/en/

World Health Organization (2014). *Global status report on alcohol and health 2014*. Geneva: WHO.

Wortley, R. (2011). *Psychological Criminology: an integrative approach*. London: Routledge.

Wortley, R. & Smallbone, S. (2014). A criminal careers typology of child sexual abusers. *Sexual Abuse: A Journal of Research and Treatment*, 26, 569–585.

Wright, A. J. (2011). *Conducting Psychological Assessment: A Guide for Practitioners*. Hoboken, NJ: Wiley.

Wright, A. M. & Holliday, R. E. (2007). Enhancing the recall of young, young-old and old-old adults with the cognitive interview and a modified version of the cognitive interview. *Applied Cognitive Psychology*, 21, 19–43.

Wright, D. B. (2007). The impact of eyewitness identifications from simultaneous and sequential lineups. *Memory*, 15, 746–754.

Wright, D. B., Boyd, C. E. & Tredoux, C. G. (2003). Inter-racial contact and the own-race bias for face recognition in South Africa and England. *Applied Cognitive Psychology*, 17, 365–373.

Wright, P. J. (2013). U.S. males and pornography, 1973–2010: consumption, predictors, correlates. *Journal of Sex Research*, 50, 60–71.

Wright, P. J., Tokunaga, R. S. & Kraus, A. (2016). A meta-analysis of pornography consumption and actual acts of sexual aggression in general population studies. *Journal of Communication*, 66, 183–205.

Wright, R., Brookman, F. & Bennett, T. (2006). The foreground dynamics of street robbery in Britain. *British Journal of Criminology*, 46, 1–15.

Wright, R. P. (2009), *Kidnap for Ransom: Resolving the Unthinkable*. Boca Raton, FL: Taylor and Francis.

Wright, R. T. & Decker, S. H. (1994). *Burglars on the Job: Streetlife and Residential Break-ins*. Boston, MA: Northeastern University Press.

Wright, R. T. & Decker, S. H. (1997). *Armed Robbers in Action: Stickups and Street Culture*. Boston, MA: Northeastern University Press.

Wyatt, W. J. (1999). Assessment of child sexual abuse: Research and proposal for a bias-free interview: Part II. *The Forensic Examiner*, 8, 24–27.

Y

Yang, B. & Lester, D. (2008). The deterrent effect of executions: A meta-analysis thirty years after Ehrlich. *Journal of Criminal Justice*, 36, 453–460.

Yang, M., Wong, S. C. P. & Coid, J. (2010). The efficacy of violence prediction: a meta-analytic comparison of nine risk assessment tools. *Psychological Bulletin*, 136, 740–767.

Yang, Y. & Raine, A. (2009). Prefrontal structural and functional brain imaging findings in antisocial, violent, and psychopathic individuals: A meta-analysis. *Psychiatry Research: Neuroimaging*, 174, 81–88.

Yardley, E., Wilson, D. & Lynes, A. (2014). A taxonomy of male British family annihilators, 1980–2012. *Howard Journal of Criminal Justice*, 53, 117–140.

Yates, P. M., Hucker, S. J. & Kingston, D. A. (2008). Sexual sadism: psychopathology and theory. In D. R. Laws & W. T. O'Donohue (eds.), *Sexual Deviance: Theory, Assessment, and Treatment*. pp. 213–230. New York, NY: Guilford Press.

Yodanis, C. L. (2004). Gender inequality, violence against women, and fear: A cross-national test of the feminist theory of violence against women. *Journal of Interpersonal Violence*, 19, 655–675.

Youngs, D., Ioannou, M. & Straszewicz, A. (2013). Distinguishing stalker modus operandi: an exploration of the Mullen, Pathé, Purcell, and Stuart (1999) typology in a law-enforcement sample. *Journal of Forensic Psychiatry and Psychology*, 24, 319–336.

Youth Justice Board (2011). http://www.justice.gov.uk/youth-justice/courts-and-orders/disposals/section-9091

Z

Zagar, R. J., Busch, K. G., Grove, W. M., Hughes, J. R. & Arbit, J. (2009). Looking forward and backward in records for risks among homicidal youth. *Psychological Reports*, 104, 103–127.

Zahn, M. A., Brownstein, H. H. & Jackson, S. L. (eds.) (2004). *Violence: From Theory to Research*. London: Matthew Bender/LexisNexis.

Zaitchik, M. C., & Mosher, D. L. (1993). Criminal justice implications of the macho personality constellation. *Criminal Justice and Behavior*, 20, 227–223.

Zajac, R. & Hayne, H. (2003). I don't think that's what *really* happened: The effect of cross-examination on the accuracy of children's reports. *Journal of Experimental psychology: Applied*, 9, 187–195.

Zajac, R. & Hayne, H. (2006). The negative effect of cross-examination style questioning on children's accuracy: Older children are not immune. *Applied Cognitive Psychology*, 20, 3–16.

Zamble, E. & Quinsey, V. (1997). *The Criminal Recidivism Process*. Cambridge: Cambridge University Press.

Zayas, V., Shoda, Y. & Ayduk, O. N. (2002). Personality in context: An interpersonal systems perspective. *Journal of Personality*, 70, 851–900.

Zhang, L., Welte, J. W. & Wieczorek, W. W. (2002). The role of aggression-related alcohol expectancies in explaining the link between alcohol and violent behavior. *Substance Use and Misuse*, 37, 457–71.

Zhao, J., Stockwell, T., Martin, M., Macdonald, S., Vallance, K., Treno, A., Ponicki, W. R., Tu, A. & Buxton, J. (2013). The relationship between minimum alcohol prices, outlet densities and alcohol attributable deaths in British Columbia, 2002 to 2009. *Addiction*, 108, 1059–1069.

Zimring, F. E., Fagan, J. & Johnson, D. T. (2010). Executions, deterrence, and homicide: A tale of two cities. *Journal of Empirical Legal Studies*, 7, 1–29.

Zimring, F. E. & Hawkins, G. (1995). *Incapacitation: Penal Confinement and the Restraint of Crime*. New York, NY: Oxford University Press.

Zucman, G. (2015). *The Hidden Wealth of Nations: The Scourge of Tax Havens*. Chicago, Il: University of Chicago Press.

Zumkley, H. (1994). The stability of aggressive behavior: a meta-analysis. *German Journal of Psychology*, 18, 273–281.

Author Index

Subject Index